高等教育出版社　中國・北京
Higher Education Press, Beijing, China

英漢實用中醫藥大全

趙樸初題

2

HE CHINESE
IATERIA
IEDICA
中藥學

THE ENGLISH-CHINESE ENCYCLOPEDIA OF PRACTICAL TRADITIONAL CHINESE MEDICINE

Chief Editor Xu Xiangcai
Assistants You Ke Kang Kai
Bao Xuequan Lu Yubin

英汉实用中医药大全

主　　编　徐象才
主编助理　尤　可　康　凯
鲍学全　路玉滨

Higher Education Press
高等教育出版社

2

中　药　学

	中文	英文
主编	邹积隆	黄奎铭
编者	赵永珍	龚修林

THE CHINESE MATERIA MEDICA

	English	Chinese
Chief Editor	Huang Kuiming	Zou Jilong
Editor	Gong Xiulin	Zhao Yongzhen

Preface

I am delighted to learn that THE ENGLISH–CHINESE ENCYCLOPEDIA OF PRACTICAL TRADITIONAL CHINESE MEDICINE will soon come into the world.

TCM has experienced many vicissitudes of times but has remained evergreen. It has made great contributions not only to the power and prosperity of our Chinese nation but to the enrichment and improvement of world medicine. Unfortunately, differences in nations, states and languages have slowed down its spreading and flowing outside China. At present, however, an upsurge in learning, researching and applying Traditional Chinese Medicine (TCM) is unfolding. In order to maximize the effect of this upsurge and to lead TCM, one of the brilliant cultural heritages of the Chinese nation, to the world for it to expand and bring benefit to the people of all nations, Mr. Xu Xiangcai called intellectuals of noble aspirations and high intelligence together from Shandong and many other provinces in China and took charge of the work of both compilation and translation of THE ENGLISH–CHINESE ENCYCLOPEDIA OF PRACTICAL TRADITIONAL CHINESE MEDICINE. With great pleasure, the medical staff both at home and abroad will hail the appearance of this encyclopedia.

I believe that the day when the world's medicine is fully

developed will be the day when TCM has spread throughout the world.

I am pleased to give it my preface.

Prof. Dr. Hu Ximing

Deputy Ministerof the Ministry of Public Health of the People's Republic of China,

Director General of the State Administrative Bureau of Traditional Chinese Medicine and Pharmacology,

President of the World Federation of Acupuncture–Moxibustion Societies,

Member of China Association of Science & Technology,

Deputy President of All–China Association of Traditional Chinese Medicine,

President of China Acupuncture & Moxibustion Society.

December, 1989

Preface

The Chinese nation has been through a long, arduous course of struggling against diseases and has developed its own traditional medicine–Traditional Chinese Medicine and Pharmacology (TCMP). TCMP has a unique, comprehensive, scientific system including both theories and clinical practice. Some thousand years since its beginnings, not only has it been well preserved but also continuously developed. It has special advantages, such as remarkable curative effects and few side effects. Hence it is an effective means by which people prevent and treat diseases and keep themselves strong and healthy.

All achievements attained by any nation in the development of medicine are the public wealth of all mankind. They should not be confined within a single country. What is more, the need to set them free to flow throughout the world as quickly and precisely as possible is greater than that of any other kind of science. During my more than thirty years of being engaged in Traditional Chinese Medicine(TCM), I have been looking forward to the day when TCMP will have spread all over the world and made its contributions to the elimination of diseases of all mankind. However it is to be deeply regretted that the pace of TCMP in extending outside China has been unsatisfactory due to the major difficulties in expressing its concepts in foreign languages.

Mr. Xu Xiangcai, a teacher of Shandong College of TCM, has sponsored and taken charge of the work of compilation and translation of The English-Chinese Encyclopedia of Practical Traditional Chinese Medicine-an extensive series. This work is a great project, a large-scale scientific research, a courageous effort and a novel creation. I deeply esteem Mr. Xu Xiangcai and his compilers and translators, who have been working day and night for such a long time, for their hard labor and for their firm and indomitable will displayed in overcoming one difficulty after another, and for their great success achieved in this way. As a leader in the circles of TCM, I am duty-bound to do my best to support them.

I believe this encyclopedia will be certain to find its position both in the history of Chinese medicine and in the history of world science and technology.

Mr. Zhang Qiwen

Member of the Standing Committee of
All-China Association of TCM,
Deputy Head of the Health Department
of Shandong Province.

March, 1990

Publisher's Preface

Traditional Chinese Medicine(TCM) is one of China's great cultural heritages. Since the founding of the People's Republic of China in 1949, guided by the farsighted TCM policy of the Chinese Communist Party and the Chinese government, the treasure house of the theories of TCM has been continuously explored and the plentiful literature researched and compiled. As a result, great success has been achieved. Today there has appeared a world-wide upsurge in the studying and researching of TCM. To promote even more vigorous development of this trend in order that TCM may better serve all mankind, efforts are required to further it throughout the world. To bring this about, the language barriers must be overcome as soon as possible in order that TCM can be accurately expressed in foreign languages.

Thus the compilation and translation of a series of English-Chinese books of basic knowledge of TCM has become of great urgency to serve the needs of medical and educational circles both inside and outside China.

In recent years, at the request of the health departments, satisfactory achievements have been made in researching the expression of TCM in English. Based on the investigation into the history and current state of the research work mentioned above, the English-Chinese Encyclopedia of Practical TCM has been published to meet the needs of extending the knowledge of TCM around the world.

The encyclopedia consists of twenty-one volumes, each dealing with a particular branch of TCM. In the process of compilation, the distinguishing features of TCM have been given close attention and great efforts have been made to ensure that the content is scientific, practical, comprehensive and concise. The chief writers of the Chinese manuscripts include professors or associate professors with at least twenty years of practical clinical and / or teaching experience in TCM. The Chinese manuscript of each volume has been checked and approved by a specialist of the relevant branch of TCM. The team of the translators and revisers of the English versions consists of TCM specialists with a good command of English professional medical translators, and teachers of English from TCM colleges or universities. At a symposium to standardize the English versions, scholars from twenty-two colleges or universities, research institutes of TCM or other health institutes probed the question of how to express TCM in English more comprehensively, systematically and accurately, and discussed and deliberated in detail the English versions of some volumes in order to upgrade the English versions of the whole series. The English version of each volume has been re-examined and then given a final checking.

Obviously this encyclopedia will provide extensive reading material of TCM English for senior students in colleges of TCM in China and will also greatly benefit foreigners studying TCM.

The assiduous efforts of compiling and translating this encyclopedia have been supported by the responsible leaders of the State Education Commission of the People's Republic of China, the State Administrative Bureau of TCM and Pharmacy, and the Education Commission and Health Department of Shandong

Province. Under the direction of the Higher Education Department of the State Education Commission, the leading board of compilation and translation of this encyclopedia was set up. The leaders of many colleges of TCM and pharmaceutical factories of TCM have also given assistance.

We hope that this encyclopedia will bring about a good effect on enhancing the teaching of TCM English at the colleges of TCM in China, on cultivating skills in medical circles in exchanging ideas of TCM with patients in English, and on giving an impetus to the study of TCM outside China.

Higher Education Press

March, 1990

Foreword

The English–Chinese Encyclopedia of Practical Traditional Chinese Medicine is an extensive series of twenty–one volumes. Based on the fundamental theories of traditional Chinese medicine(TCM) and with emphasis on the clinical practice of TCM, it is a semi–advanced English–Chinese academic works which is quite comprehensive, systematic, concise, practical and easy to read. It caters mainly to the following readers: senior students of colleges of TCM, young and middle–aged teachers of colleges of TCM, young and middle–aged physicians of hospitals of TCM, personnel of scientific research institutions of TCM, teachers giving correspondence courses in TCM to foreigners, TCM personnel going abroad in the capacity of lecturers or physicians, those trained in Western medicine but wishing to study TCM, and foreigners coming to China to learn TCM or to take refresher courses in TCM.

Because Traditional Chinese Medicine and Pharmacology is unique to our Chinese nation, putting TCM into English has been the crux of the compilation and translation of this encyclopedia. Owing to the fact that no one can be proficient both in the theories of Traditional Chinese Medicine and Pharmacology and the clinical practice of every branch of TCM, as well as in English, to ensure that the English versions express accurately the inherent meanings of TCM, collective translation measures have been taken. That is, teachers of English familiar with TCM, professional medical translators, teachers or physicians of TCM and even teachers of palaeography with a strong command of English were all invited together to co–translate the Chinese manuscripts and, then, to co–deliberate and discuss the English versions. Finally English–speaking foreigners studying TCM or teaching English in China were asked to polish the English versions. In this way, the skills of the above translators and foreigners were merged to ensure the quality of the English versions. However, even using this method, the uncertainty that the English versions will be wholly accepted still remains. As for the Chinese manuscripts, they do reflect the essence, and give a general picture, of traditional Chinese medicine and pharmacology. It is not asserted, though, that they are perfect, I whole–heartedly look forward to any criticisms or opinions from readers in order to make improvements to future editions.

More than 200 people have taken part in the activities of compiling, translating and revising this encyclopedia. They come from twenty–eight institutions in all parts of China. Among these institutions, there are fifteen colleges of TCM:Shandong, Beijing, Shanghai, Tianjin, Nanjing, Zhejiang, Anhui, Henan, Hubei, Guangxi, Guiyang, Gansu, Chengdu, Shanxi and Changchun, and scientific research centers of TCM such as China Academy of TCM and Shandong Scientific Research Institute of TCM.

The Education Commission of Shandong province has included the compilation and translation of this encyclopedia in its scientific research projects and allocated funds accordingly. The Health Department of Shandong Province has also given financial aid together with a number of pharmaceutical factories of TCM. The subsidization from Jinan Pharmaceutical Factory of

TCM provided the impetus for the work of compilation and translation to get under way.

The success of compiling and translating this encyclopedia is not only the fruit of the collective labor of all the compilers, translators and revisers but also the result of the support of the responsible leaders of the relevant leading institutions. As the encyclopedia is going to be published, I express my heartfelt thanks to all the compilers. translators and revisers for their sincere cooperation, and to the specialists, professors, leaders at all levels and pharmaceutical factories of TCM for their warm support.

It is my most profound wish that the publication of this encyclopedia will take its role in cultivating talented persons of TCM having a very good command of TCM English and in extending, rapidly, comprehensive knowledge of TCM to all corners of the globe.

Chief Editor Xu Xiangcai

Shandong College of TCM

March, 1990

Contents

Notes

CHINESE MATERIA MEDICA is the second volume of ENGLISH–CHINESE ENCYCLOPAEDIA OF PRACTICAL TRADITIONAL CHINESE MEDICINE.

As Chinese materia medica is well known as one of the most important implements for preventing and treating diseases by doctors of traditional Chinese medicine, therefore its fundamental knowledge should be studied and mastered by clinical doctors who deal with various subjects of TCM.

Concerning the contents, the book is written in two parts: Part one, General Introduction to Chinese Materia Medica; Part two, Kinds of Drugs. Part one here discusses the processing, properties, actions, indications and application of the drugs. Part two consists of nineteen chapters, in which 363 common drugs with an appendix of 57 sencondary drugs are described; and the initial part of each chapter gives a brief account of the meaning, action, indications, compatibility and remarks of the drugs concerned. Besides, in order to describe each drug briefly and plainly, a specific passage is arranged to deal with both the origin and processing together; then nomenclature used in prescriptions, action, indications, dosage, administration, notes, etc. are followed.

Some of the materials of traditional Chinese medicine referred to in this volume come from rare animals which are near extinction and of which trapping and killing has been prohibited by low. So they have lost their sources. But they have their substitutes with the same effects in both hospitals and pharmaceutical factories. Why we deal with these materials in this volume is just to the academic convenience.

An acknowledgement is expressed to Prof. Zhou Fengwu in Shandong College of TCM for his valuable revision in preparing the Chinese manuscript and to Prof. Qi Xiuheng in Taian Medical College and Prof. Fang Tianyu in Beijing University of TCM for their help in refreshing the English version of this book.

The Editor

Part One
General Introduction
to Chinese Materia Medica

1 Processing of Traditional Chinese Drugs

By processing of drugs, termed as *Paozhi* in TCM, we mean various methods of treating crude drugs according to their specific properties and medical requirements in clinical practice; or we may mean the processes of either treating crude drugs or preparing their dosage forms for use. Since most traditional Chinese drugs come from the crude plants, it is necessary for them to be processed so as to meet therapeutic requirements, ensure safety and produce satisfactory medicinal effect in clinical practice.

1.1 Purposes of Processing Drugs

The purposes of processing drugs are briefly as follows:

1. Removing or reducing the toxicity, drastic properties and side effects of some drugs

The toxicity of Radix Aconiti and Radix Aconiti Kusnezoffi will be reduced when processed; the drastic purgative property of

Fructus Crotonis will be subdued when the drug is defatted and its frostlike powder is used; and the side effect of vomiting of Radix Dichroae will be also eliminated when stir–baked with wine.

2. Promoting therapeutic effects

After being processed, the therapeutic effects of some drugs will be reinforced;for instance, the analgesic effect of Rhizoma Corydalis will be strengthened when it is prepared with vinegar; the effects of soothing the liver and relieving *Qi*–depression of Radix Bupleuri will be increased when stir–baked with vinegar; and the effect of ventilating the lung to stop cough of Flos Farfarae will be enhanced when stir–baked with honey.

3. Modifying its nature and action

The nature and action of drugs may be modified when they are cooked or processed. For instance, the crude Radix Rehmanniae is cold in nature and has effect of eliminating blood–heat; but, when processed, it will be slight warm and have effect of nourishing blood. The crude Radix et Rhizoma Rhei may have the drastic effect of diarrhea, but the processed one will only produce mild effect of relaxing bowels.

4. Facilitating preparation of forms, and storage of drugs

Most botanical drugs, when immersed in water and softened, will be easy to be cut into segments or pieces. And most minerals and shells, when calcined or quenched, will be easy to be ground into powder. For instance, there is calcined Magnetium, calcined Os Draconis, vinegar–calcined Plastrum Testudinis and vinegar–calcined Carapax Trionycis. Besides, the forms of medicines will be easily prepared and their effective components will be easily solved in the decoction when they are cut or crushed into pieces; and some drugs are to be stir–baked and dried, thus they can be kept for a long time from going moldy and rot.

5. Correcting the unpleasant flavour or tastes

The salty taste and the fishy or unpleasant smell of some drugs will be corrected or removed when they are either rinsed and washed by water, or stir–baked with honey, wine, vinegar or wheat bran. For instance, the salty taste of Sargassum and Thallus Laminariae seu Eckloniae can be eliminated by rinsing with water, and the offensive smell of Placenta Hominis removed by washing.

6. Taking away the miscellaneous substances and non–pharmaceutical parts, thus making the drugs clean and pure, and convenient for patients to take.

The muddy and sandy roots or rhizomes of the pharmaceutical plants must be washed and the miscellaneous substances must be cleared away. For instance, the hair of Folium Eriobotryae must be brushed away; the cephalic and podalic part of Periostracum Cicadae must be removed; and the center part of Radix Polygalae must be taken out before use, and so on.

1.2 Methods of Processing Drugs

There are five commonly–used methods of processing drugs:

1. Purifying and cutting

(1) Discarding miscellaneous substances

The dusty ashes, miscellaneous substances and non–pharmaceutical parts of the pharmaceutical plants should be discarded by separating, picking up, sieving, brushing or scraping, thus making the drugs clean. For instance, the twigs and leaves of

Flos Albiziae should be trimmed; the hair of the back part of Folium Eriobotryae should be brushed away; and the coarse outer covering of Cortex Magnoliae Officinalis should be scraped off.

(2) Breaking into fine pieces

Some drugs should be pounded, ground, scraped or filed so as to meet the requirements of medicinal processing or of the preparation of various forms of medicines. For instance, Os Draconis and Concha Ostreae should be pounded into small pieces for use in decocting; and Cornu Antelopis should be made into thin slices or fine powder for convenience in administration or making preparations.

(3) Cutting

By cutting drugs into pieces of certain specifications, their medicinal effective components may easily be dissolved in the decoction; in addition, it will be easier to make the drugs into preparations, or to dry and preserve them, or to weigh them as ingredients in making prescriptions. According to the medicinal properties and therapeutic requirements, there are various specifications for cutting drugs. For instance, Radix Linderae and Semen Arecae must be cut into thin slices; Rhizoma Dioscoreae and Rhizoma Atractylodis Macrocephalae into thick slices; Ramulus Cinnamomi and Radix Astragali seu Hedysari into oblique pieces; Radix Aucklandiae into short straight pieces; Folium Eriobotryae and Cortex Mori Radicis into fine pieces; Herba Ephedrae and Caulis Lonicerae into segments; Radix Puerariae and Massa Fermentata Medicinalis into small lumps.

2. Processing with water

Processing drugs with water is a kind of method of treating

pharmaceutical materials with clean water or other liquid adjuvants for the purposes of cleaning, softening, or making them easy to cut, or reducing their toxicity. The commomly–used procedures include washing and stirring, rinsing, soaking and immersing, sprinkling and softening, refining insoluble powder with water, etc. Here, only three of them are introduced.

(1) Softening

Softening, which is called *Men* or *Fu* in TCM, is a method for making the medicinal materials soft gradually through permeable action so as to make them easy to cut with no or less loss of effective components, by sprinkling, washing, infusing, immersing, soaking–with –sealing, etc., with clean water or other liquid adjuvants according to the hardness of the medicinal materials, the air temperature and equipment during processing. For instance, Herba Elsholtziae seu Moslae must be sprinkled with water; Radix Angelicae Sinensis washed with wine; Semen Arecae infused with water; Cortex Magnoliae Officinalis immersed with ginger juice; Radix et Rhizome Rhei soaked in a sealed jar filled with water, etc.

(2) Rinsing

Rinsing is a method for removing the salty elements, offensive smell, poisonous substances or non–pharmaceutical parts from the medicinal materials by putting them a certain time in a large container of water which must be running or changed frequently. For instance, Thallus Laminariae seu Eckloniae, Sargassum and pickled Herba Cistanchis must be desalted by rinsing; and the offensive smell of Placenta Hominis removed and so on.

(3) Refining insoluble powder with water

This is a method for refining and getting the fine insoluble powder by grinding the medicinal materials in water. This method is first applied to crush the medicinal materials into particals, and then to grind them in a mortar which contains a certain amount of clean water (its level above the drugs) till there is no noise during grinding; then more clean water is added into it and the content is futher stirred. Consequently, the fine particles will be floated, and the coarse ones deposited. The sediment of coarse particles will be left when the supernatant suspension is decanted, from which fine powder is precipitated, separated and then dried in the sun for use. The procedures above may be repeated until all the coarse particles are ground into fine particles and the suspension is formed. This method is suitable for those insoluble materials such as minerals and shells. In addition, it can prevent the particles from flying into the air so as to reduce the loss of medicinal materials. It can also separate the miscellaneous substasces soluble in water and purify and refine the medicinal materials, thus making them easy to be absorbed when orally taken and less irritant when externally applied. Such drugs as Cinnabaris, Talcum, Calamina and Realgar are mostly frequently treated and refined by this method.

3. Processing with fire

Medicinal processing with fire is one of the most frequently used methods which is used in treating crude drugs by direct or indirect heating (or heating with other adjuvants) with fire. Its purpose is to make crude drugs crisp, easy in preparation of dosage forms and convenient for patients to take. Besides, it can be used to correct their medicinal properties, enhance their therapeutic effects, remove or eliminate their toxicity or drastic action. This method includes these following commonly used measures——parching, stir–frying with adjuvants, calcining, roasting in ashes and burning.

(1) Parching

Parching is a frequently–used procedure in processing crude drugs by stir–baking the medicinal materials (with adjuvants or without adjuvants). The procedure of stir–baking with no adjuvants is called simple parching. According to the degrees required, parching may be divided into parching until the drugs become yellowish, parching until brownish and parching until carbonized. By parching the drugs into yellowish or brownish, they will be easy to be pounded into pieces or powder, and their properties will be moderated and the pharmaceutical components of some seeds will be apt to be dissolved in decoction; by parching until the drugs become carbonized, their properties and side effects may be moderated or checked and their effects of astringent and arresting hemorrhage will be reinforced. Besides, when drugs are stir–baked together with solid adjuvants such as mud, bran or rice, their irritant properties will be reduced while their therapeutic effects enhanced. In practice, Rhizoma Dioscoreae is often parched with mud, Cortex Ailanthi with bran and Radix Codonopsis Pilosulae with rice. The process of parching crude drugs with sand, Talcum or powder of Concha Meretricis seu Cyclinae is known as burning by which drugs can be evenly heated and crisp, and the effective components of burning–treated drugs may be dissolved easily in the decoction, or, at least, the drugs can be administered more easily. In practice, Squama Manitis is burned with sand, Colla Corii Asini with powder of Concha Meretricis seu Cyclinae, etc.

(2) Stir–baking with liquid adjuvants

This procedure, also called *Zhi* in TCM, is a method for the purpose of correcting their pharmaceutical properties, increasing their therapeutic actions or reducing their side effects through gradual increase of permeation of the liquid adjuvants into the drugs during processing. The commonly used liquid adjuvants include honey, wine, vinegar, ginger juice, salt water and sesame oil. For example, they are: honey–baked Radix Asteris or Radix Farfarae having better effects on soothing the lung and relieving cough; wine–baked Rhizoma Ligustici Chuanxiong giving stronger effect on activating the blood circulation; vinegar–baked Rhizoma Corydalis exerting more remarkable effect on relieving pain and salt–water–baked Cortex Eucommiae getting more obvious effect on reinforcing the kidney.

(3) Calcining

Calcining is a method of treating crude drugs by direct or indirect burning with strong fire. Its purposes are to make them crisp, easy to be powdered and to produce better therapeutic effect. Some crude drugs of hard minerals or shells as Concha Meretricis seu Cyclinae and Fluoritum may be burned directly till they are thoroughly reddish, then cooled and ground into pieces; and some drugs as Crinis Carbonisatus and Petiolus Trachy–carpi may be burned and carbonized indirectly in a sealed refractory container till its bottom gets fully flushed.

(4) Roasting in hot ashes

This method, called *Wei* in TCM, is a process of treating crude drugs by roasting them with mild fire. The process requires to wrap the raw medicinal materials with wet paper or dough, and heat them in smouldering ashes till the coat becomes carbonized and cracked. By this method the toxicity and drastic properties of some drugs can be reduced, such as roasted Semen Myristicae, roasted Fructus Chebulae.

4. Processing with both fire and water

It is one of the comprehensive methods for treating medicinal materials with fire and water and sometime with other adjuvants for the purposes of correcting their pharmaceutical actions, promoting their therapeutic effects and removing or reducing their toxicity or side effects. And applied by this method, the drugs will be refined and easier to be prepared. Its frequently used measures are steaming, boiling, scalding, quenching, etc.

(1) Steaming

Steaming is a method of processing crude drugs by putting them in a steaming pot or the like so as to heat them with steam. For instance, the effect of purging of Radix et Rhizoma Rhei may be moderated by steaming it after being stirred and mixed with wine. And only by repeated steaming and drying in the sun can some drugs have the required therapeutic actions: instead of the action of relaxing the bowels, Radix Polygoni Multiflori will have the actions of invigorating the liver and kidney, and replenishing vital essence and blood after being steamed repeatedly.

(2) Boiling

Boiling is a method of treating crude drugs by heating them in clean water or other liquid adjuvants at boiling temperature. For instance, boiling Flos Genkwa in vinegar will reduce its toxicity and boiling Radix Scutellariae in wine will enhance its effect of cleaning away lung heat.

(3) Scalding

Scalding is a method of treating crude drugs by putting them into boiling water, and stirring them for a short while before taking them out. This method is often used to treat such medicinal materials as seeds before being peeled and carnified and succulent drugs. For instance, Semen Armeniacae amarum and Semen Persicae are scalded so as to remove their outer coverings and Herba Portulacae and Radix Asparagi are scalded to make it easy to dry and store them.

(4) Quenching

Quenching is a method of treating crude drugs by first burning them until the drugs become red thoroughly, and then, dipping them in water or other liquid adjuvants instantly so as to make them loose and brittle. After being quenched, some adjuvants will be absorbed by them, and this will allow full play to the therapeutic actions of the drugs. For instance, Pyritum or Carapax Trionycis must be quenched with vinegar; and Calamina with concentrated of Rhizoma Coptidis.

5. Other processing methods

Besides the methods mentioned above, there are still others, such as germination, fermentation, frost–like powder making and preparing crude drugs with a series of procedures with water, Alumen, Radix Glycyrrhizae and lime, for the purpose of moderating or changing their original properties, making them produce new therapeutic action, lowering or reducing their toxicity or side effects. For instance, there are Fructus Oryzae Germinatus, Fructus Hordei Germinatus, Massa Fermentata Medicinalis, Semen Sojae Praeparatum or fermented soya bean, frost–like powder of defatted Fructus Crotonis, Rhizoma Pinelliae prepared with water in accompany with Alumen and others.

2 Properties, Actions and Indications of Traditional Chinese Drugs

This topic refers to the natures, flavours, actions and indications of traditional Chinese drugs as well as to the theory dealing with the medicinal properties. What properties mean here involves the four medicinal natures, five flavours or tastes, and the tendencies of their actions (lifting, lowering, floating and sinking), channel tropism and toxicity. All this is a conclusion drawn from long clinical practice by ancient people for the purpose of explaining how the drugs work. It is a guiding principle in clinical practice. Therefore, having a good command of this theory is most important in clinical medication.

As we know, the theory dealing with the medicinal properties is a part of the integral system of theories of traditional Chinese medicine; and it holds that every drug has its characteristics and may be cold or hot in nature, lifting or lowering in the tendency of its action, which can be employed to regulate excessive or deficient condition of *Yin*, *Yang*, *Qi* or blood so as to re-establish balance of physiological functions, the utmost goal of medical treatment. This is the fundamental principle in medication as well as the essential concept of what medicinal properties mean.

2.1 Four Natures and Five Flavours of Drugs

Four natures and five flavours of drugs are the main contents of natures and flavours of traditional Chinese medicines. Every drug has not only its nature but also its flavour, and both are closely related to its therapeutic effects. This theory is one of the main theories of traditional Chinese medicines, which is significant in guiding clinical practice.

Four natures are called four *Xing* (the Chinese sound for 'nature') in TCM. Four natures refer to cold, hot, warm and cool. The theory of four natures of drugs was summed up through long–term struggle against diseases and repeated observations in clinical practice by TCM physicians and pharmacists of various dynasties in the light of the patients' responses and the therapeutic effects of the drugs after administration of them. The drugs which can be used to treat heat syndrome are mostly cool or cold in nature; and the drugs having the therapeutic effect on cold syndrome, are warm and hot. In clinical practice, four natures of drugs—cold, hot, warm and cool—are not absolute but relative to the nature of specific syndrome whether it is cold or hot.

Drugs with cool or cold nature and drugs with warm or hot nature belong to absolutely different categories. But the difference between cool and cold or between warm and hot seems just a difference in degree; in other words, cool seems inferior to cold while warm inferior to hot. That is why we can find in classical medicinal books of various dynasties such terms as slightly cold or extremely warm; in fact, what slightly cold means is just cool while extremely warm just hot.

Although there is difference in degree between cold and cool or between warm and hot, yet cold and cool are in nature of the same category, and warm and hot are of the same category too, and each category has its own characteristics; that is, drugs cool or cold in nature have the effects of clearing away heat, purging fire, removing toxic materials, etc. and may be used to treat diseases due to invasion by pathogenic heat; while drugs warm or hot in nature have the effects of dispersing evil cold, warming the interior, invigorating vital energy, etc. and may be used to treat diseases due to invasion by cold.

Besides four natures, there is one more nature; that is, certain drugs are not remarkably cool, cold, warm or hot, it is quite mild in nature. Most drugs of this kind can be used in treating diseases due to invasion by cold or heat. Therefore, in the light of the nature of drugs, there are actually five natures, but also the four natures mentioned earlier are in common use.

The five flavours of drugs are pungent, sweet, sour, bitter and salty to the taste, which may be detected by the tongue. Besides the five flavours, there is a bland flavour; as the bland flavour is tasteless and mild, it has been affiliated with the sweet flavour; and this is why the term, bland–sweet flavour, was used in medicinal books of various dynasties. Hence the term "five flavours" "Hence the term five flavours as used in general". In the light of flavours and actions of the drugs, however, there are six flavours in reality.

Through hundreds of years of clinical practice, ancient TCM doctors found that flavours of drugs had close relation with their actions; in other words, drugs of different tastes would produce different therapeutic effects. On the basis of this, the theory of five flavours of drugs was established. The meanings and actions of the five flavours of drugs are briefly described below:

Pungent flavour

Pungent drugs include drugs of pungent taste and hot nature, and drugs of pungent taste and cool nature. These drugs can produce the effects of sweating and activating the flow of *Qi*. Most drugs having effects of perspiring and promoting circulation of *Qi* are pungent to the taste; therefore they are generally indicated in exterior syndromes due to invasion by exogenic factors or syndromes due to stagnation of *Qi* and blood.

Sweet flavour

Sweet flavour is the taste like that of sugar. Most drugs having the effects of replenishing body, regulating middle *Jiao* or relieving spasms, are sweet to the taste. They are often used to treat deficiency syndromes, relieve certain pain syndromes, or coordinate the actions of other drugs.

Sour flavour

Sour flavour can produce the effects of astringing and arresting discharge. They are often used to treat incessant sweating due to deficiency syndrome, protracted diarrhea, nocturnal emission, leukorrhea, etc. Besides, most sour drugs may be astringent to the taste at the same time. As the action of the astringent taste is somewhat similar to that of sour flavour, it is usually not considered as an entry in drug tastes.

Bitter flavour

Bitter flavour can produce effects of loosing bowels, drying or resolving dampness, reserving or consolidating *Yin*. Most drugs for clearing away heat or purging fire, treating constipation, resolving dampness or lowering the adverse *Qi* are bitter in taste; therefore they are frequently used in treating febrile diseases, constipation, fullness of stomach and abdomen due to accumulation of dampness, cough and dyspnea, vomiting and hiccup, etc. Besides, in the light of clinical experience of TCM doctors in the previous dynasties, bitter drugs may be used in reserving or consolidating vital essence; for instance, Cortex phellodendri and Rhizoma Anemarrhenae can be used to treat flaccidity syndromes due to flaring–up of prime–minister fire caused by consumption of kidney *Yin*; and this also means that *Yin* will be reserved when the fire is eliminated by these bitter drugs.

Salty flavour

Salty flavour may produce effects of descending and softening hard noddles or masses, or promoting defection, so they are used to treat scrofula, hard mass, constipation, etc.

Bland flavour

Bland flavour or tasteless taste can produce effects of inducing diuresis and eliminating dampness; and most drugs for eliminating dampness by inducing diuresis are bland to the taste. They are commonly used to treat such syndromes due to accumulation of pathogenic dampness, disorder of urination, etc.

Through a long period of clinical practice the theory of five flavours of drugs has developed and summed up, and its significance in clinical use is far beyond the boundary of the simple sense to the taste; or we can say, its field of application has been far more extended. In the light of this theory, the drugs having the effect of astringing are categorized as drugs of sour taste, and the drugs having the effect of softening hard masses are salty drugs and so on. This is why the flavours of some drugs in the medicinal books are not really coincided with those to the tastes. For instance, Holloysitum Rubrum is categorized as a sour drug; Concha Ostreae as a salty drug; and Herba Ephedra as a pungent drug. Here, the flavours of these drugs are quietly different from to the tongue's tastes, they are mainly classified and determined according to their clinical effects.

This theory of natures and flavours of traditional Chinese drugs form an important basis for discussing their clinical actions, indications and use. Each drug has its own nature and flavour, and those drugs with the same nature and flavour will be similar in their therapeutic actions. For instance, most drugs with pungent flavour and warm nature can produce the effects of sweating and dispersing cold from the exterior. That is where they are in common. On the other hand, each drug has its own characteristics; for instance, Folium et Caulis Perillae and Rhizoma Zingiberis Recens are pungent in flavour and warm in nature and can produce the effects of sweating and dispersing cold from the superficies. The former has remarkable effect of sweating and can also produce the effects on promoting the *Qi* circulation and preventing miscarriage, while the later has only mild effect of sweating but can produce the effects on warming the stomach and arresting vomiting. What is mentioned above reveals that those drugs with similar nature and flavour may be different in their therapeutic actions.

Those drugs are different in nature or flavour will be remarkably different in their therapeutic actions. For instance, Rhizoma Coptidis and Herba Spirodelae are same in cold nature, but different in flavour: the former is bitter in taste and can be used in clearing away heat and resolving dampness while the later is pungent in taste and can be used to disperse pathogenic wind−heat;. Radix Astragali seu Hedysari and Herba Dendrobii are both sweet in flavour, but they are different in nature: the former is sweet in flavour and warm in nature, and can be used to replenish *Qi* while the later is sweet in flavour and cold in nature, and can be used to replenish *Yin* and clear away asthenic heat. Besides, some drugs may be with several flavours, for instance, Ramulus Cinnamomi is pungent and sweet, Radix Curcumae is pungent and bitter, and so on. In the light of clinical use, the more flavours a drug has, the more its kinds of actions will be. So the question about the nature and flavour is very complicated. In order that we can make better use of the theory of nature and flavour of drugs in the clinical practice, we should not noly grasp the general principles and the common properties of drugs, but also have a good command of the characteristics and indications of each drug.

2.2 Lifting, Lowering, Floating and Sinking

Lifting, lowering, floating and sinking of drugs mean directions of actions of drugs in human body when being taken. Lifting indicates ascending, while lowering indicates descending; floating denotes moving outwards and dispersing, while sinking denotes moving inwards and purging. In the light of directions, lifting is somewhat like floating; and sinking, like lowering. The lifting or floating drugs moving in ascending and outward directions generally exert the effects of ascending vital energy, sweating, dispersing cold from the exterior, inducing vomiting, etc; while the lowering or sinking drugs moving in descending and inward directions may have the effects of checking exuberance of

Yang, lowering the adverse flow of *Qi*, clearing away heat evil, resolving dampness, relaxing bowels, etc. The lifting, lowering, floating and sinking of drugs used are related with the location of affected site and condition of transmission of disease. General speaking, what kinds of directions of the actions of drugs should be used are often coincidental with the location of the affected site and opposite to the direction of transmission of disease. For example, for treating disease in the upper and superficial parts, lifting and floating drugs can be used, but the lowering and sinking drugs can not; for the treatment of disease in the lower and deeper parts, lowering and sinking drugs can be used, but the lifting and floating drugs are not indicated; for the treatment of disease due to adverse ascending of pathogenic factor, the lowering drugs can be used, but the ascending drugs can not; for the treatment of disease due to invasion by evil factors sinking deeply into the interior and lowering down to the lower *Jiao*, the lifting drug can be used, but the lowering drugs can not. If we apply drugs without any considering of these factors, the unfavorable result will frequently occur. Therefore the theory of four directions of actions of drugs is useful to the clinical practice, not all of the drugs, but at least some of them.

In general, whether the drug is lifting, lowering, floating or sinking in its action has relation with its nature, flavour and weight. Most drugs with pungent or sweet flavour and in warm nature are lifting and floating in their action, while those with bitter, sour or salty and in cool or cold nature seem lowering and sinking in the therapeutic action. Most light drugs consisting of flowers and leaves such as Herba Menthae and Flos Magnoliae are lifting and floating; while most weighty drugs as roots, fruits, seeds, minerals and shells, are lowering and sinking. However, there are some exceptions; for instance, Fructus Viticis and Fructus Xanthii, consist of fruits, yet they are ascending; Flos Inulae and Folium Sennae consist of flowers or leaves, yet they are lowering. From these mentioned above, you can see in the general theory, there exists certain exceptions, and some drugs are different from the ordinary.

Since there is a close relation between the directions of the action of drugs and natures and flavours of the drugs here; in reality, the former has already resided in the latter. Each drug has its direction of action; in clinical practice, except some drugs which are still used due to certain characteristics in their directions of actions, most drugs are often used just according to their natures and flavours. Therefore, we may think the theory of the lifting, lowering floating and sinking of drugs is generalized and systematized to explain the actions of drugs from some one aspect.

Although the lifting, lowering, floating and sinking of drugs are mainly based upon natures and flavours of the drugs; yet the lifting, lowering, etc., may be changed by some medicinal processing or medicinal combination; for instance, the sinking or lowering drugs will turn into the lifting or floating ones when they are processed with wine or used in combination with a considerable amount of strong lifting or floating drugs; in the same way, the lifting or floating drugs will turn into the sinking or lowering drugs when they are processed with salt solution or used in combination with a variety of strong sinking or lowering drugs. These facts show that lifting, lowering, floating and sinking of drugs are not stable, they can be changed under some conditions.

Therefore, in clinical practice, we should not only grasp a general principle of them but should also have a good command of their variation, thus we can used them effectively and reasonably.

2.3 Channel Tropism

Channel tropism means that the drugs may often produce their therapeutic effect on some portion of a human body in preference; in other words, their therapeutic action is mainly related to some channel (viscus and its channel) or some channels in predominance. And it may seem to produce less effect or seem not related to the other channels. Thus this tells us what kinds of diseases the drugs may be indicated in .

In clinical treatment, each kind of drugs can only be used within some boundary of medicinal treatment. For instance, cold drugs, in general, have the effect of clearing away heat, yet some of them may have their remarkable effect of treating lung-heat; and some of them, treating liver-heat. Tonic drugs, in general, have the effect of replenishing or invigorating the body; yet some of them may exert their better effect of strengthening the lung; and some of them, invigorating the spleen. Therefore, in traditional Chinese medicine, all the drugs can be attributed to the twelve channels in the light of theory of *Zang-Fu* and Meridian in combination with their medicinal action. Thus the theory of channel tropism of drugs has been set up, so as to explain their specific effect on some viscera or channels.

What channel or channels a drug is attributed to is just related to the certain viscus, channel or channels on which the drug may work. Since the channels can communicate with the internal organs interiorly and the superficies exteriorly, during the time when a man is affected by pathogenic factors, they may exert influence to the interior from the superficies; and the disease of the some internal organ may also reflect in the certain portion of the body surface where the channel passes. Therefore, the disease of any portion of human body may be recognized systematically by observing the manifestations along a certain channel. For instance, cough and dyspnea may often occur when the Lung Channel is affected; hypochondriac pain or convulsion may appear when the Liver Channel is in disorder. In the light of the action of a drug having close relation with some viscus or channel, when some viscus or channel is affected, we may know what drugs can be used to treat it. For instance, Radix Platycodi and Semen Armeniacae Amarum can be used to treat cough and dyspnea, stuffiness of the chest, therefore they are attributed to the Lung Channel; Cornu Antelopis and Ramulus Uncariae cum Uncis have the effects of tranquilizing the endogenous wind and arresting convulsion, therefore they are attributed to the Liver Channel. Here, we can see the theory of Channel Tropism is mainly drawn from the therapeutic effects of drugs in practice.

It is known that some of drugs may be attributed to several channels, which means these drugs can be used to treat the disorders of these channels. For instance, Gypsum Fibrosum is attributed to the Lung and Stomach Channels, which means that Gypsum Fibrosum can be used to remove not only lung–heat but also stomach–heat; Radix Codonopsis Pilosulae is attributed to the Spleen and Lung Channels, which means that Radix Codonopsis Pilosulae can be used in invigorating spleen–*Qi* and replenishing lung–*Qi* also.

The theory of channel tropism plays an important role in

clinical treatment. For instance, for treating conjunctivitis due to invasion of the liver by heat, such drugs with effect of eliminating liver–heat can be used; for the treatment of epigastric pain due to invasion of stomach by cold, such kinds of drugs with effects of warming the stomach and relieving stomach ache can be used. By this way it is convenient for us to know how to use drugs for treating disorders of some viscera. Therefore, at the time when we have a general idea of the actions of some main drugs, it is necessary for us to know clearly what channels they are attributed in.

Besides, though the theory of channel tropism helps us know what affected portion the drug can be used for treating, conveniences for us to use it in clinical treatment, but in clinical practice, owing to frequent occurrence of transmission of disease between two organs or channels in addition to the drugs only for one channel, the drugs for the other channel are also often used. For instance, for treating lung disorders accompanied with weakness of the spleen, both the drugs for treating lung disorders and invigorating the spleen can be used, because the drugs for the spleen have the effects not only of promoting its functions of transportation and transformation but also of rehabilitating the lung disorders. In a word, only when we grasp both the channel tropism of drugs and knowledge of relationship between viscera and channels, can we apply drugs much better in clinical practice.

However, four natures and five flavours of drugs are the main theories used to elucidate actions of traditional chinese drugs; the theory of lifting, lowering, floating and sinking may serve as a reference for directions of the actions of drugs; and that of channel tropism of drugs may refer to what part of the body the drugs may exert their effects on. Yet these four natures and five flavours of drugs should not be regarded as just a sole basis in medication. And in the theory of lifting, lowering, floating and sinking and the theory of channel tropism, they are not the same in contents in medicinal books. The numbers of channels to which some drugs attribute in some books are more than those in other books, and the theory of lifting, lowering, floating and sinking of drugs has not been used widely as a universal one yet. All these theories were drawn from the experience by ancient physicians through a long time of clinical practice. Thus, we should not only pay good attention to these theories and study them hard but also explore and systematize them incessantly.

3 Application of Traditional Chinese Drugs

The application of traditional Chinese drugs mainly holds compatibility, contraindication, dosage and administration of the drugs. And only when the drugs are used according to the condition of disease, medicinal property and therapeutical requirement on the basis of knowledge of medication, can they effectively produce their therapeutic actions safely in clinical practice. This suggests that attaining a good command of application of traditional Chinese drugs is very important.

3.1 Compatibility of Drugs

During clinical pratice, we think it best to use a single drug to treat a disorder and fulfil its therapeutic purpose, because this is simple, economical and easy to apply. But, sometimes, on these occasions when the disease is accompanied by other diseases, or the disease is due to invasion of both superficies and interior by pathogenic factors, or asthenic syndrome is complicated with sthenic syndrome, or cold syndrome accompanied by heat syndrome alternatively, the single drug will fail to meet the requirement; and the several drugs in combination must be used according to their specific properties so as to meet the need of the complicated diseases and gain better therapeutic effects. Therefore, compatibility of traditional Chinese drugs refers to combination of more than two drugs according to the clinical requirement and principles of medicinal application so as to increase and reinforce the effects of these drugs due to their synergetic action in combination, or to decrease and correct the side effects of these drugs due to their mutual inhibitory action, thus obtaining better therapeutic effects. Therefore, the aim of compatibility of drugs is to meet clinical needs, take various aspects into account, make a good use of drugs and ensure safe administration.

The relationship between a single drug and the compatible ingredients was generalized previously by ancient physicians as seven aspects, namely, using a single drug, mutual reinforcing, assisting, mutual restraint, inhibition, mutual detoxication and antagonism.

Using a single drug

A single drug is used to achieve the desired therapeutic effect without any accessory drugs. Decoction of Radix Ginseng is taken as an example.

Mutual reinforcement

More than two drugs similar in action in combination can achieve remarkble reinforced synergistic effect; for example, Resina Boswelliae Carterii in combination with Resina Commiphorae Myrrhae may be used to achieve the reinforced effects on promoting the blood circulation and arresting pain.

Mutual assistance

Some main drugs are used in combination with some accessory drugs; though they are different in action, yet the therapeutic effects of the main ingredients will be increased and reinforced. For instance, when Radix Scutellariae with the effects of removing heat and purging the pathogenic fire is in combination with Radix et Rhizoma Rhei with the effects of loosening bowels and clearing away heat, the main therapeutic effects of removing intense heat and purging the pathogenic fire, produced by Radix Scutellariae, will be assisted or reinforced.

Mutual restraint

The harmful action or side effect of an ingredient may be weakened or neutralized by another one. For instance, the poisonous action of Rhizoma Pinelliae or Rhizoma Arisaematis may be decreased or eliminated by Rhizoma Zingiberis Recens. So we say there is mutual restraint between Rhizoma Pinelliae or Rhizoma Arisaematis and Rhizoma Zingiberis Recens.

Mutual detoxication

By mutual detoxicating, one drug or ingredient is used to decrease or eliminate the toxic properties of another drug or ingredient. For instance, Rhizoma Zingiberis Recens can be used to decrease or eliminate the toxic properties or side effects of Rhizoma Pinelliae or Rhizoma Arisaematis; therefore it is said that Rhizoma Zingiberis Recens is the drug or ingredient which can be used in detoxicating the toxic properties or eliminating the side effects of these drugs. From what mentioned above, we can see that mutual restraint and mutual detoxication actually refer to same thing, yet each is from its own aspect of some drugs.

Mutual inhibition

By mutual inhibition the primary action of a drug or ingredient may be weakened or eliminate when it is in combination with the other drug. For instance, Rhizoma Zingiberis can be used in inhibiting the effect of clearing away heat of Radix Scutellariae when they are both in combination.

Antagonism

It denotes that poisonous or the other severe side effects

may occur when two incompatible drugs or ingredients are used in combination. For instance, there are eighteen incompatible medicaments which are believed to give rise to serious side effects, if given in combination.

of the seven aspects in compatibility of ingredients, all refer to mutual relation among ingredients in a prescription except the use of a single drug. As resultant effects in general, they are mutual reinforcement, mutual inhibition and antagonism. Among them, the mutual reinforcement and mutual assistance are two of most frequently used kinds of ingredients with similar properties with the purpose of reinforcing each other's action; mutual restraint and mutual detoxication are two kinds of ingredients with mutual restraining or detoxicating effect with the purpose of weakening or eliminating each other's toxic action or side effects. Mutual inhibition and antagonism are two kinds of drugs or ingredients which can not be used in combination because the former may result in mutual inhibition of the drugs, thus their therapeutic action will be weakened; and the latter may lead to the severe side effects. As to drugs with antagonistic properties, although there are a few examples of these drugs used together in some old and new medical books, yet, in common, this combination of ingredients is still considered as incompatibility. Therefore antagonism should be avoided on the basis of general principles of medication. In the light of clinical experience of ancient physicians, these three kinds of combination of drugs as mutual reinforcement, mutual assistance and mutual restraint, are often used.

From these mentioned above, compatibility in a prescription may be regarded as a development of a single drug. It forms an important basis in making up a prescription, and plays an important role in medication.

3.2 Contraindication of Drugs

Drugs can produce effects not only of treating and preventing disorders but also on exerting the harmful action to human beings. For instance, cool or cold drugs, having the effect on clearing away intense heat, may be likely to damage *Yang*; pungent or hot drugs, having the effect on dispersing pathogenic cold, may damage *Yin*; drastic drugs, having the effect on removing evil factors, may damage healthy energy; tonics, having the effect on invigorating healthy energy, may retain the evil factors. Therefore we should not only know their therapeutic effects but also grasp their side action. And those drastic or poisonous drugs should be used with great care; they should be either avoided or only used after being prepared or combined with other drugs or decreased weight, thus the preponderant properties of these drugs may be corrected. And here, these unfavorable effects of medication or certain aspects we should pay attention to are used to explain what the contraindication of drugs is and why some drugs should be used with great care. Although there seems a lot in the contents of its contraindication, yet several items are listed briefly as follows:

1. Contraindication of drugs in syndromes

Drugs have their own properties, and each drug has its specific actions, indications and contraindications. For instance, Herba Ephedrae, pungent in taste and warm in nature, has the effects of sweating, dispersing wind–cold from superficies and arresting asthma; so it is indicated only in exterior syndrome in excess nature without perspiration, or exterior syndrome accompanied with cough due to invasion by exogenic factors, and due to obstruction of the lung–*Qi*; but it is contraindicated in exterior syndrome in deficiency nature with profuse sweating, or cough and asthma due to deficiency of the lung. Therefore, except a few drugs with extremely moderate nature, most drugs have their contraindications when used in certain syndromes especially those drugs with specific properties. The details will be found in the part 2 kinds of drugs.

2. Incompatibility of drugs

According to the classical medical literature some drugs can not be used together in a prescription, otherwise the therapeutic effect will be weakened or the toxic action will produce; the former is just called mutual inhibition while the latter, antagonism. And the ancient medical literature recorded in various dynesties has described the recognition and development of incompatibility of drugs, yet their points of view have not got identical. Among them, both the eighteen incompatible medicaments and the nineteen medicaments of mutual antagonism were generalized and written in Jin Kingdom and Yuan Dynasty, and they have been known and accepted widely, and have also been written into verselet for the purpose of learning easily and recitation.

(1) Eighteen incompatible medicaments

Radix Glycyrrhizae being incompatible with Radix Euphorbiae Kansui, Radix Euphorbiae Pekinensis, Sargassum and Flos Genkwa; Radix Aconiti incompatible with Bulbus Fritillariae, Fructus Trichosanthis, Rhizoma Pinelliae, Radix Ampelopsis, Rhizoma Bletillae; Rhizoma et Radix Veratri incompatible with Radix Ginseng, Radix Adenophorae Strictae,

Radix Salviae Miltiorrhizae, Radix Scrophulariae, Herba Asari and Radix Paeoniae.

(2) Nineteen medicaments of mutual antagonism

Sulfur being antagonistic to crude mirabilite; mercury to arsenic; Radix Euphorbiae Ebracteotatae to Lithargyrum; Fructus Crotonis to Semen Pharbitidis; Flos Caryophylli to Radix Curcumae; Radix Aconiti and Radix Aconiti Kusnezoffii to Cornu Rhinoceri; crystallized mirabilite to Rhizoma Sparganii; Cortex Cinnamomi to Halloysitum Rubrum; and Radix Ginseng to Faeces Trogopterorum.

As to the Eighteen Incompatible Medicaments and Nineteen Medicaments of Mutual Antagonism, they are regarded as ingredients which are incompatible; but some of them were still used in combination by some physician in various dynasties. For instance, in Decoction of Radix Glycyrrhizae and Radix Euphorbiae Kansui and Rhizoma Pinelliae, Radix Glycyrrhizae is used in combination with Radix Euphorbiae Kansui; in Jade Pot Decoction of Sargassum, Radix Glycyrrhizae is used in combination with Sargassum; in *Gan Ying* Pills, Fructus Crotonis is used in combination with Semen Pharbitidis; in the Powder of Ten Scented Drugs for Resuscitation, Flos Caryophylla is used in combination with Radix Curcumae and so on. Later, some experiments showed that in the combination of two incompatible drugs as Radix Glycyrrhizae and Radix Euphorbiae Kansui, the toxic effect was determined by the ratio of Radix Glycyrrhizae to Radix Euphorbiae Kansui; if the dosage of the former is larger than that of the latter, the toxic effect of the prescription will become remarkable. Other examples such as Radix Aconiti in combination with either Rhizoma Pinelliae or Bulbus Fritillariae

Thunbergii do not show any more drastic effect; but the combination of Herba Asari and Rhizoma et Radix Veratri can cause the death of experimental animals due to its toxic effect. The final conclusion of the eighteen incompatible medicaments and nineteen medicaments of mutual antagonism has not been confirmed although it has been researched through the extensive literature, clinical and laboratory work. So we should treat them cautiously; if we haven't any reason or experience, we should avoid using them.

(3) Contraindication of drugs in pregnancy

Since some drugs may have side effects of injuring fetus and inducing miscarriage, these drugs should be regarded as the medicines which are contraindicated in pregnant women; thus side effects of inducing abortion or miscarriage may be avoided. Drugs which are contraindicated in pregnancy involve poisonous drugs, drastic purgatives, drugs for eliminating blood stasis, drugs extremely hot in nature and aromatic stimulants.

According to the various degrees of side effect on injuring fetus, drugs may be divided into two kinds, one being contraindicated in pregnancy and the other taken with great care. The extremely poisonous or drastic medicines such as Fructus Crotonis, Mylabris, Semen Pharbitidis, Euphorbiae Pekinensis, Radix Euphorbiae Kansui, Flos Genkwa, Radix Phytolaccae, Moschus, Rhizoma Sparganii, Rhizoma Zedoariae, Hirudo and Tabanus Bivittatus, should be regarded as forbidden medicines. And drugs for eliminating blood stasis or *Qi* stagnation, hot drugs and sinking or descending drugs such as Semen Persicae, Flos Carthami, Radix et Rhizoma Rhei, Fructus Aurantii Immaturus, Radix Aconiti Praeparata, Rhizoma Zingiberis and Cortex Cinnamomi may be regarded as ones which should be used cautiously so as to meet the requirement. No matter whether the drugs are regarded as the forbidden medicines or drugs used cautiously, they should be avoided if there is no special indication, thus the untoward reaction may be avoided. But if the pregnant woman is dangerous ill, and no other drugs can be used instead, we may use the drugs mentioned above with great care according to the condition of the patient.

(4) Dietetic Restraint

Dietetic restraint is that some sorts of foods are prohibited or limited to be eaten for therapeutical purpose during medical treatment or taking certain drugs. In ancient medical books, onion is prohibited while Radix Dichroae is taken; green Chinese onion (garlic) or turnip is prohibited while Radix Rehmanniae taken; three-colored amaranth is prohibited while Carapax Trionycis taken; soft-shelled turtle is prohibited while Herba Menthae thaken; silver carp is prohibited while Radix Glycyrrhizae taken; vinegar is prohibited while Poria taken; tea is prohibited while Rhizoma Smilacis Glabrae or Fructus Quisqualis taken; green Chinese onion is prohibited while honey taken, and so on; these examples show that some sorts of foods must be prohibited while certain drugs are used. Besides, some foods must be prohibited while the patients are affected with certain diseases. For instance, greasy or sour or astringing food must be avoided while the patient is affected with exterior syndrome caused by measles; fishes, shrimps, beef, mutton, etc. must be avoided while the patient affected with furuncles or pyogenic skin infection, or pruritus; the hot or greasy food must be avoided while the patient affected with heat syndrome; cold drinking or raw fruits must be avoided while the patient affected with cold syndrome; pepper, green pepper, wine or tea must be avoided while the patient affected with frequent attacks of dizziness, insomnia and quick temper with irascibility; and the fried food must be avoided while the patient affected with indigestion.

3.3 Dosage

Since most traditional Chinese drugs are used in preparation forms, dosage here means the weight of each drug or the relative weight of each ingredient in a prescription or the actual weight of the drugs used in a preparation. In common, dosage refers to the weight of each drug or that of each ingredient in a prescription.

As the dosage of a drug has relation with its therapeutic effect, the dose of a certain drug, when used below the level of effective weight, will produce no therapeutic action; the dose of a certain drug, when used beyond the limit of weight, may produce untoward reaction. Therefore not only the compatibility of drugs but also their dose must be paid attention to. General speaking, since most traditional Chinese drugs are crude plants with fairly moderate nature and a wide–safety range of dosage, the doses of herbal medicines may not be used as strictly as those of chemicals; but the doses of those drastic or extremely poisonous drugs such as Radix Aconiti, Radix Euphorbiae Kansui and Semen Strychni must be used cautiously, thus preventing untoward reactions during treatment. In order to achieve the aim in using drugs in proper doses, we should consider following three aspects:

1. Dosage and properties of drugs

Drugs, drastic or poisonous in nature, must be used in a small amount, then gradually increased according to the conditions; but they can not be taken in an overdosage. As the disorder becomes better, the drug must be gradually decreased or not be used instantly, thus prevent toxication or side effects. Heavy drugs, such as minerals, shells, may be used in a fairly large amount; while light drugs, such as flowers, leaves or aromatic stimulants, used in a rather small amount; drugs with gelatinous or greasy in nature, used in a comparatively large amount.

2. Dosage of ingredients in a prescription

The weight of a single medicine will be usually heavier than that applied in a prescription; the weight of a drug in making decoction heavier than that in pills or power; and the weight of a drug as a main medicine in a prescription heavier than that of an accessory one.

3. Dosage and the conditions of disorder, the patients' constitution and age

For the treatment of serious, acute or protracted disease, the weight of a drug must be fairly heavy while for the mild or chronic one the weight of a drug comparatively light; for those with stunt or strong constitution, the dose must be large while for those at old age or with weak constitution, women or children, small; for the disease being newly affected the dose must be large while for a chronic disease comparatively small. Generally, for children over 6 years half a dose of an adult's is used; for the children below 5 years one fourth of an adult's used; for infant the dose must be smaller.

According to the old system of weights of traditional Chinese drugs, the weight of a drug had to do with the number sixteen; in other words, one *Jin* was equal to sixteen *Liang*; and below *Liang* the weight of a drug was weighted with decimal system. One *Liang* was equal to ten *Qian* and one *Qian* was ten *fen*. Later, the system of weight of traditional Chinese drugs has been applied with the Metric system: one kilogram is equal to one thousand grams. In order to prescribe drugs properly or to make up a prescription correctly, a relative interchangable weight system of traditional Chinese drugs is applied in practice; that is, 1 *Liang* = 30 g, 1 *Qian* = 3 g, 1 *Fen* = 0.3 g, 1 *Li* = 0.03 g.

The dosage of each drug in this book, except those with special directions, refers to the weight of the dried crude drug in a decoction taken daily for an adult; and for children the dose should be decreased according to the definite ratio with the age mentioned above.

3.4 Administration

The common administration of traditional Chinese drugs may be oral or local. Here, this article mainly deals with the methods of decocting drugs, directions and usage.

1. Methods of decocting drugs

In order to make drugs produce the better effect, we should pay attention to the method of boiling drugs. Decoction or herb broth is a medicinal solution, which is obtained by boiling drugs with an approprite amount of water for a period of time; then it is taken after the drugs are removed. It is one of most common dosage forms in clinical practice, because it is simple in making up, easily absorbed by human body and can give quick results. But the decoction is bitter in taste and often with a large amount of solution, it seems not convenient for us to carry it for use.

(1) Stewing utensils available

In making a decoction, a clay pot or earthen jar or a piece of enamelware is to be used instead of an iron one, thus the chemical change due to tannic substance or organic acids or other elements may be prevented; and the medicinal quality and therapeutic effects may be preserved well.

(2) Water available

The water available must be clean; usually the clean fountain, clear water in the stream or river, or tap water may be used. Sometimes the water in the well may also be used if its quilaty is fairly good. How much water will be used should be according to the quantity of the drugs, and the water is usually added one *Cun* over the surface of the drugs.

(3) Fire used in decocting drugs

Generally, the decoction must be first decocted with a strong fire, then with a slow fire; i.e., a strong fire is needed at the beginning period in making a decoction until the solution is boiled; then a small fire is followed until the decoction is done.

(4) Method of decocting in making a decoction

Before being decocted, drugs need immersing in water so as to make their medicinal constituents dissolved easily in the solution. Usually the drugs may be decocted for twice. In making the first decoction the level of water in the pot must be 0.5–1 *Cun* above that of the drugs; and during being heated, the drugs are stirred, and after the solution has been boiled 20–30 min., then the decoction may be decanted. In making the second decoction the water level may be just above that of the drugs, and after the solution has been boiled 20 min., the decoction may be decanted. After that, the first and second decoction are mixed, and then divided into several doses.

During stewing, not strong fire but soft fire is often used so as to make the medicinal constituents dissolved easily. A decoction of diaphoretics or aromatic stimulants must be stewed and boiled for a quite short period of time in ten minutes with not too much amount of water, so as to prevent the volatile substances from going off and preserve the medicinal action; a decoction of tonics must be stewed with a quite large amount of water for a fairly long period of time of boiling for which the time must be 10 min. Greater than that for the other drugs so as to have the effective medicinal constituents dissolved as completely as possible.

In the light of their different characteristics, different drugs should be given different following treatment in making their decoction.

(a) Being decocted first

Some kinds of mineral and shell drugs, such as Gypsum Fibrosum and Concha Ostreae, hard in nature, must be pounded into pieces and decocted first with strong fire and then boiled 15 min. Before other drugs are put in, thus making their active constituents dissolved and extracted easily. Rhizoma Arisaematis or Radix Aconiti Kusnezoffii also must be decocted first with soft fire or decocted for a rather long time, thus their poisonous actions may be lessened or eliminated.

(b) Being decocted later

Some aromatic drugs as Herba Menthae and Fructus Amomi with active volatile constituents must be added after the decoction of the other drugs has been boiled over 15 min.; then decocted from five to ten min. Thus the active volatile constituents and their therapeutic actions can be kept. Some drugs containing anthraquinone glycoside as Radix et Rhizoma Rhei and

Senna, are to be decocted later or for a short period of boiling, thus their medicinal purging action may be preserved well.

(c) Decoction of wrapped drugs

Some drugs as Semen Plantaginis containing a lot of mucilage, if decocted directly in water, will be deposited at the bottom of the pot; and some downy drugs as Flos Imulae, if decocted directly in water, will make their decoction mixed with soft hairs, which can not removed easily and can irritate the throat when the decoction is taken. Therefore these drugs must be wrapped in a piece of cloth or of gauze before they are decocted.

(d) Decoction of a single drug

Some precious drugs as Radix Ginseng and Cornu Rhinoceri, must be decocted separately so as to extract their constituents more completely and prevent them from being wasted. After the decoction has been decanted, the residue can be further added to other drugs in making decoction, and finally, the decoction of the single medicine must be mixed with other decoction to make a good use of it and produce a much better effect.

(e) Taking infusions of drugs

Some precious drugs, such as Succinum, Cinnabaris, Radix Notoginseng and Endothelium Corneum Gigeriae Galli are often used in a small dose and unsuitable to be decocted. They must be ground into fine powder and taken together with the decoction of other drugs or hot water.

Besides, some gluey or inorganic salt drugs, such as Colla Corii Asini, Natri Sulfas and maltose, are suitable to be dissolved in hot decoction of other drugs, or hot water; thus the formation of gluey substance in the decoction may be avoid. Otherwise, the gluey substance will stick on the pot bottom and not be easy to filtered, which will influence the therapeutic effect of the decoction.

2. Administration of drugs

How to take drugs is usually determined by condition of disease and their medicinal properties, and whether the administration of the drugs is correct or not has close relation with the therapeutic effect; therefore, it is necessary for us to master it.

(1) Methods of taking drugs

Generally, decoction must be taken warm. Cold syndrome can be treated by taking hot decoction with ingredients hot in nature; while heat syndrome can be treated by taking cold decoction with ingredients cold in nature. Sometimes, a patient may have more complicated manifestation by interlacing cold and heat syndromes; a patient of extreme heat inside the body may have pseudo–cold syndrome in the exterior, and vice versa; and in such case the vomiting will occur after the decoction is taken. Therefore for the treatment of pseudo–heat syndrome with extreme cold in the interior, the decoction with ingredients heat in nature must be taken cold; while for pseudo–cold syndrome with extreme heat in the interior, the decoction with ingredients cold in nature must be taken hot. For the treatmant of protracted vomiting, the decoction must be taken in small portion at frequent intervals; and for the patient with loss of consciousness or locking jaw, the decoction must be taken by nasal feeding.

Usually the solid drugs, such as pills or powder, may be taken with boiled water, except some extraordinary cases; sometimes, the pills or powder may be taken with wine because wine can produce the effect of ascending medicinal action and promoting the blood circulation; sometimes, the pills or powder may be taken with dilute salt solution because it can produce the effect of directing other drugs to act on the kidney.

(2) Time for taking drugs

Tonics must be taken usually before meals; the drugs with irritating effect on the mucosa of the stomach and intestine taken after meals; Anthelmintics or purgatives taken with an empty stomach; antimalarial drugs taken before attacks; sedatives taken at the time to go to bed. Certainly, the time for taking drugs must depend on whether the condition of the disease is acute or chronic. For the treatment of acute disease, the drugs must be taken instantly without any delay; and for the chronic, the drugs, such as pills, powder, extract or liquor, must be taken by following a strict regime of administration, three times a day, or twice a day by taking once in the morning and once at night, thus the therapeutic effect of the drugs will be produced continuously. Besides, to meet the requirement of clinical treatment, some drugs must be decocted into a solution as a tea drink and taken in small portions at frequent intervals.

Whether drugs are taken before or after meals, there must be an interval nearly one or two hours between taking them; otherwise, the therapeutic effect of the drugs will be decreased due to interference from food materials.

Generally, A decoction of traditional Chinese drugs may be diveded into two or three doses for use; a chronic patient may take two doses a day, one dose in the morning and the other at night; an acute one must continue to take decoction, a dose for every four hours, thus the drugs may produce the therapeutic effects continuously on eliminating manisfestations and syndromes.

Diaphoretics or purgatives, if strong in action, must be used according to whether the patients are strong or weak; usually, taking drugs must be stopped when the patients get sweating or bowel movement, thus the overdosage of such drugs can be avoided, and the damage of healthy *Qi* may be prevented, too.

Part Two
Kinds of Drugs

I Diaphoretics or Drugs for the Treatment of Exterior Syndrome

Drugs which have the effects of dispersing evils from the superficies and relieving the exterior syndrome by perspiration (or mild perspiration) are called diaphoretics.

Most diaphoretics are pungent in taste, and mainly attributed to the Lung and Urinary Bladder Channels. Since drugs with pungent taste can be used to disperse evils from superficies; the Lung Channel is externally related with the skin and hair, and the Urinary Bladder Channel dominates the superficies of the body. Therefore diaphoretics are good at working at muscles and superficies and likely to cause sweating in varying degrees, and disperse evils from the superficies; they are suitable for treatment of the exterior syndrome caused by invasion of evils. Their indications are as follows:

1. Exterior syndrome due to invasion by pathogenic evils, marked by fever, chills, headache, stiffness of nucha, general soreness, anhidrosis, floating pulse, etc.

2. Cough and dyspnea due to obstruction of Lung-*Qi*

caused by invasion of pathogenic evils.

3. With the function of relieving pain, some diaphoretics may be used to treat headache and pantalgia due to invasion by external factors and arthralgia or *Bi* syndrome due to invasion by wind–dampness.

4. With the function of promoting eruption of measles, some diaphoretics may be used to treat rubella or measles with lingering exogenic evils or in want of eruption.

5. Since diaphoretics have the effect of sweating and relieving edema, and some of them may also have function of promoting the circulation of body fluid; they can be used to treat edema, edema with exterior syndrome or edema occurring above the lumbar region.

Most of the diaphoretics are pungent to the taste and have the function of dispersing evils from the superficies. Some of them are cool in nature while some warm; therefore they can be used to treat different exterior syndromes. In other words, they may divided into two kinds, one with pungent–warm property and the other with pungent–cold property. The former is indicated in the patients with the exterior syndrome marked by heavy chills with moderate fever, and the latter is indicated in them with the exterior syndrome marked by mild chills with high fever. Which kind of diaphoretics will be selected is dependent on the differentiation of clinical syndromes.

Diaphoretics can often be used to treat the exterior syndrome by sweating, yet profuse sweating will consume *Yang* and body fluid; therefore, they are contraindicated or should be used with great care for treating spontaneous sweating due to deficiency of the exterior, fever due to deficiency of *Yin*, later stage of febrile disease with deficiency of body fluid and syndrome of losing blood.

1.1 Diaphoretics With Pungent and Warm Properties

Diaphoretics with pungent and warm properties which are also termed as drugs for dispersing wind-cold, are pungent to the taste and warm in nature. Since they have remarkable function of dispersing evils from superficies, they are indicated in patients with the exterior syndrome caused by wind-cold, which characterized by chills, fever, anhidrosis, headache, pantalgia, thin and white tongue coating, floating and tense pulse. Besides, some of them may be used to treat cough and dyspnea, edema, skin pyogenic infection with the exterior syndrome of wind-cold, and arthralgia.

Most of the drugs may have potent function of sweating; therefore, those with weak constitution should take them with great care.

Ephedra (麻黄 *Mahuang*)
Herba Ephedrae

The drug consists of the dried perennial herbaceous stems and twigs of Ephedra sinica Stapf, Ephedra intermedia Schrenk et C. A. Meyer or Ephedra equisetina Bunge; it is dried in shade and cut into pieces. Either its crude one or prepared one with honey is often used.

Nomenclature Used in Prescriptions: *Sheng Mahuang*, *Zhi Mahuang*

Properties and Channel Distribution: The drug is pungent, somewhat bitter to the taste, warm in nature, and is distributed to the Lung and Urinary Bladder Channels.

Action and Indications:

1. Sweating and dispersing exopathogens from superficies of the body

It is used as a diaphoretic for the disorder due to attack of wind and cold, charaterized by fever, headache and general soreness, obstruction of nose, no perspiration, floating and tight pulse; and its perspiratory effect will be reenforced if combined with Ramulus Cinnamomi.

2. Ventilating the lung and stopping asthma

It is often combined with Semen Armeniacae Amarum for enhancing effects on relieving cough and asthma due to invasion of superficies by wind and cold, and sluggishness of lung–energy; with Rhizoma Zingiberis, Herba Asari, Fructus Schisandrae, Ramulus Cinnamomi, etc., for treating cough due to lung–coldness which is characterized by cough and dyspnea with profuse watery sputum by warming the lung and resolving the stasis of fluid; and with Gypsum Fibrosum, for cough due to lungheat.

3. Promoting Diuresis and eliminating edema

It is often combined with Rhizoma Atractylodis Macrocephalae and used for edema which is related to excess syndrome of retention of fluid and associated with other exterior syndromes.

Besides, the drug with its warming property and the effect of expelling cold may be combined with other drugs and used for arthralgia, cold abscess and so on.

Dosage and Administration: Generally, its dosage is 1.5 to 5 g. The crude drug with its potent perspiratory action is used to disperse exopathogens and promote diuresis; the drug with its mild action of perspiration and soothing effect, after baked and mixed with honey, is used for cough and asthma.

Notes: Since the drug has the strong action of perspiration, the weight used can not be excessive; and it should be avoided if the patient is affected with deficiency syndrome in the exterior accompanied with spontaneous sweating, palpitation, insomnia, or if the patient is affected with hypertension.

Cinnamon Twigs (桂枝 *Guizhi*)
Ramulus Cinnamomi

The drug consists of the dried slender twigs of Cinnamomum cassia Presl (Family Lauraceae); it is often dried either in shade or in the sun, then is cut into pieces or segments for use.

Nomenclature Used in Prescription: *Guizhi*, *Chuan Guizhi*, *Nan Guizhi*

Properties and Channel Distribution: The drug is pungent and sweet to the taste, warm in nature, and distributed to the Heart, Lung and Urinary Bladder Channels.

Action and Indications:

1. Sweating and dispersing exopathogens from the muscles

It can be used as a diaphoretic for the syndrome due to attack by wind and cold, whether the patient perspires or not. It is often combined with Radix Paeoniae Alba to treat the asthenia–syndrome of the superficies with spontaneous perspiration by mediating *Ying* and *Wei* systems; and it can also be combined with Herba Ephedrae to reinforce each other's actions for sthenic syndrome of the superficies with anhidrosis.

2. Warming the channels and arresting pain

It is often combined with such antirheumatics as Rhizoma seu Radix Natopterygii, Radix Ledebouriellae and Radix Paeoniae Alba, Radix Aconiti Praeparata, Rhizoma Atractylodis Macrocephalae and Rhizoma Anemarrhenae for the treatment of arthralgia syndrome due to attack of the upper limbs by cold and dampness. For instances, it is often used with Radix Aconiti Praeparata for the treatment of syndrome due to invasion of superficies by cold and wind, and deficiency of *Yang* in the exterior; with Radix Astragali seu Hedysari, Radix Paeoniae Alba, etc., for the syndrome of arthralgia due to blood disorder manifested as numbness of the extremities; with Radix Paeoniae Alba, maltose, etc., for epigastric or abdominal pain due to invasion of the stomach by cold; and with such drugs for promoting blood flow and regulating menstruation as Radix Angelicae Sinensis, Radix Paeoniae Alba, Rhizoma Ligustici Chuanxiong, Semen Persicae, Cortex Moutan Radicis, etc. for irregular menstruation due to blood stasis caused by invasion of cold, or for amenorrhea with abdominal pain.

3. Promoting *Yang* and reinforcing vital energy

It is often combined with Rhizoma Atractylodis Macrocephalae and Poria for the treatment of cough and expectoration of watery phlegm due to retention of dampness-phlegm in the lung and a blockage in the passage of *Qi*; with Poria, Polyporus Umbellatus, Rhizoma Alismatis, etc. for disorder of urination caused by dysfunction of the urinary bladder; and with Fructus Trichosanthis, Bulbus Allii Macrostemi for angina pectoris or thoracic pain; with Radix Glycyrrhizae, Radix Ginseng, Colla Corii Asini, etc., for palpitation with knotted or intermittent pulse by promoting thoracic-*Yang* and restoring the normal pulse.

Dosage and Administration: Generally, its dosage is 3–10 g and it is often decocted in water for oral administration.

Purple Common Perilla (紫苏 *Zisu*)
Folium et Caulis Perillae

The drug consists of the dried herbs of annual plant, Perilla Frutescens (L.) Britt. (family Labiatae); it is to be dried in shade and cut into segments for being used as medicine, its leaves are called Folium Perillae and its stems, Caulis Perillae.

Nomenclature Used in Prescriptions: *Zisuye*, *Suye*, *Lao Sugeng*.

Properties and Channel Distribution: The drug is pungent to the taste and warm in nature, and distributed to the Lung, Spleen and Stomach Channels.

Action and Indications:

1. Dispelling pathogenic wind and cold from the superficies

It is often combined with Herba Schizonepetae, Radix Ledebouriellae, Rhizoma Zingiberis Recens, etc. and used for the treatment of cold due to attack of pathogenic wind and cold, charaterized by chilliness and fever, headache and obstruction of the nose, etc.; and with Semen Armeniacae Amarum, Radix Peucedani, etc to reinforce their effects on ventilating the lung and arresting cough; and with Rhizoma Cyperi, Pericarpium Citri Reticulatae, etc., for those with stuffiness in the chest due to stagnation of chest–*Qi*.

2. Promoting the flow of *Qi* and regulating the function of the stomach

The drug can be used in treating fullness in the epigastrium, stuffiness of the chest and vomiting. For the treatment of those patients with cold syndromes, it should be often combined with Herba Agastachis, Rhizoma Pinelliae, Rhizoma Zingiberis Recens and so on; for those with heat syndromes, it should be combined with Rhizoma Coptidis and Caulis Bambusae in Taeniam; for those with syndrome of *Qi*–stagnation and sputum–stasis, it should be combined with Rhizoma Pinelliae and Cortex Magnoliae Officinalis; for those with disorder of *Qi*–flow, marked by over movement of fetus, stuffiness of the chest and abdominal distention, vomiting and nausea, it is often combined with Pericarpium Citri Reticulatae, Fructus Amomi, etc., thus reinforcing the effects on arresting vomiting and preventing miscarriage. However, the drug is regarded as an ingredient frequently used in regulating *Qi*–flow and preventing miscarriage.

3. Detoxifying poisonous substance of fishes and crabs

For the treatment of fish poisoning or crab poisoning, characterized by vomiting, diarrhea, abdominal pain, etc., it is often combined with Herba Agastachis, Pericarpium Citri Reticulatae, Rhizoma Zingiberis Recens, etc.

Dosage and Administration: Usually, the drug, 6–12 g in weight, is decocted; yet sometimes, 30–60 g of the drug may be used for the treatment of fish or crab poisoning. During treatment, either its leaves or its stems are often used in separation; the former has better function in dispelling cold from the superficies, while the latter, regulating the flow of *Qi* and preventing miscarriage; therefore, in treating syndrome of invasion of cold and wind, the leaves can be used; and in treating disorder of *Qi*–flow and abnormal condition of fetus, its stems used.

Schizonepeta (荆芥 *Jingjie*)
Herba Schizonepetae

The drug consists of dried aerial parts of the annual herbaceous plant, Schizonepeta tenuifolia Briq. (family Labiatae). Usually, they are first bundled up and dried in the sun, then its stems, leaves and ears are all cut into segments, or only its ears cut for use; generally, either crude one or carbonized one is used for medicine.

Nomenclature Used in Prescriptions: *Jingjie*, *Jingjietan*, *Jingjiesui*, *Chaojiesui*, *Jiesuitan*.

Properties and Channel Distribution: The drug is pungent to the taste and slightly warm in nature, and distributed to the Lung and Liver Channels.

Action and Indications:

1. Sweating and dispelling the exogenous wind

The drug with neutral property, slightly warm and not dry in nature, can be used for wind–cold and wind–heat syndrome and used for treating diseases due to pathogenic wind, marked by chilliness with fever, anhidrosis and headache, etc. For the treatment of affection with wind and cold, it is often combined with Radix Ledebouriellae, Radix Angelicae Dahuricae, Rhizoma Zingiberis Recens, etc.; for the treatment of affection with wind and heat, it is often combined with Herba Menthae, Flos

Lonicerae, Fructus Forsythiae and so on. Besides, in treating patients with conjunctivitis, sore throat due to invasion of wind and heat it can be combined with Herba Menthae, Fructus Arctii, Radix Bupleuri, Radix Platycodi, Radix Glycyrrhizae, etc.

2. Facilitating eruption, dispelling evils from superficies

For the treatment of measles with retarded eruption, urticaria at beginning stage, or pyogenic infection of skin, it is often combined with Radix Ledebouriellae, Periostracum Cicadae, Fructus Arctii, Radix Sophorae Flavescentis, etc. according to the different symptoms.

3. Removing blood stasis and arresting bleeding

With other hemostatics, it is indicated in spitting blood, epistaxis, hematochezia, etc. Besides, for the treatment of syndrome due to invasion of exogenic evils in postnatal stage, charaterized by stiffness of nucha, locked jaw, the drug has the effects of dispersing the evil wind, regulating blood and arresting clonus, its powder, 6 g in weight, can be taken singly, or with wine or boy's urine.

Dosage and Administration: Its dosage is 3–10 g for decoction; in arresting bleeding the carbonized drug is used, while in dispersing the evil wind from the superficies the crude is indicated.

Ledebouriella Root (防风 *Fangfeng*)
Radix Ledebouriellae

The drug consists of the dried root of perennial herbaceous plant, Ledebouriella divaricata (Turcz.) Hiroe (family Umbelliferae). The crude plant is first cut into sections, then dried for being used for medicine.

Nomeclature used in Prescription: *Fangfeng*, *Qingfangfeng*, *Koufangfeng*.

Properties and Channel Distribution: The drug is pungent and sweet to the taste, slight warm in nature, and distributed to the Urinary Bladder, Lung and Liver Channels.

Action and Indications:

1. Dispelling pathogenic wind and dispersing exopathogens from superficies of the body

It is used in treating the exterior syndromes especially for those patients with severe headache and pantalgia. The drug is slightly warm in nature but without dryness, and moderate sweet in taste with mild effects; it is considered as one of the medicines for dispersing the wind but with moisturizing effect; it can be indicated in exterior syndrome either with wind-cold or with wind-heat. For the treatment of syndrome of wind-cold, it is often combined with Herba Schizonepetae; for that of wind-heat, with Herba Menthae, Folium Mori; for the treatment of urticaria, skin itching, with Herba Schizonepetae, Fructus Arctii, Fructus Tribuli, etc.

2. Resolving dampness and arresting soreness

It can be used in treating syndrome of arthralgia due to invasion of pathogenic wind, cold and dampness in combination with Rhizoma seu Radix Notopterygii, Radix Angelicae Pubescentis, Rhizoma Ligustici Chuanxiong, etc.; and by this combination its functions of resolving dampness and dispersing wind will be reenforced.

3. Dispersing wind and arresting convulsion

It can be used to treat tetanus, marked by opisthotonus,

locked jaw, local spasm or general convulsion, etc. in combination with Rhizoma Arisaematis, Rhizoma Gastrodiae, Rhizoma Typhonii, etc.

Besides, it is recorded in the old medical books that the drug can be indicated in relieving Arsenicum poisoning when it is combined with Radix Glycyrrhizae.

Dosage and Administration: Usually, its dosage is 3–10 g for decoction.

Notopterygium Root (羌活 *Qianghuo*)
Rhizoma seu Radix Notopterygii

The drug consists of the dried rhizomes and roots of the perennial herbaceous plant, Notopterygium incisium Ting or Notopterygium forbesii Boiss (family Umbelliferae); and the plant is cut into pieces and dried in the sun for being used.

Nomenclature Used in Prescriptions: *Qianghuo, Chuanqianghuo, Xiqianghuo.*

Properties and Channel Distribution: The drug is pungent and bitter to the taste and warm in nature, and distributed to the Urinary Bladder, Liver and Kidney Channels.

Action and Indications:

1. Dispelling pathogenic wind and dispersing cold from the superficies

It is indicated in the exterior syndromes due to invasion of wind and cold, maked by chilliness and fever, headache and pantalgia when it is combined with Radix Ledebouriellae, Herba Asari, Rhizoma Ligustici Chuanxiong, etc.

2. Dispelling wind and resolving dampness

It is used in treating *Bi* syndrome, arthralgia of shoulder, back and upper limbs or pantalgia of the muscles of the upper part of body or with sensation of cold contraction and aversion of cold. The drug has good effects of dispelling evil wind, resolving dampness, expelling cold and arresting soreness, when it is combined with Radix Angelicae Pubescentis, Radix Ledebouriellae, etc.

Dosage and Administration: Usually, its dosage is 3–10 g for decoction; in treating cold it is used in fairly light weight; in treating arthralgia it is used in comparatively large weight. Generally speaking, the dosage used in clinical practice should not be too large.

Asarum Herb (细辛 *Xixin*)
Herba Asari

The drug consists of the dried entire herb of the perennial herbaceous plant, Asarum heterotropoides Fr. var. mandshuricum (Maxim.) Kitag. or Asarum sieboldi Miq. (family Aristolochiaceae); usually, it is first dried in the shade and cut into pieces for being used.

Nomenclature Used in Prescriptions: *Xixin*, *Liaoxixin*, *Beixixin*.

Properties and Channel Distribution: The drug is pungent to the taste and warm in nature, and is distributed to the Lung and Kidney Channels.

Actions and Indications:

1. Dispersing the wind–cold from the superficies

For the treatment of cold due to weak constitution, marked

by chilliness and fever, episodes of bad chills and mild fever, tongue coating moisturized and smooth and deep pulse, it is often combined with Herba Ephedrae, Radix Aconiti Praeparata, thus promoting vital energy and dispersing evils from superficies.

2. Expelling wind and arresting pain

For the treatment of vertigo and headache, it may be combined with Rhizoma seu Radix Notopterygii, Radix Ledebouriellae, Rhizoma Ligustici Chuanxiong, Radix Angelicae Dahuricae and so on; for those with toothache due to invasion of wind and cold, with Radix Aconiti 1.5 g, Olibanum 3 g, Radix Angelicae Dahuricae 3 g; and for this purpose mentioned above, 3 g of this Herba Asari and the other 3 ingredients are mixed and powdered, and a little amount of the powder is used locally for each time, several times a day. For toothache due to wind–heat, the drug 3 g and Gypsum Fibrosum 30 g are decocted; for arthralgia due to wind, cold and dampness, it can be with Rhizoma seu Radix Notopterygii, Radix Angelicae Pubescentis, Radix Ledebouriellae, Radix Gentianae Macrophyllae, etc.

3. Dispelling the interior cold from the lung and removing the stasis of fluid

For the treatment of cough and dyspnea with retention of fluid, marked by profuse watery sputum, it can be combined with Rhizoma Zingiberis, Rhizoma Pinelliae, Herba Ephedrae and so on.

4. Removing the obstruction of the nose

For the treatment of sinusitis, marked by obstruction of the nose with headache, episodes of running nose, it can be used in combination with Radix Angelicae Dahuricae, Flos Magnoliae,

Herba Menthae and so on.

Besides, it can be used locally for the treatment of aphtha and tongue sore; for this purpose, its powder mixed with water may be applied to umbilicus; at the same time, the affected area, the mouth or tongue, can be applied with the concentrated decoction of Rhizoma Coptidis.

Dosage and Administration: 1–3 g of the drug is used for decoction; for local administration its powder form can be applied by insufflating into the nose cavity for sinusitis or by local smearing.

Notes: It is contraindicated in patients with headache due to hyperactivity of liver–*Yang* or with cough due to deficiency of lung–*Yin* and invasion of lung–heat. Generally, the weight of the drug used can not be too large. Besides, it is antagonized by Rhizoma et Radix Veratri.

Dahurian Angelica Root (白芷 *Baizhi*) Radix Angelicae Dahuricae

The drug consists of the dried root of the perennial herbaceous plant, Angelica Dahurica (Fisch. ex Hoffm.) Benth. et Hook. f. or Angelica Dahurica (Fisch. ex Hoffm.) Benth. et Hook. f. var. formosana (Boiss.) Shan et Yuan; usually, it is first dried in the sun and then cut into pieces for use.

Nomenclature Used in Prescriptions: *Baizhi*, *Hangbaizhi*, *Xiangbaizhi*.

Properties and Channel Distribution: The drug is pungent to the taste and warm in nature, and distributed to the Lung and Stomach Channels.

Action and Indications:

1. Dispersing evil cold from superficies

In treating cold due to invasion of wind and cold, with headache over the frontal part of the head, the drug is often combined with Herba Schizonepetae, Radix Ledebouriellae, Fructus Viticis, Rhizoma seu Radix Notopterygii, etc.

2. Dispelling wind and arresting pain

It is indicated in vertigo, Migraine, supraorbital neuralgia, headache with nasosinusitis, toothache. For the treatment of vertigo or headache due to invasion of wind, it can be used as a single medicine or combined with Rhizoma Ligustici Chuanxiong, Flos Chrysanthemi, Radix Ledebouriellae and Rhizoma seu Radix Notopterygii; for headache due to nasosinusitis, with Fluctus Xanthii, Flos Magnoliae; for toothache due to invasion of wind and cold, with Herba Asari; for toothache due to invasion of wind and fire, with Gypsum Fibrosum.

3. Relieving swelling and letting out pus

It is indicated in furuncle or pyogenic infection; besides, it can be used to relieve swelling and disperse evils when the local lesion is at its beginning; it can be used to let the pus out after the lesion has been ruptured; therefore it is commonly used in the field of traditional Chinese surgery. For the treatment of mastitis, it is often combined with Fructus Trichosanthis, Bulbus Fritillariae Thunbergii, Herba Taraxaci etc.; for the treatment of other carbuncles or pyogenic infection, with Flos Lonicerae, Fructus Forsythiae and so on.

4. Resolving dampness and relieving leucorrhagia

For the treatment of leucorrhagia due to invasion of cold and dampness, marked by white watery vaginal dischage, it is often combined with Rhizoma Atractylodis Macrocephalae, Poria, Os Sepiellae seu Sepiae and so on.

Dosage and Administration: Usually, its dosage is 3–9 g for decoction.

Ligusticum Root (藁本 *Gaoben*)
Rhizoma Ligustici

The drug consists of the dried rhizoma and roots of Ligusticum sinense Oliv. or Ligusticum jeholense Nakai et Kitag. (family Umbelliferae). The crude plant is first dried in the sun and cut into pieces for being used as medcine.

Nomenclature Used in Prescription: *Gaoben*, *Chuangaoben*.

Properties and Channel Distribution: The drug is pungent to the taste and warm in nature, and distributed to the Urinary Bladder Channel.

Action and Indications:

1. Dispersing cold from superficies

It is indicated in cold due to affection by wind and cold, marked by headache, chills, anhidrosis, it is often combined with Rhizoma seu Radix Notopterygii, Radix Ledebouriellae, Herba Asari, etc.

2. Dispelling wind and resolving dampness

It is indicated in headache over the vertex and occipital region due to affection by wind and cold, or headache due to affection by wind and dampness, or wind syndrome of head; therefore it is a drug frequently used to treat headache especially that over the vertex region. The drug is likely to communicate with the *Du* Channel and to get to the vertex region of the head; for such headache it is often combined with Radix Angelicae Dahuricae, Rhizoma Ligustici Chuanxiong, Herba Asari, etc. For the treatment of arthralgia or soreness of limbs due to invasion of wind–cold, it is often combined with Rhizoma seu Radix Notopterygii, Radix Angelicae Pubescentis, Radix Ledebouriellae, Radix Clematidis and so on.

Dosage and Administration: 3–10 g for decoction.

Notes: It is contraindicated in headache due to blood deficiency or that not due to affection by wind–cold and dampness.

Xanthium Fruit (苍耳子 *Cangerzi*)
Fructus Xanthii

The drug consists of the dried ripe fruit involving the whole bud of the annuel herbaceous plant, Xanthium sibiricum Patr. (family Compositae); it is baked and stirred for being used as medicine after its thorns are removed.

Nomenclature Used in Prescriptions: *Cangerzi*

Properties and Channel Distribution: The drug is pungent and bitter to the taste, warm and a little poisonous in nature, and distributed to the Lung Channel.

Action and Indications:

1. Dispersing wind and removing the obstruction of the orifices

It is indicated in headache due to affection by wind–cold or wind–syndrome of head, or indicated in nasosinusitis. For the treatment of headache due to affection by wind–cold or wind–syndrome of head it is often combined with Radix Ledebouriellae, Radix Angelicae Dahuricae, Rhizoma Ligustici, etc. The drug is regard as a main medicine in treating nasosinusitis, characterized by headache with sinusitis, episodes of running nose, loss of smelling; and for the treatment of nasosinusitis it is often combined with Flos Magnoliae and Radix Angelicae Dahurica.

2. Resolving dampness and arresting soreness

It is indicated in rheumatic arthralgia, numbness of muscles and often combined with Rhizoma seu Radix Notopterygii, Radix Ledebouriellae, Radix Angelicae Sinensis, Radix Achyranthis Bidentatae, etc.

Dosage and Administration: 3–10 g for decoction.

Notes: The drug is a little poisonous in nature, over dose taken will lead to drug intoxication, marked by stuffiness of the episgastrium, nausea and vomiting, sometimes accompanied with abdominal pain and diarrhea, headache and restlessness, etc.

Appendix:

1. Herba Xanthii

The drug consists of the entire plant of Xanthium sibiricum Patr., dried in the sun and cut into pieces for being used. It is bitter and pungent in taste and slight cold, and poisonous in nature. Its action and indications are nearly the same as Fructus Xanthii, but its effect of detoxifying the toxic materials seems more remarkable; therefore it can be used to treat such diseases as various kinds of furuncles, carbuncles and boils, pyogenic skin infections, eczema, bee or wasp sting, snake or insect bite, etc. by local smearing with the herb after being washed and pounded to pieces, or by taking its soft extract (*Wan Ying Gao*) which is usually made by cutting the herbs to pieces, stewing them in water to a concentrated decoction, then filtrating it and heating the solution with the slow fire, and concentrating the solution to the soft extract. During treatment, the soft extract (*Wan Ying Gao*) can be applied by taking 1.5−3 g by the mouth or by local smearing. Usually 5−10 g of the dried herbs are taken as a dose, and 10−15 g of the herbs will be used if they are fresh; the weight used above is for the preparation of decoction, and for the local use a proper amount will be used.

2. Worm in the stem of Xanthium sibiricum Patr. (*Cangerchong*)

The drug consists of a kind of larva of an insect, parasitizing in the stem of the plant, Xanthium sibiricum Patr. Generally after being collected, the worms are reserved in sesame oil as a medicated preparation. The worm, having the functions of removing the toxic materials and relieving swelling and congestion, can be used in treating furuncles, carbuncles and pyogenic skin infections. During treatment, 1−2 worms are applied on the affected site and covered with an adhensive plaster.

Magnolia Flower (辛夷 *Xinyi*)
Flos Magnoliae

The drug consists of the flower buds of the deciduous bush, Magnolia liliflora Desr. (family Magnoliaceae). The crude drug is usually dried in the sun and pounded for being used.

Nomenclature Used in Prescriptions: *Xinyi, Xinyibao*

Properties and Channel Distribution: The drug is pungent to the taste, warm in nature, and distributed to the Lung Channel.

Action and Indications:

1. Dispersing wind and cold from the superficies

For the treatment of cold due to invasion by evil wind and cold, marked by headache, obstruction of the nose, etc., It may be combined with Radix Angelicae Dahuricae, Radix Ledebouriellae, Rhizoma Ligustici Chuanxiong, etc.

2. Removing obstruction of nose

It is indicated in sinusitis and headache, accompanied with obstruction of the nose, purulent nasal discharge, loss of smelling; usually it is regarded as a medicine specially for the treatment of sinusitis. For the treatment of nasosinusitis due to invasion by wind–cold, it may be combined with Radix Angelicae Dahuricae, Herba Asari, etc.; for that due to wind–heat, it may be combined with Herba Menthae, Radix Scutellariae, etc.

Now, it is often used for chronic rhinitis, allergic, rhinitis, and maxillary sinusitis. And for this purpose, besides its decoction, medicated oil or emulsion, and medicinal powder are often used for local administration by dripping, insufflating or smearing; they often reveal satisfactory effects.

Dosage and Administration: 3–9 g of the drug are taken as a dose; and a proper amount of its powder is applied for local administration to the nasal cavity.

Fresh Ginger (生姜 *Shengjiang*)
Rhizoma Zingiberis Recens

The drug consists of the fresh rhizoma of the perennial herbaceous plant, Zingiber officinale (Willd.) Rosc. (family Zingiberaceae). The crude drug Should be washed and cut into pieces and used when it is fresh. Succus Zingiberis consists of the juice of ginger, which is collected by crushing the fresh plant;

Exocarpium Zingiberis Recens consists of the exocarp of the plant; and the plant prepared by roasting in hot ashes is called roasted ginger.

Nomenclature Used in Prescriptions: *Shengjiang*, *Xian Shengjiang*.

Properties and Channel Distribution: The drug is pungent to the taste, slightly warm in nature, and distributed to the Lung, Spleen and Stomach Channels.

Action and Indications:

1. Promoting perspiration and dispersing wind–cold from superficies

It is often used for the treatment of cold due to invasion of wind–cold. Since its action of perspiration seems mild, it is frequently used as an accessory ingredient in the prescription for reinforcing the effect of sweating of pungent–warm drugs. For the treatment of moderate common cold, either its decoction with brown sugar or infusion with boiling water can be taken.

2. Warming the stomach to arrest vomiting

In treating vomiting due to the stomach attacked by cold, it is usually combined with Rhizoma pinelliae; and some drugs are sometimes prepared with ginger juice to strengthen their effect of arresting vomiting.

3. Dispelling evil cold from the lung to relieve cough

For the treatment of cough due to invasion of the lung by wind–cold, marked by expectoration of white and watery sputum, it is often combined with such drugs for dispelling cold of the lung to relieve cough.

4. Relieving poisoning

It can be used to relieve the poisonous action of crude

Rhizoma Pinelliae, Rhizoma Arisaematis, marked by tingling and paralysis of tongue and epiglottis, with its juice taken with water or its decoction

Dosage and Administration: Generally, 3–10 g are used as a dose for decoction.

Appendix:

1. Succus Zingiberis

It can be used in treating wind stroke or loss of conciousness due to invasion of the heart by phlegm, marked by lockjaw, syncope, persistent attacks of vomiting, etc.; since it with its taste and effect of dispersing evil cold, has the actions of resolving phlegm and arresting vomiting. 3–10 drops of the juice are taken as a dose after pouring water over it.

2. Exocarpium Zingiberis Recens

It is pungent to the taste and cold in nature; it has the effect of promoting the circulation of the body fluid; therefore it is often used in treating edema. 3–6 g are taken as a dose.

3. Rhizoma Zingiberis (roasted)

It is prepared by wrapping the drug in wet paper and baked in hot ashes till the paper turns black. The effect of its pungent taste on dispersing cold seems weaker than that of Rhizoma Zingiberis Recens, but its actions of warming middle *Jiao* and arresting vomiting are stronger; therefore it is indicated in the cold syndrome of the spleen and stomach of the deficiency type, marked by abdominal pain, vomiting, watery stools, etc. Usually 3–10 g are taken as a dose.

Fistular Onion Stalk (葱白 *Congbai*)
Bulbus Allii Fistulosi

The drug consists of the white stalk of the perennial herbaceous plant, Allium fistulosum L. (family Liliaceae); usually the fresh stalk near the root is used as medicine.

Nomenclature Used in Prescriptions: *Congbai. Congbaitou*

Properties and Channel Distribution: The drug is pungent to the taste, warm in nature, and distributed to the Lung and Stomach Channels.

Action and Indications:

1. Promoting perspiration to disperse the evils from superficies

It is often combined with Semen Sojae Praeparatum or Rhizoma Zingiberis Recens for cold due to invasion by cold-wind, especially at the beginning stage of a mild one.

2. Dispelling evil cold from the interior and regulating *Yang*

It is often combined with Rhizoma Zingiberis and Radix Aconiti Praeparata for the treatment of cold syndrome in the interior due to invasion by abundance of evil *Yin*-cold, accompanied with adverse rising of athenic *Yang*, which is characterized by cold limbs, watery stools, flushed face and thready pulse; and for epigastric or abdominal pain due to retention of cold and stagnation of *Qi*, or retention of urine, the stir-baked drug can be applied on umbilicus or lower abdomen for warming the local region.

Dosage and Administration: Generally, 3–10 g or 3–5 pieces of the drugs are used for decoction; a proper amount of the drug is used for local administration.

Notes: It can not be taken with honey.

Chinese Tamarisk tops (柽柳 *Chengliu*)
Cacumen Tamaricis

The drug consists of the young green twigs of the deciduous bush or a kind of arbor, Tamarix chinensis Lour., Tamarix juniperina Bge. or Tamarix ramossima Ledeb. (family Tamaricaceae). Generally, it is cut into sections for being used.

Nomenclature used in Prescriptions: *Cheng Liu, Chi Cheng Liu, Xi He Liu, San Chun Liu.*

Properties and Channel Distribution: The drug is pungent to the taste, even in nature, and distributed to the Lung, Stomach and Heart Channels.

Action and Indications: Inducing persperation to disperse the evils from superficies and promoting eruption.

For treating measles especially at its beginning stage with failure of eruption, retarded or suspending eruption due to wind, it is often combined with Radix Puerariae, Fructus Arctii, Periostracum Cicadae and Herba Lophatheri. Since it has functions of dispersing the evils from the superficies with its pungent taste and of effectively removing the toxic materials in the blood as well, it is regarded as an indispensable medicine for facilitating eruption of measles.

Besides, it can also be used in treating pruritus or the itch due to other causes by bathing with its decoction since it has the functions of dispelling evil wind and arresting itching.

Dosage and Administration: 3–10 g of the dried drugs or

6–20 g of the fresh are considered for decoction; a proper amount of the drug may be used as fumigant or for decoction for local bath. For the local administration, the drug is put into the mixture of wine and water and then decocted; or into the boiling mixture of wine and water, and further boiled for once or twice, then the steam of the decoction can be used to fume limbs and the chest of the patient. The decoction can be also used to wash limbs, thus inducing slightly sweating and promoting eruption. Usually, the head and face are not washed; thus prevent these regions from over eruption.

Notes: It should be avoided for those with measles which has come out completely. Its dose for oral taking can not be excessive; otherwise it will lead to restlessness.

Herb of Haichow Elsholtzia (香薷 *Xiangru*)
Herba Elsholtziae seu Moslae

The drug consists of the aerial parts of the perennial herbaceous plant, Elsholtzia splendens Nakai ex F. Maekawa (family Labiatae) Usually, its crude plant is cut into pieces for being used.

Nomenclature Used in Prescriptions: *Xiangru, Xiangru.*

Properties and Channel Distribution: The drug is pungent to the taste, slightly warm in nature, and distributed to the Lung, Spleen and Urinary Bladder Channels.

Action and Indications:

1. Inducing perspiration to disperse evils from superficies, regulating the spleen to resolve dampness

It is indicated in the illness due to invasion of the exterior by the evil cold as well as invasion of the interior by dampness, remarked by chilliness and fever, heaviness of head and headache, stuffiness of the chest, anhidrosis, abdominal pain with diarrhea, etc. Generally, this illness is caused by living at cool place or over taking fruits or cool melons, thus the vital energy is inhibited by such *Yin* evils; then the syndrome of both the exterior and interior occurs. For the treatment of this illness, it is often combined with Dolichos lablab L. and Cortex Magnoliae Officinalis.

2. Promoting diuresis to relieve edema

It is indicated in edema of the head and face, chill and anhidrosis, dysuria. For treating such diseases, 500 g of the drug are decocted with water in a pot, and concentrated into soft extract, in which 250 g of the powder of Rhizoma Atractylodis Macrocephalae are added; thus the pill is formed. Usually, 9 g of the pills are regarded as a dose, they are taken with water, twice or thrice per day.

Dosage and Administration: 3–10 g of the drug are often prescribed for decoction. And for dispersing cold from superficies, decocting should take a short time; for eliminating edema, take a long time comparatively. The drug has a fragrant odour. If its decoction is taken hot, it may cause vomiting; therefore it should be taken cool.

Notes: It is contraindicated in such syndrome due to invasion by summer–heat in summer, characterized by high fever with remarkable thirst, profuse sweating; usually, such syndrome is known as *Yang* summer–heat syndrome.

1.2 Diaphoretics with Pungent and Cold Properties

Diaphoretics with pungent and cold properties, termed as drugs for dispersing wind–heat, are pungent and bitter to the taste and cold (or cool) in nature. Since they can induce moderate sweating, they are indicated in the beginning stage of the exterior syndrome due to invasion by wind– heat, characterized by moderate chills and high fever, thirst with perspiration or anhidrosis; thin, white and dry or thin and yellowish tongue coating; floating and rapid pulse and so on. Some of the drugs, having the function of promoting eruption, are indicated in rubella, measles, etc. The drugs are combined with antipyretics or drugs for clearing up internal heat during clinical pratice.

Peppermint (薄荷 *Bohe*)
Herba Menthae

The drug consists of the aerial parts of the perennial herbaceous plant, Mentha haplocalyx Briq. (family Labiatae); usually, the crude drug or the fresh one is cut into sections for being used.

Nomenclature Used in Prescriptions: *Bohe*, *Bohegeng*, *Boheye*, *Xianbohe*.

Properties and Channel Distribution: The drug is pungent to the taste, cold in nature, and distributes to the Lung and Liver Channels.

Action and Indications:

1. Dispersing evil wind–heat from superficies

For either exterior syndrome due to wind–heat which is

marked by fever with slight chill, headache and anhidrosis, or exterior syndrome of seasonal febrile disease at its beginning stage, Herba Menthae is often combined with Flos Lonicerae, Fructus Forsythiae, etc.; for high fever, with Gypsum; for syndrome of summer–heat in summer which is marked by dizziness, fever, thirst, scanty and dark urine, with Talcum, Radix Glycyrrhizae.

2. Clearing away the evil factors in the head, brightening the eyes and soothing the throat

For treating cold due to wind–heat or such symptoms as headache with red eyes, sore throat, etc., due to invasion of the head by wind–fire, it is combined with Herba Schizonepetae, Flos Chrysanthemi, Radix Ledebouriellae, Fructus Arctii, Radix Platycodi, Radix Glycyrrhizae, etc.

3. Promoting eruption and arresting itching

It is often combined with Fructus Forsythiae, Periostracum Cicadae, Fructus Arctii, Herba Schizone–petae, Radix Ledebouriellae, etc. for the treatment of measles at its beginning stage and with retardation of eruptions, or measles with failure of letting out skin eruptions due to invasion of the super–ficies and muscles by wind–heat, and urticaria, pruritus, etc.

Besides, it is also indicated in depression of liver–*Qi*, distention and pain of the chest and hypochon–driac region; for this purpose, a proper amount may be added to the other ingredients of the prescription for soothing the liver.

Dosage and Administration: 3–10 g of the dried plants or 15–30 g of the fresh are taken. Since it contains the volatile oils, the decocting should not be long. Usually its stems and twigs are used in dispersing wind–heat from superficies, and its leaves used in soothing the liver.

Arctium Fruit (牛蒡子 *Niubangzi*)
Fructus Arctii

The drug consists of the ripe fruit of the biennial herbaceous plant, Arctium lappa L. (family Compositae); usually, it is slightly bake–stirred and pounded for being used.

Nomenclature Used in Prescriptions: *Niubangzi*

Properties and Channel Distribution: The drug is pungent and bitter to the taste, cold in nature, and distributed to the Lung and Stomach Channels.

Action and Indications:

1. Dispersing wind–heat from the superficies

It is often combined with Herba Schizonepetae, Radix Platycodi, Radix Glycyrrhizae, etc., for the treatment of cold caused by wind–heat, accompanied with itching throat and cough, expectoration of scanty and sticky sputum, etc.

2. Soothing the throat and dispersing the mass due to retention of evils

For the treatment of sore throat due to invasion by wind–heat, it is often combined with drugs for dispersing wind–heat; for that due to fire, it is often used in combination with those drugs with effects of purging fire and removing toxic materials; for the treatment of sore throat due to abundant wind–fire and virulent heat–evil, with both the drugs for dispersing wind–heat and those for purging fire and dispelling virulent heat.

3. Ventilating the lung and facilitating eruption

It is often combined with Radix Ledebouriellae, Herba

Schizonepetae, Flos Lonicerae and others for dispersing wind, promoting eruption and removing toxic materials for the treatment of measles with retardation of eruption, urticaria, etc.

4. Removing toxic materials and relieving pyogenic infection of the skin

It is often combined with the drugs for dispelling evil heat and removing toxic materials of carbuncle or pyogenic infection of the skin, accompanied with either syndrome of wind-heat or constipation.

Dosage and Administration: 5–19 g of the drug are used as a dose for decoction.

Notes: In treating those with watery stools it should be used with care because the drug has the effects on lubricating the intestines and facilitating defecation.

Mulberry Leaf (桑叶 *Sangye*) Folium Mori

The drug consists of the leaves of the deciduous arbor, Morus alba L. (family Moraceae)

Nomenclature in used Prescriptions: *Sangye*, *Shuangsangye*, *Dongsangye*

Properties and Channel Distribution: The drug is bitter and sweet to the taste, cold in nature, and distributed to the Lung and Liver Channels.

Action and Indications:

1. Dispersing wind-heat from superficies

It is often combined with Flos Chrysanthemi, Fructus Forsythiae, Herba Menthae, Semen Armeniacae Amarum, etc.

and is used for treating cold due to invasion by wind–heat accompanied with headache and red eyes, or for wind–warm syndrome characterized by fever, cough, and so on.

2. Clearing away evil heat in the lung to arrest coughing

It is often combined with Semen Armeniacae Amarum, Bulbus Fritillariae Thunbergii, Radix Ophiopogonis, Gypsum Fibrosum, etc., for the treatment of cough and dryness of the throat due to invasion of the lung by dryness–heat.

3. Dispelling liver–fire and brightening the eyes

For treating the blood–shot eyes with pain and swelling due to an attack by pathogenic wind–heat, it is often combined with Flos Chrysanthemi, Semen Cassiae, etc.; for treating dizziness and blurred vision due to uprising of liver–*Yang*, with Flos Chrysanthemi, Ramulus Uncariae cum Uncis, etc.; For treating blurred vision due to deficiency of *Yin* of liver and kidney, 500 g of the drug and 150 g of Semen Sesami may be used by grinding them into powder and making them into pills mixed with honey; and the pills can be taken for a long time.

Dosage and Administration: 6–12 g of the drug are for decoction.

Chrysanthemum Flower (菊花 *Juhua*)
Flos Chrysanthemi

The drug consists of the flower–head of the perennial herbaceous plant, Chrysanthemum morifolium Ramat. (family Compositae); usually it is dried in the shade for use.

Nomenclature Used in Prescription: *Ganjuhua*, *Hangjuhua*, *Chujuhua*, *Huangjuhua*, *Baijuhua*.

Properties and Channel Distribution: The drug is sweet, slightly bitter to the taste, slightly cold in nature, and distributed to the Lung and Liver Channels.

Action and Indications:

1. Dispersing wind–heat from the superficies

It is often combined with Folium Mori, Herba Menthae, Fructus Forsythiae, etc. for treating exterior syndrome due to wind–heat which is marked by fever, headache; combined with Radix Ledebouriellae, Fructus Tribuli, for blood–shot eyes.

2. Calming liver–*Yang* and brightening the eyes

For treating syndrome of uprising of liver–*Yang*, marked by headache, dizziness or vertigo, etc., it can be combined with Concha Haliotidis, Ramulus Uncariae cum Uncis, Radix Rehmanniae, Radix Paeoniae Alba, etc.; for blurred vision due to deficiency of *Yin* of the liver and spleen, and failure of supply of blood, with Rhizoma Rehmanniae Preparata, Fructus Lycii, etc.

Dosage and Administration: 9–15 g of the drug are used for decoction. *Hangjuhua* or *Huangjuhua* is often used for dispersing wind–heat; while *Chujuhua* or *Baijuhua*, for soothing or calming the liver and brightening the eyes.

Appendix: Flos Chrysanthemi Indici (野菊花 *Yejuhua*)

The drug consists of the dried flower–head of the perennial herbaceous plant, Chrysanthemum indici L. (family Compositae); usually either it is dried in the sun or the fresh one is collected for being used. The drug is bitter and pungent in taste, slightly cold in nature, indicated in furuncle, carbuncle and the pyogenic infection of the skin, sore throat, blood–shot eyes, etc. It is often combined with these drugs for dispelling evil heat and removing the toxic materials, brightening the eyes and soothing the throat;

it can be used orally and locally. Generally, 10–15 g of the drug are decocted; sometimes 30 g of the drug may be used if necessary. For local administration, it can be pounded to smear on the affected site or be decocted for a skin wash; for this purpose a proper amount of the drug is used.

Fruit of Shrub Chastetree (蔓荆子 *Manjingzi*)
Fructus Viticis

The drug consists of the fruit of the deciduous shrub or arbor, Vitex rotundifolia L. or V. trifolia L. (family Verbenaceae); it is often dried in the shade, and bake–stirred untill it becomes brown in colour.

Nomenclature Used in Prescriptions: *Manjingzi.*

Properties and Channel Distribution: The drug is pungent and bitter to the taste, slightly cold in nature, and distributed to the Urinary Bladder and Liver and Stomach Channels.

Action and Indications:

1. Dispersing wind–heat from superficies

For the treatment of cold due to wind–heat, charaterized by headache and dizziness, or for treating head–wind syndrome marked by painful attacks involving head, teeth and cheek, etc., it may be combined with Flos Chrysanthemi, Herba Menthae, Rhizoma Ligustici Chuanxiong, Ramulus Uncariae cum Uncis, Radix Ledebouriellae or Gypsum Fibrosum, some of which may be chosen according to what symptoms occur.

2. Dispelling evils from the head and the eyes

For treating blood–shot eyes due to wind–heat or dizziness with blurred vision, it is often combined with Flos Chrysanthemi,

Semen Cassiae, etc.

Dosage and Administration: 6–12 g of the drug are taken as a dose for decoction.

Pueraria Root (葛根 *Gegen*)
Radix Puerariae

The drug consists of the roots of the perennial deciduous liana, Pueraria lobata (Willd.) Ohwi (family Leguminosae); usually, the roots are dried in the sun for being used, and the crude flowers can also be used for medicine.

Nomenclature Used in Prescriptions: *Gegen*, *Fengegen*.

Properties and Channel Distribution: The drug is sweet and pungent to the taste, cold in nature, and is distributed to the Spleen and Stomach Channels.

Action and Indications:

1. Expelling the evils in the muscles andrelieving fever

It is indicated in exterior syndrome marked by fever, anhidrosis, headache, stiffness of the nucha and back. For treating the patient with remarkable chilliness, it may be combined with Herba Ephedrae, Ramulus Cinnamomi, Radix Paeoniae Alba, etc.; for the patient with high fever, combined with Radix Bupleuri, Radix Scutellariae and Gypsum Fibrosum, etc.

2. Promoting the production of body fluid and arresting thirst

For treating the exterior syndrome of febrile disease accompanied with thirst, or treating diabetes, it is often used as a single medicine or combined with the drugs for dispelling evil heat and promoting the production of body fluid.

3. Promoting eruption for measles

For treating measles at the early stage or with retardation of eruption it may be combined with Rhizoma Cimicifugae, Radix Paeoniae Alba, etc.

4. Ascending spleen–energy and relieving diarrhea

For treating diarrhea due to deficiency of spleen–energy it is often combined with Radix Codonopsis Pilo–sulae, Rhizoma Atractylodis Macrocephalae, Poria, etc.; for treating diarrhea or dysentery due to heat and accompanied with the exterior syndrome, with Rhizoma Coptidis, Radix Scutellariae, etc.

Besides, it is also indicated in hypertensive cerebropathy and used to relieve such symptom as headache, dizziness, stiffness of the nucha, etc.; and it may also be used to treat angina pectoris due to coronary heart disease, and the effects are fairly good.

Dosage and Administration: 6–15 g of the drug are used as a dose for decoction

Appendix: Flos Puerariae

The drug consists of the flower–bud of Pueraria lobata (Willd.) Ohwi; usually it is dried in the sun for being used. It is sweet in taste and even in nature. The drug has the functions of regulating the stomach, relieving thirst and neutralizing the toxic materials of the wine or spirits, it can be used for treating vomiting of the drunk and thirst, etc.; during treatment, it is often combined with Fructus Amomi, Semen Myristicae, Rhizoma Alismatis, Rizoma Atractylodis Macrocephalae, Poria, Polyporus Umbellatus, etc. 6–15 g of the drug are taken for decoction.

Bupleurum Root (柴胡 *Chaihu*)
Radix Bupleuri

The drug consists of the dried root or the herb of the Perennial herbaceous plant, Bupleurum chinense Dc. or B. scozonerifolium Willd. (family Umbelliferae); sometime, it is stir-baked with vinegar for use.

Nomenclature Used in Prescriptions: *Chaihu*, *Beichaihu*, *Nenchaihu*, *Chunchaihu*, *Cuchaihu*.

Properties and Channel Distribution: The drug is bitter and pungent to the taste, slightly cold in nature, and is distributed to the Liver and Gall Bladder Channels.

Action and Indications:

1. Dispersing evil heat from the superficies

For treating cold with fever, it is often combined with Radix Puerariae, etc., thus dispersing evil heat from the superficies; for treating the syndrome of alternating episodes of chills and fever, with Radix Scutellariae, thus mediating *Shaoyang* disease. This drug is effective in eliminating the evil located in the half-superficies and half-interior, hence an indispensable medicine for *Shaoyang* disease. Besides, for malaria marked by alternating episodes of chills and fever, it is often combined with Radix Scutellariae, Radix Dichroae, Fructus Tsaoko, etc.

2. Lifting up the vital energy of middle-*Jiao*

For the treatment of prolapse of rectum, or of uterus, or gastroptosis due to deficiency of *Qi* of middle-*Jiao*, it is often combined with drugs for lifting *Yang-Qi*, such as Radix Ginseng, Radix Astragali seu Hedysari and Rhizoma Cimicifugae.

Dosage and Administration: 3–10 g of the drug are taken as a dose. For treating fever, 15–30 g of the drug may be used sometimes. And the drug should be stewed for a long duration, thus making a concentrated decoction. When the drug is bake–stirred with vinegar, its function of dispersing evils will be weakened, but its function of relieving soreness and pain will be strengthened.

Notes: Since it has the function of lifting up *Yang–Qi*, it is contraindicated in tinnitus, deafness, dizziness, headache, etc., due to uprising of liver–*Yang* and a flare–up of fire caused by deficiency of *Yin*.

Bugbane Rhizome (升麻 *Shengma*)
Rhizoma Cimicifugae

The drug consists of the rhizome of the perennial herbaceous plant, Cimicifuga foetida L. or Cimicifuga dahurica (Turcz.) Maxim. or Cimicifuga heracleifalia Komar.; usually, it is cut into sections and dried in the sun for being used; the crude drug or the drug bake–stirred with honey is often used.

Nomenclature Used in Prescription: *Shengma*, *Lushengma*, *Zhishengma*

Properties and Channel Distribution: The drug is pungent and sweet to the taste, slight cold in nature, and is distributed to the Lung, Spleen, Stomach and large intestine Channels.

Action and Indications:

1. Dispersing evils from the superficies and promoting eruption

For treating measles at its beginning stage with retadation of eruption, it is often combined with Radix Puerariae; for treating profuse eruption due to invasion of abundant virulent heat, with Fructus Arctii, Radix Arnebiae seu Lithospermi, etc.

2. Dispelling evil heat and expelling the virulent factors

It is indicated in headache and toothache caused by stomach–heat, sore throat and aphtha. For treating aphtha and toothache, it is often combined with Gypsum Fibrosum, Rhizoma Coptidis, etc.; for treating sore throat, with Radix Scrophulariae, Fructus Arctii, Radix Platycodi, etc.; for treating headache, with Gypsum Fibrosum, Radix Angelicae Dahuricae, etc.

3. Ascending *Yang–Qi* or the vital energy of the spleen

For treating prolapse of rectum, prolapse of uterus, etc. it is often combined with Radix Ginseng, Radix Astragali seu Hedysari, Radix Bupleuri, thus ascending *Yang–Qi*.

Dosage and Administration: 3–9 g of the drug are taken for decoction; usually, the crude drug is used to disperse evils from superficies while the drug prepared with honey is used to ascend *Qi* of middle *Jiao*.

Cicada Slough (蝉蜕 *Chantui*)
Periostracum Cicadae

The drug consists of the slough shed by the cicada, Cryptotympana pustulata Fabr. (family Cicadidae); the crude drug is dried in the sun for being used.

Nomenclature Used in Prescriptions: *Chantui*, *Chanyi*, *Chantui*

Properties and Channel Distribution: The drug is sweet to the taste, cold in nature, and is distributed to the lung and Liver

Channels.

Action and Indications:

1. Dispersing wind–heat from the superficies

For treating cold due to wind–heat or seasonal febrile disease at the beginning stage and accompanied by the exterior syndrome, it is often combined with Herba Menthae, Radix Glycyrrhizae, Gypsum Fibrosum, etc.; for treating sore throat accompanied with hoarse voice due to wind–heat, it can be used as a single medicine or may be combined with Semen Sterculiae Scaphigerae; for treating infantile cold marked by fever, irascibility or nocturnal crying with restlessness, etc. with Ramulus Uncariae cum Uncis, Medulla Funci, Herba Menthae, etc.

2. Promoting eruption and relieving itching

At the beginning stage of measles with retardation of eruption, it may be with Radix Puerariae, Fructus Arctii, Herba Menthae, Fructus Forsythiae.

3. Resolving nebula and brightening the eyes

For treating blood–shot eyes due to wind–heat, or nebula with poor vision, it is often combined with Flos Chrysanthemi, Flos Eriocauli, etc.

4. Dispelling evil wind and relieving pain

For treating tetanus marked by lockjaw, opisthotonus, it is often combined with Rhizoma Gastrodiae, Scorpic and other drugs for dispelling wind and relieving convulsion; for treating infantile convulsion with fever, with Ramulus Uncariae cum Uncis, Radix Scutellariae, Cornu Antelopis, etc.

Dosage and Administration: 3–9 g are usually taken for decoction; for the treatment of dispelling wind and relieving convulsion 15–30 g of the drug may be used.

Spirodela (浮萍 *Fuping*)
Herba Spirodelae

The drug consists of the entire plant of the herbaceous plant, Spirodela Polyrrhiza (L.) Schleid. or Lemna minor L. (family Lemnaceae). Usually, the crude drug is dried in the sun for use.

Nomenclature Used in Prescription: *Fupingcao*, *Zibeifuping*.

Properties and Channel Distribution: The drug is pungent to the taste, cold nature, and is distributed in the Lung and Urinary Bladder Channels.

Action and Indications:

1. Dispersing evils from the superficies and promoting eruption

For treating exterior syndrome due to wind–heat, marked by fever and anhidrosis,it may be combined with Herba Schizonepetae, Radix Ledebouriellae, Herba Menthae, Fructus Forsythiae, etc.; for treating measles with retardation of eruption, with Fructux Arctii, Herba Menthae, Flos Lonicerae, Tamarix chinese Lour., Herba Lophatheri, etc.; for treating urticaria due to wind–heat and pruritus, with Herba Schizonepetae, Radix Ledebouriellae, Periostracum Cicadae, Fructus Tribuli Fructus Kochiae, Cortex Dictamni Radicis, etc.

2. Promoting diuresis and relieving edema

It is effectively indicated in edema, scanty urine, accompanied with exterior syndrome; for this purpose it is often combined with Semen Plantaginis, Exocarpium Benincasae, Semen Phaseoli, Fructus Forsythiae, etc. It may also be used as a single medicine, pounded into powder and taken with water.

Dosage and Administration: 3–10 g of the drug or 15–30 g of the fresh drug are taken for decoction.

Prepared Soybean (淡豆豉 *Dandouchi*)
Semen Sojae Praeparatum

The drug consists of the prepared Semen Sojae Nigrum, the black seed of the annual plant, Glycine max (L.) Merr. (family Leguminosae). Prepared usually in summer, the black soybean is washed and steamed; then it is put evenly on the straw mat and covered with Folium Mori and fresh Herba Artemisiae Chinghao, untill it is fermented and becomes brown in color; then the fermented soybean is put into the jar with clean water, and the jar is sealed. After the jar is put on the ground in the sun for three weeks, then the soybean is taken out from it and dried in the sun for use. This process of the preparation for making drugs is often used.

Nomenclaclature Used in Prescriptions: *Dandouchi*, *Douchi*, *Xiangdouchi.*

Properties and Channel Distribution: The drug is pungent, sweet and slight bitter to the taste, cold in nature, and is distributed to the Lung and Stomach Channels.

Action and Indications:

1. Dispersing evils from the superficies

It is indicated in cold marked by chilliness, headache, fever, etc. For treating cold due to wind–cold, it is often combined with Bulbus Allii Fistulosi; for treating cold due to wind–heat, with Herba Menthae, Fructus Forsythiae, etc.

2. Relieving restlessness

For treating febrile disease at the later stage or before its convalescent stage, lingling with mild fever, stuffiness in the chest with restlessness, it may be combined with Fructus Gardeniae, and stewed together to make decoction.

Dosage and Administration: 9–15 g of the drug are taken for decoction.

Appendix: Sprouted black soybean (*Dadou Huangjuan, Qingshui Doujuan*).

When prepared, the black soybeans are soaked, sprouted, and then dried in the sun. the drug is sweet to the taste and even in nature, and is distributed to the Stomach Channel. It has the functions of resolving dampness and clearing up evil heat, dispersing evils from the superficies; therefore it is indicated in summer–heat dampness syndrome, dampness–heat syndrome, or syndrome of damp–heat in the interior, marked by fever with scanty perspiration, stuffiness of the chest and uneasiness, arthralgia due to wind, dampness and heat, soreness of knee joints and of tibia etc. 15–30 g are regarded as a dose for decoction.

2 Antipyretics or Drugs for Clearing Away Internal Heat

Drugs whose main function is reducing internal heat, are called antipyretics or drugs for clearing away internal heat. With their cold or cool property, they are chiefly used to treat febrile diseases, pestilence, carbuncle, pyogenic infection and hot eyes, sore throat, and other syndromes of internal heat.

In order to have a good command of the characteristics of each of these drugs, we divide the drugs into the six groups according to their peculiarities:

1. Drugs for reducing intense heat in the interior and purging evil fire. Most of these drugs exert their therapeutic effect on the troubles of *Qi* system, so they are used to treat intense heat syndrome of *Qi* system by clearing away heat and purging evil fire.

2. Drugs for reducing intense heat in the interior to brighten vision. These drugs have the functions of clearing away liver–fire and brightening the eyes; so they are often indicated in flaring–up of liver–fire, painful conjunctival congestion, etc.

3. Drugs for eliminating evil heat from blood. These drugs mainly exert their effect on troubles of blood system; therefore they are indicated in intense heat syndrome of blood system by clearing away evil heat from blood.

4. Drugs for eliminating heat and dampness. Generally, these

drugs are bitter in taste and dry in nature. They have the functions of clearing away evil heat and resolving dampness, so they are indicated in dampness–heat syndrome.

5. Drugs for eliminating heat–toxicant. These drugs have the functions of clearing away evil heat and removing toxicants; they are indicated in syndrome caused by heat–toxicant.

6. Drugs for eliminating asthenic heat. These drugs have the functions of clearing asthenia–heat and relieving hectic fever due to *Yin* deficiency, so they are often used to treat afternoon fever, lingering of low fever, etc.

Drugs of different groups may be combined properly according the condition of the disease. What drug should be used first as a main role must depend upon the clinical condition; for instance, the heat syndrome in the interior accompanied with exterior syndrome should be treated first with the drugs for dispersing evils from the superficies or treated simultaneously with the drugs for dispersing evil from the superficies and the drugs for clearing away the internal heat; for treating heat syndrome of *Qi* system accompanied with heat syndrome of blood system both, the drugs for reducing heat in the *Qi* system and the drugs for treating heat in blood system can be used; for treating heat syndrome of *Qi* system without invasion of *Ying* or blood system by evil heat, in no case can the drugs for clearing away heat from blood be used hastily.

Most drugs for clearing away internal heat are cool or cold in nature, and they are likely to hurt *Yang–Qi* of human body; so these drugs should be used with great care for those with dysfunction of the spleen and stomach due to deficiency of *Yang–Qi*.

2.1 Drugs for Reducing Intense Heat in the Interior and Purging Evil Fire

Heat involving fire is one of the six exogenous factors; heat actually acts as the mild fire at its beginning stage and fire actually is derived from abundant heat at its stage when fire goes to its extreme; therefore the difference between them lies in their degree. Drugs that have the effect on reducing heat are the medicines for clearing away fire.

Drugs for reducing and purging heat are those that mainly deal with heat or fire of *Qi* system; so they are indicated in the syndrome of heat in *Qi* system, marked by high fever with thirst, irri–tability; or in the syndrome of intense heat in the interior, delirium, yellow or dry fur, full and forceful pulse, etc.

For treating patients with weak constitution, the drugs should be used with care not to hurt healthy energy; if necessary, they may be combined with drugs for invigorating it. And during practice the drug should be used according to its nature and action and its indications (to clear away liver–heat or lung–heat or stomach heat).

Gypsum (石膏 *Shigao*)
Gypsum Fibrosum

The drug consists of a kind of soft mineral of hydrated calcium sulfate called Gypsum ($CaSO_4 \cdot 2H_2O$) (monoclinic system); the crude drug may be pounded or calcined for being used as a medicine.

Nomenclature Used in Prescriptions: *Shengshigao, Duanshigao.*

Properties and Channel distribution: The drug is pungent and sweet to the taste and very cold in nature, and distributed to the Lung and Stomach Channels.

Action and Indications:

1. Reducing intense heat and purging fire, relieving fidgets and arresting thirst

It is indicated in seasonal febrile disease due to invasion of *Qi* system by evil factors, marked by high fever with fidgets, thirst with longing for water drinking, perspiration, full purse, even with delirium; for treating the disease mentioned above, it is often combined with Rhizoma Anemarrhenae, Radix Glycyrrhizae, etc.; for treating eruptions letting out in dark or dark violet color due to abundant heat toxicants , with Cornu Rhinoceri, Radix Scrophularize; for the later stage of seasonal febrile disease, marked by lingering of mild fever, iracibility with thirst, red tongue with scanty fur, with Herba Lophatheri, Radix Ophiopogonis; for thirst due to invasion of stomach by heat, or headache or toothache due to flare–up of stomach–fire, with Rhizoma Rehmanniae Praparatae, Rhizoma Anemarrhenae, etc; for treating toothache, with Herba Asari; and for asthma or dyspenia due to attack by lung–heat accompanied with irascibility and thirst, with Herba Ephedrae, Semen Armeniacae Amarum, etc.

2. Promoting tissue regeneration and wound healing

Its calcined powder is indicated in wound, ulcer, scald or burn, marked by failure of tissue regeneration or wound healing. For treating wound, it is often mixed with Hydrargyri Oxydum Rubrum (Gypsum Fibrosum to Hydrarguri Oxydum Rubrum ratio, 9:1), which is called *Jiuyi* powder; or it may be mixed with the powder of such ingredientis as Os Draconis, Calamina, Olibanum, Resina Commiphorae Myrrhae, Resina Draconis, and other drugs for resolving dampness, promoting blood circulation and tissue regeneration.

Dosage and Administration: 15–60 g of the drug are taken for decoction; sometimes, 120 g may be used as a large dose. A proper amount of the drug is used externally; the crude drug is used for purging fire while the calcined one is used for promoting tissue regeneration and wound healing. For decocting it is suitable to be decocted first.

Anemarrhena Rhizome (知母 *Zhimu*)
Rhizoma Anemarrhenae

The drug consists of the dried rhizome of a perennial herbaceous plant, Anemarrhena asphodeloides Bge. (family Liliaceae); usually, the crude drug is dried or bakestirred with salt solution for use.

Nomenclature Used in Prescriptions: *Zhimu*, *Yanzhimu*.

Properties and Channel Distribution: The drug is bitter and sweet to the taste, cold in nature, and distributed to the Lung, Stomach and Kidney Channels.

Action and Indications:

1. Clearing away intense heat to purge fire; For treating seasonal febrile disease due to invasion of *Qi* system by evils, marked by high fever, fidgets and thirst, it is often combined with Gypsum Fibrosum; for cough due to lung–heat or unproductive cough or cough with expectoration of scanty sputum due to deficiency of lung–*Yin*, it is often with Bulbus Fritillariae Cirrhosae.

2. Nourishing vital essence to relieve dryness:

For treating hectic fever, nocturnal emmision, night sweating, etc., due to deficiency of *Yin* and flare–up of fire, it is often combined with Cortex Phellodendri, Radix Rehmanniae, etc.; for sore throat or aphtha due to the same cause, with Radix Rehmanniae, Radix Scrophulariae.

3. Promoting the production of body fluid and arresting thirst: The drug can be used to treat thirst due to stomach–heat, or diabetes in combination with Radix Trichosanthis, Radix Ophipogonis, Radix Puerariae, etc.

Dosage and Administration: 3–12 g of the crude drug are used as a dose; for treating illness due to kidney–fire, the drug should be prepared with salt solution, by this way, its effect can be conducted to the kidney on reducing fire.

Capejasmine Fruit (栀子 *Zhizi*)
Fructus Gardeniae

The drug consists of the riped fruits of the evergreen deciduous shrubs, Gardenia jasminoides Ellis. (family Rubiaceae); besides the crude one, it can be bake–stirred either to brown or with ginger juice; occasionally its peel and seed may be used in separation.

Nomenclature Used in Prescriptions: *Zhizi, Shengzhizi, Shengshanzhi, Chaozhizi,Jiangzhizi, Zhizitan, Heishanzi, Zhiziren, Zhizipi.*

Properties and Channel Distribution: The drug is bitter to the taste, cold in nature, and distributed to the Heart, Liver, Lung, Stomach and *Sanjiao* Channels.

Action and Indications:

1. Clearing away intense fire and relieving fidgets: For the treatment of febrile disease with fidgets or irascibility, restlessness, it is often combined with Semen Sojae Preparatum, for the combination of these two drugs has the effect on reducing heart–fire and relieving fidgets. For the treatment of febrile disease with unconciousness and delirium due to abundance of heat–toxicant, it is often combined with the drugs for reducing heat, purging fire and relieving toxicants, such as Rhizoma Coptidis, Radix Scutellariae and Cortex Phellodendri; for hot eyes, dry mouth and thirst, fidgets, with Flos Chrysanthemi, Radix Scutellariae, Radix Glycyrrhizae, etc.

2. Clearing away heat and resolving dampness: The drug, having the functions of facilitating the flow of the bile and relieving jaundice, is indicated in jaundice due to damp–heat, accompanied with scanty urine in dark color; and for the treatment of jaundice, it is often with Herba Artemisiae Scopariae, Cortex Phellodendri, etc.; for the treatment of stranguria with bloody urine, painful micturition with hot sensation and with urine in dark color, with Radix Rehmanniae, Caulis Akebiae, Semen Plantaginis, etc.

3. Reducing heat in the blood and arresting haemorr–hagia: For the treatment of spitting blood, epistaxis, dysentery with hematochezia, painful urination with hematuria, etc., it is often combined with drugs for reducing heat in the blood.

Besides, its powder mixed with vinegar can be used to treat injury or sprain, hematoma with pain and swelling; and it is often mixed with white of eggs and is used to treat scald and burn.

Dosage and Administration: 3–10 g of the drug are used for decoction. The crude drug acts as a medicine for clearing away heat and purging fire; and the bake-stirred drug is less cold in its nature than the crude one. The drug bake-stirred to brown is often used to arrest bleeding, while the drug with ginger juice is used to treat vomiting and fidgets.

Notes: It is contraindicated in poor appetite with watery stools due to asthenia-cold syndrome of spleen and stomach.

Trichosanthes Root (天花粉 *Tianhuafen*)
Radix Trichosanthis

The drug consists of the root of perennial plant, herbaceous vine of perennial root, Trichosanthes kirilowii Maxim. The crude drug is peeled and cutted into pieces for use.

Nomenclature Used in Prescriptions: *Tianhuafen*, *Huafen*, *Gualougen*

Properties and Channel Distribution: The drug is sweet and slightly bitter to the taste, slightly cold in nature, and distributed to the Lung, Stomach Channels.

Action and Indications:

1. Clearing away heat and promoting the production of the body fluid: For the treatment of deficiency of the body fluid with fidgets and thirst, due to febrile disease or diabetes, it is often combined with Radix Adeno-phorae strictae, Radix Ophiopogonis, Rhizoma Anemarrhenae, etc. The drug, having functions of clearing away lung-heat and moisturizing lung-dryness, can be used to treat cough due to lung-heat or lung-dryness; and for the treatment of cough mentioned above it is often combined with Bulbus Fritillariae Cirhosae, Radix Adenophorae

Strictae, Radix Ophiopogonis, Rhizoma Anemarrhenae, etc.

2. Relieving swelling and congestion and letting pus out: For the treatment of carbuncle or skin pyogenic infection or skin lesion with congestion, redness and pain and hot sensation, it is combined with Flos lonicerae, Bulbus Fritillariae Thunbergii, etc.; besides its powder can be used externally.

Dosage and Administration: 10–15 g of the drug may be taken for decoction: and a proper amount of the drug, for external administration.

Reed Rhizoma (芦根 *Lugen*)
Rhizoma Phragmitis

The drug consists of the dried or fresh underground rhizomes of perennial herbaceous plant, Phragmites communis Trin. (family Gramineae); the fresh of the crude one may be used as medicine after it has been cut into segments.

Nomenclature Used in Prescription: *Lugen*, *Xianlugen*, *Huolugen*, *Ganlugen*, *Weigen*, *Weijing*.

Properties and Channel Distribution: The drug is sweet to the taste, cold in nature, and distributed to the Lung and Stomach Channels.

Action and Indications:

1. Clearing away heat and promoting production of the body fluid: For the treatment of febrile disease with consuming body fluid, thirst, dryness of the tongue and deficiency of saliva, it is often combined with Radix Trichosanthis, Radix Ophipogonis, etc.

2. Clearing away lung–heat: For the treatment of lung abscess marked by cough and expectoration of purulent sputum

with foul smell or bloody sputum, it is often combined with Semen Coicis, Semen persicae, Semen Benincasae, Herba Houttuyniae, etc.; for the treatment of cold due to wind–heat with cough and dryness of mouth and tongue, with Flos Lonicerae, Fructus Forsythiae, etc.

3. Reducing stomach–heat to arrest vomiting: For the treatment of syndrome of stomach–heat marked by nausea, vomiting, regugitation, hiccup, etc., it is often combined with Caulis Bambusae in Taeniam, Folium Eriobotryae, etc.; when it is combined with Caulis Bambusae in Taeniam, ginger juice, japonica rice, and water for decoction, it is used specially to treat regurgitation and vomiting.

Besides, it is indicated in measles at its beginning stage with retardation of eruption. It has the effects of dispersing evils and letting out eruption; so it can be used as a single medicine or combined with others having the effects on dispersing evils and letting eruption out.

Dosage and Administration: 15–60 g of the drug are taken as a dose. The effect of the drug will be better when the drug is used in its fresh state. The drug is usually for decoction.

Lophatherum (淡竹叶 *Danzhuye*)
Herba Lophatheri

The drug consists of the entire plant of a perennial herb, Lophatherum gracile Brongn. (family Gramineae); the crude drug may be cut into segments for being used.

Nomenclature Used in Prescriptions: *Danzhuye.*

Properties and Channel Distribution: The drug is sweet and blunt to the taste and cold in nature, and is distributed to the Heart, Lung, and Small Intestine Channels.

Action and Indications:

1. Reducing heart–fire and relieving fidgets: For the treatment of febrile disease with fidgets and thirst, it is often combined with Radix Trichosanthis, Rhizoma Phragmitis, and others for clearing away heat and promoting the production of the body fluid; for the treatment of nocturnal crying due to heat of the heart, with Ramulus Uncariae cum Uncis, Herba Menthae, Periostracum Cicadae, Medulla Funci, etc.

2. Promoting diuresis and relieving stranguria: For the treatment of scanty urine in dark color, painful stranguria or aphtha and tongue sore, it is often combined either with Radix Rehmanniae, Caulis Akebiae, etc., or with Medulla Funci, Semen Plantaginis, etc.

Dosage and Administration: 6–12 g of the drug are taken for decoction.

Appendix: Hanon Bamboo (*Zhuye*, *Zhuyejuanxin*)

The drug consists of the dried or fresh leaves of a kind of perennial evergreen bamboolike arbor or shrub, Phyllostachys nigra (Lodd.) Munro var, henonis (Mitf.) ex Rendle (family Gramineae). The slender young leaves are like rolls in shape, which are called *Zhuyejuanxin*. Usually, the fresh ones are more effective; and the effect of this drug is nearly the same as that of Herba Lophatheri, yet its effects on clearing away heart–fire and relieving fidgets seems stronger than that of Herba Lophatheri, and its effect on promoting diuresis seems weaker. The young rolllike leaves of Hanon Bamboo are mainly used to treat evil heat in the heart, they act as a main ingredient of "Decoction for

Clearing Away Evil Heat of *Yingfen* Syndrome". The drug can be used for the treatment of unconsiousness and delirium of febrile disease. Its dosage and administration are the same as those of Herba Lophatheri.

2.2 Drugs for Reducing Intense Heat in the Interior to Brighten Vision

This kind of drugs, having the effects on clearing away liver–fire and relieving nebula, is indicated in flare–up of liver–fire marked by hot eyes, nebula, etc.; and some of the drugs may be used to treat syndrome of hyperactivity of liver–*Yang*.

Prunella Spike (夏枯草 *Xiakucao*)
Spica Prunellae

The drug consists of the spike of the perennial herbaceous plant, Prunella vulgaris L. (family Labiatae); usually, the drug is dried in the sun for being used.

Nomenclature Used in Prescriptions: *Xiakucao*.

Properties and Channel Distribution: The drug is bitter and pungent to the taste and cold in nature, and distributed to the Liver and Gall Bladder Channels.

Action and Indications:

1. Reducing Liver–fire to brighten vision: For treatment of bloodshot eyes due to liver–fire, it is with Flos Chrysanthemi, Herba Taraxaci, etc.; for painful sensation of the eye–ball more severe at night, with Rhizoma Cyperi 30 g, Radix Glycyrrhizae 6 g, and 6 g of their powder may be taken as a dose, twice a day; for painful sensation of the eye–balls due to deficiency of liver–*Yin*,

with Radix Angelicae Sinensis, Radix Paeoniae Alba, etc.; for syndrome of hyperactivity of liver–*Yang* or flare–up of liver–fire, marked by headache and vertigo, irascibility, fever and restlessness and insomnia, as a medicine frequently used, it may be used singly or combined with drugs for reducing heat, pacifying liver–*Yang* as Semen Cassiae, Flos Chrysanthemi Indici, Concha Haliotidis, Radix Scutellariae, etc.

2. Clearing away evil fire and resolving mass: For the treatment of Scrofula, goiter, mastitis, mumps, etc. due to accumulation and retention of evil factor as phlegm–fire, it may be used as a single medicine for preparation of soft extract taken for a duration of time, or combined with Radix Scrophulariae, Bulbus Fritillariae Thunbergii, Thallus Laminariae seu Eckloniae, etc., which may be selected according to the syndrome of the specific patient.

Now, it is often indicated in hypertension, goiter, tuberculosis of lymph nodes, hyperplasia of the mammary gland, etc. Besides, it can also be used to treat pulmonary tuberculosis, lymphosarcoma, tumour of mediastinum, etc.

Dosage and Administration: 10–12 g of the drug may be taken as a dose for decoction.

Cassia Seed (决明子 *Juemingzi*)
Semen Cassiae

The drug consists of the ripe seed of the annuel herba–ceous plant, Cassia tora L. (family Leguminosae). The drug is bake–stirred for a short time and pounded for being used.

Nomenclature Used in Prescriptions: *Juemingzi*, *Caojueming*.

Properties and Channel Distribution: The drug is sweet and bitter to the taste, slightly cold in nature, and is distributed to the Lung and Kidney Channels.

Action and Indications:

1. Reducing liver–heat to brighten the eyes: It is indicated in bloodshot eyes with aversion of light and an overflow of tears due to liver–heat or attack on the liver channel by wind–heat. For the treatment of syndrome of liver–heat, it may be combined with Spica Prunellae, Fructus Gardeniae; for syndrome of wind–heat, with Folium Mori, Flos Chrysanthemi. It is also used to treat advanced optic atrophy, internal oculopathy, blurred vision, eyes without luster; in these cases, it is often combined with Radix Rehmanniae, Fructus Lycii, Radix Scrophulariae, Rhizoma Dioscoreae, etc.

2. Lubricating the intestines and relieving constipation: For the treatment of constipation due to the dryness of intestines, it can be used as a single medicine, or combined with Fructus Cannabis, Semen Pruni, etc.

Besides, it is also often used to treat headache, as one of the symptoms of hypertension due to hyperactivity of liver–*Yang*, and it has got effects.

Dosage and Administration: 6–10 g of the drug may be taken for decoction; it can also be used singly by pouring hot water on it, and after a while the solution is taken.

Notes: It is contraindicated in diarrhea or watery stools.

Seed of Feather Corkscomb (青葙子 *Qingxiangzi*) Semen Celosiae

The drug consists of the matured seeds of an annuel herbaceous plant, Celosia argentea L. or Celosia cristata L. (family Amaranthaceae); the seed of Celosia argentea is similar to the seed of Celosia cristata in shape and nature, the former is called the wild of the latter.

Nomenclature Used in Prescriptions: *Qingxiangzi.*

Properties and Channel Distribution: the drug is bitter to the taste, slightly cold in nature, and is distributed in the Liver Channel.

Action and Indications:

Reducing liver–fire to brighten eyes and relieving nebula: For the treatment of syndrome of flare–up of liver fire, marked by red eyes, nebula, blurred vision, etc., it is often combined with Semen Cassiae, Spica Prunellae, etc.

Besides, it is often used to treat hypertension with dizziness due to hyperactivity of liver–*Yang* in combination with Semen Cassiae, Spica Prunellae, Ramulus Uncariae cum Uncis, etc.

Dosage and Administration: 6–10 g of the drug are taken as a dose for decoction.

Notes: The drug, having the effects of clearing away heat and dilating the pupil, is contraindicated in asthenic eye disease and glaucoma.

Flower of Pale Butterflybush (密蒙花 *Mimenghua*) Flos Buddlejae

The drug consists of the dried flower bud and spike of a deciduous bush, Buddleja officinalis Maxim. (family Loganiacea). the drug is processed by first being immersed in wine, dried in the sunshine, then mixed with honey and steamed.

Nomenclature Used in Prescriptions: *Mimenghua.*

Properties and Channel Distribution: The drug is sweet to the taste, slightly cold in nature, and is distributed to the Liver Channel.

Action and Indications:

Reducing liver-heat and soothing the liver, brightening vision and relieving nebular: For the treatment of bloodshot eyes with a lot of gum due to invasion of liver-heat, it may be combined with Concha Haliotidis, Flos Chrysanthemi, etc.; for blurred vision, dryness of the eyes or nebula, with Fructus Lycii, Semen Cuscutae, etc. The drug is indicated in the eye disease either with sthenic syndrome or with asthenic syndrome, esp. in that due to deficiency of *Yin* of liver and kidney accompanied by heat.

Dosage and Administration: 6～10 g of the drug are taken as a dose for decoction.

Flower of Buerger Pipewort (谷精草 *Gujingcao*) Flos Eriocauli

The drug consists of the dried spike of the annual herbaceous plant, Eriocaulon buerferianum Koern. (family Eriocaulaceae). Usually, it is cut into segments for being used.

Nomenclature Used in Prescriptions: *Gujingcao*, *Gujingzhu.*

Properties and Channel Distribution: The drug is pungent and sweet to the taste, even in nature, and is distributed to the Liver and Stomach Channels.

Action and Indications:

Dispersing wind-heat, relieving nebula and brightening vision: For treatment of such diseases due to wind–heat, marked by bloodshot eyes with aversion of light or nebula, it is often combined with Flos Chrysanthemi, Semen Cassiae, Herba Equiseti Hiemalis, Spica Prunellae, etc.; for nebula after measles, with pig's liver, powder of Concha Meretricis seu Cyclinae.

Dosage and Administration: 6 ~ 12 g of the drug are taken for decoction.

Herb of Common Scouring Rush (木贼 *Muzei*) Herba Equiseti Hiemalis

The drug consists of the entire plant of the evergreen perennial herbaceous plant, Equisetum hiemale L. Cut into segments, It is dried in the sun for use.

Nomenclature Used in Prescriptions: *Muzei*, *Muzeicao*.

Properties and Channel Distribution: The drug is sweet and bitter to the taste, even in nature, is distributed to the Lung and Liver Channels.

Action and Indications:

Dispersing wind–heat, brightening vision and relieving nebula: For the treatment of bloodshot eyes with presence of nebula, it is often combined with Flos Eriocauli, Periostracum Cicadae, etc.; for blurred vision with an overflow of tears, it may be combined with Rhizoma Atractylodis, Radix Ledebouriellae, Spica Prunellae, etc.

Dosage and Administration: 3–10 g of the drug are used for decoction.

Notes: It is not suitable for persistent nebula of blood deficiency; and if taken in an overdosage, it will be likely to cause congestion of the eyes.

2.3 Drugs for Eliminating Evil Heat from Blood

The drugs are indicated in spitting blood or epistaxis due to extravasation of blood caused by blood–heat, eruption of macule or papule, irascibility and restlessness due to invasion of the heart by abundance of heat, and crimson tongue and impairment of conciousness.

When evil heat attacks *Yingfen* or blood system, the vital essence or the body fluid seems likely to be consumed. In the drugs Radix Rehmanniae and the like have the functions of nourishing the vital essence and replenishing the body fluid; besides, for the treatment of febrile disease with *Yin*–defeciency or *Yang*–exhaustion, this kind of drugs may be combined with drugs for replenishing *Yin*, such as Radix Scrophulariae, Radix Ophiopogonis; by this way, both the exterior symptoms and the cause of disease can be treated.

This kinds of drugs are usually indicated in the heat syndrome in blood system. For treating syndrome due to both *Qi* and blood system being attacked by abundance of evils, they may be combined with the drugs for clearing away heat and purging fire; for syndrome of abundance of virulent–fire evil, with the drugs for eliminating heat–toxicant.

Rhinoceros Horn (犀角 *Xijiao*)*
Cornu Rhinoceri

The drug consists of the horn of Rhinoceros unicornis L. or Rhinoceros sondaicus Desmarest or Rhinoceros sumatrensis (Fischer) or the other. Besides these origins there are two other kinds; the one consisting of the horn of Rhinocerus bicornis L.or R. simus Burchell. and the another consisting of the bud on the tip of the horn; of these two kinds, the former is called *Guangjiao* and the latter is called *Xiaoxijiao* or *Mogutou* in TCM. After the rhinocerus has been caught, the horn is cut off for being used as a medicine imported; the drug may be prepared in the form of stick, pieces or powder; sometimes its suspension may be taken by being ground it with water.

Nomenclature Used in Prescriptions: *Xijiaopian(hua)*, *Xijiaofen*, *Quangjiaopian*, *Quangjiaofen*.

Properties and Channel Distribution: The drug is bitter, salty to the taste, cold in nature, and is distributed to the Heart, Liver and Stomach Channels.

Action and Indications:

1. Reducing the evil heat in the heart to calm the mind: For the treatment of febrile disease with delirium due to invasion of the heart by evil heat, it may be combined with Radix Rehmanniae, Radix Scrophulariae, Fructus Forsythiae.; for con-

---

* Please see Notes. We deal with these materials in this volume is just to the academic convenience

vulsion due to invasion of the heart and liver by evil heat, with Calculus Bovis or Cornu Antelopis or others for arresting convulsion and restoring the mind.

2. Eliminating heat from blood to arrest bleeding:

For the treatment of spitting blood or epistaxis due to extravasation of blood caused by blood–heat, it is often combined with Radix Rehmanniae, Cortex Moutan Radicis, Radix Paeoniae, etc.

3. Removing toxic materials and resolving eruptions: For the treatment of seasonal febrile disease due to abundant pirulent heat marked by eruptions in dark or purple color, it may be combined with Gypsum Fibrosum.

Dosage and Administration: 1.5–6 g of the drug are taken for decoction; usually the drug in powder form is often used; and the drug may also be used as single medicine for decoction taken together with other preparations; usually, 1–3 g of the powder are taken with water. The horn of Rhinocerus bicornis L. (*guangjiao*) seems weaker in its effects and cheaper in price, than Cornu Rhinoceri, its weight should be doubled. Now, the drug is often replaced by Cornu Bubali.

Notes: It should not be used or used with care to treat such disease when *Ying*–Blood system has not been invaded by evil heat; and the pregnant woman should used with care. Besides, it can not be used with Radix Aconiti, or Radix Aconiti Kusnezoffii.

Appendix: Buffle Horn (水牛角 *Shuiniujiao*) Cornu Bubali

The drug consists of the horn of Bubalus bubalis L. (family Bovidae). The therapeutic action of Cornu Bubali is similar to that of Cornu Rhinocerus, it is used to treat acute febrile disease marked by high fever, eruptions, delirium, convulsion, etc. During treatment, it is advisable to be used in a large amount; the weight of this drug used is 8–10 times as many as that of Cornu Rhinoceri, that is 30–150 g of the drug are often used by first filing it into powders, secondly stewing. And 1.5–6 g of its powders are taken as a dose. Compendium of Meteria Medica (*Li Shizhen*) says that Cornu Bubali can be used to treat seasonal febrile disease with headache; besides, its decoction can be used to treat convulsion and high fever due to pirulent heat evil. Lately, some articles have revealed that Cornu Bubali has been used to treat seasonal febrile disease and infantile febrile disease instead of Cornu Rhinoceri, and the therapeutic effect of the drug has proved fairly satisfactory and its pharmacological action is nearly similar to that of Cornu Rhinoceri.

Rehmannia Root (生地黄 *Shengdihuang*)
Radix Rehmanniae

The drug consists of the dried tuberous root of a perennial herbaceous plant, Rehmannia glutinosa (Gaertn) Libosch or Rehmannia glutinosa Libosch F. hueichingensis (Chao et Schih) Hsiao. (family Scrophulariaceae). The crude drug is cut into pieces and dried in the sun for being used; and the fresh one or the carbonized one also may be used.

Nomenclature Used in Prescriptions: *Shengdihuang*, *Ganshengdi*, *Shengdi*, *Shengditan*, *Xiandihuang*

Properties and Channel Distribution: The drug is sweet and bitter to the taste, cold in nature, and is distributed to the Heart, Liver and Kidney Channels.

Action and Indications:

1. Reducing heat and nourshing *Yin*: For the treatment of seasonal febrile disease at the stage when *Yingfen* or blood system has been invaded by evil heat, marked by fever and thirst, red or crimson tongue, etc., it is often combined with Radix Scrophulariae, Cornu Rhinoceri, etc.; for syndrome of abundance of heat with deficiency of *Yin*, marked by constipation due to deficiency of the body fluid, with a heavy weight of Radix Rehmanniae, Radix Scrophulariae, Radix Ophiopogonis, etc.; for the late stage of the febrile disease with lingering fever or for chronic disease with fever due to deficiency of *Yin*, with Herba Artemisiae Chinghao, Carapax Trionycis, Cortex Lycii Radicis, Rhizoma Anemarrhenae, etc.

2. Reducing heat from blood to arrest bleeding: For the treatment of syndrome of blood–heat with extravasation of blood, marked by spitting blood, epistaxis, bloody urine, hematochezia, metrorrhagia, etc., it is often combined with drugs for reducing blood–heat and arresting bleeding such as Cacumen Biotae, Radix Rubiae, etc.; for eruptions in dark or purple color due to abundant blood–heat, with Cornu Rhinoceri, Cortex Moutan Radicis and other drugs for eliminating blood–heat and removing toxic materials.

3. Promoting the production of the body fluid to relieve thirst: For the treatment of febrile disease with consuming of the body fluid, marked by redness and dryness of the tongue or thirst with dry lips, it is often combined with Radix Ophiopogonis, Rhizoma Polygonati Odorati, Radix Adenophorae Strictae and other drugs for invigorating stomach and promoting the production of the body fluid; for diabetis marked by thirst with eager-

ness of drinking, it may be combined with Radix Asparagi, Fructus Lycii, Rhizoma Dioscoreae, Fructus Corni and other drugs for replenishing vital essence of the liver and kidney.

Besides, for the treatment of urticaria and other tinea or tinea–like diseases due to blood heat, it may be combined with Fructus Tribuli, Cortex Dictamni Radicis, Radix Ledebouriellae, etc.

Dosage and Administration: 10–30 g of the drug are taken for decoction; the crude drug is usually used for reducing heat and promoting vital essence while the carbonized one is used for arresting bleeding.

Notes: It is contraindicated in syndrome of weakness of the spleen due to dampness, marked by fullness of the abdomen and watery stools.

Moutan bark (牡丹皮 *Mudanpi*)
Cortex Moutan Radicis

The drug consists of the bark of the root of a perennial deciduous shrub, Paeonia suffruticosa Andr. (family Ranunculaceae). The crude drug is cut into pieces and dried in the sun, then baked and stirred with wine or carbonized for being used.

Nomenclature Used in Prescriptions: *Mudanpi, Fendanpi, Jiudanpi, Danpitan.*

Properties and Channel Distribution: The drug is bitter and pungent to the taste and slightly cold in nature, and is distributed to the Heart, Liver and kidney Channels.

Action and Indications:

1. Eliminating evil heat from blood: For the treatment of seasonal febrile disease with eruption, spitting blood and epistaxis due to blood–heat, it is often combined with Radix Rehmanniae, or with Cornu Rhinoceri if the disease is very serious; for the later stage of the disease with lingering heat attacking on *Yingfen* marked by night fever, with Herba Artemisiae Chinghao, Carapax Trionycis or Radix Rehmanniae and Fructus Corni; for asthenia–heat or fever before menstruation of women, with Fructus Gardeniae, Radix Angelicae Sinensis, Radix Rehmanniae, Radix Paeoniae Rubra, Rhizoma Ligustici Chuanxiong, etc. when necessary.

2. Promoting blood circulation to remove blood–stasis: For the treatment of amenorrhea, dysmenorrhea due to blood stasis or abdominal mass due to accumulation of stasis of blood, it may be often combined with Ramulus Cinnamomi, Poria, Radix Paeoniae, Semen Persicae, etc.; for injury due to accident (esp. contusion of the chest or abdomen), marked by pain and blood–stasis, it is often combined with Radix Paeoniae Rubra, Olibanum, Resina Commiphorae Myrrhae, etc.; for the intestinal abscess with abdominal pain and constipation, it is often combined with Radix et Rhizoma Rhei, Semen Persicae, Semen Benincasae, etc. Besides, it can be used to treat carbuncle, abscess or skin pyogenic infection in combination with the other drugs.

Moreover, it can be used to treat hypertension and arteriosclerosis in combination with Flos Chrysanthemi Indici, Concha Haliotidis, Caulis Lonicerae, etc.

Dosage and Administration: 5–10 g of the drug are taken for decoction; usually, the crude one is for eliminating heat from blood; the drug bake–stirred with wine, for promoting the circulation of blood and removing blood–stasis; and the carbonized one, for arresting bleeding.

Notes: It is not suitable to be taken by women with menorrhagia or pregnancy.

Red Peony Root (赤芍 *Chishao*)
Radix Paeoniae Rubra

The drug consists of the roots of a perennial herbaceous plant, Paeonia, lactiflora pall. or P. obovata Maxim or Paeonia veitchii Lynch (family Ranunculaceae). Usually, the root is cut into pieces and dried in the sun for being used.

Nomenclature Used in Prescriptions: *Chishaoyao, Chishao.*

Properties and Channel Distribution: The drug is bitter to the taste, slightly cold in nature, and is distributed to the Liver Channel.

Action and Indications:

1. Eliminating heat from blood and promoting the circulation of the blood: For the treatment of amenorrhea or dysmenorrhea due to blood–stasis accompanied with invasion of blood by heat, it is often combined with Radix Angelica Sinensis, Radix Salviae Miltiorrhizae, Semen Persica, Flos Carthami, etc.; for carbuncles due to blood heat, accompanied with congestion, swelling and pain, with Radix Angelica Sinensis, Rhizoma Ligustici Chuanxiong, Flos Lonicerae, Fructus Forsythiae, etc.; for spitting blood or epistaxis or eruptions in dark color, due to blood–heat, with Radix Rehmanniae, Cortex Moutan Radicis, etc.

2. Removing blood stasis and relieving pain: for the treat-

ment of mass in the abdomen due to blood stasis or abdominal pain due to blood stasis after labor, it is often combined with Radix Angelica Sinensis, Rhizoma Ligustici Chuanxiong, etc.; for syndrome of remarkable blood stasis, with Semen Persica, Flos Carthami; for abdominal pain after labor due to blood stasis, with Rhizoma Zingiberis roasted in hot ashes and drugs for warming the interior to promote the circulation of blood; for injury due to accidents, accompanied with swelling and pain due to blood stasis with Olibanum, Resina Commiphorae Myrrhae, Radix Angelica Sinensis, Semen Persica, etc.

3. Reducing liver-heat to brighten vision: For the treatment of red eyes due to liver-heat, it is often combined with Flos Chrysanthemi, Herba Menthae, etc.

Dosage and Administration: 6–12 g of the drug are taken for decoction.

Notes: It can not be used in combination with Rhizoma et Radix Veratri.

Arnebia or Lithoeperm Root (紫草 *Zicao*)
Radix Arnebiae seu Lithospermi

The drug consists of the roots of a perennial herbaceous plant, Lithospermum erythrorhizon Sieb. et Zucc. or Arnebia euchroma (Royle) Johnst. or Onosma Paniculatum Bur. et Franch.; usually, it is dried in the sun and cut into segments for use.

Nomenclature Used in Prescriptions: *Zicao*, *Zicaogen*.

Properties and Channel Distribution: The drug is sweet to the taste, cold in nature, and distributed to the Heart and Liver

Channels.

Action and Indications:

1. Eliminating blood–heat and promoting circulation of the blood, removing toxic materials and letting eruptions out: For the treatment of retardation of eruption or eruptions in dark or purple color or in dull color due to abundance of virulent heat evil, it may be combined with Radix Paeoniae Rubra, Periostracum Cicadae, etc.; for furuncle, carbuncle, eczema, dermatitis, pruritus vulvae, scald and burn, etc., its medicated oil may be used externally and the medicated oil can be prepared by immersing the powder into the vegetable oil (3:6) for several days and then filtering the oil out for being used as medicine. To treat various kinds of carbuncles, deep–root carbuncles, skin pyogenic infections it may be combined with Radix Angelicae Sinensis, Radix Angelicae Dahuricae, Resina Draconis, Calomelas, etc., for being prepared and used as an ointment for local application.

2. Promoting diuresis and facilitating defecation: For the treatment of stranguria or constipation due to abundant blood–heat, it may be combined with the drugs for reducing evil heat and removing toxic materials; or may be used as a single medicine in the form of powder taken with water.

Dosage and Administration: 3–10 g of the drug may be taken for decoction; a proper amount of the drug may be used externally.

2.4 Drugs for Eliminating Heat and Dampness

This kind of drugs are usually bitter in taste and cold in nature; as the drugs with bitter taste are often used to resolve dampness; and the drugs with cold nature, to reduce heat. They are indicated in internal syndrome of damp–heat or in heat syndrome due to accumulation of dampness, marked by fever with iracibility, bitterness of mouth, stuffiness of the chest, jaundice, diarrhea or dysentery, or carbuncles and skin pyogenic infection, urine in dark tan color, etc.

In thes division there are drugs, as Radix Scutell–ariae, Rhizoma Coptidis, Cotex Phellodendri, Radix Gentianae, etc., which are also commonly–used drugs for eliminating heat–toxics; therefore, they should be used according to the specific syndrome.

Although this kind of drugs can be used to treat syndrome due to heat of fire, yet they with bitterness and dryness in properties are likely to consume *Yin* and hurt the stomach; therefore they are not indicated in syndrome due to consuming of the body fluid or asthenia syndrome of the spleen and stomach. When used, they should be combined with the drugs for nourishing essence and invigorating the stomach.

Scutellaria Root (黄芩 *Huangqin*)
Radix Scutellariae

The drug consists of the dried root of a perennial herbaceous plant, Scutellaria baicalensis Georgi (family Labiatae). Usually, cut into pieces and dried in the sun, the crude one, bake–stirred one with wine or the carbonized one, may be used.

Nomenclature Used in Prescriptions: *Huangqin*, *Jiuhuangqin*, *Kuqin*, *Tiaoqin*, *Ziqin*, *Huangqintan*.

Properties and Channel Distribution: The drug is bitter taste, cold in nature, and is distributed to the Lung, large Intestine and

Small Intestine, Spleen and Gall Bladder Channels.

Action and Indications:

1. Eliminating heat and resolving dampness: For the treatment of diarrhea or dysentery due to damp–heat accompanied with tenesmus, it is often combined with Radix Paeoniae Rubra, Radix Glycyrrhizae; for diarrhea, with Radix Puerariae, Rhizoma Coptidis, etc.; for jaundice due to invasion of damp–heat, it is used as an assistant drug in combination with Herba Artemisiae Scopariae, Fructus Gardeniae, etc.; for painful urination and stranguria due to invasion of the urinary bladder by damp–heat, with Radix Rehmanniae, Caulis Akebiae, etc.

2. Purging fire and removing toxic materials: For the treatment of acute febrile disease marked by high fever and irascibility, yellow fur, rapid pulse, etc., it is often combined with Rhizoma Coptidis, Fructus Gardeniae, etc.; for cough due to invasion of the lung by evil heat, marked by cough with expectoration of purulent yellow sputum, with Cortex Mori Radicis, Rhizoma Anemarrhenae, Radix Ophiopogonis, etc.; for carbuncle or skin pyogenic infection or scald or burn, with the drugs for purging fire and removing toxic materials and they may be taken by mouth or used locally.

3. Eliminating heat and calming fetus: For the treatment of threatened abortion with over fetal movement due to invasion of fetus by heat it is often combined with Rhizoma Atractylodis Macrocephalae, Radix Angelicae Sinensis, etc.

Besides, it can also be used to treat spitting blood, epistaxis, hematochezia, metrorrhagia, etc., due to abundant heat and presence of extravasation of blood; to treat arteriosclerosis, hypertension due to hyperactivity of Liver–*Yang*, marked by headache, bitterness of the mouth, flush face, fidgets, etc., it may be combined with Spica Prunellae, Flos Chrysanthemi, Concha Haliotidis, etc.

Dosage and Administration: 3–12 g of the drug are taken for decoction. Usually, the crude drug is used to eliminate heat; the drug bake–stirred, to calm the fetus; the drug prepared with wine, to clear away heat from upper *Jiao*; the carbonized drug, to arrest bleeding.

Notes: It is not suitable to be used to treat asthenia–cold syndrome of the spleen and stomach, marked by poor appetite and watery stools.

Coptis Root (黄连 *Huanglian*)
Rhizoma Coptidis

The drug consists of the dried rhizomes of a perennial herbaceous plant, Coptis chinensis Franch. or C. deltoidea C. Y. Cheng et Hsiao or C. teetoides C. Y. Cheng (family Rananculaceae). Usually, it is first dried in the sun, then it can be used for medicine, or bake–stirred or prepared with wine or bake–stirred with ginger juice or bake–stirred with decoction of Fructus Euodiae. The drug is usually pounded for use.

Nomenclature Used in Prescription: *Huanglian, Chuanhuanglian, Chuanyalian, Chaohuanglian, Jianglian, Jiulian, Yulian*

Properties and Channel Distribution: The drug is bitter to the taste and cold in nature, and is distributed to the Heart, Stomach, Liver, Gall Bladder and Large Intestine Channels.

Action and Indications:

1. Eliminating heat and resloving dampness: it having func-

tions of clearing the intestine–heat and relieving dysentery, is used to treat syndrome of damp–heat attacking on the intestine and stomach, marked by diarrhea or dysentery, tesnesmus in combination with Radix Aucklandiae, Radix Scutellariae, Radix Pulsatillae, etc.; to treat dysentery with bloody stools and fever in the superficies, it may be combined with Radix Puerariae, Radix Scutellariae; to treat damp–heat syndrome of intestine and stomach, marked by fullness of epigastrium and abdomen, nausea and vomiting, with Radix Scutellariae, Rhizoma Pinelliae, Rhizoma Zingiberis Recens, etc.; to treat abdominal pain with nausea or vomiting due to retention of heat in the chest, cold in the intestine, and presence of disharmony of cold and heat, with Rhizoma Zingiberis, Ramulus Cinnamomi, Rhizoma Pinelliae, etc.

2. Purging fire and removing virulent factors and toxic materials: For the treatment of acute febrile disease due to flare–up of evil fire, marked by high fever with irascibility, unconsciousness and delirium or syndrome of flaming of heart fire, marked by stuffiness and hotness of the chest, fidgets and insomnia or aphtha and tongue sore, it is often combined with Radix Scutellariae, Fructus Gardeniae, etc.; for the treatment of spitting blood or epistaxis accompanied with constipation and urine in dark color, with Radix et Rhizoma Rhei, Radix Scutellariae and the others for reducing heat from blood and arresting bleeding; for fidgets and insomnia, with Cinnabaris, Semen Ziziphi Spinosae or Colla Corii Asini, etc; besides, it having the functions of reducing liver–heat and brightening vision, can be used to treat bloodshot eyes with aversion of light and overflow of tears due to ascending of liver–fire, it may be combined with Radix

Scutellariae, Fructus Gardeniae, Flos Chrysanthemi, Herba Menthae, etc., or used as a single medicine by immersing its pieces into human milk, and the medicated milk may be used as the eye drops, twice or three times a day. For the treatment of vomiting of bitter fluid and regurgitation of acid due to stomach–heat, it is often used as a medicine for clearing stomach–heat and arresting vomiting in combination with Fructus Euodiae or Folium Perillae; for nail–like boil or carbuncle, aphtha and tongue sore, eczema or pruritus, etc., it can be used internally or externally.

Dosage and Administration: 1.5–4.5 g of the drug are taken for decoction; and 0.6–1.5 g of its powder are taken as a dose, 2–3 times a day; a proper amount of the drug is used externally. The crude drug is suitable for the treatment of syndrome of invasion of the heart or the large intestine by evil fire; the drug decocted with decoction of fructus Euodiae, suitable for the clearing up of liver–fire and gall bladder fire; the drug prepared with wine, suitable for the reducing of the fire of upper *Jiao*; the drug prepared with ginger juice, suitable for treating vomiting due to stomach fire. Usually, the drug prepared with certain drug or medicinal juice or other materials not only can be reinforced in its therapeutic effects but also can be modulated in its bitter and cold properties; therefore the drug must be processed specifically and used according to the clinical syndromes, yet it seems not suitable to process such drugs excessively.

notes: It is contraindicated in asthenia–cold syndrome of spleen and stomach without invasion by damp–heat or intense fire.

Bark of Chinese Corktree (黄柏 *Huangbai*)
Cortex Phellodendri

The drug consists of the bark of a deciduous arbor, Phellodendron amurense Rupr. or P. chinense Schneid. (family Rutaceae). Usually, the crude drug is cut into pieces or further bake–stirred with salt solution for use.

Nomenclature Used in Prescription: *Huangbai*, *Yanhuangbai*.

Properties and Channel Distribution: The drug is bitter to the taste, cold in nature, and is distributed to the Kidney, Urinary Bladder and Large Intestine Channels.

Action and Indications:

1. Reducing heat and resolving dampness: For the treatment of dysentery due to damp–heat accompanied with fever and tenesmus, it is often combined with Radix Pulsatillae, Cortex Fraxini, etc.; for jaundice with fever due to damp–heat, with Fructus Gardeniae and others for reducing heat and resolving dampness; for yellow and thick leukorrhea due to damp–heat with Semen Euryales, Semen Ginkgo, etc.; for the treatment of the low extremities affected with hotness and pain due to the descending of damp–heat, with Rhizoma Atractylodis, Radix Achyranthis Bidentatae; for stranguria with hot sensation or painful urination with dark urine, with Fructus Gardeniae, Semen Plantaginis, etc.

2. Purging fire and eliminating virulent evil factors:

For the treatment of eczema and skin pyogenic infection due to virulent heat, it may be used internally or externally: for eczema, it can be used with Herba Schizonepetae, Radix Sophorae

Flavescentis; for skin pyogenic infection, it can be used internally in combination with Rhizoma Coptidis, Fructus Gardeniae, etc. and used externally by mixing its powder with pig's bile.

3. Eliminating asthenia–heat: For the treatment of hectic fever, nocturnal emmision, night sweating, due to deficiency of *Yin* leading to flare–up of fire, it is often combined with Rhizoma Anemarrhenae.

Dosage and Administration: 3–10 g of the drug are used for decoction: a proper amount of the drug may be used externally and the drug bake–stirred with salt solution may be used internally; and the crude drug is often used for local administration.

Notes: It is not suitable for those patients with asthenia–cold syndrome of the spleen and stomach.

Chinese Gentian (龙胆草 *Longdancao*)
Radix Gentianae

The drug is consists of the root and rhizome of a perennial plant, Gentiana scabra Bge. or G. triflora Pall. (family Gentianaceae). Usually, it is cut into segments for use.

Nomenclature used in Prescriptions: *Longdancao*, *Dancao*.

Properties and Channel Distribution: The drug is bitter to the taste, cold in nature, and is distributed to the Liver and Gall Bladder Channels.

Action and Indications:

1. Reducing heat and resolving damphess: The drug is one of the medicines frequently used for eliminating damp–heat from the liver, gall bladder and lower *Jiao*. For the treatment of jaundice due to damp–heat, it can be combined with Herba

Artemisiae Scopariae, Radix Curcumae, Cortex Phellodendri, etc.; for the treatment of pruritus of the vulvae of scrotum due to the decending of damp–heat, with Semen Plantaginis, Talcum, etc. which are medicines for eliminating damp–heat.

2. Eliminating intense fire from the liver: For the treatment of sthenia–fire syndrome of the liver and gall bladder, marked by headache and feeling of distention in the head, bloodshot eyes, deafness and swelling of the ears, hypochondriac pain and bitterness of the mouth, etc., it is often combined with Radix Scutellariae, Fructus Gardeniae, etc.; for the treatment of persistent high fever accompanied with convulsion due to stirring of wind caused by liver–heat, with drugs for eliminating liver heat such as Concha Haliotidis, Aloe, Ramulus Uncariae cum Uncis.

Dosage and Administration: 3–6 g of the drug are taken as a dose in making a decoction.

notes: It is not suitable for the treatment of asthenia–cold syndrome of spleen and stomach.

Flavescent Sophora Root (苦参 *Kushen*)
Radix Sophorae Flavescentis

The drug consists of the dried root of a perennial deciduous plant, a kind of sub–shrub, Sophora flavescens Ait. (family Leguminosae). The crude drug is usually dried in the sun, cut into segments for use.

Nomenclature Used in Prescriptions: *Kushen*

Properties and Channel Distribution: The drug is bitter to the taste and cold in nature, and is distributed to the Heart, Liver, Large Intestine, Gall Bladder Channels.

Action and Indications:

1. Clearing away heat and resolving dampness: For the treatment of dysentery due to invasion by damp–heat, it may be combined with Radix Scutellariae, Herba Portulacae or Radix Puerariae and Fructus Crataegi; for bloody stools or hemorrhoids, with Radix Sanguisorbae, Fructus Sophorae.

2. Killing parasites and stopping itching: For the treatment of scabies or tinea, eczema, pruritus, etc., it is often combined with Cortex Dictamni Radicis, Fructus Cnidii, etc.; for seborrheic dermatitis, impetigo, etc., 60 g of the drug in combination with 45 g of Radix Angelicae Sinensis may be used by making them into pills with honey, and it is advisable that the pills should be taken for a long time; for trichomonas vaginitis, pruritus valvae with leukorrhagia, it is often combined with Radix Pulsatillae, Fructus Cnidii, etc.; for leprosy, with Semen Hydnocarpi, Fructus Xanthii, etc.

Besides, it can be used to treat jauntice. And since it has the function of promoting diuresis, it can also be used to treat stranguria or disorder of urination due to accumulation and retention of damp–heat.

Dosage and Administration: 3–10 g of the drug are taken for decoction; and a proper amount is used for local administration.

Dittany Bark (白蘚皮 *Baixianpi*)
Cortex Dictamni

The drug consists of the bark of the old root of a perennial herbaceous plant, Dictamnus dasycarpus Turcz. (family Rutaceae). The drug is usually dried and cut into pieces for use.

Nomenclature Used in Prescriptions: *Baixianpi.*

Properties and Channel Distribution: The drug is bitter and cold to the taste and nature respectively, and is distributed to the Spleen, Stomach and Urinary Bladder Channels.

Action and Indications:

Clearing away evil heat and resolving dampness, dispelling wind and relieving itching: For the treatment of suppurative inflammation of skin due to damp-heat, urticaria or scarbies or ringworm, pruritus, etc., it is often combined with Radix Sophorae Flavescentis, Periostracum Cicadae, Fructus Kochiae, Radix Ledebouriellae, etc.; for pruritus valvae with leukorrhagia, with Radix Sophorae Flavescentis, Fructus Cnidii and Pericarpium Zanthoxyli for wash.

Besides, it can also be used to treat jaundice or arthragia due to damp-heat, etc.

Dosage and Administration: 6–15 g of the drug are taken for decoction; a proper amount is used for local administration.

Ash Bark (秦皮 *Qinpi*)
Cortex Fraxini

The drug consists of the bark of a deciduous arbor, Fraxinus rhynchophylla Hance. or F. bungeana DC. or F. paxiana Lingelsh. (family Oleaceae); it is usually dried in the sun and cut into pieces used for medicine.

Nomenclature Used in Prescriptions: *Qinpi*, *Beiqinpi*

Properties and Channel Distribution: The drug is bitter and astringent to the taste, cold in nature, and is distributed to the Liver, GallBladder, Large Intestine Channel.

Actions and Indications:

1. Reducing heat and resolving dampness: For the treatment of acute dysentery due to damp–heat, it is often used in combination with Radix Pulsatillae, Rhizoma Coptidis, Cortex Phellodendri or Radix Sophorae Flavescentis, Radix Aucklandiae; for chronic dysentery, with Radix Sanguisorbae, Cortex Ailanthi, etc.

2. Clearing away liver–heat and brightening vision, relieving red eyes and nebula: For the treatment of bloodshot eyes with nebula it can be used for wash. For acute inflammation of the eyes with swelling and pain, with Herba Lophatheri, Rhizoma Coptidis, or with 6 g of Rhizoma Coptidis and 12 g of Talcum, which are pounded into powder and immersed in the hot water, and then used for fumigant and wash.

Dosage and Administration: 6–10 g of the drug are used for decoction, and a proper amount of the drug is used as medicine for local application.

2.5 Drugs for Eliminating Heat-toxicant

Here, heat–toxicant or virulent heat implies a variety of pyogenic infections, carbuncles or purulent skin infections, accompanied with swelling in red color, hot and pain, due to abundance of evil fire or heat, which may also be called fire–toxicant or virulent fire. This kind of drugs has the functions of clear away evil fire or heat and relieving swelling and removing heat–toxics, the functions of anti–inflammation and anti–infection (antibacterial or antiviral actions); therefore, they are classified into the category of the drugs for eliminating heat–toxics.

There are different syndromes due to invasion of the different internal organs, channels, parts by virulent heat; and this kind of drugs has their specific indications, indications in treating carbuncles, furuncles, eruptions, erysipelas, acute febrile diseases, sore throat with somewhat obstruction, dysentery, etc. Therefore, in the clinical practice it is necessary to select the indispensable drug or drugs according to different syndromes due to invasion by virulent heat, or to use some of this kind in combination with the other drugs; for instance, to treat virulent heat in the blood, This kind of drugs is combined with the drugs which have the function of eliminating heat in the blood; to treat flare–up of virulent–heat, with the drugs having the function of purging evil fire; to treat virulent heat with dampness, with the drugs having the function of resolving dampness or promoting diuresis; to treat carbuncles or pyogenic skin infections with deficiency in nature, with certain tonics. Besides, for the treatment of purulent skin infection, carbuncles or sore throat with obstruction, they should be in combination for local use.

This kind of drugs is cold or cool in nature; therefore, they are not indicated in such diseases as carbuncles or skin infections, sore throat, dysentery, eruptions which are of *Yin* or cold nature.

Honeysuckle Flower (金银花 *Jinyinhua*)
Flos Lonicerae

The drug consists of the flower–bud of a perennial semi–evergreen twined shrub, Lonicera japonica Thunb. (family Caprifoliaceae); the crude buds are dried in the shade for use.

Nomenclature Used in Prescriptions: *Jinyinhua*, *Yinhua*, *Shuanghua*, *Erbaohua*, *Rendonghua*.

Properties and Channel Distribution: The drug is sweet to the taste, cold in nature, and distributed to the lung, Heart and Stomach Channels.

Action and Indications:

1. Reducing intense heat and eliminating heat–toxics: The drug is indicated in treating febrile diseases at their beginning stages, marked by fever with slight aversion of wind, eruptions, etc. The drug also has the functions of dispelling wind and dispersing evil heat, it can often combined with Fructus Forsythiae, Semen Sojae Praeparatum, Herba Menthae, etc. For the treatment of syndrome of serious virulent heat, accompanied with sore throat, mumps, with Radix Scutellariae, Radix et Rhizoma Rhei, Cotex Phellodendri, Radix Isatidis, etc.; for pyogenic skin infection or carbuncle due to virulent heat or inflammation of throat, with Fructus Forsythiae; for either dispelling the skin infection, carbuncle with obvious pain and swelling or letting their pus out, with Squama Manitis, Spina Gledisiae, etc.; for nail–like boil or furunculosis, with Herba Violae, Herba Taraxaci, Flos Chrysanthemi Indici, etc.; for sore throat, with Radix Sophorae Subprostratae, Herba Menthae, etc.; for pyogenic infection of intestines, with Semen Coicis, Radix Scutellariae, Radix Angelicae Sinensis, etc.

2. Dispelling heat in the blood and relieving dysentery: For the treatment of dysentery due to invasion of virulent heat, accompanied with purulent and bloody stool, it can be combined with Radix Scutellariae, Radix Paeoniae Rubra, etc.; for the disease mentioned above, it can be used as a single medicine for the preparation of the concentrated decoction.

Dosage and Administration: 10–15 g of the drug are often used as a dose; for syndrome of serious virulent heat 30–60 g of the drug are needed for decoction.

Appendix: Honey–suckle Stem (忍冬藤 *Rendongteng*); Caulis Lonicerae

The drug consists of the dried stems, branches of Lonicera japonica Thunb. (family Caprifoliaceae); it is also called *Yinhuateng* in Chinese. Before used, it is cut into segments and dried in the sun. Its actions and indications are like that of Flos Lonicerae, and it also has the function of dispersing wind–heat from the channels; therfore it is often used to treat carbuncle or skin pyogenic infections, sore throat, arthritis, arthralgia and other disorders of the channels. Usually, 15–30 g are used for decoction.

Forsythia Fruit (连翘 *Lianqiao*)
Fructus Forsythiae

The drug consists of the dried fruits of the deciduous shrub, Forsythia suspensa (Thunb.) Vahl (family Oleaceae); it is to be dried for use.

Nomenclature Used in Prescriptions: *Lianqiao*, *Qinglianqiao*, *Lianqiaoke*, *Lianqiaoxin*

Properties and Channel Distribution: The drug is bitter to the taste, slightly cold in nature, and distributed to the Heart and Small intestine Channels.

Action and Indications:

1. Reducing intense heat and eliminating virulent substances: It is used to treat the febrile diseases at beginning stage accompanied with fever, slight aversion of wind, eruptions and so on.

The drug being light in its weight and having functions of reducing evil heat and dispersing the evil heat from superficies, is often in combination with such drugs for eliminating virulent heat or dispersing heat from the superficies as Flos Lonicerae, Herba Menthae, etc; to treat heat syndrome due to invasion of the chest and diphragm by evil heat accompanied with fidgets, it can be combined with Radix Scutellariae; to treat those with fever, fidgets and unconsciousness, it may be combined with Cornu Rhinoceri or Flos Lonicerae, Folium Isatidis, Radix Scutellariae, etc.; to treat pyogenic skin infections or mastitis, etc., with Flos Lonicerae, Herba Violae, Herba Taraxaci, Flos Chrysanthemi Indici, etc. In short, the drug is an indispensible drug for treating diseases due to virulent heat, and often combined with Flos Lonicerae in clinical pratice.

2. Eliminating fire and dispersing mass: To treat scrofula due to tuberclosis, it is often combined with Radix Scrophulariae, Spica Prunellae, etc.

Besides, it is also used to treat anaphylactic purpura in combination with Radix Paeoniae Rubra 10 g, Herba Ephedrae 6 g, Radix Glycyrrhizae 6 g, for decoction.

Dosage and Administration: 6–15 g of the drug are taken as a dose for decoction.

Appendix: Seeds of Forsythia fruit, *Lianqiaoxin* in TCM, is bitter in taste, slightly cold in nature. It has the function of eliminating heat syndrome of the heart, and is often used to treat seasonal febrile diseases with delirium and unconsciousness due to invasion of the pericardium by evil heat. And it is often combined with the central portion of Radix Scrophulariae, Radix Ophiopogonis with leaf bud, Plumula Nelumbinis, etc. 3–6 g of the drug are used for decoction.

Isatis Leaf (大青叶 *Daqingye*)
Folium Isatidis

The drug consists of the dried leaves of a kind of herbaceous biennial plant, Isatis indigotica Fort. (family Cruciferae); the drug is dried in sun or the drug is fresh for use.

Besides, the drug may also consist of the leaves of herbaceous annual plant, Clerodendron cyrtophyllum Turcz. (Verbenaceae) or Polygonum tinctorium Ait.

Nomenclature Used in Prescrsptions: *Daqingye*

Properties and Channel Distribution: The drug is bitter to the taste, cold in nature, and distributed to the Heart, Liver and Stomach Channels.

Action and Indications:

1. Reducing intense heat and removing virulent factors or toxic materials: For the treatment of pestilence or seasonal febrile diseases with high fever and headache or sore throat, aphtha, pyogenic skin infection, erysipelas, etc., due to virulent heat, it can be used singly or with Gypsum Fibrosum, Radix Scutellariae, Radix Scrophulariae, and Flos Lonicerae, Fructus Gardeniae, etc.

2. Eliminating intense heat in the blood and relieving eruptions: It can be used to treat eruptions due to virulent heat or spitting blood and epistaxis due to blood-heat in combination with Cornu Rhinoceri, Fructus Gardeniae, etc.

At present, it is often used for the treatment of the infection of the upper respiratory tract, influenza, etc., marked by fever, congestion of the throat, swelling of the tonsils; it can also be used to treat epidemic cephalitis, epidemic mumps, viral hepatitis, viral pneumonia, etc., effectively; besides, it is an indispensable drug for eliminating virulent heat or removing toxic materials.

Dosage and Administration: 9−15 g of the drug are taken as a dose for decoction.

Appendix: Radix Isatidis (板蓝根 *Banlangen*).

The drug consists of the root of Isatidis indigotica Fort.; and it is often cut into pieces for use. It is bitter to the taste and cold in nature, and has the functions like that of Folium Isatidis; and it has good effects on eliminating virulent heat and dispersing mass. Therefore, it is often used to treat epidemic disease with swollen head, marked by redness and swelling of the head and face or inflammation of the throat, scarlet fever, etc., in combination with Folium Isatidis, Gypsum Fibrosum, Radix Scutellariae, Rhizoma Coptidis, and Flos Lonecerae, Fructus Forsythiae, Radix Scrophulariae, etc., according to the syndrome of the patient. At present, it is commonly used to treat epidemic cephalitis type B, mumps, influenza, viral hepatitis, etc. 9−15 g of the drug are taken as a dose for decoction.

Viola Herb (紫花地丁 *Zihuadiding*)
Herba Violae

The drug consists of the dried herb of the herbaceous perennial plant, Viola yedoensis Makino (family Violaceae). Usually it is cut into pieces, and dried in the sun for use; its fresh plant is also used.

Besides, in other regions the drug consists of the herb of the herbaceous perennial plant, Gueldenstaedtia multiflora Bge., G. Pauciflora (Rall.) Fisch. (family Leguminosae) or the herb of the herbaceous annual, Viola japonica Langsd(family Violaceae).

Nomenclature Used in Prescriptions: *Zihuadiding*, *Diding*.

Properties and Channel Distribution: The drug is bitter and pungent to the taste, cold in nature, and distributed to the Heart and Liver Channels.

Action and Indications:

Reducing intense heat and eliminating heat toxics.

Since the drug has good effect in treating furuncle, carbuncle and skin pyogenic infections, it is often used to treat such kinds of diseases mentioned above. with Herba Taraxaci, Flos Lonicerae, Fructus Foreythiae, etc. Or the fresh herbs may be pounded to gets its juice for internal administration or the fresh pounded drug is applied on the local area; for the treatment of poisonous snake bite, the pounded fresh herbs may be applied on the local area; for the treatment of pyogenic infection of the internal organ, it can be used with other drugs according to the specific syndromes.

Dosage and Administration: 10 30 g of the drug or a large amount, 30−60 g can be used if necessary; for external application a proper amount is used.

Dandelion Herb (蒲公英 *Pugongying*) Herba Taraxaci

The drug consists of the herb of a perennial plant, Taraxacum mongolicum Hand.−Mazz. or Taraxacum sinicum Kitag. or other genuses of the same family (family Compositae).

Usually, the fresh or crude plant is cut and used as medicine.

Nomenclature Used in Prescriptions: *Pugongying*, *Gongying*

Properties and Channel Distribution: The drug is sweet and bitter to the taste, cold in nature, and distributed to the Liver and Stomach Channels.

Action and Indications:

1. Reducing intense heat and eliminating heat toxics: To treat mastitis, funruncles, carbuncles, lung abscess. intestinal abscess, etc., it is often used with Herba Violae for mutual reinforcement; both of them are common drugs frequently in treating pyogenic diseases, esp. mastitis. At the beginning stage of mastitis, red and swelling and hard, for this purpose, the drug can be used in combination with Flos Lonicerae, Fructus Forsythiae, Squama Manitis (baked and stirred), Radix Trichosanthis, etc.. To treat the intestinal abscess with abundant virulent heat, it can be used with Flos Lonicerae, Radix et Rhizoma Rhei, Semen Persicae, etc.; to treat, furuncle, with Herba Violae, Flos Chrysanthemi Indici, Flos Lonicerae, etc.; to treat other pyogenic infections or carbuncles, with other drugs for reducing heat and eliminating heat toxicants.

2. Clearing away liver fire and improving vision: To treat bloodshot eye due to flare–up of liver fire, it can be used with Radix Scutellaroae, Flos Chrysanthemi, Spica Prunellae, etc. The drug may be used singly or with Flos Chrysanthemi to boil with water for being as fumigant and wash.

Besides, the drug has the effect of promoting urination, therefore it is often used to treat the infections of the urinary tract, jaundice due to damp–heat. It can also be used to treat the infections of the upper respiratory tract, acute tonsillitis, chronic gastritis, etc.

Dosage and Administration: 15–30 g of the drug are taken generally; if necessary, a rather large amount, 60 g, can be used for decoction; if used too often or in a large amount, it may induce mild loose bowels.

Patrinia Herb (败酱草 *Baijiangcao*) Herb Patriniae

The drug consists of the entire plant of the perennial herb, Patrinia scabiosaefolia Fisch. ex Link. or P. villosa Juss. (family Valerianaceae). Generally, it is dried in the shade and cut into pieces for use.

Moreover, in the north of our country the entire plant of the perennial, Sonchus brachyotus DC. (family Compositae) is used; while in the south the entire plant with fruit of the perennial, Thlaspi arvens L. (family Cruciferae) is used.

Nomenclature Used in Prescriptions: *Baijiang, Baijiangcao*

Properties and Channel Distribution: The drug is pungent and bitter to the taste, slightly cold in nature, and distributed to the Stomach and large Intestine and Liver Channels.

Action and Indications: Reducing intense heat, eliminating heat toxic, removing stasis and letting pus out

To treat intestinal abscess, according the old prescription, it is used with Semen Coicis, Radix Aconiti Praeparata; now, it is often used with Semen Coicis, Semen Benincasae, Semen Persicae for reducing intense heat and eliminating heat toxics such as Flos Lonicerae, Fructus Forsythiae, etc. To treat lung abscess, with Herba Houttuyniae, Rhizoma Phragmitis, Radix Platycodi, etc.;

to treat furuncles and skin pyogenic infections due to heat toxics, it can be used singly for decoction, or with Flos Lonicerae, Fructus Forsythiae, Herba Violae, etc., and its fresh plant can be pounded for local use. the drug has good effect of treating the abscess of the internal organ, so it is regarded as an indispensary drug for intestinal abscess, whether there is pus or not. To treat pain syndrome of the chest or abdomen due to heat in blood or blood stasis, it can be used as a single medicine in decoction or used with Radix Angelicae Sinensis, Rhizoma Ligustici Chuanxiong, Olibanum, etc.

Besides, it can be used to treat acute enteritis, dysentery, icteric hepatitis, liver abscess, etc.

Dosage and Administration: 10–30 g of the drug are used as a dose in decoction.

Stem of Sargentgloryvine (红藤 *Hongteng*) Caulis Sargentodoxae

The drug consists of the stem of a deciduous woody vine, Sargentodoxa cuneata Rehd. et Wils. (family Lardizabalaceae). It is to be cut when fresh and to be dried in the sun for use.

Nomenclature in Used Prescriptions: *Hongteng*, *Shengteng*, *Daxueteng*.

Properties and Channel Distribution: The drug is bitter to the taste, even in nature, and distributed to the Stomach and Large Intestine Channels.

Action and Indications:

1. Reducing heat and removing heat toxics, dispersing carbuncles and eliminating mass: The drug, an indispensary medi-

cine, is used to treat intestinal abscess or appendicitis; it is often used for treating intestinal abscess in combination with Flos Lonicerae, Fructus Forsythiae, Radix et Rhizoma Rhei, Cortex Moutan Radicis, etc.; to treat acute mastitis, it is used with Herba Taraxaci, Radix Trichosanthis Flos lonicerae, Bulbus Fritillariae Thunbergii, etc.

2. Promoting the circulation of blood and regulating menstruation, dispelling wind and resolving dampness: To treat amenorrhea due to blood stasis it can be used in combination with Radix Angelicae Sinensis, Herba Leonuri, Rhizoma Cyperi, etc., in decoction taken with brown sugar; to treat arthritis or arthralgia due to wind and dampness, numbness and contracture of limbs, it can be used in combination with Cortex Acanthopanacis Radicis, Radix Clematidis, etc.

Dosage and Administration: 10–15 g are used as a dose generally.

Houttuynia (鱼腥草 *Yuxingcao*)
Herba Houttuyniae

The drug consists of the dried aerial parts of a perennial herb, Houttuynia cordata Thunb. (family Saururaceae). The fresh drug or the drug dried in the shade is generally used.

Nomenclature Used in Prescription: *Yuxingcao*.

Properties and Channel Distribution: The drug is pungent to the taste, slightly cold in nature, and distributed to the Lung Channel.

Action and Indications:

1. Reducing heat and eliminating heat toxicants, dispersing

carbuncles and evacuating pus: To treat lung abscess with abundant phlegm–heat and expectoration of purulent and bloody phlegm, it is used in combination with Radix Platycodi, Rhizoma Phragmitis, Semen Benincasae, etc.; to treat cough due to lung–heat with expectoration of yellow and sticky sputum, with Radix Scutellariae, Bulbus Fritillariae Thunbergii, Cortex More Radicis, etc.; to treat carbuncles or skin pyogenic infections, it can be used for decoction or the fresh drug may be pounded to apply on the local area; and to treat hemorrhoids, it can be boiled with water used as wash. although the drug can be used to treat both internal and external abscesses, yet it seems as an indispensable medicine for the treatment of lung–abscess.

2. Having diuretic effect and eliminating stranguria: To treat stranguria due to invasion by damp–heat with painful sensation, it is often used with Caulis Akebiae, Talcum, Semen Plantaginis, etc.

At present, it is often used for the treatment of Lung abscess, pneumonia, acute or chronic bronchitis, the infections of the urinary tract, etc.

Dosage and Administration: 15–30 g of the drug are taken; the double weight will be used if the drug is fresh. Generally it is stewed in water for a short period of time for local use.

Belamcanda Rhizome (射干 *Shegan*)
Rhizoma Belamcandae

The drug consists of the rhizome of a perennial herb, Belamcanda chinensis (L.) DC. (family Iridaceae). Generally, the crug drug is dried by the sun and cut for use.

Nomenclature Used in Prescriptions: *Shegan, Sheganpian*

Properties and Channel Distribution: The drug is bitter to the taste, cold in nature, and distributed to the Lung Channel.

Action and Indications:

1. Removing virulent heat and soothing the throat: The drug is regarded as an indispensable medicine for sore throat; to treat sore throat with swelling and pain due to phlegm-heat, it is a quick remedy when used with Caulis Lonicerae, Lasiosphaera seu Calvatia, Radix Platycodi, Radix Glycyrrhizae, etc.

2. Resolving phlegm to disperse mass: The drug is often used for the treatment of expectoration of abundant phlegm and cough due to perverse ascending of lung-*Qi*. To treat cough due to wind-heat with expectoration of a lot of phlegm, it can be used with Radix Peucedani, Semen Armeniacae Amarum, Bulbus Fritillariae Thunbergii; to treat cough with expectoration of a lot of phlegm due to wind-cold or asthma and dyspnea with cough, difficulty in breathing, appearance of wheezing due to wind-cold or retention of cold phlegm, it can be used with Herba Ephedrae, Herba Asari, Rhizoma Zingiberis Recens, Fructus Schisandrae, etc.

Dosage and Administration: 3-10 g are taken as a dose in decoction.

Puff-ball (马勃 *Mabo*)
Lasiosphaera seu Calvatia

The drug consists of the fruiting bodies (mushrooms) of Lasiosphaera fenzlii Reich. or Calvatia gigantea (Batsch ex Pers.) Lloyd or Calvatia lilacina (Mont. et Berk.) Lloyd. (family

Lycoperdaceae). It is generally dried in the sun for use.

Nomenclature Used in Prescriptions: *Mabo, Qingmabo, Maborong*.

Properties and Channel Distrebution: The drug is pungent to the taste, even in nature, and distributed to the Lung Channel.

Action and Indications:

1. Reducing lung–heat to soothe throat, Removing heat–toxics to eliminate swelling: To treat sore throat, cough and dysphonia, due to flare–up of lung–fire, it can be used with Radix Scrophulariae, Radix Platycodi, Radix Isatidis, Radix Glycyrrhizae, etc.

2. Astringing wounds and arresting bleeding: To treat wound with bleeding or cold injury, the pollen of the fruiting bodies can be used to apply on the wound; to treat spitting blood or epistaxis, it can be used with other drugs for reducing intense heat and arresting hemorrage.

Dosage and Administration: 2–3 g of the drug are taken and wrapped in gauze in making decoction; a proper amount of the drug is needed for local administration.

Calyx or Fruit of Franchet Groundcherry
(锦灯笼 *Jindenglong*)
Calyx seu Fructus Physalis

The drug consists of the calyx or the calyx with fruit of the perennial herbal plant, Physalis alkekengi L. var. franchetii (Mast.) Makino (family Solanaceae). The fresh drug or the crude drug dried by the sun is used.

Nomenclature Used in Prescriptions: *Jindenglong*,

Jindenglong, *Guajindeng*

Properties and Channel Distribution: The drug is bitter to the taste, cold in nature, and distributed to the Heart, Lung and Urinary Bladder Channels.

Action and Indications:

1. Reducing intense heat to remove heat-toxics, soothing throat to relieve swelling: The drug is regarded as a drug commonly used in treating sore throat, and often combined with Rhizoma Belamcandae, Fructus Arctii, Radix Platycodi, Radix Scrophulariae, etc.

2. Descending perverse lung-*Qi* and resolving phlegm: To treat cough due to wind-heat, expectoration of much phlegm with ascending of lung-*Qi*, it is used with Semen Armeniacae Amarum, Radix Platycodi, Radix Peucedani, etc.

3. Promoting urination to relieve stranguria: To treat painful urination due to heat, urine in dark color with difficulty in discharge, it is often used with Semen Plantaginis, Caulis Akebiae, Herba Lophatheri, etc.

Dosage and Administration: 6–12 g of the drug are decocted in making a decoction.

Root of Tonkin Sophora (山豆根 *Shandougen*) Radix Sophorae Subprostratae

The drug consists of the root and rhizome of a kind of trailing short and small shrub, Sophora tonkinensis Gapnep. (family Leguminosae); it is generally cut and dried in the sun for use.

Nomenclature Used in Prescriptions: *Shandougen*

Properties and Channel Distribution: The drug is bitter to the taste, cold in nature, and distributed to the Lung and Stomach Channels.

Action and Indications:

Reducing intense heat to remowe heat toxics, soothing throat to relieve swelling: To treat sore throat or gingivitis, it can be decocted with Radix Scrophulariae, Radix Platycodi or ghizoma Belamcandae, Fructus Arctii, etc., in making decoction or a mouth wash. It is usually known as a indispensable medicine for sore throat caused by invasion by heat toxics.

Besides, it is often used to treat stomatitis, cervicitis or skin ulcer whether its decoction or powder is applied on the local region.

Dosage and Administration: 3–10 g of the drug are taken as a dose. A proper amount of that is for local administration.

Chinese White Olive (青果 *Qingguo*)
Fructus Canarii

The drug consists of the ripe fruit of the evergreen tree, Canarium album (Lour.) Raeusch. (family Burseraceae); the fresh fruit of the crude fruit dried in the shade is for use.

Nomenclature Used in Prescriptions: *Qingguo, Ganqingguo, Ganlan*

Properties and Channel Distribution: The drug is sweet, astrigent and sour to the taste, even in nature, and distributed to the Lung Channel.

Action and Indications:

1. Reducing lung–heat to soothe the throat: To treat sore throat or cough due to lung–heat, it is often with Flos Lonicerae,

Senen Sterculiae Scaphigerae, Semen Armeniacae Amarum, Radix Platycodi, Radix Flycyrrhizae, etc.; to prevent people from catching the infectious sore throat caused by wind-fire, the fresh Fructus Cannarii and fresh turnip are decocted.

2. Removing poisonous substances: To treat puffer poisoning, turtle poisoning or alcoholism, the fresh olive juice can be taken in small dose repeatedly at short intervals, or the olives may also be decocted for use.

Appendix: Radix Tinosporae (金果榄 *Jinguolan*)

The drug consists of the root tuber of the evergreen small vine, Tinospora capillipes Gagnep. (family Menispermaceae). It is similar to olive, thus named. The drug is bitter in taste, cold in nature; it has the effects of removing poisonous substances and soothing the throat. It is suitable to be used in treating sore throat, cough due to lung-heat, carbuncles or skin pyogenic infections. 3-10 g are decocted.

Root of Uniflower Swisscentaury or of Broadleaf Globe thistle (漏芦 *Loulu*)
Radix Rhapontici seu Echinopsis

The drug is the root of the perennial herb, Rhaponticum uniflorum (L.) DC. or Echinops Latifolius Tausch. (family Compositae). The crude drug is dried in the sun and cut into pieces for use.

Nomenclature in Used prescriptions: *Loulu*

Properties and Channel Distribution: The drug is bitter to the taste, cold in nature, and distributed to the Stomach Channel.

Action and Indications:

Reducing heat and removing heat toxics, relieving carbuncles and facilitating lactation

It is often used in treating carbuncles, skin pyogenic infections, and difficulty in discharging milk. To treat epidemic disease or erysipelas, infectious scarlet fever, it can be used with Rhizoma Cimicifugae, Folium Isatidis, Radix et Rhizoma Rhei, etc. to treat mastitis at its beginning stage, with Fructus Trichosanthis, Herba Taraxaci, Flos Lonicerae, Radix Angelicae Dahuricae, etc.; to treat difficulty in lactation, with Semen Vaccariae, Squama Manitis, etc.

Dosage and Administration: 6–12 g of the drug are decocted.

Male Fern Rhizome (贯众 *Guanzhong*)
Rhizoma Drypteris Crassirhizomae

The drug consists of the rhizome and the base of the frond of the perennial herb, Dryopteris crassirhizoma Nakai (family Dryopteris) or Lunathyrium acrostichoides (Sw.) Ching or Matteuccia struthiopteris (L.) Todaro or Osmunda japonica Thunb or Blechnum orientale L. or Brainia insignis (Hook) J. Sm. or Woodwaradia japonica (L. f.) Sw. and etc. Generally it is dried in the sun and cut into pieces, the crude or carbonized drug is used.

Nomenclature Used in Prescriptions: *Guanzhong*, *Guanzhong*, *Guanzhongtan*.

Properties and Channel Distribution: The drug is bitter to the taste, slightly cold and poisonous in nature, and distributed to the Liver, Kidney, Lung and Stomach Channels.

Action and Indications:

1. Reducing intense heat and removing toxics or virulent heat: To treat skin pyogenic infections due to damp-heat, mumps, etc., its powder mixed with vegetable oil can be used; to prevent epidemic disease during the time when the epidemic disease is communicated, it can be dipped into the drinking water with Rhizoma Acori Graminei, Rhizoma Atractylodis, Realgar, etc.; to prevent or treat measles, 10 g of the drug and 15 g of Retinervus Luffae Fructus can be decocted as a drink.

2. Cooling blood-heat to arrest bleeding: To treat metrorrhagia or spot vaginal bleeding or uterine bleeding after labor, its carbonized form can be decocted, or its powder can be taken with water, or it can be used with Herba Ecliptae, Colla Corii Asini, etc.; besides, it can be used in treating bloody dysentery, bloody stools, etc.

3. Killing parasites and removing stagnation of food: To treat ascariasis enterobiasis, teniasis solium, ancylostomiasis, etc., with abdominal pain, itching of the anus or pruritus over the anal region, it is used with drugs having effects of killing intestinal parasites.

Besides, for preventing influenza, 10 g of the drug are decocted and taken per day, or 1.5–3 g of the powder of the drug taken with water three times a day, or used with Flos Lonicerae, Radix Glycyrrhizae in making decoction. In preventing epidemic meningitis, it can be used with Radix Glycyrrhizae, Flos Chrysanthemi Indici in decoction for 3–7 days.

Dosage and administration: 3–10 g of the drug are used in making decoction; to eliminate virulent epidemic evils the crude drug is to be used, while to arrest bleeding the carbonized one is used.

Smilax Glabra Rhizome (土茯苓 *Tufuling*)
Rhizoma Smilacis Glabrae

The drug consists of the rhizome of the perennial climbing shrub, Smilax glabra Roxb. Generally the fresh plant or the fresh drug cut and dried in the sun is used.

Nomenclature Used in Prescriptions: *Tufuling*

Properties and Channel Distribution: The drug is sweet and tasteless to the taste, even in nature, and distributed to the Liver and Stomach Channels.

Action and indications:

Resolving dampness and eliminating virulent factors or poisonous substances

The drug has the functions in eliminating blood-heat and removing poisonous substances and has good effect on contracture of the bone and tendon due to syphillis, so it is known as an indispensable medicine for treating syphillis. Besides, it can be used to treat contraction of the limbs due to mercurial or Cinnabaris poisoning. In clinical pratice to treat syphilis or syphilis with contracture of the bones or limbs after taking mercurial, it can be used alone in large doses for decoction, or with Flos Lonicerae, Cortex Dictamni Radicis, Radix Clematidis, Radix Glycyrrhizae, etc; to treat contracture of limbs due to taking mercurials, it may be used in large dose with 3 g of Fructus Gleditsiae Sinensis and 3 g of Semen Pharbitidis; to treat carbuncles or furuncles or chronic protracted ulcers, it can be used with Flos lonicerae, Fructus Forsythiae, Herba Taraxaci, etc.; to treat chronic eczema, with Radix Rehmanniae, Radix

Paeoniae Rubra, Fructus Kochiae, etc.

Besides, it can be used to treat psoriasis, for which 30 g of the drug are decocted as a drink sometimes, it may be used in treating arthralgia.

Paris Rhizome (蚤休 *Zaoxiu*)
Rhizoma Paridis

The drug consists of the rhizome of the perennial herb, Paris polyphylla Smith or Paris chinensis Franch. (family Liliaceae). The drug is dried in the sun and cut for use.

Nomenclature in Prescriptions: *Zaoxiu, Chonglou, Qiye Yizhihua.*

Properties and Channel Distribution: The drug is slightly bitter to the taste, cold in nature, slightly poisonous in property, and distributed to the Liver Channel.

Action and Indications:

Reducing intense heat and removing toxic materials, eliminating swelling and pain: The drug can be used in treating various kinds of furuncles and carbuncles, sore throat, snake–bite or snake venum poisoning, etc.; to treat furuncles or pyogenic infections of skin, its juice mixed with vinegar may be used locally or it may be used with Flos Lonicerae, Rhizoma Coptidis, Periostracum Cicadae, Bombyx Batryticatus, etc.; to treat snake venum poisoning, 3 g of its powder may be used as a dose, 2–3 times a day, and its juice mixed with vinegar may be used for local administration.

Besides, to treat infantile convulsion due to high fever, 1 g of its powder may be taken with boiled water, or used with others drugs having functions in reducing heat and removing virulent factors or with drugs having functions in dispelling wind and arresting convulsion.

It is often combined with Folium Isatidis, Radix Isatidis and others for reducing heat and removing heat toxics to treat epidemic encephalitis B, mumps, etc.; and the result is quite satisfactory.

Dosage and Administration: 5—10 g of the drug are decocted; a proper amount is used locally.

Portulaca (马齿苋 *Machixian*)
Herba Portulacae

The drug consists of the entire herb of an annual carnified herbaceous plant, Portulaca oleracea L. (family Pottulacaceae). The crude drug is dried in the sun and cut into pieces for use; or the fresh one is used.

Nomenclature Used in Prescriptions: *Machixian*

Properties and Channel Distribution: The drug is acidic to the taste, cold in nature, and is distributed to the Heart and Large Intestine Channels.

Action and Indications:

Reducing intense heat to remove heat toxics, relieving dysentery and treating furuncles or sores: To treat dysentery due to heat evil or with bloody stools, the drug can be used for decoction, or its juice of the drug may be taken with honey; it can also be used in preventing bacillary dysentery. To treating carbuncles or furuncles, it can be decocted, and the fresh drug may be used by smearing on the affected area.

Besides, it can be used in treating uterine functional bleeding, metrorrhagia or vaginal spot bleeding or postnatal bleeding; generally it is used with Herba Leonuri, Radix Sanguisorbae, Radix Rubiae and the others for arresting hemmorage. To treat whooping cough, 60 g of the drug may be decocted and divided into three doses.

Dosage and Administration: 15–30 g of the drug may be decocted; the fresh drug should be used in 30–60 g;the proper amount is applied to the local affected area.

Pulsatilla Root (白头翁 *Baitouweng*)
Radix Pulsatillae

The drug consists of the root of the perennial herb, Pulsatilla chinensis (Bge.) Regel (family Ranunculaceae). The drug is dried in the sun and cut for use.

Nomenclature Used in Prescriptions: *Baitouweng*

Properties and Channel Distribution: The drug is bitter to the taste, cold in nature, and is distributed to the Stomach and Large Intestine Channels.

Action and Indications:

Reducing intense heat to remove heat toxics, eliminating heat in the blood to relieve dysentery

It can often be used to treat dysentery with bloody stools and abdominal pain due to virulent heat; to treat dysentery with tenesmus it is often with Rhizoma Coptidis, Cortex Fraxini, etc.; to treat dysentery with deficiency of blood or this same disease after labor, with Colla Corii Asini, Radix Glycyrrhizae.

It has got good effects in treating bacillary or amebic dysentery, and it can also be used to treat vaginal trichomoniasis in combination with Radix Sophorae Flavescentis, Fructus Cnidii as fumigant and wash, and the result is quite good.

Dosage and Administration: 10–15 g of the drug are decocted, and a proper amount for local use.

Green Chiretta (穿心莲 *Chuanxinlian*)
Herba Andrographitis

The drug consists of the entire plant or leaf of an annual herb, Androgaphis paniculata (Burm.f.) Nees (family Acantheceae). It is cut and dried in the sun for use.

Nomenclature Used in Prescriptions: *Chuanxinlian*, *Yijianxi*, *Lanhelian*.

Properties and Channel Distribution: The drug is bitter to the taste, and cold in nature, and distributed to the Lung, Stomach and Large Intestine Channels and Urinary Bladder Channels.

Action and Indications:

1. Reducing intense heat to remove heat toxics: To treat cough and dyspenia due to lung–heat, lung abscess or sore throat, it may be used in combination with Flos Lonicerae, Radix Scutellariae, etc.; to treat furuncles, carbuncles or skin pyogenic infections, with Flos Lonicerae, Flos Chrysanthemi indici, Rhizoma of Helminthostachys zeylanica (L.), Herba Oldenlandiae Diffusae, etc.

2. Reducing intense heat and resolving dampness: The drug can be used to treat diarrhea or dysentery due to damp–heat, stranguria due to heat, eczema, etc. To treat dysentery due to damp–heat, it can be used singly or in combination with

Rhizoma Coptidis Radix Scutellariae, Herba Portulacae, etc.; to treat pain urination with dribbling, with Semen Plantaginis, Spora Lygodii, Folium Pyrrosiae, etc. having the effects of promoting diuresis and relieving stranguria; to treat eczema, the powder of the drug mixed with glycerin may be used.

The drug has been found and used as an effective new species of reducing intense heat to remove heat toxics and treating infection; therefore it can be widely used in treating various infections of respiratory system, digestive system, urinary system or pyogenic skin infections.

Dosage and Administration: 6–15 g of the dry drug are decocted; 1.5–3 g of its powder are used as a dose, 3 times a day; since its powder is sharply bitter in taste, it is suitable to be packed in capsule to be taken with sugar solution. For the time being, 6–8 tablets are taken, 3 times a day.

Notes: The drug is sharply bitter in taste, so it is not suitable to be taken in a large dose or for a long time; otherwise it will hurt or injure vital energy of the stomach.

Oldenlandia (白花蛇舌草 *Baihuasheshecao*)
Herba Oldenlandiae

The drug consists of the entire plant of an annual herb, Oldenlandia diffusa (Willd.) Roxb. (family Rubiaceae). It is dried in the sun and cut into pieces for use.

Nomenclature Used in Prescriptions: *Baihuasheshecao*

Properties and Channel Distribution: The drug is sweet and bland to the taste, cool in nature, and distributed to the Stomach, Lung, Large Intestine and Urinary Bladder Channels.

Action and Indications:

1. Reducing intense heat to remorve heat toxics, removing stasis to eliminating carbuncles: It can be used in treating appendicitis, lung abscess, furuncles, carbuncles, snake–bite by poisonous snake, etc. by oral or local administration; to treat appendicitis, it can be used with Flos Lonicerae, Caulis Sargentodoxae, etc.; to treat lung abscess, with Herba Houttuyniae, Radix Platycodi, Rhizoma Phragmitis, etc.; to treat furuncles or carbuncles, with Flos Lonicerae, Fructus Forsythiae, Flos Chrysanthemi Indici, etc.; to treat snake–bite, it can be used as a local medicine or with Herba Violae, Herba Lobeliae Radicantis, etc., in making decoction.

2. Promoting diuresis to relieve stranguria: It can be used to treat stranguria with painful urination in combination with Flos Lonicerae, Herba Plantaginis, Cortex Phellodendri, Folium Pyrrosiae, etc.

Besides, to treat acute nephritis with edema and proteinuria, it can be used in 15 g and with Herba Plantaginis 15 g, Rhizoma Imperatae 30 g, Fructus Gardeniae 9 g, Folium Perillae 6 g in decoction; this decoction has got good effect on nephritis of children especially on the symptom of edema. Moreover, it has been tried to treat various cancers including the cancers of the stomach, esophagus, rectum or the other organs; yet the effect of treatment is waiting for further identification.

Root of Japanese Ampelopsis (白蔹 *Bailian*)
Radix Ampelopsis

The drug consists of the root of the perennial trailing liana,

Ampelopsis japonica (Thunb.) Mak. (family Vitaceae). It is cut into pieces along the oblique line and dried in the sun for use.

Nomenclature Used in Prescriptions: *Bailian, Bailiangen*

Properties and Channel Distribution: The drug is bitter and pungent to the taste, slightly cold in nature, and distributed to the Heart, Liver and Stomach Channels.

Action and Indications:

Reducing intense heat to remove heat toxics, eliminating swelling and promoting healing. To treat carbuncles or pyogenic skin infections without formation of pus, it may be used with Radix Paeoniae Rubra, Fructus Forsythiae; or its powder may be used locally. To treat carbuncles with pus, with Radix Angelicae Dahuricae, Radix Trichosanthis; to treat carbuncles after the pus is completely discharged, and the wounds fail in theirs healing, with Radix Angelicae Sinensis, Olibanum, etc. having the functions in nourishing blood and promoting healing; to treat scald or burn, its powder can be applied to the affected area by mixing with some water or mixing with powder of Semen Phaseoli and egg white, the drug may also be used in decoction.

Besides, 30 g of this drug can be used to treat inguinal hernia with abdominal pain for being decocted with brown sugar.

Dosage and Administrarion: 3—10 g of the drug are used as a dose; if necessary, 30 g of the drug in large dose may be decocted. For external administration a proper amount may be used.

Notes: The drug is antagonized by Radix Aconiti.

Radical Lobelia (半边莲 *Banbianlian*)
Herba Lobeliae Radicantis

The drug consists of the entire plant of an perennial trailing herb, Lobelia chinensis Thunb. (family Campanulaceae). The drug is dried in the sun or shade, or the fresh plant is for use.

Nomenclature Used in Prescriptions: *Banbianlian*

Properties and Channel Distribution: The drug is sweet and tasteless to the taste, slightly cold in nature, and distributed to the Lung, Liver and Kidney Channels.

Action and Indications:

1. Reducing heat and removing poisonous substances: It is often used in treating snake–bite, centipede–bites, bee–stings or scorpionism; to treat snake–bite, 120 g of the fresh plant are pounded and its juice is mixed with rice wine or warm boiled water for oral administration, and after taking the medicine the patient should stay in bed with quilts covered to let out mild perspiration.

Generally it is taken once a day, and for serious cases taken twice a day; besides, the fresh plant pounded and mixed with some salt may be applied to the swelling region and around the affected spot, the fresh plant can also be used and its decidue may be applied to the affected area. To treat bee–stings or scorpionism, the fresh plant may be used by pounding and applying to the affected area.

2. Promoting discharge of urine to eliminate edema: It is used in treating edema or ascites or oliguria or with others having the function in promoting the discharge of urine.

At present, it is often used in treating ascites due to schistosomiasis or due to hepatocirrhosis. To treat acute otitis media, its juice mixed with a little bit of spirit may be used as ear drop. For the time being it is used in treating cancer in clinical pratice for medical researches.

Dosage and Administration: 15–30 g of the drug or 30–60 g of the fresh may be used in decoction.

2.6 Drugs for Eliminating Asthenic Heat

Most drugs of this kind are cold or cool in nature and have the functions in eliminating blood–heat and clearing asthenic heat; therefore they are indicated in hectic fever due to deficiency or lingering of low fever, etc.

In clinical practice they are often combined with *Yin* tonics, thus the syndrome and its cause may be both treated at the same time.

Sweet Wormwood (青蒿 *Qinghao*)
Herba Artemisiae Chinghao

The drug consists of the aerial part of an annual or biennial herb, Artemisia apiacea Hance or Artemisia annua L. (family Compositae). The drug is dried in the shade and cut into pieces for use.

Nomenclature Used in Prescriptions: *Qinghao, Nenqinghao*

Properties and Channel Distribution: The drug is bitter and slightly pungent to the taste, and cold in nature, and distributed to the Liver and Gall Bladder Channels.

Action and Indications:

1. Clearing asthenia heat to relieve hectic fever: To treat the syndrome of invasion of *Yingfen* by heat in the later stage of febrile disease, characterized by presence of fever at night, no perspiration after fever has been subsided, it can be used with Carapax Trionycis, Radix Rehmanniae, Rhizoma Anemarrhenae, etc.; to treat hectic fever or night sweating due to *Yin* defficiency, it is often with Carapax Trionycis, Cortex Lycii Radicis, etc. It is often used to help *Yin* tonics with the function in clearing asthenic heat.

2. Reducing heat to relieve summer–heat syndrome: To treat febrile disease due to summer–heat, marked by fever with perspiration, it can be used with Fructus Forsythiae, Talcum, Radix Glycyrrhizae, etc.; to treat children with fever in summer, with Cortex Lycii Radicis, Radix Ampelopsis, Rhizoma Anemarrhenae, etc.

3. Clearing heat in the Gall Bladder Channel to relieve malaria: To treat malaria with alternating attacks of chilliness and fever, a quite large amount of its juice of the fresh drug may be taken with water. Since the drug has the function in relieving summer–heat syndrome, it has been used in treating malaria accompanied with syndrome of summer–heat for a long time. to treat malaria with syndrome of summer–heat, marked by fever with irracibility, stuffiness in the chest with sticky tongue coating, it is often with Radix Scutellariae, Caulis Bambusae in Taeniam, the reddish part of Poria, etc.

4. Eliminating blood heat to arrest hemorrhage: It can be used to treat epistaxis and purpura. For the treatment of epistaxis, its juice of the fresh drug can be taken with cold boiled water; for purpura with Rhizoma Cimicifugae, Carapax

Trionycis, Radix Angelicae Sinensis, Radix Rehmanniae, etc.

Dosage and Administration: 6–15 g of the drug are taken usually; when used in a large amount, 18–30 g may be decocted. Its juice can also be used.

Notes: The drug should be boiled only in a short duration of time.

Swallowwort Root (白薇 *Baiwei*)
Radix Cynanchi Atrati

The drug consists of the root and rhizome of a perennial herb, Cynanchum atratum Bge. or Cynanchum versicolor. Bge. (family Asclepiadaceae). It is dried in the sun and cut into pieces.

Nomenclature Used in Prescriptions: *Baiwei, Xianbaiwei.*

Properties and Channel Distribution: The drug is bitter and salty to the taste, cold in nature, and distributed to the Stomach and Liver Channels.

Actions and Indications:

1. Clearing away blood heat and relieving hectic fever: To treat the syndrome of heat in the blood due to deficiency of blood, marked by afternoon fever, lingering of low fever or hectic fever or asthenic fever without any known cause it is often used with Radix Rehmanniae, Herba Artemisiae Chinghao, Cortex Lycii Radicis, etc.; to treat fever only due to deficiency of *Yin* , with *Yin* tonics. For the treatment of fever due to blood deficiency after labor or fainting, with Radix Angelicae Sinensis, Radix Ginseng, Radix Glycyrrhizae.

2. Promoting the discharge of urine to relieve stranguria: To treat stranguria due to heat, stranguria with bloody urine or pain-

ful urination with red urine and hot sensation, it is often used in combination with Caulis Akebiae, Talcum, Folium Pyrrosiae, etc.

Besides, it is also used in treating mastitis, furuncles and snake-bite, a proper amount of the entire plant of this drug (Radix Cynanchi Atrati) may be pounded and applied to the local area, or it may be used in combination with the other drugs having functions in clearing away heat and removing heat toxics or poisonous materials.

Dosage and Administration: 6–15 g of the drug are taken in decoction; or it may be used in pills or powder.

Stellaria Root (银柴胡 *Yinchaihu*)
Radix Stellariae

The drug consists of the root of a perennial herb, Stellaria dichotoma L.var. lanceolata Bge. (family Caryophyllaceae). It is often dried in the sun and cut into pieces for use.

Nomenclature Used in Prescriptions: *Yinchaihu* , *Yinhu* .

Properties and Channel Distribution: The drug is sweet to the taste, slightly cold in nature, and distributed to the Liver and Stomach Channels.

Action and Indications:

1. Clearing away blood-heat to relieve hectic fever: To treat syndrome of blood invaded by heat due to deficiency of blood or hectic fever, it is often used with Herba Artemisiae Chinghao, Carapax Trionycis, Cortex Lycii Radicis, etc.; to treat chronic and protracted malaria, low grade fever or lingering of fever in the later stage of the febrile disease, with other drugs according to the specific syndromes. The drug has good function in treating

asthenic fever, therefore it is considered as an indispensable drug in treating asthenic fever.

2. Relieving fever due to infatile malnutrition: To treat infantile malnutrition with being emaciated and thirsty and restlessness. it can be used with Rhizoma Picrorhizae, Endothelium Corneum Gigeriae Galli, Radix Codonopsis Pilosulae, Rhizoma Atractylodis Macrocephalae, etc.

Dosage and administration: 3−10 g of the drug are decocted.

Notes: It is contraindicated in the syndrome of fever due to invasion of pathogenic wind−cold or in the syndrome of blood−deficiency without fever.

Wolfberry Bark (地骨皮 *Digupi*)
Cortex Lycii Radicis

The drug consists of the root−bark of a deciduous trailing bush, Lycium chinense Mill. (family Solanaceae). The crude drug is dried in the sun and cut into pieces for use.

Nomenclature Used in Prescriptions: *Digupi*

Properties Used in Prescriptions: The drug is sweet to the taste, cold in nature, and distributed to the Lung and Kidney Channels.

Action and Indications:

1. Clearing away blood−heat to relirve hectic fever: It can be used to treat syndrome of blood−heat due to *Yin* deficiency, marked by hectic fever and night sweating, or the syndrome of infantile malnutrition with fever. The drug has the function in treating asthenic heat and it is often used with Carapax Trionycis, Rhizoma Anemarrhenae, etc.

2. Clearing and purging lung−fire: To treat cough and

dyspenia or expectoration of bloody sputum due to invasion of lung by heat evil, it may be used with Cortex Mori Radicis, Radix Glycyrrhizae, etc.

Besides, it is used in treating diabetes mellitus, characterized by thirsty and polyuria in combination with feverish sensation and restlessness.

Dosage and Administration: 6–12 g of the drug are taken as a dose in making decoction.

Rhizoma of Figwortflower Picrorhiza
(胡黄连 *Huhuanglian*)
Rhizoma Picrorhizae

The drug consists of the rhizome of a perennial herb, Picrorrhiza scrophulariaeflora Punnell (family Scrophulariaceae). the crude drug is dried in the sun and cut into pieces for use.

Nomenclature Used in Prescriptions: *Huhuanglian* .

Properties and Channel Distribution: The drug is bitter to the taste, and cold in nature, and distributed to the Heart, Liver, Stomach, and Large Intestinal Channels.

Action and Indications:

1. Clearing blood–heat and relieving hectic fever: To treat syndrome of fever due to deficiency of *Yin* , hectic fever, it is often used with Radix Stellariae, Cortex Lycii Radicis, etc.

2. Eliminating afternoon fever and relieving malnutrition: To treat infantile malnutrition with fullness of abdomen, afternoon fever, it is used with Radix Codonopsis Pilosulae, Rhizoma Atractylodis Macrocephalae, Fructus Quisqualis, Fructus

Crataegi, etc. or with mass of fermentation of the seed of Ulmus macrocarpa Hance and dried Gekko Swinhoana; to treat eye disease due to infantile malnutrition, poor vision, it can be used with chicken liver by steaming.

3. Reducing intense heat to solve dampness: To treat dysentery due to invasion by damp-heat, it can be used and its effects are similar to the effects of Rhizoma Coptidis. It can also be used in treating hemorrhoids with pain and swelling by oral or local administration.

Dosage and Administration: 3–10 g of the drugs are decocted.

3 Cathartics

Drugs which have the effects of inducing diarrhea (or lubricating bowels), and facilitating defecation are called cathartics.

Cathartics are indicated in the interior excessive syndrome, they can exert three main functions as follows:

1. Removing retention of undigested food and dried feces and other harmful materials from human body by defecation;

2. Reducing intense heat and purging fire, thus discharging heat toxics from our body;

3. Expelling the retained water and relieving edema.

Moreover, cathartics may be indicated in several kinds of disorders as follows:

1. It can be used for treating congestion or hemorrhage of the upper part of the body with constipation by means of inducing loosing bowels, which is called the method of treating disorders of the upper by purging the lower;

2. It can be used in treating dysentery at its beginning stage, accompanied with tenemus, loosing bowels yet discharging the feces unsmoothly, which is called the method of relieving dysentery by using the drugs for inducing defecation and purging toxic materials;

3. Recently the cases of acute abdomen have been treated by means of combination of traditional Chinese medicine with Western medicine. In the light of the principles of TCM: "obstruction induces pain", "pain will be cured when obstruction is re-

moved" and "free going in passages is necessary for six hollow organs for carrying out their functioning", acute abdomen due to intense internal heat is treated by purging undigested food and feces in the interior, and reducing the intense heat and fire. The result is quite good, thus most cases have got free from painful surgical operations.

According to their specific actions they may be divided into three kinds: purgatives, drastic purgatives for expelling retained water and aperients. Purgatives and drastic purgatives have the instant effect of loosing bowels; and of them, drastic purgatives are radical, and likely to injure healthy *Qi*. Therefore purgatives and drastic purgatives are not indicated in chronic illness with deficiency of healthy *Qi*, old and weak patients with weak constitution, pregnant or postnatal women, or women during menstruation. Aperients are mild, they can be used in treating constipation or difficult defecation by lubricating the intestines; yet they are not likely to cause severe diarrhea, therefore, they are indicated in the senile and weak patients, women with constipation during pregnancy or after labor due to intestinal driness and deficiency of blood or body fluid.

In practice, several points should be noted:

1. There exists the relationship between the intensity of its action in causing diarrhea and its dosage taken. To treat the severe interior excessive syndrome with constipation which is meeded to be treated by urgent purgation, the drastic purgatives may be used in large dose, thus the instant effect can appear; to treat the mild case that needs to be treated by mild loosing bowels, the dose of the purgatives should not be large, they are often used in pill form; mild purgative, if used in a large dose, will produce ef-

fect which is similar to that of the drastic one, or vice versa. Therefore it is important for cathartics to be used in proper dosage.

2. The pharmaceutical effects of the purgatives may be different in a large degree if prepared by different way; therefore we should pay good attention to their processing and decocting.

3.1 Purgatives

Most purgatives are bitter in taste and cold in nature, and have remarkable function in inducing defecation. They are indicated to treat various interior excess syndrome due to food retention and constipation. Since purgatives are cool (or cold) in nature and can produce effects of reducing intense heat and purging fire, they are suitable to be used to treat interior excess syndrome due to invasion by heat, accompanied with constipation or difficult defecation caused by dry and solid feces; to treat costipation due to accumulation by cold, it is used with drugs for warming the interior; to treat constipation with fullness of abdomen due to stagnation of *Qi* , with drugs for regulating the flow of *Qi* ; to treat weak patients with constipation who can not stand loosing bowels induced by purgatives, with tonics. Being applied purging method together with reenforcing method, such weak patients' healthy energy will not be injured even by loosing bowels. In treating excess syndrome of the interior accompanied with exterior syndrome, the latter should be treated first, then the former is to be treated; if necessary, purgatives can be used with the drugs for dispersing the pathogenic evils from the exterior, thus the disorders of the interior and exterior are both treated, and the pathogenic evils will be prevented from sinking into the interior.

Rhubarb (大黄 *Dahuang*)
Radix et Rhizoma Rhei

The drug refers to the root and rhizome of the perennial herb, Rheum palmatum L. or R. tanguticum Maxim. ex Reg. or R. officinale Baill. (family Polygonaceae). The crude drug is often cut into pieces or lumps for use. The drug may be steamed with wine and honey, or bake-stirred with wine or carbo-nized if necessary.

Nomenclature Used in Prescriptions: *Shengdahuang*, *Shudahuang*, *Jiudahuang* , *Dahuangtan* .

Properties and Channel Distributions: The drug is bitter in taste, cold in nature, and distributed to the Stomach, Large Intestine, Spleen, Liver and pericardium Channels.

Action and Indications:

1. Purging feces to remove stagnation: It is used to treat retention of the undigested food and constipation with dried feces. The drug is bitter in taste, cold in nature, and of descending in property; with strong actions travelling in all directions, it has remarkable effect on inducing defecation and considered as an indispensable drug in treating constipation due to retention of undigested food and dried feces. With its bitter taste and cold property, it has the effect of purging the evil fire, it is suitable to be used for constipation due to accumulation of heat evil. In practice, to treat constipation caused by accumulation of heat evil, accompanied with lingering of high fever, irritability and delirium, it is often used with Natrii Sulfas, Fructus Aurantii Immaturus, Cortex Magnoliae Officinalis; to treat the interior excess syndrome with deficiency of *Qi* and blood, with Radix

Ginseng, Radix Angelicae Sinensis and others for reinforcing *Qi* and nourishing blood; to treat the syndrome of accumulation of heat and deficiency of *Yin,* with Radix Rehmanniae, Radix Scrophulariae, Radix Ophiopogonis and others for nourishing *Yin* and promoting the production of the body fluid; to treat constipation due to deficiency of spleen *Yang* and accumulation of cold, with Radix Codonopsis Pilosulae, Radix Aconiti Praeparata, Rhizoma Zingiberis and others for reinforcing *Qi* and warming *Yang* ; to treat dysentery due to invasion of the intestine and stomach by damp–heat or to treat watery stools with tenesmus, with Radix Paeoniae, Radix Scutellariae, Rhizoma Coptidis and Radix Aucklandiae. The syndrome will be treated effectively by the method called treating disease by removing the retention (or stagnation) of the evils.

2. Purging evil fire and removing heat toxics

To treat spitting blood, epistaxis (both due to extravasation of blood caused by blood–heat) or sore throat, gingivitis and bloodshot eyes (all due to flare–up of evil fire), it may be used with Radix Scutellariae, Rhizoma Coptidis; to treat aphthae, its powder with the powder of dried Alumen may be used together locally; to treat carbuncles or pyogenic skin infections, its powder mixed with vinegar can be applied to the local area. For the treatment of other diseases, it can be used with drugs for reducing intense heat and removing heat toxics; to treat scald or burn, its powder mixed with the same amount of powder of Radix Sanguisorbae is applied locally by mixing with sesame oil; to treat appendicitis, it may be used with Natrii Sulfas, Cortex Moutan Radicis, Semen Persicae and so on.

3. Removing blood stasis and regulating menstruation

To treat amenorrhea due to blood stasis or abdominal pain due to that after labor, it can be used with Semen Persicae, Eupolyphaga seu Steleophaga; to treat wound or injury from falling down, or pain and swelling due to blood stasis, its powder can be orally taken with same amount of powder of Radix Angelicae Sinensis.

Besides, as it has the function of eliminating damp–heat, it can be used in treating stranguria and jaundice due to invasion by damp–heat; to treat stranguria, the drug is used with Caulis Akebiae, Semen Plantaginis and fruit of Gardenia Jasminoides; to treat jaundice, it is often in combination with Herba Artemisiae Scopariae and fruit of Gardenia Jasminoides.

Dosage and Administration: 3–15 g of the drug are taken for decoction and a proper amount is used locally. A large amount will be used for removing retention of food and inducing defecation, while a small smount for promoting the circulation of blood to remove blood stasis. The crude drug is radical in its action while the prepared is mild; so the crude form is used for those who are to be treated by inducing defecation. It should be decocted later in making decoction or it may be taken being infused in boiling water. The drug prepared with wine may be used in treating the disease of the upper part due to evil heat or fire, and the carbonized form is used for treating blood stasis and arresting hemorrhage.

Notes: To treat pregnant women or women during the periods of menstruation, labor, and puerperium, it should be used cautiously or not be used.

Mirabilite (芒硝 *Mangxiao*)
Natrii Sulfas

The drug consists of the refined crystalline sodium sulphate, usually made from natural sources. In the period between autumn and winter the mineral substance containing Natrii Sulfas is first dissolved in the hot water, and filtered; then the crystalline sodium sulphate is crystallized by cooling. The crystalline sodium sulphate at this time is called *Poxiao* or *Pixiao* ; then *Poxiao* is decocted in the water with pieces of turnips, and the upper part of the decoction is taken out and treated by cooling, the refined sodium sulphate can be crystallized out, which is called *Mangxiao* (some time the crystal is like the tooth of the horse, it is called *Yaxiao*).

Nomenclature Used in Prescriptions: *Mangxiao*, *Fenghuaxiao*.

Properties and Channel Distribution: The drug is bitter and salty in taste, cold in nature, and is distributed to the Stomach and Large Intestine Channels.

Action and Indications:

1. Softening dried feces to induce defecation

To treat constipation due to dried feces caused by accumulation of intense heat in the stomach and intestine, it is often used with Radix et Rhizoma Rhei and Radix Glycyrrhizae.

2. Clearing away intense heat and Purging fire

To treat the swelling and sores of the throat or aphtha it can be used with Borneolum Syntheticum, Borax; to treat mastitis it can be used as a local medicine, it has the effect on dispersing mass; besides, it can be used to stop milk secretion by local application.

Moreover, 30 g of the drug and 30 g of Alumen can be used to treat eczema and urticaria by dissolving in hot water as a wash.

Dosage and Administration: 3–10 g of the drug are used to be added in the other decoction; a proper amount may be used for local application.

Appendix: Natrii Sulfas Exsiccatus (玄明粉 *Xuanmingfen*)

Consisted of the dehydrated white powder of Mirabilite after being prepared with Radix Glycyrrhizae. It is sweet, salty and slightly bitter in taste, cold in nature. It has the actions like Mirabilite, yet its actions are slightly milder than those of Mirabilite, Its powder form with Borneolum Syntheticum, Borax, etc. is mainly used locally for aphtha, sore throat, bloodshot eyes, wounds and sores; and its solution form is used for eye drops, local smearing and wash. Usually 3–10 g of the drug are taken as a dose and a proper amount is used locally. Besides, it is contraindicated in the pregnant women.

Senna leaf (番泻叶 *Fanxieye*)
Folium Sennae

The drug consists of the leaflets of a herbaceous short shrub, Cassia angustifolia Vahl or Cassia acutifolia Delile (family Leguminosae). The crude drug is for use.

Nomenclature Used in Prescriptions: *Fanxieye* , *Xieye* , *Xieyeca* .

Properties and Channel Distribution: The drug is sweet and bitter in taste, cold in nature, and distributed to the Large Intestine Channel.

Action and Indications:

1. Clearing away heat by inducing loosing bowels

To treat stagnation of undigested food due to accumulation of heat, and constipation due to dryness of the intestine, it can be combined with Fructus Aurantii Immaturus, Cortex Magnoliae Officinalis, or it may be used singly after being infused in hot water or mixed with honey in pills.

2. Promoting the discharge of water to relieve ascites

To treat ascites with fullness and distention it is more safe than Radix Euphorviae Kansui and is often used with Semen Pharbitidis, Pericarpium Arecae or used singly in boiling water as a drink.

Dosage and Administration: 1–2 g of the drug are used for inducing loosing bowels and 3–6 g of the drug are for drastic diarrhea; it is often added later for being decocted with others, or infused in hot water as a drink. Its effect is mild if it is used in the form of pills.

Notes: It is contraindicated in those women with pregnancy, menstruation, lactation, or vaginal bleeding; if the dose is too large, it will produce the side effects of vomiting, nausea, abdominal pain, etc.

Aloes (芦荟 *Luhui*)
Aloe

The drug consists of the juice of the base of the leaf of a perinnial evergreen plant, Aloe ferox Mill. or Aloe vera L. var. chinensis (Haw.) Berger (family Liliaceae), and the juice is futher concentrated and made into a kind of black of dark green and transparent or semitransparent hard extract. Usually the hard extract is ground into powder for use.

Nomenclature Used in Prescriptions: *Luhui*

Properties and Channels Distribution: The drug is bitter in taste, cold in nature, and distributed to the Liver, Stomach and Large Intestine Channels.

Action and Indications:

1. Clearing away the intense heat by inducing loosing bowels

To treat the syndrome due to invasion of the liver and gall bladder by heat evil, accompanied with constipation, it is often used with Radix Gentianae, Fructus Gardeniae, Radix Scutellariae, etc.; to treat constipation due to invasion of the intestine by heat evil, accompanied with deficiency of *Yin* and irascibility, 22 g of the drug and 15 g of Cinnabaris are ground into powder in making pills by mixing with wine; and 3 g of the pills are taken with boiled water.

2. Killing the intestinal parasites to relieve malnutrition

To treat infantile ascariasis, infantile malnutrition it can be used with Rhizoma Picrorhizae, medicated leaven of fruit of Ulmus macrocarpa Hance (Fructus Gardeniae), Radix Aucklandiae, etc.

Now it is used to treat leukemia in combination with Indigo Naturalis, Radix Angelicae Sinensis and others for reducing heat and nourishing blood; by this method, quite satisfactory result has been got.

Dosage and Administration: 1–2 g of the drug are used for making pills or powder; usually it is not used for decoction.

Notes: The drug is contraindicated in those with cold syndrome of the Spleen and Stomach in deficiency nature or in those with pregnancy.

3.2 Drastic Purgatives

Most drugs of this kind can produce rather drastic effect of inducing serious diarrhea, thus a lot of water is discharged by defecation and urination, and edema gets cured.

They are indicated in the excess syndrome, marked by dyspnea and fullness of the chest or abdomen, accompanied by hiccup or vomiting, due to hydrothorax, ascites or retention of phlegm or water in the serious stage of edema. Recently it is used in treating ascites in the later stage of schistomiasis, and it has got good result on relieving the symptoms of the disease.

Most drugs of this kind are drastic in their actions and poisonous in nature, so they can not be taken in over dose or in large weight. All of their processing, combination, dosage, administration and indication should be used cautiously, thus they can be used safely.

When used to treat ascites, the drugs should be used in combination with tonics according to the specific syndromes; in clinical practice, the method of applying purgative should be followed by the reinforcing method once more; Usually, the purgative method and reinforcing method are used in combination at the same time or used alternately, thus the healthy *Qi* will be reserved or kept.

Kansui Root of Gansui (甘遂 *Gansui*)
Radix Euphorbiae Kansui

The drug consists of the tuberous root of a perennial carnified herb, Euphorbia Kansui Liou (family Euphorbiaceae).

It is usually bake–stirred with vinegar or wheat bran for use.

Nomenclature Used in Prescriptions: *Chaogansui* , *Zhigansui* , *Gansui*

Properties and Channel Distribution: The drug is sweet in taste and cold in nature, slightly poisonous in property, and distributed to the Liver, Spleen and Kidney Channels.

Action and Indications:

1. Removing the retained water by purgation

To treat the excess syndrome due to internal retention of water in the thorax or abdomen, marked by thoracic or hypochondric pain, cough and dyspenia, fullness and solidness of the epigastric region, fullness and distension with ascites, it is used with Radix Euphorbiae Pekinensis, Folium et Flos Wikstroemiae Chamaedaphnis, Semen Sinapis Albae, Semen Pharbitidis, Radix Aucklandiae, etc.

2. Relieving swelling and dispersing mass

To treat skin inflamation due to damp–heat, its powder is mixed with water for local smearing.

At present, it is used to treat intestinal obstruction with remarkable retention of fluid in the intestinal cavity in combination with Radix et Rhizoma Rhei, Cortex Magnoliae Officinalis, Semen Persicae, etc.

Dosage and Administration: 0.6–1.5 g of the drug are used; usually the drug is added into others as an ingredient in pills or powder. A proper amount of the crude drug is for local use.

Notes: It is contraindicated in those with pregnancy or weak constitution; besides, it is antagonized by Radix Glycyrrhizae.

Peking Spurge Root (大戟 *Daji*)
Radix Euphorbiae Pekinensis

The drug consists of the root of a perennial herb, Euphorbia pekinensis Rupr. (family Euphorbiaceae) or of a perennial herb, Knoxia valerianoides Thorel (family Rubiaceae); usually the drug is prepared with vinegar or cooked with bean curd for use.

Nomenclature Used in Prescriptions: *Daji* , *Hongya Daji* .

Properties and Channel Distribution: The drug is bitter in taste, cold in nature, poisonous in property, and distributed to the Lung, Spleen and Kidney Channels.

Action and Indications:

1. Inducing urination to remove retention of phlegm

It is often used to treat the syndrome of retention of water or phlegm in the thorax or abdomen, marked by cough and dyspenia due to retention of phlegm, thoracodynia and hypochondric pain, fullness of abdomen due to ascites, in combination with Radix Euphorbiae Kansui, Flos Genkwa.

2. Relieving swelling to disperse mass

It is used to treat pyogenic skin infection or scrofula, etc. in soft extract form for local use.

Dosage and Administration: 0.6–1.5 g of the drug are taken, which are often used as an ingredient in pills or powder.

Notes: It is contraindicated in those with weak constitution or pregnancy; and the drug is antagonized by Radix Glycyrrhizae.

Genkwa Flower (芫花 Yuanhua)
Flos Genkwa

The drug consists of the flower–bud of a deciduous shrub, Daphne genkwa Sieb. et Zucc. (family Thymelaeaceae). The drug is usually bake–stirred or cooked with vinegar.

Nomenclature Used in Prescriptions: *Cuyuanhua*, *Chenyuanhua*, *Yuanhua* .

Properties and Channel Distribution: The drug is pungent and bitter in taste, and cold in nature, poisonous in property, and distributed to the Lung, Spleen and Lidney Channels.

Action and Indications:

1. Inducing urination to remove retention of phlegm

It is often used to treat cough and dyspnea due to retention of phlegm, thoracodynia and hypochondric pain, fullness of abdomen and ascites, in combination with Radix Euphorbiae Kansui, Radix Euphorbiae Pekinensis.

2. Killing skin parasites and relieving tinea or wound

It is used in treating tinea ficosa, pyogenic scalp infection, tinea capitis, etc. or in combination with Realgar in powder mixed with lard for local use; in treating cold injury, it with Radix Glycyrrhizae is used locally as a wash for local use.

Dosage, Administration and Notes:

Pharbis Seed (牵牛子 *Quianniuzi*)
Semen Pharbitidis

The drug consists of the seed of annual trailing herb, Pharbitis nil(L.) Choisy or Pharbitis purpurea (L.) Voigt (family Convolvulaceae). The crude seed or the seed bake–stirred may be used as medicine after it is pounded or ground into powder.

Nomenclature Used in Prescriptions: *Quianniuzi* , *Heichou* , *Baichou* , *Heibaichou* , *Erchou* .

Properties and Channel Distribution: The drug is bitter in taste, cold in nature, poisonous in property, and distributed to the Lung, Kidney and Large Intestine Channels.

Actions and Indications:

1. Inducing urination to remove retention of phlegm

It is used in treating edema and local fullness, oliguria and constipation in combination with brown sugar, Radix Glycyrrhizae, Fructus Ziziphi Jujubae; in treating constipation due to accumulation of damp–heat, it can be used in powder form for oral administration with decoction of Radix Glycyrrhizae; besides, it can be used with Semen Lepidii seu Descurainiae, Semen Armeniacae Amarum and Cortex Magnoliae Officinalis for treating cough and dyspnea due to retention of phlegm.

2. Killing parasites and removing stagnation of evils

To treat abdominal pain due to ascariasis, the drugs, Semen Arecae and Radix et Rhizome Rhei are used in powder form in equal amount and the powder 2–3 g is taken twice a day, one in the morning and the other in the evening, when the belly is empty; to treat enterobiasis, the drug 9 g, Omphalia 9 g and Radix et Rhizome Rhei 3 g are powdered and divided into three doses, one dose per day, usually the powder is taken with water before sleep.

Dosage and Administration: 3–9 g of the drug are decocted, and 1.5–4.5 g of the peeled drug are used in pill or powder form.

Notes: It is contraindicated in the pregnant women, and it is antagonized by Fructus Crotonis.

Phytolacca Root (商陆 *Shanglu*)
Radix Phytolaccae

The drug consists of the root of a perennial herb, Phytolacca acinosa Roxb. (family Phytolaccaceae). The crude drug or the drug cooked with vinegar is for use.

Nomenclature Used in Prescriptions: *Shanglu* , *Shanglugen* .

Properties and Channel Distributions: The drug is bitter in taste cold in nature, poisonous in property, and distributed to the Lung, Spleen and Kidney Channels.

Action and Indications:

1. Promoting discharge of water to relieve edema by diuresis

To treat general edema, fullness and distension of the chest and abdomen, disorders of urination and defecation, it can be used with the outer cover layer of Poria, Semen Zanthoxyli, Semen Arecae, Semen Phaseoli, etc. or with lean pork by steaming together.

2. Removing heat–toxics to relieve swelling

To treat carbuncles or pyogenic skin infection, the fresh drug is mixed with salt, then pounded for local use.

Dosage and Administration: 2–4.5 g of the drug are decocted as a dose, a proper amount is for local use. For internal use, it is cooked with vinegar; while for external use, the crude drug is often used.

Notes: It is contraindicated in those with deficiency syndrome characterized by edema, or with pregnancy.

Croton Seed (巴豆 *Badou*)
Fructus Crotonis

The drug consists of the ripe seed of the evergreen tree, Croton tiglium L. (family Euphorbiaceae). The drug is de–fatted by grinding and pounding, and then the white–powder like substance is used. Or the carbonized drug may be used.

Nomenclature Used in Prescriptions: *Badoushuang* , *Jiaobadou* .

Properties and Channel Distribution: It is pungent in taste, hot in nature, drastic poisonous in property, and distributed to the Stomach, Large Intestine Channels.

Action and Indications:

1. Removing accumulation of cold in the intestine by loosing bowels

To treat constipation due to accumulation of cold evil, fullness and distension of abdomen, even with collapse and shortness of breath, it can be used with Rhizoma Zingiberis and Radix et Rhizoma Rhei in their equal amount in pill form which are as large as the seeds of Chinese parasol tree; and 0.6–0.9 g are used as a dose taken with water. To treat retention of phlegm or indigested food of children, it is used with Rhizoma Arisaema prepared with bile, Massa Fermentata Medicinalis, etc.

2. Promoting the discharge of water to relieve abdominal distension

To treat abdominal distension due to ascites, 90 pieces of carbonized Semen Crotonis and 60 pieces of Semen Armeniacae Amarum bake–stirred are used in pill form, and 0.3–0.6 g of the pills are taken repeatedly with water till the patient has got loosing bowels. At present, to treat ascites due to hepatocirrhosis in the later stage of schistomiasis, 9 g of the white powder of Semen Crotonis and 30 g of Calcined melanterite in making pills as large as small beans by mixing with Massa Fermentata Medicinalis, and 1–1.5 g of the pills are taken with water, once a day.

3. Resolving phlegm and removing the obstruction in the throat

To treat sore throat accompanied with retension of phlegm in the throat, breathlessness, short of breath due to asphyxia, the drug can be used since it can produce the effects of resolving phlegm to remove the obstruction in the throat; to treat such disease mentioned above, a little amount of the white powder of Semen Crotonis can be taken with water drop by drop; or it can be bake–stirred with Alumen, and Alumen is prepared and singly ground into powder for oral administration with water or for local use by being puffed on the surface of the throat, thus promoting the discharge of the phlegm to remove obstruction in the throat.

4. Removing heat toxics to relieve skin infections

To treat pyogenic skin infections or furuncles, with pus inside before diabrosis, carbonized Semen Crotonis and Olibanum are used in paste form by pounding for local use; or carbonized

Semen Crotonis, Realgar and Radix et Rhizoma Rhei are used in equal amount in making pills as large as the small beans for internal use, 2–4 pills are taken with water as a dose, twice a day.

At present, to treat obstruction in the throat due to diphtheria or inflammation of the throat, the white powder of Semen Crotonis may be used by puffing on the local area, thus inducing discharge either of the phlegm by vomiting or of stools; by this way the obstruction may be removed.

Dosage and Administration: 0.1–0.2 g are used in pills or powder as an ingredient; for local use, a proper amount is applied; in clinical practice the carbonized drug may produce the effect of moderate loosing bowels, while the white powder of the crude drug may produce the effect of drastic diarrhea.

Notes: Hot porridge or hot water should not be taken with Semen Crotonis at the same time, otherwise the drastic effect of purgation will be exagerated. Hot food or drinking will promote its effect of purgation, so the hot or warm porridge is indicated in those patients who have not got effective purgation though they have already taken Semen Crotonis; or the cool porridge or cold drinking will be needed if its purgative effect is too drastic and the patient has got very severe diarrhea. If the patient is intoxicated by the drug and looses his bowels drastically and continuously with abdominal pain, the decoction of Rhizoma Coptidis or Semen Phaseoli Radiatus will urgently need to be taken. Besides, it is contraindicated in those with weak constitution or pregnancy.

3.3 Aperients

Most drugs of this kind consist of seeds of plants; they are full of oil and have the effects of lubricating the intestinal walls and feces, and facilitating the loosing bowels. Therefore they are indicated in those with constipation due to senial age and deficiency of body fluid, deficiency of blood after labor, deficiency of the body fluid after disease or due to loss of blood.

For the treatment of constipation due to lack of body fluid caused by abundant heat, they may be combined with *Yin* tonics; for constipation with deficiency of blood, with blood tonics; for constipation with stagnation of *Qi* , with the drugs having the effect of regulating the flow of *Qi* .

Hemp Seed (火麻仁 *Huomaren*) Fructus Cannabis

The drug consists of the fruits of as annual herb, Cannabis sativa L. (family Moraceae); then the seeds of the fruits are gathered, mildly bake–stirred and pounded into pieces for use.

Nomenclature Used in Prescriptions: *Huomaren* , *Damaren* , *Maziren* .

Properties and Channel Distribution: It is sweet in taste, even in nature, and distributed to the Spleen, Stomach and the large Intestine Channels.

Action and Indications:

Moistening and loosening the bowels, replenishing body fluid and nourishing *Yin*

To treat constipation due to dryness and heat of the intestine and stomach of the old man or those with weak constitution, it is often used with Radix et Rhizoma Rhei, Fructus Aurantii Immaturus, etc; to treat constipation due to postnatal blood deficiency or senial age, with Herba Cistanchis, Radix Angelicae Sinensis, etc.

Besides, it can be used in treating habitual constipation or constipation due to hemorrhoids.

Dosage and Administration: 10–15 g of the drug are decocted for decoction.

Notes: It is not suitable to take the drug in over dose; 60–120 g of the drug, if taken as a dose, will be poisonous and induce vomiting and diarrhea, numbness of limbs and even drowsiness and dullness of consciousness.

Bush–cherry Seed (郁李仁 *Yuliren*)
Semen Pruni

The drug consists of the seeds of a deciduous bush, Prunus humilis Bge. or P. japonica Thunb. (family Rosaceae); the seeds are treated by cutting away their follicles and are prepared by being mildly bake–stirred and pounded into pieces for use.

Nomenclature Used in Prescriptions: *Yuliren*

Properties and Channel Distribution: The drug is pungent and bitter in taste, even in nature, and distributed to the Large Intestine, Small Intestine and Spleen Channels.

Action and Indications:

1. Moistening and loosening the bowels

To treat constipation due to dryness of the intestine and lack of body fluid, it is often used with Semen Armeniacae Amarum, Semen Biotae, etc.

2. Promoting the circulation of water to relieve edema

To treat ascites with fullness and distension of the abdomen, it can be used with Semen Pharbitidis, Radix Euphorbiae Kansui, etc; to treat edema due to beriberi, disorders of urination and defecation, 10 g of the drug and 30 g of Semen Coicis may be used for decoction.

Dosage and Administration: 6–12 g of the drug are decocted as a dose.

Notes: To treat those patients with pregnancy it should be used cautiously.

4 Antirheumatics or Drugs for Relieving Rheumatism

Drugs which can produce the effects of eliminating wind–dampness evil from muscles, channels and collaterals, tendons and bones, and relieving arthralgia are called Antirheumatics or drugs for relieving rheumatism.

The arthralgia–syndrome occurs when there is obstruction of channels and stagnation of *Qi* and blood due to invasion of human body by wind, cold or dampness. Its main manifestations are general soreness or painful joints, aching and numbness, heaviness, contracture of the tendons and muscles. Of pathogenic factors, wind, cold and dampness, one of them may be more prominent than the others, therefore the syndrome of the patient seems also different; wandering arthralgia–syndrome may occur if the wind is the predominant; the manifestations are wondering soreness and contracture of tendons. Painful arthralgia–syndrome may occur if the cold evil is predominant; the manifestations are remarkable soreness and pain. Fixed arthralgia–syndrome may occur if the damp evil is predominant, and its manifestations are numbness, swelling and soreness, and the manifestations are immovable. Besides, there is hot arthralgia–syndrome, an arthralgia due to pathogenic heat which is derived from the other evils such as wind, cold and dampness.

This kind of drugs may have their speciffic functions, such as dispelling wind, dispersing cold, resolving dampness, promoting the circulation of the channels, relieving arthralgia–syndrome, arresting soreness and pain. And some drugs may also have the effects of replenishing the liver and kidney, strengthening tendons and bones. Therefore the drugs should be selected according to the differentiation of syndromes.

Since arthralgia–syndrome is complicated, the drugs should be used with other drugs according to the specific manifestations, thus their therapeutic effects can be reinforced; to treat arthralgia with evils as wind, cold and dampness in superficies with diaphoretios, thus these evils can be eliminated; to treat arthralgia syndrome due to wind, cold and dampness, which stay in the tendons, bones or channels, other drugs for promoting the circulation of blood and channels may be used with these drugs, thus the evils may be eliminated easily; to treat arthralgia mainly due to wind, other drugs for expelling wind and stopping pain should be used with these drugs; to treat arthralgia mainly due to cold, other drugs for dispersing cold with pungent taste and warm nature should be used with these drugs; to treat arthralgia mainly due to dampness, other drugs for resolving dampness should be combined with these drugs;to treat arthralgia mainly due to heat, other drugs with bitter taste and cold nature for clearing away the heat evil should be combined with these drugs; to treat arthralgia with deficiency of blood and *Qi* due to long duration of illness, the drugs for reinforcing *Qi* and nourishing blood should be combined with the drugs in order to strengthen the healthy energy and disperse evils from human body. These principles of compatibility should be followed in clinical practice.

Most antirheumatics are pungent in taste and dry in nature; they can injure vital essence and consume blood, so they should be used cautiously to treat those patients with deficiency of *Yin* and blood.

Pubescent Angelica Root (独活 *Duhuo*)
Radix Angelicae Pubescentis

The drug consists of the root of a perennial herb, Angelica pubescens Maxim. f. biserrata Shan et Yuan. or Angelica pubescens Maxim. (family Umbelliferae). The drug is dried in the sun and cut into cross sections for use.

Nomenclature Used in Prescriptions: *Duhuo* , *Chuanduhuo* .

Properties and Channel Distribution: The drug is pungent and bitter in taste, slightly warm in nature, and distributed to the kidney and liver Channels.

Action and Indications:

1. Dispelling wind, resolving dampness and relieving pain

To treat arthralgia due to wind and dampness, with heaviness of lumbar regions and lower limbs, it is often used with Ramulus Loranthi, Radix Gentianae Macrophyllae, Radix Achyranthis Bidentatae, etc. The drug can produce the effect of treating wind in the interior of the lower portion of the human body, so it is suitable to be used in treating arthralgia of the muscles and joints in the lower portion.

2. Dispelling cold by perspiration

To treat cold due to wind-cold with headache and general soreness, it may be used with Rhizoma seu Radix Notopterygii, Radix Ledebouriellae, Radix Angelicae Dahuricae, Rhizoma Ligustici Chuanxiong, Radix Glycyrrhizae, Rhizoma Zingiberis Recens, etc.

Dosage and Administration: 3–10 g of the drug are decocted as a dose.

Large–leaf Gentian Root (秦艽 *Qinjiao*)
Radix Gentianae Macrophyllae

The drug consists of the roots of a perennial herb, Gentiana macrophylla Pall. or G. straminea Maxim. or G. crassicaulis Duthie ex Burk. (family Gentianaceae); the crude drug is cut into pieces for use.

Nomenclature Used in Prescriptions: *Qinjiao* , *Xiqinjiao* , *Zuqinjiao* .

Properties and Channel Distribution: The drug is bitter and pungent in taste, even in nature, and distributed to the Stomach, Large Intestine, Liver, and Gall Bladder Channels.

Action and Indications:

1. Dispelling wind to relieve pain

To treat either arthralgia due to wind and dampness, marked by contracture of joints, disorder of the movement of the tendons and bones, or arthralgia due to invasion by wind, it is often used with Radix Angelicae Pubescentis, Radix Ledebouriellae, Rhizoma Ligustici Chuanxiong, Radix Stephaniae Tetrandrae, Cortex Erythrinae, etc.

2. Relieving asthnic heat to treat hectic fever

To treat hectic fever, it is often used with Herba Artemisiae Chinghao, Cortex Lycii Radicis, Carapax Trionycis, etc.

Besides, the drug can produce the effects of resolving damp–heat and facilitating urination and defecation, therefore it can be used in treating jaundice due to damp–heat and relieving fresh bloody stools.

Dosage and Administration: 6–12 g of the drug are decocted as a dose.

Clematis Root (威灵仙 *Weilingxian*)
Radix Clematidis

The drug consists of the root and rhizome of the perennial trailing shrub, Clematis chinensis Osbeck. or C. hexapetala Pall. or C. manshurica Rupr. (family Ranunculaceae). Either the crude drug or the drug dried in the sun and cut into pieces may be used.

Nomenclature Used in Prescriptions: *Weilingxian*, *Tielingxian.*

Properties and Channel Distribution: The drug is pungent and salty in taste, warm in nature, and distributed to the Urinary Bladder Channel.

Action and Indications:

1. Dispelling wind and resolving dampness, reactivating channels.

To treat arthralgia with contracture and pain due to cold and preponderant wind, it can be used with drugs having the effects on dispelling wind and promoting blood circulation; to treat stuffiness and breathlessness due to invasion of abdomen by serious beriberi wuth abundant cold and dampness, its powder 6 g can be taken with wine.

2. Regulating the flow of *Qi* to remove *Qi* stagnation

To treat women with abdominal pain due to stagnation of *Qi* and blood, it can be used with Radix Angelicae Sinensis, Cortex Cinnamomi, etc.

Besides, to treat sticking in the throat by fish bone or other bones, it can be decocted singly, or with vinegar and brown sugar and taken hot slowly after the decoction being filtered.

Dosage and Administration: 6–10 g of the drug are decocted as a dose.

Pieces of Rhizome of Aromatic Turmeric (片姜黄 *Pianjianghuang*) Rhizoma Curcumae

The drug consists of the rhizome of a perennial herb with perennial root, Curcuma aromatica Salisb. (family Zingiberaceae). Sometimes it is also called *Pianzijianghuang* , *Maojianghuang* , or *Wenezhu* . It is dried in the sun for use.

Nomenclature Used in prescriptions: *Pianjianghuang*

Properties and Channel Distribution: The drug is pungent and bitter in taste, warm in nature, and distributed to the Liver and Spleen Channels.

Action and Indications:

Warming channels to dispel cold, expelling wind and resolving dampness, promoting the circulation of *Qi* to stop pain

It can produce the effect of facilitating the movement of tendons and muscles in the limbs; therefore it is often used in combination with Rhizoma seu Radix Notopterygii, Radix Angelicae Sinensis, Radix Paeoniae Rubra, etc. to treat arthralgia-syndrome due to wind and dampness; besides, it is often in combination with Radix Angelicae Sinensis Radix Paeoniae alba, Rhizoma Ligustici Chuanxiong, Rhizoma Zedoariae, Flos Carthami, etc. to treat various pain syndromes in the chest, hypochondric region, epigastric region or abdomen due to stagnation of *Qi* and blood, or to treat abdominal mass due to amenorrhea caused by stasis of blood.

Dosage and Administration: 3–10 g of the drug are decocted as a dose.

Chaenomeles Fruit (木瓜 *Mugua*)
Fructus Chaenomelis

The drug consists of the fruit of a deciduous shrub, Chaenomeles lagenaria (Loisel.) Koidz. (family Rosaceae). The drug is immersed and softened, then steamed and cut into pieces for use.

Nomenclature Used in Prescriptions: *Mugua*, *Xuanmugua*, *Chenmugua*.

Properties and Channel Distribution: The drug is sour in taste, warm in nature, and distributed to the Liver and Spleen Channels.

Action and Indications:

1. Relieving rigidity of muscles and activating collaterals:

It is often used in treating wet beriberi syndrome due to dampness, marked by swelling of the ankle joints, lumbar soreness and aching knee, swollen joints, contracture of tendons and weakness of lower limbs. To treat beriberi due to cold–dampness, it is often used with Folium Perillae, Fructus Evodiae, Rhizoma Zingiberis Recens, etc.; to treat beriberi due to dampheat, with Cortex Phellodendri, Rhizoma Dioscoreae Hypoglaucae, Herba Dendrobii, etc.; to treat lumbar soreness and aching knees, with Radix Dipsaci, Cortex Eucommiae, etc.

2. Resolving dampness and regulating the stomach

To treat syndrome due to summer–heat in the summer season, and irregular food taking, characterized by vomiting, diarrhea like cholera, even with painful legs accompanied with contracture of muscles and tendons, it is often used either with Herba Agastachis, Cortex Magnoliae Officinalis, Rhizoma Pinelliae, etc. or with Fructus Euodiae, Caulis Perillae, etc. Since the drug can produce the effects of resolving dampness and removing the accumulation of damp evil with its warm nature, and soothing muscles and tendons to treat contracture and pain limbs, the drug can be used in treating wet beriberi, and various kinds of contracture of muscles and tendons or painful legs.

Besides, it can be used in treating indigestion and relieving thirst since it with its sour taste has the effects of regulating middle *Jiao* , resolving dampness and promoting the production of body fluid.

Dosage and Administration: 6–10 g of the drug are decocted as a dose.

Tetrandra Root (防己 *Fangji*)
Radix Stephaniae Tetrandrae

The drug consists of the tuberous root of a perennial trailing vine, Stephania tetrandra S. Moore (family Menispermaceae) or the tuberous root of a perennial trailing vine, Aristolochia fangchi Wu (family Aristolochiaceae). The drug is peeled, and then cut into pieces for use.

Nomenclature Used in Prescriptions: *Fangji* , *Hanfangji* , *Mufangji* .

Properties and Channel Distribution: The drug is bitter and pungent in taste, cold in nature, and distributed to the Urinary Bladder, Spleen and Lung Channels.

Action and Indications:

1. Dispelling wind to stop pain (the root of Aristolochia is indicated)

To treat arthralgia–syndrome due to wind and dampness, marked by painful joints, it can be used with Rhizoma Atractylodis Macrocephalae, Cortex Cinnamomi, Radix Aconiti, Rhizoma Zingiberis Recens, etc.; to treat painful joints due to damp–heat leading to the obstruction of channels or to treat beriberi with edema and soreness, with Radix Achyranthis Bidentatae, Cotex Phellodendri, Fructus Chaenomelis, Semen Coicis, etc.

2. Promoting the discharge of water by urination to treat edema (the root of Stephania tetrandra is indicated)

It is used in treating the syndrome of invasion of lower *Jiao* by damp–heat, edema, ascites, disorder of urination, etc. To treat general edema with superficial pulse and general heaviness, perspiration accompanied by aversion of wind, it can be used with Radix Astragali seu Hedysari, Rhizoma Atractylodis Macrocephalae, Radix glycyrrhizae; to treat disorder of urination with edema of extremities, with Poria, Radix Astragali, Ramulus Cinnamomi and Radix Glycyrrhizae. In case of phlegm–retention syndrome with fullness and distension of the abdomen due to water–retension in the intestine, yet accompanied with dryness of the mouth and tongue, it can be with Semen Zanthoxyli, Semen Lepiddii seu Descurainiae and Radix et Rhizoma Rhei; and an equal amount of each drug is mixed and powdered for honeyed pills. The pills 6 g are taken as a dose, three times a day.

Dosage and Administration: 6–9 g of the drug are decocted as a dose.

Notes: Since the drug is sharply bitter in taste and badly cold in nature, it can not be used in a large dose; otherwise it will injure Stomach–*Qi* . Besides, it is contraindicated in those with weak constitution and deficiency of *Yin* or with poor appetite.

Mulberry Twig (桑枝 *Sangzhi*)
Ramulus Mori

The drug consists of the slender twigs of a short arbor, Morus alba L. (family Moraceae); the crude drug is cut into pieces for use.

Nomenclature Used in Prescriptions: *Sangzhi* , *Nensangzhi* .

Properties and Channel Distribution: The drug is bitter and sweet in taste, even in nature, and distributed to the Liver Channel.

Action and Indications:

Expelling wind and reactivating channels.

To treat arthralgia–syndrome due to wind–dampness, marked by numbness of hand and arm, it is often used with Radix Clematidis, Radix Stephaniae Tetrandrae, Radix Angelicae Sinensis, etc.; to treat hot arthralgia–syndrome, it is often used in combination with Caulis Trachelospermi, Caulis Lonicerae, Lumbricus, etc.

Dosage and Administration: 15–30 g are decocted as a dose.

Mulberry Mistletoe (桑寄生 *Sangjisheng*) Ramulus Loranthi

The drug consists of the foliferous stems and branches of a short shrub, a kind of a parasitic plant, Viscum coloratum (Kom.) Nakai or Loranthus parasiticus (L.) Merr. (family Loranthaceae). The drug in crude state is often cut into pieces or segments for use.

Nomenclature Used in Prescriptions: *Sangjisheng* .

Properties and Channel Distribution: The drug is bitter and sweet in taste, even in nature, and distributed to the Liver and Kidney Channels.

Action and Indications:

1. Dispelling wind-damp evil and strengthening tendons and bones

It is often used in treating arthralgia-syndrome marked by lumbar soreness and aching knee. Since the drug has good effects of invigorating the liver and kidney, and strengthening the tendons and bones, it is used with Radix Angelicae Pubescentis, Cortex Eucommiae, Radix Achyranthis Bidentatae, Radix Angelicae Sinensis, etc. to treat chronic arthralgia, complicated with impairment of both the functions of the liver and Kidney, and movement of the tendons and joints with lumbar soreness and aching knee.

2. Invigorating the liver and kidney, nourishing blood and preventing miscarriage.

To treat threatened abortion with spot vaginal bleeding or restlessness of fetus due to deficiency of the liver and kidney, and impairment of the *Chong* and *Ren* Channels, it is often used in combination with Radix Angelicae Sinensis, Colla Corii Asini, Radix Dipsaci, etc. The drug is good at dispelling pathogenic evils, but it is too weak to invigorate the internal organs: therefore it is not suitable to be as a tonic in practice.

Besides, the drug can produce the effect of relieving hypertension.

Dosage and Administration: 15—30 g are decocted as a dose.

Acanthopanax Bark (五加皮 *Wujiapi*)
Cortex Acanthopanacis Radicis

The drug consists of the root bark of a duciduous short shrub, Acanthopanax gracilistylus W. W. Smith (family Araliacea); the drug is usually called *nanwujiapi*. The crude drug is cut into pieces for use.

Nomenclature Used in Prescriptions: *Wujiapi*

Properties and Channel Distribution: The drug is pungent and bitter in taste, warm in nature, and distributed to the Liver and Kidney Channels.

Action and Indications:

1. Dispelling wind and resolving dampness

To treat arthralgia mainly due to dampness, marked either by soreness, heaviness, edema and pain of the lumbar region and lower limbs or by contracture of the tendons and bones, it is often decocted with Fructus Chaenomelis, Lignum Pini Nodi, Radix Achyranthis Bidentatae, etc. or 60 g of the drug are dipped into 500 CC of white spirit for seven days, and then filtered, a proper amount of the medicated wine may be taken, three times a day.

2. Strengthening tendons and bones

To treat weakness of tendons and bones, weakness of the lower limbs with retardation of walking or injury with fracture of bone, it can be used with other drugs having effects on soothing tendons and promoting the circulation of channels.

Besides, it can also produce the effects of facilitating the discharge of water and relieving edema; therefore it can be used in treating edema.

Dosage and Administration: 6–10 g of the drug can be decocted and a proper amount may be used for local application. usually it is often dipped in the spirit in making extract for use.

Tiger Bone (虎骨 *Hugu*)*
Os Tigris

The drug consists of the bones of the skeleton of a vertebrate, Panthera tigris L. (family Felidae); the bone is fried in the sesame oil thoroughly or bake–stirred with sand till it becomes brown, then the hot brown bone is cooled with vinegar for use.

Nomenclature Used in Prescriptions: *Zhihugu* , *Hujinggu* .

Properties and Channel Distribution: The drug is pungent in taste, warm in nature, and is distributed to the Liver and kidney Channels.

Action and Indications:

---

* Please see Notes. We deal with these materials in this volume is just to the academic convenience.

Expelling pathogenic wind to stop pain, strengthening tendons and bones

To treat arthralgia due to either wind-cold or dampness marked by soreness and aching of the tendons and bones, it is often used with Fructus Chaenomelis, Radix Angelicae Sinensis, Radix Achyranthis Bidentatae, Radix Gentianae Macrophyllae, etc.; to treat weakness of tendons and extremities, etc., it may be combined with Rhizoma Rehmanniae Praeparatae, Rhizoma Anemarrhenae, Cortex Phellodendri, etc.

Dosage and Administration: 3-10 g of the drug are decocted as a dose; usually the drug is used as an ingredient in pills or powder or used singly in medicated liquor.

Appendix: Leopard Bone (豹骨 *Baogu*); Os Pardi

The drug consists of the bones of the skeleton of a vertebrate, Panthera Pardus L. (family Felidae); the bones are bake-stirred with sand and adjunvant for use. The properties, actions and indications, dosage and administrations are similar to those of Os Tigris, but its actions are weaker than those of Os Tigris.

Long-noded Pit Viper (白花蛇 *Baihuashe*) Agkistrodon Acutus

The drug consists of the dried body of Agkistrodon acutus(Guenther) (family Crotalidae); the dried body is first dipped into wine for three days, then the meat of the body is for use.

Nomenclature Used in Prescriptions: *Baihuashe* , *Qisherou*

Properties and Channel Distribution: The drug is sweet and salty in taste, warm in nature, poisonous in property, and distributed to the Liver Channel.

Action and Indications:

Expelling wind and reactivating channels, relieving convulsion and stopping pain

To treat arthralgia–syndrome due to wind and dampness, marked by numbness of muscles and painful joints, etc., it may be used with Rhizoma seu Radix Notopterygii, Radix Gentianae Macrophyllae, Cortex Acanthopanacis Radicis, etc.; to treat leprosy with numbness of extremities, with Zaocys, Realgar, etc.; to treat tetanus, with Scolopendra, etc.

Dosage and Administration: 3–6 g of the drug are used as an ingredient in pills, powder, medicated liquor and extract; usually it is not used in decoction.

Appendix: Black–tailed Snake (乌梢蛇 *Wushaoshe*);

Zaocys

The drug consists of the dried body, Zaocys dhumnades (Cantor) (family Colubridae); the viscera of the snake are taken out from the body, then the body is dried for use. It is sweet in taste, even in nature, poisonousless in property; its actions are weaker than those of Akistroden. 3–12 g of the drug are decocted as a dose.

Erythrina Bark (海桐皮 *Haitongpi*)
Cortex Erythrinae

The drug consists of the dried bark of the evergreen tree, Erythrina variegata L. var. orientalis(L.) Merr. (family Leguminosae). Usually it is dried in the sun and cut into pieces for use.

Nomenclature Used in Prescriptions: *Haitongpi*

Properties and Channel Distribution: The drug is bitter and pungent in taste, even in nature, and distributed to the Liver and Kidney Channels.

Action and Indications:

1. Dispelling wind and dampness, reactivating channels

To treat arthralgia due to wind-dampness, lumbar soreness and aching knee, contracture of the extremities, etc., it is often used with Radix Angelicae Pubercentis, Rhizoma Ligustici Chuanxiong, Radix Achyranthis Bidentatae, Radix Angelicae Sinensis, etc. having effects on reactivating channels and blood.

2. The drug can produce the effects of killing parasites and relieving itching, and be decocted as a wash or ground in making powder for treating scabies, tinea and eczema.

Dosage and Administration: 6–10 g of the drug are decocted as a dose; a proper amount is used for local application.

Siegesbeckia Herb (豨莶草 *Xixiancao*)
Herba Siegesbeckiae

The drug consists of the whole plant of an annual herb, Siegesbeckia orientalis L. var. pubescens Mak. or S. glabrescens Mak. (family Campositae). The crude drug is dried in the sun and cut into sections or is steamed with wine for use.

Nomenclature Used in Prescriptions: *Xixiancao*.

Properties and Channel Distribution: The drug is pungent and bitter in taste, cold in nature, and is distributed to the Liver and Kidney Channels.

Action and Indications:

1. Expelling wind and dampness, strengthening tendons and bones (prepared drug is used)

To treat soreness and pain of the tendons and bones, numbness of the extremities, weakness of lumbar region and knee joints, it is powdered and steamed with wine in making honeyed bolus and each is 9 g in weight; take one bolus as a dose, twice or three times a day; to treat arthralgia due to wind marked by wandering pain or hemiplegia, it can be used with Fructus Xanthii, Cortex Acanthopanacis Radicis, Caulis Piperis Futokadsurae, Radix Angelicae Sinensis, etc.

2. Resolving damp–heat and relieving itching caused by wind (the crude drug is indicated in this disease)

To treat urticaria rubella, and itching due to eczema, it can be used with Cortex Dictamni Radicis, Fructus Xanthii, etc.

besides, Since it can produce the effect of relieving hypertension, it may be used in treating this disease.

Dosage and Administration: 10–15 g are decocted as a dose.

Twig and Leaf of Harlequin Glorybower
(臭梧桐 *Chouwutong*)
Ramulus et Folium Clerodendri Trichotomi

The drug consists of the slender twigs and leaves of a deciduous shrub or short tree, Clerodendron trichotomum Thumb. (family Verbenaceae). The crude drug is for use.

Nomenclature Used in Prescriptions: *Chouwutong* , *Bajiaowutong*

Properties and Channel Distribution: The drug is pungent and bitter in taste, even in nature, and distributed to the Liver Channels.

Action and Indications:

Dispelling wind–damp: To treat disorder of movement of tendons and muscles of limbs due to wind and dampness or hemiplegia caused by wind stroke, it can be used with Herba Siegesbeckiae in pills; to treat general itching caused by wind evil, it can be decocted as a wash.

Besides, the drug has the effect on lowering the blood pressure, so it can be powdered and taken a long time, or decocted as an ingredient in a prescription for treating hypertension due to hyperativity of liver–*Yang* marked by vertigo and headache. It is suitable to be collected before its flowers bloom; in this way, its good therapeutic effect can be reserved. Moreover, it is not suitable to be decocted for a long time at high temperature with violent fire; otherwise, its anti–hypertension effect will be weakened.

Dosage and Administration: 10–15 g of the drug are decocted as a dose in decoction; 3 g of its powder are used as a dose; and a proper amount, for local application.

Club–moss (伸筋草 *Shenjincao*)
Herba Lycopodii

The drug consists of the entire plant of a perennial evergreen herb of trailing stem, Lycopodium clavatum L. (family Lycopodiaceae); the entire herb is dried in the sun and cut into sections for use.

Nomenclature Used in Prescriptions: *Shenjincao* .

Properties and Channel Distribution: The drug is pungent and bitter in taste, warm in nature, and distributed to the Liver and Kidney Channels.

Action and Administrations:

Dispelling wind and reactivating channels.

To treat arthralgia caused by wind–damp, marked by soreness of the limbs and joints with impairment of their movement, and numbness of the skin, etc., it can be used in a compound prescription according to the specific syndromes.

Futokadsura Stem (海风藤 *Haifengteng*)
Caulis Piperis Futokadsurae

The drug consists of the stem of an evergreen trailing vine, Piper kadsura (Choisy) Ohwi (family Piperaceae); the crude drug is cut into pieces for use.

Nomenclature Used in Prescriptions: *Haifengteng*

Properties and Channel Distribution: The drug is pungent and bitter in taste, slightly warm in nature, and distributed to the Liver Channel.

Action and Indications:

Dispelling wind–damp and reactivating channels.

To treat arthralgia due to wind, cold and dampness, marked by painful joints and contracture of the tendons and muscles, it is often used with Rhizoma seu Radix Notopterygii, Radix Angelicae Pubercentis, Radix Angelicae Sinensis, Ramulus Cinnamomi, etc.

Dosage and Administration: 10–15 g are decocted as a dose.

Chinese Starjasmine (络石藤 *Luoshiteng*)
Caulis Trachelospermi

The drug consists of the foliferous stem of an evergreen trailing shrub, Trachelospermum jasminoides(Lindl.) Lem. (family Apocynaceae). The crude drug is cut into pieces for use.

Nomenclature Used in Prescriptions: *Luoshiteng*

Properties and Channel Distribution: The drug is bitter in taste, slightly cold in nature, and distributed to the Heart and Liver Channels.

Action and Indications:

1. Dispelling wind and reactivating channels.

To treat arthralgia due to wind–damp accompanied with soreness and aching of tendons and bones, it can be with Rhizoma Homalomenae, Radix Angelicae Pubescentis, Radix Clematidis, Radix Stephaniae Tetrandrae, Radix Ledebouriellae, Radix Gentianae Macrophyllae, etc.; to treat arthralgia due to wind, damp and heat, marked by redness and swelling of the joints, with Caulis Lonicerae, Radix Cynanchi Atrati, Radix Salviae Miltiorrhizae, Cortex Zanthoxyli, Rhizoma Atractylodis, Cortex Phellodendri, Radix Achyranthis Bidentatae, etc.

2. Clearing away blood–heat and relieving swelling and inflammation

To treat carbuncles, furuncles and skin pyogenic infections, it can be used with Spina Gleditisiae, Olibanum, etc.; to treat sore throat with obstruction, it can be used with Radix Platycodi, Rhizoma Belamcandae, Caulis Akebiae, etc. or decocted singly in 30 g for being drunk slowly.

Dosage and Administration: 15–30 g are decocted as a dose.

Root–Bark of Chinese Hydrangeavine
(钻地风 *Zuandifeng*)
Cortex Schizophragmatis Integrifolii Radicis

The drug consists of the bark of the root of a deciduous woody vine, Schizophragma integrifolium (Franch.) Oliv. (family Saxifragaceae); the drug is dried in the sun and cut into pieces for use.

Nomenclature Used in Prescriptions: *Zuandifeng* , *Zhuidifeng* , *Difeng* .

Properties and Channel Distribution: The drug is tasteless, cool in nature, and distributed to the Liver and Kidney Channels.

Action and Indications:

Dispelling wind and resolving dampness, soothing tendons and promoting blood circulation

To treat arthralgia marked with soreness and aching of the tendons and bones, and weakness and numbness of the knee joints or the lower limbs, etc., it is often used with Rhizoma Homalomenae; to treat painful joints of the limbs, Cortex Schizophragmatis Integrifolii Radicis 750 g, Rhizoma Homalomenae 250 g, Cortex Acanthopanacis Radicis 250 g, Radix Salviae Miltiorrhizae 250 g and Radix Achyranthis Bidentatae 180 g and Herba Ephedrae 15 g are reserved with 12 *Jin* of wine in a sealed pot by indirect heating in a pan filled with water for 4 hours, then the medicated solution 100 CC. may be taken as a dose, twice a day; when the medicated solution is used up, 10 *Jin* of wine may be added into the jar, then the preparation can be repeated as before and a proper amount will be taken.

Dosage and Administration: 6–12 g of the drug are decocted as a dose.

Rhizome of Obscured Homalomina
(千年健 *Qiannianjian*)
Rhizoma Homalomenae

The drug consists of the carnified rhizome of a perennial herb, Homalomena occulta (Lour.) Schott (family Araceae). The drug in crude state is cut into pieces for use.

Nomenclature Used in Prescriptions: *Qiannianjian* , *Qiannianjian* , *Nianjian* .

Properties and Channel Distribution: The drug is bitter and pungent in taste, warm in nature, and distributed to the Liver and Kidney Channels.

Action and Indications:

Dispelling wind–damp and strengthening tendons and bones.

To treat arthralgia due to wind, cold and damp, marked by soreness and aching of the tendons and bones, contracture and numbness of limbs, it may be used with Cortex Schizophragmatis Integrifolii Radicis.

Besides, In treating sciatica due to wind–cold, it is often used in combination with Ramulus Cinnamomi, Radix Paeoniae, Radix Aconiti Praeparata, Herba Lycopodii, Cortex Schizophragmatis Integrifolii Radicis, Radix Achyranthis Bidentatae, Radix Angelicae Sinensis, Radix Glycyrrhizae, Rhizoma Zingiberis, Fructus Ziziphi Jujubae, etc.; and the effect seems good, esp. in treating those senial patients.

Dosage and Administration: 6–12 g of the drug are decocted as a dose, but it seems more effective if its medicated liquor is used.

Nodular Branch of Pine (松节 *Songjie*)
Lignum Pini Nodi

The drug consists of the nodular branches of an evergreen tree, Pinus tabuleaformis Carr. (family Pinaceae). The crude drug is cut into pieces for use.

Nomenclature Used in Prescriptions: *Songjie* , *Yousongjie* .

Properties and Channel Distribution: The drug is bitter in taste, warm in nature, and distributed to the Liver and Kidney Channels.

Action and Indications:

Dispelling wind and resolving dampness.

To treat arthralgia due to wind–damp of tendons, bones and joints, it is often used singly to be immersed in the white spirit for medicated liquor or in combination with Rhizoma seu Radix Notopterygii, Radix Angelicae Pubescentis, Radix Ledebouriellae, Caulis Piperis Futokadsurae, Ramulus Mori, Radix Angelicae Sinensis, Rhizoma Ligustici Chuanxiong, etc.

Dosage and Administration

10–15 g of the drug are decocted as a dose; the drug is suitable to be immersed in spirit to form medicated liquor.

Silkworm Faeces (蚕砂 *Cansha*)
Faeces Bombycis

The drug consists of the dried faeces of the mulberry Silkworm, Bombyx Mori L. (family Bombycidae); the crude drug is dried for use.

Nomenclature Used in Prescriptions: *Cansha* , *Wancansha* .

Properties and Channel Distribution: The drug is sweet and pungent in taste, warm in nature, and distributed to the Liver, Spleen and Stomach Channels.

Action and Indications:

1. Dispelling wind and resolving dampness.

To treat protracted arthralgia due to wind, cold and dampness, accompanied with painful joints, it can be used with Agkistrodon, Cortex Schizophragmatis Integrifolii Radicis, Eupolyphaga seu Steleophaga, Scorpio, etc.; or it can be singly filled into two pakages and used as local hot compress after the two pakages are steamed hot alternately.

2. Regulating the stomach and promoting digestion and transformation of indigested food.

To treat vomiting, diarrhea, abdominal pain even with convulsion due to irregularity of taking food or taking too much raw or cold food, it can be used with Semen Coicis, Rhizoma Pinelliae, Fructus Chaenomelis, etc.

Dosage and Administration: 6—10 g of the drug are wrapped with a cloth and decocted for local use.

Paniculate Swallowwort Root (徐长卿 *Xuchangqing*) Radix Cynanchi Paniculati

The drug consists of the root of a perennial herb, Cynanchum paniculatum (Bge.) Kitag. (family Aslepiadaceae); usually the crude drug is dried in the shade and cut into pieces for use.

Nomenclature Used in Prescriptions: *Xuchangqing*

Properties and Channel Distribution: The drug is pungent in taste, warm in nature, and distributed to the Lung, Stomach, Liver and Kidney Channels.

Action and Indications:

Dispelling wind and arresting pain or itching.

To treat arthralgia–syndrome with lumbar soreness and aching knee, it can be used with Radix Stephaniae Tetrandrae; to treat injury with hematoma, it can be decocted as a decoction or as a wash; to treat stomachache, abdominal pain, 1.5–3 g of the powder of the drug can be used singly or with 1.5–3 g of Rhizoma Corydalis in powder form and taken with water, or it may be decocted with Rhizoma Cyperi; to treat toothache due to dental caries, 10 g of the drug can be decocted as a wash for rincing out the mouth cavity; to treat urticaria, general pruritus, protracted tinea, it can be decocted for oral or local use, or used with a small amount of Alumen in the hot water for bath.

Besides, it can be decocted singly in treating chronic asthma; to treat mountain sickness or motion sickness, 1.5 g of its powder may be taken with water. Moreover, it has effect of relieving snake poisoning; to treat snake bite, it can either be decocted with

Herba Scutellariae Radicantis or be used locally as a paste.

Dosage and Administration: 10–15 g of the drug are taken as a dose in making decoction.

Herb of Wooly Dutchmonspipe (寻骨风 *Xungufeng*)
Herba Aristolochiae Mollissimae

The drug consists of the entire plant and its rhizome of a perennial trailing herb, Aristolochia mollissima Hance (family Aristolochiae); the crude drug is dried in the sun and cut into segments for use.

Nomenclature Used in Prescriptions: *Xungufeng*

Properties and Channel Distribution: The drug is pungent and bitter in taste, even in nature, and distributed to the Liver Channel.

Action and Indications:

Dispelling wind–damp and reactivating channels to relieve pain.

To treat rheumatic arthralgia with painful joints, dysfunction of the tendons and bones, injury and wounds with swelling and pain, it can be used singly in making decoction, medicated liquor, liquid extract or tablets for use; or it can be used in combination with other drugs having the effect of relieving arthralgia.

Besides, it can also be used in treating stomachache, hernia, and swelling and pain of testis.

Dosage and Administration: 15–30 g of the drug are decocted as a dose; and a proper amount of the drug is used for local administration.

5 Drugs with Fragrant Odour for Resolving Dampness

Drugs which can produce the effects of resolving dampness and regulating the function of the spleen are generally called drugs with fragrant odour for resolving dampness.

The drugs are aromatic in odour, warm and dry in nature, which have the effects on regulating the circulation of *Qi* , resolving dampness and invigorating the spleen and stomach; therefore they can be used in treating such symptoms as fullness and distension of epigastrium and abdomen, poor appetite and lassitude, vomiting and acid regurgitation, sweet taste with a lot of saliva, watery stools and white and sticky tongue coating, etc. due to invasion of middle *Jiao* by evil dampness, and dysfunction of the spleen and disorders of transportation and transformation; it may also be used for treating dampness–heat syndrome, summer– heat–dampness syndrome, etc.

In clinical practice, it should be used with other drugs according to specific properties of dampness and its complications. To treat cold–dampness syndrome, it is used with drugs for warming the interior or dispelling cold from the interior; to treat damp–heat syndrome, used with drugs for clearing away heat evil and resolving dampness; to treat damp syndrome due to deficiency of the spleen, with drugs for invigorating the spleen; to treat syndrome due to retention of phlegm–dampness, with drugs for resolving phlegm and dampness; to treat syndrome of retention of dampness and stagnation of *Qi* , with drugs for regulating the flow of *Qi* .

Since this kind of drug are pungent in taste, aromatic in odour, warm and dry in nature. They are likely to consume vital essence and vital energy, they should be used cautiously for treating patients with deficiency of *Yin* and body fluid, red tongue and deficiency of *Qi* . Since the drugs are aromatic, fragrant and contain volatile oil, it should be decocted later for a short time, otherwise their effects will be weakened.

Atractylodes Rhizome (苍术 *Cangzhu*)
Rhizoma Atractylodis

The drug consists of the rhizome of a perennial herb, Atractylodes lancea(Thunb.) DC. or A. chinensis (DC.) Koidz. (family Compositae); the crude drug is dried by heating near fire, then softened by water, cut into pieces, and cooked thoroughly with water in which rice has been washed, then baked and stirred until it becomes light tan for use.

Nomenclature Used in Prescriptions: *Zhicangzhu* , *Cangzhu* , *Maocangzhu*

Properties and Channel Distribution: The drug is pungent and bitter in taste, warm in nature, and distributed to the Spleen and Stomach Channels.

Action and Indications:

1. Resolving dampness to invigorate the Spleen.

To treat syndrome of retension of dampness of middle *Jiao* , marked by dysfunction of the spleen due to invasion by dampness, fullness and distension of epigastrium and abdomen or diarrhea, turbid and sticky tongue coating, it is often used with Cortex Magnoliae Officinalis. Pericarpium Citri Reticulatae. It can be used to treat syndrome of retension of phlegm or edema due to invasion of the spleen by predominant dampness according to the specific syndromes.

2. Dispelling wind–dampness.

It can be used in treating arthralgia marked by general soreness or painful joints due to invasion by wind and dampness or by wine and cold. In treating arthralgia due to invasion by wind, cold and dampness, it can be used with Rhizoma seu Radix Notopterygii, Radix Ledebouriellae, Ramulus Cinnamomi, Radix Gentianae Macrophyllae, etc.; in treating hot arthralgia, with Cortex Phellodendri, Radix Cyathulae Officinalis, etc.

3. Dispersing cold evil from the superficies.

To treat those with cold due to pathogenic wind and cold accompanied with headache and anhidrosis, it can be used with Rhizoma Ligustici, Radix Angelicae Dahuricae, etc.

Besides. the drug has the effects of removing nebula, brightening eyes and improving vision, therefore it can be used in treating the internal or external nebula, glaucoma, night blindness, etc. it can be used singly or with the liver of pig, or black sesame.

Dosage and Administration: 6–10 g of the drug are decocted as a dose.

Notes: It is contraindicated in those with syndrome of heat in the interior due to insufficiency of *Yin* or with perspiration due to deficiency of *Qi* .

Magnolia bark (厚朴 *Houpo*)
Cortex Magnoliae Officinalis

The drug consists of the barks of the trunk, roots and twigs of a deciduous tree, Magnolia officinalis Rehd et Wils. or Magnolia biloba (Rehd. et Wils) cheng (family Magnoliaceae). The crude drug is dried in the sun and cut into pieces for use; or its pieces, mixed with the pieces of Rhizoma Zingiberis for use; or its pieces, bake–stirred with juice of Rhizoma Zingiberis for use.

Nomenclature Used in Prescriptions: *Houpo* *Chuanpo* , *Zhichuanpo* , *Jianghoupo* .

Properties and Channel distribution: The drug is bitter and pungent in taste, warm in nature, and distributed to the Spleen, Stomach, Lung and Large Intestine Channels.

Action and Indications:

1. Regulating the flow of *Qi* and resolving dampness.

It can be used in treating syndrome due to invasion of the spleen by dampness or stagnation of food and *Qi* with either fullness and distension of epigastrium and abdomen or abdominal pain with diarrhea, etc. In treating cold–dampness syndrome of the spleen and stomach with fullness and distension of the thorax and abdomen, it can be used with Rhizoma Zingeberis Recens, Rhizoma Pinelliae, etc.; in treating damp–heat syndrome of the intestine and stomach with fullness and distension of abdomen (due to stagnation of *Qi* and constipation), it can be used with Fructus Aurantii Immaturus, Radix et Rhizoma Rhei.

2. Warming middle *Jiao* to stop pain

To treat epigastric and abdominal pain due to accumulation

of cold, it can be used with Rhizoma Zingiberis, Semen Alpiniae Katsumadai, Radix Aucklandiae, etc.

3. Lowering the adverse ascending of *Qi* to relieve asthma

To treat cough and asthma or dyspnea due ot accumulation of damp–phlegm in the lung, it can be used with Semen Armeniacae Amarum, Herba Ephedrae, Rhizoma Pinelliae, etc.

Dosage and Administration: 3–10 g of the drug are taken as a dose in making decoction.

Appendix: Flower of Officinal Magnolia (厚朴花 *Houpohua*); Flos Magnolia Officinalis

The drug consists of the flower–bud of Magnolia Officinalis Rehd. et Wils.; its taste and nature are similar to those of Cortex Magnoliae Officinalis. It can produce the effects of invigorating the stomach to stop stomachache and regulating flow of *Qi* to relieve the stuffiness of the chest; therefore it can be used in treating syndrome of stagnation of *Qi* of the liver and stomach accompanied with fullness and distension of the chest and abdomen, etc. Its dosage is the same as the dosage of Cortex Magnoliae Officinalis.

Agastache (藿香 *Huoxiang*)
Herba Agastachis

The drug consists of the aerial parts of a perennial herb, Pogestemon cablin (Blanco) Benth. or Agastache rugous (Fisch. et Mey) O. Ktze. (family Labiatae); the crude drug is usually dried in the sun and cut into sections for use; sometimes, the fresh herb, or its twigs and leaves may be used.

Nomenclature Used in Prescriptions: *Guanghuoxiang* ,

Huoxiangyi, *Houxianggeng*, *Xianhuoxiang*.

Properties and Channel Distribution: The drug is pungent in nature, slightly warm in nature, and distributed to the Spleen, Stomach and Lung Channels.

Action and Indications:

1. Removing dampness and arresting vomiting

To treat the syndrome due to invasion of the middle *Jiao* by accumulation of cold–dampness with vomiting, it can be used with Rhizoma Pinelliae and Pericarpium Citri Reticulatae; to treat dampness–heat syndrome with lassitude and stuffiness of the chest, with Rhizoma Pinelliae, Cortex Magnoliae Officinalis, Semen Armeniacae Amarum, etc.; to treat those with *Qi* –deficiency, with Radix Codonopsis and Rhizoma Atractylodis Macrocephalae; to treat those with heat in predominance, with Rhizoma Coptidis; to treat those pregnant women with morning sickness and vomiting sour fluid (due to influence of fetal energy), it can be used with Fructus Amomi and Rhizoma Cyperi.

2. Dispersing evils from the superficies and clearing away summer–heat

To treat headache, chilliness and fever, stuffiness of the chest and abdominal distension with nausea, vomiting or diarrhea, etc. (due to over eating of cold food or raw vegetables, or invasion by wind and cold in summer), it is usually used with Folium et Caulis Perillae, Rhizoma Pinelliae, Cortex Magnoliae Officinalis, Pericarpium Arecae, Poria, etc.; to treat syndrome due to summer–heat, it can be used with Herba Eupatorii, Herba Menthae and infused in hot water to make a drink, thus manifestations of summer–heat syndrome such as fullness and heaviness in the head with stuffiness of the chest accompanied with nausea, feeling of stickiness in the mouth, poor appetite, etc will be likely to be cured. Usually the fresh drugs reveal the remarkable effects.

3. Activating the flow of *Qi* to stop pain

To treat syndrome of stagnation of *Qi* of the spleen and stomach with distension and pain of the epigastrium and abdomen, it can be used with Cortex Magnolia Officinalis, Fructus Amomi, Pericarpium Citri Reticulatae, Radix Aucklandiae, Fructus Aurantii Immaturus, etc

Besides, it can be used in treating rhinorrhea in making decoction mixed with bile of pig.

Dosage and Administration: 6–12 g of the drug are decocted as a dose; and 15–30 g of the fresh are used. The leaves of the drug can produce the effect of dispersing evils from superfices; the twigs can produce the effect of regulating middle *Jiao* ; and the fresh plant has the remarkable effects on clearing away summer–heat, resolving dampness evil, and preventing human body from the affection due to invasion by pathogenic or virulent factors. In making decoction, it is not suitable to be decocted for a long time.

Eupatorium (佩兰 *Peilan*)
Herba Eupatorii

The drug consists of the aerial parts of a perennial herb, Eupatorium fortunei Turcz. (family Compositae). The crude drug is usually dried in the sun and cut into segments for use, or the fresh herb may be used.

Nomenclature Used in Prescriptions: *Peilan* , *Nanpeilan* , *Xiangpeilan* , *Xianpeilan* .

Properties and Channel Distribution: The drug is pungent in taste, even in nature, and distributed to the Spleen, Stomach and Lung Channels.

Action and Indications:

Resolving dampness and clearing away summer–heat, invigorating the Spleen and regulating middle *Jiao* .

To treat stuffiness of the chest and distension of the abdomen accompanied with sweet taste in the mouth, foul smell and sticky tongue coating, etc. (due to invasion of middle *Jiao* by dampness), it is often used with Herba Agastachis, Rhizoma Pinelliae Praeparatae, Cortex Magnoliae Officinalis, Pericarpium Citri Reticulatae, etc.; to treat fever and headache, stuffiness of the chest and poor appetite due to summer–heat in summer, with Herba Agastachis, Cortex Magnoliae Officinalis, Folium Nelumbinis, etc.

Dosage and Administration: 6–12 g of the drug are decocted as a dose while the fresh can be used in 15–30 g. The drug is not suitable to be decocted for a long time.

Amomum Fruit (砂仁 *Sharen*)
Fructus Amomi

The drug consists of the fruit of a perennial herb, Amomum villosum Lour. or A. langiligulave T.L.Wu or A. xanthioides Wall (family Zingiberaceae). Usually the ripe fruit is crushed into pieces just before use.

Nomenclature Used in Prescriptions: *Sharen* , *Chunsharen* , *Suosharen* , *Yangchunsha* .

Properties and Channel Distribution: The drug is pungent in taste, warm in nature, and distributed to the Spleen, Stomach and Kidney Channels.

Action and Indications:

1. Resolving dampness and activating the flow of *Qi*

To treat abdominal pain with fullness and distension due to invasion of middle *Jiao* by dampness and stagnation of *Qi* of the spleen and stomach, it is often used with Radix Aucklandiae and Fructus Aurantii Immaturus; to treat deficiency of the spleen with stagnation of *Qi* , with Radix Codonopsis Pilosulae, Rhizoma Atractylodis Macrocephalae, etc.

2. Warming stomach to arrest vomiting

To treat athenia–cold syndrome of spleen and stomach, and syndrome of obstruction of *Qi* in the chest with vomiting, it is often used with Radix Aucklandiae, Rhizoma Pinelliae Praeparatae, Pericarpium Citri Reticulatae, etc.; to treat morning sickness, 1.5–3 g of the drug are powdered as a dose, three times a day, taken with decoction of Rhizoma Zingiberis recens.

3. Warming Spleen to relieve diarrhea

To treat diarrhea or dysentery due to syndrome of deficiency of *Yang* of Spleen accompanied with accumulation of cold–damp, it is used with Rhizoma Zingiberis, Semen Myristicae, Fructus Chebulae, etc.

Besides, it can produce the effect of relieving threatened abortion with excessive fetal movement; therefore, it can be used with Rhizoma Atractylodis Macrocephalae, Ramulus Loranthi, Radix Dipsaci, etc. in treating the excessive fetal movement due to stagnation of *Qi* .

Dosage and Administration: 3–6 g of the drug are decocted as a dose; it, however, is suitable to be powdered for making pills, and its powder is also often taken together with the decoction of other drugs. When it is used as an ingredient in decoction, it is usually decocted later.

Appendix: The peel of Fructus Amomi is tasteless in taste and slightly warm in nature; it seems slightly effective in treating *Qi*–obstruction in the chest and poor appetite because it has the mild effects of activating the *Qi* flow of middle *Jiao* and invigorating stomach. The dosage of the drug used is the same as that of Fructus Amomi.

Round Cardamom (白豆蔻 *Baidoukou*) Amomum Kravanh Pirre ex Gagnep

The drug consists of the fruit of a perennial herb, Amomum cardamomum L. (family Zingiberaceae); usually, the crushed fruit and seeds are prepared for use before decoction is made.

Nomenclature Used in Prescriptions: *Baidoukou*, *Baikouren*, *Zikou*, *Kongbaikou*.

Properties and Channel Distribution: The drug is pungent in taste, warm in nature, and distributed to the Lung, Spleen and Stomach Channels.

Action and Indications:

1. Resolving dampness and activating the flow of *Qi*

To treat syndrome due to invasion of middle *Jiao* by dampness and stagnation of *Qi* of the spleen and stomach, marked by fullness of the chest and epigastrium, it can be used with Cortex Magnoliae Officinalis, Pericarpium Citri Reticulatae, Fructus Amomi, etc; to treat damp–warm syndrome at its beginning stage with stuffiness of the chest, poor appetite, turbid and sticky tongue coating, it is often used with Semen Coicis, Semen Armeniacae Amarum, Cortex Magnoliae Officinalis, etc.

2. Warming the stomach to stop vomiting

It is often used in treating cold syndrome of the spleen and stomach in nature of deficiency, accompanied with nausea and vomiting, hiccup and regurgitation of air, etc. To treat regurgitation of acid and vomiting, it can be decocted with Herba Agastachis, Pericarpium Citri Reticulatae, etc. or with the juice of Rhizoma Zingeberis Recens in making pills.

Besides, the drug can be used in treating alcholism; therefore, to treat those who have lost their consciousness due to over drinking, it can be used.

Dosage and Administration: 3–6 g of the drug are decocted as a dose. Usually, it is suitable to be powdered and added to other medicinal pills or powder, or its powder may be taken with the decoction of other drugs. Used as an ingredient in making decoction, it should be decocted later.

Appendix: Peel of Round Cardamom (豆寇壳 *Doukouke*); Pericarpium Amomi Rotundus

The drug consists of the peel of the herb, Round Cardamom. it is tasteless in taste, weak in flavour, slightly warm and dry in property. It can produce the effects of soothing middle *Jiao* and activating the flow of *Qi* , regulating stomach and resolving the turbid. Its dosage is similar to that of Amomum Kravanh Pirre ex Gagnep.

Seed of Katsumada Galangal (草豆蔻 *Caodoukou*)
Semen Alpiniae Katsumadai

The drug consists of the dried ripe seeds of a perennial herb, Alpinia Katsumadai Hayata (family Zingiberaceae); usually, the drug is dried and pounded just before use.

Nomenclature Used in Prescriptions: *Caodoukou*

Properties and Channel Distribution: The drug is pungent in taste and warm in nature, and distributed to the Spleen and Stomach Channels.

Action and Indications

Resolving dampness, warming stomach, arresting vomiting and activating the flow of *Qi*

To treat the syndrome of accumulation of cold–damp in middle *Jiao* with fullness, distension and pain of the epigastrium and abdomen, and vomiting, it is often used with such drugs having effects of warming the stomach and dispersing internal cold in middle–*Jiao* as Rhizoma Alpiniae Officinarum, Rhizoma Zingiberis Recens, Rhizoma Pinelliae, Fructus Evodiae, etc.; to treat syndrome due to invasion of the spleen and stomach by asthenic cold, marked by poor appetite, loosing bowels with thick and sticky tongue coating, it can be used with Cortex Magnoliae Officinalis, Fructus Amomi, Pericarpium Citri Reticulatae, Rhizoma Atractylodis, etc.

Dosage and Administration: 3–6 g of the drug are decocted as a dose in making decoction. It should be decocted later when used as an ingredient to be added to the decoction of other drugs.

Caoguo (草果 *Caoguo*)
Fructus Tsaoko

The drug consists of the fruit of a perennial herb, Amomum tsao–ko Crevost et Lemaire (family Zingiberaceae); the fruit is crushed and the seed is pounded just before use.

Nomenclature Used in Prescriptions: *Caoguoren* , *Weicaoguo* .

Properties and Channel Distribution: The drug is pungent in taste, warm in nature, and distributed to the Spleen and Stomach Channels.

Action and Indications:

1. Resolving dampness and warming middle *Jiao*

To treat syndrome of cold–damp accumulating in the interior with pain and distension of the chest and abdomen, it can be used with Rhizoma Alpiniae Officinarum, Flos Caryophylli, Cortex Magnoliae Officinalis, etc.; to treat syndrome of accumulation of dampness in middle *Jiao* with pain and distension of episgatrium and abdomen or vomiting, with Rhizoma Atractylodis, Cortex Magnoliae Officinalis, etc.; to treat syndrome of retension of damp–phlegm, marked by headache and back pain, nausea and vomiting after meal, with Rhizoma Pinelliae Praeparatae, Pericarpium Citri Reticulatae, Rhizoma Arisaematis, etc.

2. Arresting onset of malaria

The drug can produce the effects of resolving dampness, dispersing cold and relieving malaria, especially due to predominant cold–dampness. To treat cold syndrome of spleen with malaria with heavy chilliness and lower fever, or with only chilliness but no fever, or diarrhea and anorexia, etc., it can be used with Radix

Aconiti Praeparata, Rhizoma Zingiberis Recens, Fructus Ziziphi Jujubae; to treat quotidian or tertian malaria with alternating chilliness and fever, accompanied with headache and flush face and thirst, it can be used with Radix Bupleuri, Radix Scutellariae, Radix Dichroae, etc.

Dosage and Administration: 3–6 g are decocted as a dose.

Notes: It is contraindicated in those patients with *Yin* –deficiency, and deficiency syndrome of the spleen and stomach not caused by cold–dampness.

6 Drugs for Inducing Diuresis and Resolving Dampness

Drugs with the main functions of promoting the flow in the water passage and removing dampness are called drugs for inducing diuresis and resolving dampness. Since they can promote discharge of urine and cause increase in its volume, they are also referred to as drugs for inducing diuresis. And they are mostly tasteless.

This kind of drugs can be generally divided into three categories: The first one is used to induce diuresis and relieve edema and has the functions of removing dampness and inducing diuresis, they are mainly used to treat retention of dampness, dysuria and edema; the second one is used to induce diuresis to treat stranguria and is used to treat difficulty and pain in urination or stranguria with turbid urine; the third one is used to remove dampness and to treat jaundice, thus it can be used to treat jaundice and lithiasis due to damp–heat. Some of the drugs can also be used to treat retention of phlegm, sore, eruption, arthralgia, diarrhea, etc. In short, this kind of drugs are usually used to remove retention of fluid and induce urination.

This kind of drugs can cause damage of *Yin* and consumption of body fluid, and therefore should not be used alone for those with dysuria or scanty urine due to deficiency in the source of urine, edema of asthenic type, and seminal emission without presence of damp-heat.

6.1 Drugs for Inducing Diuresis and Relieving Edema

Poria (茯苓 *Fuling*)
Poria

This drug consists of the dried sclerotium of the fungus, Poria cocos (schw.) wolf (family Polyporaceae). The crude drug is cut into slices or pieces for use. The external layer of the drug is called "poria peel,"; the light red part beneath the peel is called "red poria,"; the drug with it host wood, usually root of Pinus species attached, is called "poria with hostwood"; and the white part is called "white poria", i.e. the drug proper. Since the drug grown in Yunnan Province is most famous, it is also called *yunling* in TCM.

Nomenclature Used in Prescriptions: *Fuling* , *Baifuling* , *Yunling*

Properties and Channel Distribution: This drug is sweet and tasteless in taste and neutral in nature, and is distributed to the Heart, Spleen, Lung and Kidney Channels.

Action and Indications:

1. Inducing diuresis and removing dampness

In treating dysuria, edema, etc. due to retention of water, the drug is often used with Rhizoma Atractylodis Macrocephalae, Polyporus Umbellatus, Rhizoma Alismatis, Pericarpium Arecae, etc.

2. Invigorating the spleen and tonifying the middle warmer

In treating retention of phlegm, loose stool, etc. due to failure in transportation and transformation of water as a result of deficiency of the spleen, the drug is often used with Radix Codonopsis Pilosulae, Rhizoma Atractylodis Macrocephalae, Rhizoma Dioscoreae, etc.

3. Calming the mind

In treating palpitation and insomnia due to deficiency of the heart and spleen, the drug is often used with Radix Codonopsis Pilosulae, Arillus Longan, Semen Ziziphi Spinosae, etc.; in treating palpitation and insomnia (due to internal obstruction by turbid phlegm or breakdown of the normal physiological coordination between the heart and kidney), the drug is often used with Rhizoma Acori Graminei, Radix Polygalae, etc.

Dosage and Administration: Usually, 10–30 g of the drug is used in decoction.

Appendix: Poria peel (茯苓皮 *Fulingpi*)

This drug is similar to Poria in properties but is especially effective in inducing diuresis and relieving edema. It is often used to treat edema of the skin. The dosage is the same as that of Poria.

Umbellate Pore (猪苓 *Zhuling*)
Polyporus Umbellatus

This drug consists of the sclerotium of the fungus, Polyporus umbellatus (Pers.) Fries (family Polyporaceae). The crude drug is thoroughly moistened and softened, dried in shade and cut into slices for use.

Nomenclature Used in Prescriptions: *Zhuling* , *Fenzhuling* .

Properties and Channel Distribution: This drug is sweet and tasteless in taste and neutral in nature, and is distributed to the Kidney and Urinary Bladder Channels.

Action and Indications:

Inducing diuresis and removing dampness: This drug can be used to treat dysuria, painful stranguria, edema, diarrhea, leukorrhea, etc. This drug is especially effective for discharging water, with stronger effect of inducing diuresis and removing dampness than Poria. Since it is slightly cool in nature, it is usually used to treat disorders due to retention of water and dampness, accompanied with heat. The drug is often used with Poria, Rhizoma Alismatis, etc.

This drug may be used alone. For example, in treating edema of low limbs during pregnancy, the drug powder can be taken with warm water.

Dosage and Administration: Usually, 10–15 g of the drug is used in decoction.

Alismatis Rhizome (泽泻 *Zexie*)
Rhizoma Alismatis

This drug consists of the tuber of the perinnial marsh plant, Alisma Plantago–aquatica L. var. orientale (Sam.) Juzep. (family Alismataceae). The drug is cut into slices and dried in the sun. The crude drug or the drug parched with bran or salt is used.

Nomenclature Used in Prescriptions: *Zexie* , *Yanzexie* .

Properties and Channel Distribution: This drug is sweet and tasteless in taste and cold in nature, and is distributed to the Kidney and Urinary Bladder Channels.

Action and Indications:

Inducing diuresis, removing dampness and eliminating heat: This drug can be used to treat dysuria, edema, diarrhea, fluid retention, etc. In treating dysuria and edema, the drug is often used in combination with Polyporus Umbellatus and Poria. In treating fluid retention and dizziness, 24 g of the drug and 30 g of Rhizoma Atractylodis Macrocephalae can be decocted and taken. In treating diarrhea, the drug is often used with Rhizoma Atractylodis Macrocephalae, Polyporus Umbellatus, Semen Plantaginis, etc.

Dosage and Administration: Usually, 10–15 g of the drug is decocted. The drug parched with salt water is usually used.

Coix Seed (薏苡仁 *Yiyiren*)
Semen Coicis

This drug consists of the ripe seed of the annual or perennial herb, Coix lacryma-jobi L. var. ma-yuen (Roman) Stapf. (family Gramineae). The crude or parched drug is used.

Nomenclature Used in Prescriptions: *Yiyiren* , *Shenyiren* , *Chaoyiren*

Properties and Channel Distribution: This drug is sweet and tasteless in taste and slightly cold in nature, and is distributed to the Spleen, Lung and Kidney Channels.

Action and Indications:

1. Inducing diuresis and removing dampness

In treating dysuria, edema, beriberi, etc., the drug can be used with Radix Stephaniae Tetrandrae, Rhizoma Atractylodis, Semen Pruni, etc.

2. Removing dampness to treat arthralgia

In treating arthralgia due to damp-heat, the drug is often used with Rhizoma Atractylodis, Caulis Lonicerae, Cortex Phellodendri, etc.

3. Evacuating pus to treat abscess

In treating pulmonary abscess and periappendicular abscess, the drug can be used with Semen Persicae, Cortex Moutan Radicis, Rhizoma Phragmitis, etc. for the former, and Semen Persicae, Cortex Moutan Radicis, Caulis Sargentodoxae, Flos Lonicerae, etc. for the latter.

4. Invigorating the spleen to arrest diarrhea

In treating diarrhea due to dampness formed as a result of deficiency of the spleen, the drug is often used with Rhizoma Atractylodis Macrocephalae, Poria, Rhizoma Dioscoreae, etc. In treating leukorrhea due to excess of dampness, with Rhizoma Dioscoreae, Semen Euryales, etc.

Dosage and Administration: Usually, 15-30 g of the drug is decocted. The crude drug is used to remove damp-heat, and the parched drug can be used to arrest diarrhea. The drug can also be cooked into a thick soup or gruel with polished nonglutinous rice and eaten at the meals as a medicated diet.

Plantain Seed (车前子 *Cheqianzi*)
Semen Plantaginis

This drug consists of the ripe seed of the perennial herb, Plantago asiatica L. or P. depressa Willa. (family Plantaginaceae). The drug is dried in the sun and the crude drug or the drug parched with salt water is used.

Nomenclature Used in Prescriptions: *Cheqianzi*, *Chaocheqian*

Properties and Channel Distribution: This drug is sweet in taste and slightly cold in nature, and is distributed to the Liver, Kidney, Lung and Small Intestine Channels.

Action and Indications:

1. Inducing diuresis to treat stranguria

In treating edema, dysuria, stranguria with burning pain and blood, etc., the drug is often used with Herba Dianthi, Caulis Akebiae, Herba Polygoni Avicularis, Talcum, etc.

2. Removing dampness to arrest diarrhea

In treating vomiting and diarrhea due to summer–heat, and dysuria, the drug is often used with Herba Elsholtziae seu Moslae, Poria, Polyporus Umbellatus, etc.

3. Clearing away heat from the liver and improving vision

In treating conjunctival congestion due to liver–heat, the drug can be used with Flos Chrysanthemi, Flos Buddlejae, Radix Scutellariae, Radix Gentianae, etc.

4. Clearing away heat from the lung and resolving phlegm

In treating cough with profuse sputum, the drug can be used in combination with Radix Platycodi, Semen Armeniacae Amarum, Radix Asteris, etc.

Dosage and Administration: Usually, 9–15 g of the drug is decocted.

Waxgourd Peel (冬瓜皮 *Dongguapi*)
Exocarpium Benincasae

This drug consists of the exocarp of the annual herb, Benincasa hispida (Thunb.) Cogn. (family Cucurbitaceae). The crude drug is used.

Nomenclature Used in Prescriptions: *Dongguapi*

Properties and Channel Distribution: This drug is sweet in taste and slightly cold in nature, and is distributed to the Lung and Small Intestine Channels.

Action and Indications:

Clearing away heat, inducing diuresis and relieving edema: In treating skin edema, distention and dysuria, the drug is often used with Poria, Semen Plantaginis, etc.

Dosage and Administration: Usually, 15–30 g of the drug is used in decoction.

Appendix: Semen Benincasae (冬瓜子 *Dongguazi*)

This drug consists of the seeds of waxgourd. The crude or parched drug is broken for use. The drug is similar to waxgourd peel in taste and nature. It has the effect of clearing away heat in the lung to resolve phlegm, removing dampness to evacuate pus and relieving diarrhea, and can be used to treat cough due to lung–heat, pulmonary abscess, periappendicular abscess, stranguria, leukorrhea, etc. The dosage is 15–30 g.

Red Bean (赤小豆 *Chixiaodou*)
Semen Phaseoli

This drug consists of the ripe seed of the annual climbing herbage, Phaseolus calcaratus Roxb. or P. angularis Wight (family Leguminosae). The crude drug is dried in the sun for use.

Nomenclature Used in Prescriptions: *Chixiaodou, Hongxiaodou*

Properties and Channel Distribution: This drug is sweet and sour in taste and neutral in nature, and is distributed to the Heart and Small Intestine Channels.

Action and Indications:

1. Inducing diuresis and relieving edema

In treating edema, dysuria, beriberi, etc., the drug is often cooked with carp and taken. In treating edema of deficiency type, the drug is often decocted in combination with peanuts, Fructus Ziziphi Jujubae, etc. and taken for a long time.

2. Removing toxin and evacuating pus

In treating carbuncle at the initial stage manifested by redness, swelling and burning pain, the drug powder can be mixed with water or vinegar and applied to the local area. The drug can also be taken orally.

Besides, the drug is also used to treat jaundice due to damp–heat. Nowadays, it is used to treat nephritic edema, ascites due to cirrhosis, and edema due to malnutrition.

Dosage and Administration: Usually, 15–30 g of the drug is decocted. Proper amount of the drug can be used in external treatment.

6.2 Drugs for Inducing Diuresis to Treat Stranguria

Prostrate Knotweed (萹蓄 *Bianxu*)
Herba Polygoni Avicularis

This drug consists of the whole plant of the annual herb, Polygonum aviculare L. (family Polygonaceae). The crude drug is cut into pieces for use.

Nomenclature Used in Prescriptions: *Bianxu* , *Bianxucao*

Properties and Channel Distribution: This drug is bitter in taste and slightly cold in nature, and is distributed to the Urinary Bladder Channel.

Action and Indications:

1. Inducing diuresis to treat stranguria

In treating scanty dark urine, dribbling urination and burning pain of the urethra, the drug is often used with Herba Dianthi, Talcum, Caulis Akebiae, etc.; in treating stranguria with blood, with Herba seu Radix Cirsii Japonici, Herba Cephalanoploris, Rhizoma Imperatae, etc.

2. Destroying parasite and relieving itching

In treating eczema, Trichomonas vaginalis and pruritus genitalium, the drug decoction can be used to wash the local area.

Dosage and Administration: Usually, 10–30 g of the drug is used in decoction.

Chinese Pink Herb (瞿麦 *Qumai*)
Herba Dianthi

This drug consists of the whole plant (with flower) of the perennial herb, Dianthus Superbus L. and Dianthus chinensis L. (family Caryophyllaceae). The crude drug is cut into pieces for use.

Nomenclature Used in Prescriptions: *Qumai* , *Qumaisui*

Properties and Channel Distribution: This drug is bitter in taste and cold in nature, and is distributed to the Heart and Small Intestine Channels.

Action and Indications:

1. Inducing diuresis to treat stranguria

In treating stranguria due to heat, dribbling urination with burning pain or hematuria, the drug is often used in combination with Herba Polygoni Avicularis Fructus Gardeniae, Talcum, etc.

2. Activating blood circulation to restore menstrual flow

In treating amenorrhea due to stasis of blood, the drug can be used in combination with Radix Salviae Miltiorrhizae, Radix Paeoniae Rubra, Herba Leonuri, Flos Carthami, etc.

Dosage and Administration: Usually, 10–30 g of the drug is used in decoction.

Notes: This drug is contraindicated in pregnant women.

Manshurian Aristolochia Stem (木通 *Mutong*) Caulis Aristolochiae Manshuriensis

This drug consists of the stem of the deciduous woody liana, Akebia trifoliata (Thunb.) Koidz. var. australis (Diels) Rehd. (family lardizabalaceae), the liana, Hocguartia manshuriensis (Komar.) Nakai (family Aristolochiaceae), or the evergreen climbing thrub, Clematis armandii Franch and C. montana Buch.–Ham. (family Ranunculaceae). The crude drug is cut into slices for use.

Nomenclature Used in Prescriptions: *Mutong*, *Ximutong*

Properties and Channel Distribution: This drug is bitter in taste and cold in nature, and is distributed to the Heart, Lung, Small Intestine and Urinary Bladder Channels.

Action and Indications:

1. Removing fire and inducing diuresis

In treating dribbling urination with blood and burning pain, sores or the mouth and lip, vexation, etc., the drug is often used with Radix Rehmanniae, Herba Lophatheri and the tip of Radix Glycyrrhizae; In treating flaccidity and edema of the feet and dysuria, with Polyporus Umbellatus, Folium Perillae, Semen Arecae, etc.

2. Removing obstruction in the blood vessels

In treating galactostasis, the drug can be used with Medulla Tetrapanacis, Radix Rhapontici seu Echinopsis, Semen Vaccariae, pig's trotters, etc.; In treating amenorrhea due to stasis of blood, with Radix Salviae Miltiorrhizae, Radix Achyranthis Bidentatae, Semen Persicae, Pollen Typhae, etc.; in treating arthralgia due to damp–heat, with Caulis Lonicerae, Cortex Erythrinae, Ramulus Mori, etc.

Dosage and Administration: Usually, 3–6 g of the drug is used in decoction.

Notes: According to the clinical report, administration of large dosage (60 g) may cause acute renal failure. Therefore, overdosage is forbidden. Pregnant women should take the drug cautiously.

Ricepaper Pith (通草 *Tongcao*)
Medulla Tetrapanacis

This drug consists of the pith of the shrub, Tetrapanax papyriferus (Hook.) K. Koch. (family Araliaceae). The crude drug is dried in the sun and cut into slices for use.

Nomenclature Used in Prescriptions: *Tongcao*, *Baitongcao*, *Fangtongcao*.

Properties and Channel Distribution: This drug is sweet and tasteless in taste and cold in nature, and is distributed to the Lung and Stomach Channels.

Action and Indications:

1. Clearing away heat and inducing diuresis

In treating dysuria due to damp–heat, the drug is often used in combination with Herba Lophatheri, Talcum, etc.

2. Promoting lactation

In treating galactostasis, the drug is often used with pig's trotters, Squama Manitis, Rhizoma Ligustici Chuanxiong and Radix Glycyrrhizae.

Dosage and Administration: Usually, 6–10 g of the drug is used in decoction.

Notes: This drug is contraindicated in pregnant women.

Rush Pith (灯心草 *Dengxincao*) Medulla Junci

This drug consists of the pith of the perennial herb, Juncus effusua L. var. decipiens Buchen. (family Juncaeae). The crude drug is cut into segments for use.

Nomenclature Used in Prescriptions: *Dengxincao* , *Dengxin* , *Dengcao* .

Properties and Channel Distribution: This drug is sweet and tasteless in taste and slightly cold in nature, and is distributed to the Heart, Lung and Small Intestine Channels.

Action and Indications:

1. Clearing away heat and inducing diuresis

In treating stranguria due to heat, the drug can be used in combination with Fructus Gardeniae, Talcum, the tip of Radix Glycyrrhizae, etc. Since this drug is quite mild in its effect, it is only used for mild cases, or used with other drugs for clearing away heat and inducing diuresis.

2. Clearing away heat in the heart to relieve vexation

In treating vexation and night crying of children due to heart–heat, this drug can be used with Herba Lophatheri, put into boiling water and drunk instead of tea.

Dosage and Administration: Usually, 3–5 g of the drug is used in decoction.

Broom Cypress Fruit (地肤子 *Difuzi*)
Fructus Kochiae

This drug consists of the fruit of the annual herb, Kochia scoparia (L.) Schrad. (family Chenopodiaceae). The crude drug is used.

Nomenclature Used in Prescriptions: *Difuzi*

Properties and Channel Distribution: This drug is pungent and bitter in taste and cold in nature, and is distributed to the Kidney and Urinary Bladder Channels.

Action and Indications:

1. Removing damp–heat and inducing diuresis

In treating dysuria due to damp–heat, the drug is often used in combination with Herba Dianthi, Polyporus Umbellatus, Talcum, Radix Glycyrrhizae, etc.

2. Dispelling wind to relieve itching

In treating pruritus, eczema, urticaria, scabies, etc., the drug is often used in combination with Cortex Dictamni Radicis, Periostracum Cicadae, Herba Menthae, Herba Schizonepetae, etc.; in treating vaginitis and vulvitis, the decoction of the drugs,

Fructus Kochiae, Fructus Cnidii, Radix Sophorae Flavescentis, Alumen and Pericarpium Zanthoxyli, can be used to wash the local area.

Dosage and Administration: Usually, 10–12 g of the drug is used in decoction. A proper amount of the drug can be used in external treatment.

Cluster Mallow Fruit (冬葵子 *Dongkuizi*)
Fructus Malvae Vertillatae

This drug consists of the fruit of the annual or perennial herb, Malva verticillata L. (family Malvaceae). The crude drug is broken into pieces for use.

Nomenclature Used in Prescriptions: *Dongkuizi*

Properties and Channel Distribution: This drug is sweet in taste and cold in nature, and is distributed to the Small Intestine and Large Intestine Channels.

Action and Indications:

1. Inducing diuresis to treat stranguria

In treating dysuria and stranguria with pain, the drug can be used with Poria, Semen Plantaginis, Caulis Akebiae, etc.; in treating stranguria caused by urinary stone, with Talcum, Lumbricus, etc.; in treating edema, heaviness in the limbs and dysuria during pregnancy, with Poria.

2. Promoting lactation

In treating galactostasis with distention and pain of the breast, 12 g of the drug, 12 g of Semen Vaccariae, 15 g of Radix Rhapontici seu Echinopsis and two pig's trotters are cooked together, and the soup can be drunk and the trotters eaten.

Besides, this drug can also moisten the intestine and therefore is used to treat constipation.

Dosage and Administration: Usually, 10–15 g of the drug is decocted.

Pyrrosia Leaf (石苇 *Shiwei*)
Folium Pyrrosiae

This drug consists of the leaf of the perennial evergreen herb, Pyrrosia lingua (Thunb.) Farw., Pyrrosia sheareri (Bak.) Ching, or P. petiolosa (christ) Ching. (family Polypodiaceae). The crude drug is cut into pieces for use.

Nomenclature Used in Prescriptions: *Shiwei*

Properties and Channel Distribution: This drug is sweet and bitter in taste and slightly cold in nature, and is distributed to the Lung and Urinary Bladder Channels.

Action and Indications:

1. Inducing diuresis to treat stranguria

In treating stranguria due to heat, hematuria, uropsammus, etc., the drug is often used with Semen Plantaginis, Talcum, Caulis Akebiae, Herba Dianthi, etc.

2. Clearing away heat and arresting bleeding

In treating metrorrhagia, metrostaxis and hemoptysis due to blood–heat, 30 g of the drug can be decocted and taken.

In addition, the drug decocted alone with addition of crystal sugar can be used to treat cough and asthma due to lung–heat, bronchitis and bronchial asthma, with some effect.

Dosage and Administration: Usually 6–10 g of the drug is decocted.

Climbing Fern Spore (海金沙 *Haijinsha*)
Spora Lygodii

This drug consists of the ripe spore of the perennial climbing fern, Lygodium japonicum (Thunb.) Sw. (family Lygodiaceae). The crude drug is used.

Nomenclature Used in Prescriptions: *Haijinsha*

Properties and Channel Distribution: This drug is sweet and salty in taste and cold in nature, and is distributed to the Urinary Bladder and Small Intestine Channels.

Action and Indications:

Inducing diuresis to treat stranguria: This drug can be used to treat galacturia, uropsammus, stranguria from urolithiasis, stranguria due to heat, etc. This drug is especially effective in removing obstruction in the water passages and therefore is a main drug for treating stranguria with painful urination. It can be used in combination with Talcum, Radix Glycyrrhizae, Herba Lysimachiae, etc.

Besides, the drug is also used nowadays to treat nephritic edema.

Dosage and Administration: Usually, 6–12 g of the drug is used in decoction. The drug is wrapped in cloth before being decocted.

Seven-lobed Yam (萆薢 *Bixie*)
Rhizoma Dioscoreae Septemlobae

This drug consists of the rhizome of the perennial twining

liana, Dioscorea hypoglauca palib. and Dioscorea officinalis Tsi. mss. (family Dioscoriaceae). The crude drug is cut into slices and dried in the sun for use.

Nomenclature Used in Prescriptions: *Bixie* , *Fenbixie* .

Properties and Channel Distribution: This drug is bitter in taste and neutral in nature, and is distributed to the Kidney and Stomach Channels.

Action and Indications:

1. Removing dampness and treating turbid urine

In treating turbid urine from galacturia, dribbling urination, frequent urination and leukorrhea due to hyperactivity of dampness, the drug is often used in combination with Poria, Rhizoma Acori Graminei, Radix Linderae, etc.

2. Relieving arthralgia

In treating arthralgia due to wind–dampness and pain of the joints and muscles of the loin and spine, the drug can be used in combination with Radix Achyranthis Bidentatae, Rhizoma Atractylodis Macrocephalae, Radix Aconiti Praeparata, etc.

Dosage and Administration: Usually, 6–10 g of the drug is used in decoction.

Talc (滑石 *Huashi*)
Talcum

This drug consists of a soft mineral composed mainly of hydrous magnesium silicate (monoclinic system). The mineral is ground into powder or refined with water for use.

Nomenclature Used in Prescriptions: *Huashi* , *Feihuashi*

Properties and Channel Distribution: This drug is sweet and tasteless in taste and cold in nature, and is distributed to the Urinary Bladder and Stomach Channels.

Action and Indications:

1. Inducing diuresis to treat stranguria

In treating stranguria due to heat and stranguria caused by urinary stone, the drug can be used in combination with Caulis Akebiae, Spora Lygodii, Herba Lysimachiae, etc.

2. Clearing away summer–heat

In treating vexation, thirst, dribbling urination or watery diarrhea due to invasion of summer–heat, the drug is often used with Radix Glycyrrhizae.

3. Removing dampness to treat eczema

In treating eczema, the drug is often ground into powder with Alumen, Cortex Phellodendri, etc. and applied to the local area. This drug is also a main ingredient in the prickly–heat powder.

This drug can be used to treat lithiasis of the urinary system. It is cold and slippery in nature and therefore may facilitate removal of stones.

Dosage and Administration: Usually, 10–15 g of the drug is decocted. In treating urolithiasis, the dosage may increase up to 24–30 g. Proper amount of the drug can be used locally.

6.3 Drugs for Removing Dampness to Treat Jaundice

Oriental Wormwood (茵陈蒿 *Yinchenhao*)
Herba Artemisiae Capillaris

This drug consists of the young shoot of the perennial herb, Artemisia capillaris Thunb, or Artemisia scoparia Waldst. et Kit. (family Compositae). The crude drug is dried in the sun for use.

Nomenclature Used in Prescriptions: *Yinchenhao* , *Yinchen* , *Mianyinchen*

Properties and Channel Distribution: This drug is bitter in taste and slightly cold in nature, and is distributed to the Spleen, Stomach, Liver and Gall Bladder Channels.

Action and Indications:

Clearing away heat, removing dampness and treating jaundice

This drug is used to treat jaundice due to damp–heat. The drug is especially effective in clearing away heat, removing dampness and treating jaundice and is the main drug for jaundice. If the disease is due to damp–heat and manifested by bright yellow body and eye, fever and scanty dark urine, the drug can be used in combination with Fructus Gardeniae, and Radix et Rhizoma Rhei; if the disease is due to cold–dampness and manifested by dark yellow body, poor appetite, stuffy epigastrium, listlessness and aversion to cold, the drug can be used with Radix·Aconiti Praeparata, Rhizoma Zingiberis, etc.

Besides, the drug can also be used to treat eczema with itching sensation and discharge of yellow water, and is often used with Radix Sophorae Flavescentis, etc.

This drug is used nowadays to treat acute or chronic infectious icterohepatitis, hepatocirrhosis, cholelithiasis, cholecystitis, etc. It has the effect of normalizing functioning of the gall bladder and therefore can be used with Fructus Mume to treat biliary ascariasis.

Dosage and Administration: Usually, 15–30 g of the drug is decocted.

Lysimachia (金钱草 *Jinqiancao*)
Herba Lysimachiae

This drug consists of the whole plant of the perennial herb, Lysimachia christinae Hance (family Primulaceae). The fresh plant or the plant dried and cut into pieces is used.

Nomenclature Used in Prescriptions: *Jinqiancao*

Properties and Channel Distribution: This drug is sweet and tastelessness in taste and neutral in nature, and is distributed to the Liver, Gall Bladder, Kidney and Urinary Bladder Channels.

Action and Indications:

1. Removing dampness to treat jaundice

In treating jaundice due to damp–heat, the drug can be used in combination with Herba Artemisiae Capillaris, Fructus Gardeniae, etc.

2. Treating stranguria and removing stones

This drug can be used to treat stranguria due to heat, stranguria from urolithiasis and stranguria caused by urinary stones. This drug is the main drug for lithiasis of the urinary system. In treating lithiasis of the urinary bladder and ureter, 60 g of the drug can be decocted and taken frequently everyday instead of tea, or the drug can be used with Spora Lygodii, Talcum, Endothelium Corneum Gigeriae Galli, etc.; in treating renal lithiasis, the drug can be used with Folium Pyrrosiae, Asteriscus Pseudosciaenae, cortex Eucommiae, Semen Juglandis, etc. This drug has the effect of normalizing functioning of gall bladder and removing stones, and therefore is often used with Herba Artemisiae Scopariae, Radix Curcumae, Fructus Gardeniae, etc. to treat hepatolith; in treating lithiasis, the drug should be taken persistently for at least one month.

3. Removing toxin and subduing swelling

In treating furuncle and pyogenic infection, a small cup of the juice of the drug (about 50 ml.) prepared by pounding the fresh drug can be drunk (25 ml of the juice at a time); in treating scald and burns, the juice can be applied to the local area.

Dosage and Administration: Usually, 30–60 g of the drug, or 150–300 g of the fresh drug, is used in decoction. The maximum dosage is 120–150 g. A proper amount of the drug can be used locally.

7 Drugs for warming the Interior

Drugs with the functions of warming the interior to dispel cold and supplementing fire to restore yang are called drugs for warming the interior; or drugs for dispelling cold in the interior.

This kind of drugs are pungent in taste and heat in nature and has the functions of warming the middle *Jiao* to dispel cold and warming the kidney to restore yang. They are used to treat diseases due to internal cold. Internal cold involves two aspects: The first refers to invasion of the interior by cold, which affects *Yang–Qi*, thus cold syndrome of the internal organs occurs and is manifested by hiccups, vomiting, diarrhea, coldness and pain of the chest and abdomen, poor appetite, etc., for which the method of warming middle *Jiao* to dispel cold and regulate preponderant *Yin* should be used; the second refers to that the Kidney–*Yang* is weak and the internal cold forms, thus syndrome of exhaustion of *Yang* and collapse occur and is then manifested by sweating, aversion to cold, feeling of cold air breathed out during respiration, diarrhea, cold limbs, feeble pulse, etc., for which the method of warming the kidney to restore *Yang* should be used to supplement the source of fire.

In using this kind of drugs, proper compatibility of drugs should be considered in accordance with different disease conditions. For example, for diseases due to invasion of exogenous cold into the interior, both this kind of drugs and drugs for relieving exterior syndrome should be used; for diseases due to accumulation of cold and stasis of *Qi*, drugs for promoting flow of *Qi* should also be used; for diseases due to internal accumulation of cold–dampness, drugs for invigorating the spleen and resolving dampness should also be used; for diseases due to deficiency of *Yang* of the spleen and kidney, drugs for warming and tonifying the spleen and kidney should also be used; for diseases due to exhaustion of yang and collapse of *Qi*, drugs for tonifying the primordial *Qi* should also be used.

This kind of drugs are warm, hot, dry and drastic in nature and may exhaust *Yin* and assist fire. Therefore, they should not be used for diseases due to hyperactivity of *Yang* and deficiency of *Yin*, or diseases with real internal heat but false exterior cold. Also, the dosage of this kind of drugs should vary with the climatic conditions.

Prepared Aconite Root (附子 *Fuzi*) Radix Aconiti Praeparata

This drug consists of the processed secondary root of the perennial herb, Aconitum carmichaeli Debx. (family Ranunculaceae). The crude drug is cut into slices for use.

Nomenclature Used in Prescriptions: *Shufuzi*, *Paofuzi*, *Chuanfuzi*, *Danfuzi*, *Shengfuzi*

Properties and Channel Distribution: This drug is pungent in taste and greatly hot in nature with toxicity, and is distributed to the Heart, Kidney and Spleen Channels.

Action and Indications:

1. Recuperating depleted *Yang* and rescuing the patient from collapse

In treating syndrome of exhaustion of *Yang* and collapse, manifested by cold limbs, feeble pulse, cold sweating, severe vomiting or severe diarrhea, the drug is often used in combination with Rhizoma Zingiberis and Radix Glycyrrhizae; in treating cold limbs, abdominal pain, vomiting, diarrhea, etc. due to invasion of cold into the interior, the drug can be used with Rhizoma Zingiberis, Cortex Cinnamomi, Radix Ginseng, etc. In treating persistent cold sweating due to failure of superficial defence as a result of exhaustion of *Yang*, the drug can be used with Radix Astragali seu Hedysari Praeparata. In treating prostration due to bleeding and exhaustion of *Yang*, the drug can be used in combination with Radix Ginseng.

2. Reenforcing *Yang* and inducing diuresis

In treating exhaustion of kidney–*Yang* manifested by general edema (more severe below the loin), pain, soreness and heaviness of the loin, oliguria, etc., the drug is often used with Rhizoma Atractylodis Macrocephalae, Poria, etc.; in treating deficiency of spleen–*Yang* manifested by edema of limbs, abdominal distention, loose stool, etc., the drug is often used with Rhizoma Zingiberis, Rhizoma Atractylodis Macrocephalae, Fructus Tsaoko, etc.

3. Dispelling cold to relieve pain

In treating arthralgia due to wind, cold and dampness, the drug is often used in combination with Ramulus Cinnamomi, Rhizoma Atractylodis Macrocephalae, etc.; in treating hyperactivity of internal cold and coldness and pain of the epigastrium and abdomen, with Rhizoma Zingiberis, Radix

Codonopsis Pilosulae, Rhizoma Atractylodis Macrocephalae, etc.

Dosage and Administration: Usually, 3–12 g of the drug is decocted. The crude drug is rather drastic and is used to recuperate depleted *Yang* to rescue the patient from collapse.The processed drug has less powerful toxicity and is used to supplement *yang* and dispel cold. The drug (crude or prepared) should be decocted for at least one hour to reduce its toxicity.

Notes: This drug is rather drastic and therefore should not be taken by those without hyperactivity of *Yin* and deficiency of *Yang* or with deficiency of *Yin* and internal heat, or by pregnant women. The drug is antagonized by Rhizoma Pinelliae, Fructus Trichosanthis, Radix Ampelopsis, Rhizoma Bletillae, Bulbus Fritillariae Thunbergii and Cornu Rhinoceri.

Appendix: Radix Aconiti, Radix Aconiti Kusnezoffii(川乌头, 草乌头 *Chuanwutou, Caowutou*)

They are the tuberous roots of the perennial herb, Aconitum carmichaeli Debx., and A. kusnezoffii Reichb. (family Ranunculaceae) respectively. The processing method for them is the same as that for Radix Aconiti praeparata. Radix Aconiti is similar to Radix Aconiti praeparata in properties and actions, being less effective in supplementing *Yang* but more effective in dispelling wind to treat arthralgia. There is therefore such an ancient saying, "Radix Aconiti Praeparata is used to dispel cold while Radix Aconiti, to dispel wind." It is quite effective in treating arthralgia with soreness, pain and numbness due to wind, cold and dampness, and coldness and pain of the epigastrium and stomach. It has strong toxicity (Radix Aconiti Kusnezoffii has even stronger toxicity) and therefore should be used with care. The dosage is 3–9 g. The dosage and notes are the same as those for Radix Aconiti praeparata.

Dried Ginger (干姜 *Ganjiang*)
Rhizoma Zingiberis

This drug consists of the rhizome of the perennial herb, Zingiber officinale Rosc. (family Zingiberaceae). The drug may be either cut into slices, or cut into pieces and baked till it turns brown, for use.

Nomenclature Used in Prescriptions: *Ganjiang*, *Danganjiang*, *Ganjiangpian*

Properties and Channel Distribution: This drug is pungent in taste and hot in nature, and is distributed to the Heart, Lung, Spleen and Stomach Channels.

Action and Indications:

1. Warming the middle *Jiao* to restore *Yang*

In treating deficiency of *Yang* of the spleen and stomach, manifested by diarrhea with undigested food in the stool, cold limbs, feeble pulse, flushed face and vexation, the drug can be used in combination with Radix Aconiti Praeparata and Bulbus Allii Fistulosi; in treating diarrhea due to cold syndrome of deficiency type of the spleen and stomach with loose and odourless stool, borborygmus and abdominal pain, equal amount of the drug and Rhizoma Alpiniae Officinarum can be made into pills with water, and 3–6 g of the pills can be taken with warm water, or the drug can be used with Radix Codonopsis Pilosulae, Rhizoma Atractylodis Macrocephalae and Radix Glycyrrhizae.

2. Warming the lung and resolving phlegm

In treating cough and asthma due to accumulation of cold,

the drug is often used in combination with Herba Ephedrae, Rhizoma Pinelliae, Herba Asari, Fructus Schisandrae, etc.

Dosage and Administration: Usually, 3–10 g of the drug is used in decoction.

Notes: This drug should not be taken by those with heat syndrome and deficiency of *Yin*, or by pregnant women.

Appendix: Baked Ginger (炮姜 *Paojiang*)

This drug is also called *Heijiang* and *Paojiangtan* in TCM. It is bitter in taste and warm in nature with milder effect. It has the effect of warming the channels and arresting bleeding, and can be used to treat hematemesis, hemafecia, metrorrhagia, etc. due to cold of deficiency type. The drug should not be taken by those with bleeding due to hyperactivity of blood–heat as a result of deficiency of *Yin*. The dosage is 1.5–6 g.

Cinnamon Bark (肉桂 *Rougui*)
Cortex Cinnamomi

This drug consists of the bark of the evergreen arbor, Cinnamomum cassia Presl (family Lauraceae). The drug is cut into slices or ground into powder for use.

Nomenclature Used in Prescriptions: *Rougui*, *Ziyougui*, *Guixin*

Properties and Channel Distributions: This drug is pungent and sweet in taste and greatly hot in nature, and is distributed to the Liver, Kidney, Heart, Spleen and Stomach Channels.

Action and Indications:

1. Supplementing fire and assisting *Yang*

In treating exhaustion of kidney–*Yang* manifested by aversion to cold, cold limbs, flaccidity of loin and feet, impotence, dysuria, etc., the drug is often used in combination with Radix Aconiti Praeparata, Radix Rehmanniae Praeparata, Rhizoma Dioscoreae, Fructus Corni, etc.; in treating abdominal pain and diarrhea due to deficiency of *Yang* of the spleen and kidney, with Rhizoma Zingiberis, Radix Aconiti Praeparata, Semen Myristicae, Poria, etc.

2. Dispelling cold and relieving pain

In treating gastralgia, abdominal pain, hernia, etc. due to cold syndrome of deficiency type, the drug can be ground into powder and taken, or the drug can be used with other drugs for warming the middle *Jiao* to dispel cold; in treating dysmenorrhea due to cold of deficiency type, with Radix Angelicae Sinensis, Rhizoma Zingiberis, Radix Rehmanniae Praeparata, etc.

In addition, small amount of the drug can be used in prescriptions for treating deficiency of *Qi* and blood, to invigorate *Qi* and blood. Examples of the prescriptions are "Ginseng Nutrition Decoction" and "Decoction of Ten Powerful Tonics," which are used to treat deficiency of *Qi* and blood, "Powder for Removing Toxin" and "*Yang*–Activating Decoction," which are used to treat longlasting sores and ulceration, and "Tongguan Pill," which is used to treat dysuria due to damp–heat in the lower warmer.

Dosage and Administration: Usually, 2–5 g of the drug is used in decoction. The drug is usually ground into powder and taken with water. When used in decoction, the drug should be decocted after other drugs are decocted for some time.

Notes: This drug should not be taken by those with deficiency of *Yin* and hyperactivity of fire, excess heat in the interior, or hyperactivity of blood–heat, or by pregnant women.

Galangal Rhizome (高良姜 *Gaoliangjiang*)
Rhizoma Alpiniae Officinarum

This drug consists of the rhizome of the perennial herb, Alpinia officinarum Hance (family Zingiberaceae).The crude drug is cut into slices for use.

Nomenclature Used in Prescriptions: *Gaoliangjiang*, *Liangjiang*, *Liangjiangpian*

Properties and Channel Distribution: This drug is pungent in taste and hot in nature, and is distributed to the Spleen and Stomach Channels.

Action and Indications:

1. Dispelling cold and relieving pain

In treating intermittent gastralgia due to cold, the drug can be made into pills with equal amount of Rhizoma Cyperi, and 6 g of the pills can be taken with water; in treating coldness and colicky and stabbing pain of the epigastrium and abdomen and distention of the hypochondrium, the drug is often used with Cortex Magnoliae Officinalis, Lignum Cinnamomi, etc., or with Faeces Trogopterorum. In treating hernia with abdominal pain due to cold, the drug can be used with Fructus Foeniculi.

2. Warming the middle warmer to arrest vomiting

In treating hiccups due to stomach cold, vomiting of clear water, cold limbs, etc., 6 g of the drug and 6 Chinese dates can be decocted and taken.

Dosage and Administration: Usually, 3–6 g of the drug is decocted.

Evodia Fruit (吴茱萸 *Wuzhuyu*)
Fructus Euodiae

This drug consists of the nearly matured fruit of the evergreen thrub or arbor, Evodia rutaecarpa (Juss). Benth. (family Rutaecae). The drug is bake–stirred either with salt water or decoction of Radix Glycyrrhizae for use.

Nomenclature Used in Prescriptions: *Wuzhuyu*, *Wuyu*, *Danwuyu*

Properties and Channel Distribution: This drug is pungent and bitter in taste and hot in nature, and is distributed to the Liver. Kidney, Spleen and Stomach Channels.

Action and Indications:

1. Dispelling cold and arresting diarrhea

In treating frequent attacks of cold ness and pain of the head which lasts a long time accompanied by salivation, the drug is often used with Radix Codonopsis Pilosulae, Rhizoma Zingiberis Recens, etc.; in treating painful hernia due to cold, 5 g of the drug, 6 g of Fructus Foeniculi, 9 g of Fructus Meliae Toosendan and 3 g of Radix Aucklandiae can be decocted and taken; in treating abdominal pain, vexation and mental confusion due to ascending of cold–dampness of beriberi, the drug can be used with Fructus Chaenomelis, Semen Arecae and Rhizoma Zingiberis Recens.

2. Sending down *Qi* to arrest vomiting

In treating cold syndrome of deficiency type of the stomach manifested by vomiting after meals, abdominal pain or retching with salivation, the drug is often used with Radix Codonopsis

Pilosulae and Rhizoma Zingiberis Recens; in treating acid regurgitation after meals and coldness and pain of the chest and abdomen, the drug can be ground into powder with an equal amount of baked ginger; in treating hypochondriac pain, acid regurgitation, vomiting, etc. due to attack of liver–fire on the stomach, the drug is often made into pills with Rhizoma Coptidis.

Besides, the drug powder can be mixed with vinegar and applied to the sole to induce fire to go down. This method can be used to treat sores of the mouth and lip.

Dosage and Administration: Usually, 1–5 g of the drug is used in decoction.Proper amount of the drug can be used in external treatment. Generally, the drug is parched with the decoction of Radix Glycyrrhizae for use; and the drug parched with salt water is used to treat hernia.

Common Fennel Fruit (小茴香 *Xiaohuixiang*) Fructus Foeniculi

This drug consists of the ripe fruit of the perennial herb Foeniculum Vulgare Mill. (family Umbelliferae). The drug is parched with salt water for use.

Nomenclature Used in Prescriptions: *Xiaohuixiang*

Properties and Channel Distribution: This drug is pungent and sweet in taste and warm in nature, and is distributed to the Liver, Kidney, Spleen and Stomach Channels.

Action and Indications:

1. Dispelling cold and relieving pain

In treating abdominal pain and hernia due to cold, the drug

can be used with Cortex Cinnamomi, Lignum Aquilariae Resinatum, Radix Linderae, etc.; in treating hernia with swelling of the testis, which is extremely painful, the drug can be used with Semen Litchi, Fructus Meliae Toosendan, etc. In treating edema of scrotum and swelling of testis, 30 g of the drug, 30 g of Semen Plantaginis and 6 g of table salt can be ground into fine powder, and 6 g of the powder is to be taken with millet wine at a time, twice a day.

2. Regulating the flow of *Qi* in the stomach

In treating abdominal pain due to cold in the stomach, hiccups and poor appetite, 30 g of the drug and 60 g of ginger can be parched till they turn brown, ground into powder, mixed with wine and made into pills, and 6 g of the pills can be taken at a time, twice a day.

Dosage and Administration: Usually, 6–10 g of the drug is used in decoction.

Notes: This drug should not be taken by those with deficiency of *Yin* and hyperactivity of fire.

Cloves (丁香 *Dingxiang*)
Flos Caryophylli

This drug consists of the flower and fruit of the evergreen arbor, Syzygium aromaticum (L.) Merr. et Perry (family Myrtaceae). The crude drug is used.

Nomenclature Used in Prescriptions: *Gongdingxiang*, *Mudingxiang*

Properties and Channel Distribution: This drug is pungent in taste and warm in nature, and is distributed to the Lung, Stomach, Spleen and Kidney Channels.

Action and Indications:

1. Warming the middle *Jiao* and sending down *Qi*

This drug is the main drug for treating hiccups due to cold of deficiency type.In treating vomiting and hiccups due to cold syndrome of the stomach, infantile vomiting of milk, etc., 1.5 g of the drug, 5 persimmon calyxes, 9 g of Radix Codonopsis Pilosulae and 9 g of ginger can be decocted and taken; in treating vomiting, diarrhea and poor appetite due to cold of deficiency type of the spleen and stomach, the drug can be used with Fructus Amomi, Rhizoma Atractylodis Macrocephalae, etc.

2. Sending down *Qi* and relieving pain

In treating sensation of gas rushing with pain of the chest and abdomen, the drug can be used with Fructus Schisandrae and Rhizoma Zedoariae; In treating painful hernia in the hypogastrium due to cold, the drug can be used with Radix Aconiti Praeparata, Fructus Meliae Toosendan, Fructus Foeniculi, etc.

3. Warming the kidney to strengthen *Yang*

In treating cold feeling of external genitals, impotence, etc., the drug can be used with drugs for warming the kidney and strengthening *Yang* such as Bombyx mori (male), Fructus Foeniculi, Radix Aconiti Praeparata, Cortex Cinnamomi, etc.

Besides, the drug powder can be used to treat female cracked nipple, being mixed with sesame oil and applied to the nipple.

Dosage and Administration: Usually, 1–3 g of the drug is used in decoction.

Notes: This drug should not be taken by those with heat syndrome. It is antagonized by Radix Curcumae.

Pricklyash Peel (花椒 *Huajiao*)
Pericarpium Zanthoxyli

This drug consists of the pericarp of the deciduous shrub or arbor, Zanthoxylum bungeanum Maxim., or Zanthoxylum schinifolium Sieb. et Zucc. (family Rutaceae).The drug grown in Sichuan Province is call "chuanjiao" in Chinese. The drug is slightly parched and deprived of the kernal for use.

Nomenclature Used in Prescriptions: *Chuanjiao*, *Shujiao*, *Huajiao*

Properties and Channel Distribution: This drug is pungent in taste and warm in nature with slight toxicity, and is distributed to the Spleen, Stomach and Kidney Channels.

Action and Indications:

1. Warming the middle *Jiao* and relieving pain

In treating coldness and pain of the epigastrium and abdomen and vomiting with inability to taken in food due to cold syndrome of deficiency type of the spleen and stomach, the drug can be used with Rhizoma Zingiberis, Radix Codonopsis Pilosulae, etc.; in treating abdominal pain and diarrhea with white foam due to cold, 6 g of the drug, 9 g of Radix Aconiti Praeparata and 6 g of Rhizoma Zingiberis can be decocted and taken; in treating coldness and pain of the stomach which affects the back, 5 g of the drug, 9 g of Radix Aconiti Praeparata and 9 g of Rhizoma Pinelliae can be made into pills, and 6 g of the pills can be taken with warm water, twice a day.

2. Destroying parasite and relieving itching

This drug can be used to treat abdominal pain and vomiting

caused by ascariasis, vomiting of ascaris, etc.If the above diseases are due to cold, 6 g of the drug, 9 g of Fructus Mume, 9 g of Rhizoma Zingiberis Recens and 9 g of Semen Torreyae can be decocted and taken; if the diseases are due to heat, 6 g of the drug, 9 g of Fructus Mume, 3 g of Rhizoma Coptidis, 9 g of Cortex Phellodendri and 6 g of Fructus Aurantii Immaturus can be decocted and taken. In treating itchy eczema, the drug can be decocted with Radix Sophorae Flavescentis, Fructus Kochiae and Alumen, and the decoction can be used to wash the local area to destroy parasites and relieve pain.

Dosage and Administration: Usually, 2–6 g of the drug is used in decoction. Proper amount of the drug can be used in external treatment.

Appendix: Semen Zanthoxyli (椒目 *Jiaomu*)

This drug consists of the seed of Zanthoxylum bungeanum Maxim. It is bitter and pungent in taste and cold in nature with slight toxicity, and is distributed to the Spleen and Urinary Bladder Channels. It has the effects of inducing diuresis and relieving asthma. It is used to treat the excess syndromes of edema and cough and asthma due to retention of phlegm

Long Pepper (荜茇 *Biba*)
Fructus Piperis Longi

This drug consists of the unripe fruit–spike of the perennial liana, piper longum L. (family Piperaceae). The crude drug is dried in the sun for use.

Nomenclature Used in Prescriptions: *Biba*, *Bibo*

Properties and Channel Distribution: This drug is pungent in taste and hot in nature, and is distributed to the Stomach and Large Intestine Channels.

Action and Indications: Warming the middle warmer and relieving pain

In treating abdominal pain, vomiting and diarrhea due to stomach cold, the drug can be made into pills with Cortex Cinnamomi, Rhizoma Alpiniae Officinarum, etc.

Besides, the drug can also be used to treat headache and toothache due to accumulation of cold in the exterior and accumulation of fire in the interior: 6 g of the drug, 3 g of Herba Asari, 6 g of Rhizoma Cimicifugae and 9 g of Radix et Rhizoma Rhei can be decocted and taken. The drug powder can also first be applied locally and then decoction of Fructus Xanthii is used to rince the mouth; this is the other method for toothache.

Dosage and Administration: Usually, 1.5–6 g of the drug is decocted. Proper amount of the drug can be used locally.

Notes: This drug should not be taken by those with heat of excess type turning into fire, or with deficiency of *Yin* and hyperactivity of fire.

Litsea Cubebs (荜澄茄 *Bichengqie*)
Fructus Litseae

This drug consists of the fruit of the evergreen climbing liana, Piper cubeba L. (family Piperaceae), or the deciduous arbor or thrub, Litsea cubeba (Lour.) Pers. (family Lauraceae). The crude drug is broken into pieces for use.

Nomenclature Used in Prescriptions: *Bichengqie*

Properties and Channel Distribution: This drug is pungent in taste and warm in nature, and is distributed to the Spleen, Stomach, Kidney and Urinary Bladder Channels.

Action and Indications:

1. Warming the middle *Jiao*, dispelling cold, promoting flow of *Qi* and relieving pain

In treating gastralgia and vomiting due to stomach cold, poor appetite, etc., the drug can be used with Fructus Euodiae, Rhizoma Pinelliae, etc.; in treating periumbilical colic due to cold, with Fructus Euodiae, Rhizoma Cyperi, etc.; in treating dysuria due to cold of deficiency type of the lower warmer, with Semen Zanthoxyli, Ramulus Cinnamomi, etc. In treating frequent micturition due to cold syndrome of deficiency type of the urinary bladder, with Radix Linderae, Semen Euryales, etc.

Dosage and Administration: Usually, 1.5–6 g of the drug is used in decoction.

Pepper (胡椒 *Hujiao*)
Fructus Piperis nigri

This drug consists of the fruit of the evergreen woody liana, Piper nigrum L. (family Piperaceae). This commercial drug is of two kinds, namely, "black pepper," which consists of the unripe dried fruit, and "white pepper," which consists of the dried ripe fruit with the peel removed. The former is more effective. The crude drug is ground into powder for use.

Nomenclature Used in Prescriptions: *Hujiao*, *Baihujiao*

Properties and Channel Distribution: This drug is pungent in taste and hot in nature, and is distributed to the Stomach and Large Intestine Channels.

Action and Indications:

Warming the middle *Jiao*, dispelling cold, promoting flow of *Qi* and relieving pain

In treating coldness and pain of the stomach, the drug can be used in combination with Flos Syzygii Aromatici, Radix Aucklandiae, Faeces Trogopterorum, etc.; in treating vomiting and diarrhea due to cold syndrome of stomach, with Rhizoma Zingiberis, Flos Syzygii Aromatici, Rhizoma Pinelliae, Pericarpium Citri Reticulatae, etc.; in treating abdominal pain and diarrhea due to cold, the drug can be made into plaster and applied to the umbilicus.

This drug is also a flavouring and may whet the appetite if used in a small amount.

Dosage and Administration: Usually, 1.5–3 g of the drug is decocted. When the drug is ground into powder, 0.3–0.6 g of the drug is taken at a time. Proper amount of the drug can be used in external treatment.

8 Drugs for Regulating Flow of *Qi*

Drugs with the functions of regulating the *Qi* system and promoting flow of *Qi* are generally called drugs for regulating flow of *Qi*.

This kind of drugs are mostly pungent and bitter in taste, aromatic in odour and warm in nature, characterized by moving, dispersing and descending properties. They have the functions of regulating flow of *Qi* to invigorate the spleen, promoting flow of *Qi* to relieve pain, sending down adverse flow of *Qi*, soothing the depressed liver, relieving stagnation of *Qi*, etc. They can be used to treat stagnation of *Qi*, adverse flow of *Qi*, etc. caused by disturbance of the functional activity of *Qi*.

Disorders of the *Qi* system are often related to the liver, spleen (stomach), and lung. Since the lung is in charge of *Qi*, the liver is responsible for maintaining free flow of *Qi* and the spleen (stomach) regulates flow of *Qi*, improper diet, climatic changes, mental depression, melancholy and anxiety may lead to depression of liver–*Qi*, disturbance of spleen–*Qi* (stomach–*Qi*) and stagnation of lung–*Qi*, resulting in various kinds of *Qi* stagnation. Other factors such as phlegm–dampness, diet, stasis of blood, etc. may also affect the functional activity of *Qi*. The manifestations of stagnation of *Qi* may vary with its degree and locations. Generally speaking. a mild case of stagnation of *Qi* is manifested by stuffiness, a more severe case is manifested by distention and a severe case is manifested by pain. Stagnation of spleen–*Qi* is manifested by distention of epigastrium and abdomen, belching, acid regurgitation, nausea, vomiting, and constipation or diarrhea; stagnation of liver–*Qi* is manifested by distention and pain of the hypochondrium, stuffy chest, painful hernia, distention of the breast, irregular menstruation, etc.; stagnation of lung–*Qi* is manifested by stuffy chest, cough, dyspnea, etc.

In using this kind of drugs, proper combination of drugs should be considered. For example, for those with damp–heat affecting the spleen, drugs for clearing away heat and removing dampness should be used; for those with cold–dampness affecting the spleen, drugs for warming the middle warmer and removing dampness should be used; for those with stagnation of food, drugs for promoting digestion should be used; for those with deficiency of the spleen and stomach, drugs for invigorating the spleen should also be used. Stagnation of the liver–*Qi* have various clinical manifestations and therefore drugs for nourishing and invigorating the liver, relieving pain, or activating blood to regulate menstruation, etc. should be used according to different conditions. For those with disorder of free–going of lung–*Qi* accompanied by retention of phlegm, drugs for dispelling phlegm should also be used.

Drugs for regulating flow of *Qi* are mostly pungent in taste, aromatic in odour and warm and dispersing in nature. Although they can be used to relieve *Qi* stagnation, they are likely to exhuast *Qi* and damage *Yin*. Therefore, they should be used with care for those with deficiency of *Yin* or *Qi*.

Nutgrass Flatsedge Rhizome (香附 *Xiangfu*) Rhizoma Cyperi

This drug consists of the dried rhizome of the perennial herbage Cyperus rotundus L. (family Cyperaceae.) The crude drug or the drug parched with vinegar is used.

Nomenclature Used in Prescriptions: *Sheng Xiangfu*, *Zhi Xiangfu*, *Xiangfu Zi*, *Xiangfu Mi*

Properties and Channel Distribution: This drug is pungent, slightly bitter and slightly sweet in taste and neutral in nature, and is distributed to the Liver and the Triple Warmer Channels.

Action and Indications:

1. Soothing the liver and regulating flow of *Qi*:

In treating stuffy chest and hypochondrium, pain of the epigastrium and abdomen, etc. due to depression of liver–*Qi*, the drug is often used in combination with other drugs for regulating flow of *Qi*.

2. Regulating menstruation to relieve pain:

It is a chief drug for irregular menstruation and dysmenorrhea, and is especially effective when the diseases are due to depression of liver–*Qi*. It is often used in combination with Radix Angelicae Sinensis, Rhizoma Ligustici Chuanxiong, Radix Paeoniae or Folium Artemisiae Argyi, etc.

Dosage and Administration: Usually, 6–12 g of the drug is used in decoction, The crude drug is used to regulate *Qi* and relieve depression and the prepared drug can be used to regulate menstruation to relieve pain.

Aucklandia Root (木香 *Muxiang*)
Radix Aucklandiae

This drug consists of the root of the perennial or biennial herbage Saussurea lappa Clarke or Vladimiria souliei (Franch.) Ling (family Compositae). The drug is broken into pieces and the crude or roasted drug is used.

Nomenclature Used in Prescriptions: *Muxiang*, *Yunmuxiang*, *Guangmuxiang*, *Weimuxiang*

Properties and Channel Distribution: This drug is pungent and bitter in taste and warm in nature, and is distributed to the Spleen, Stomach, Large Intestine and Triple Warmer Channels.

Action and Indications:

1. Promoting flow of *Qi* to relieve pain: This drug can be used to treat distention and pain of the epigastrium and abdomen, diarrhea, dysentery, tenesmus, etc. due to stagnation of *Qi* in the stomach and intestine. In treating distention and pain of the epigastrium and abdomen, vomiting, etc., the drug is often used in combination with Fructus Amomi, Herba Agastachis, Flos Syzygii Aromatici, etc. In treating stagnation of food, stasis of *Qi*, distention of the epigastrium and abdomen, constipation or diarrhea and dysentery with tenesmus, etc., the drug is often used in combination with Rhizoma Coptidis, Semen Arecae, Radix et Rhizoma Rhei, etc.

2. Invigorating the stomach to promote digestion: In treating indigestion, poor appetite, vomiting, chronic diarrhea, etc. the drug is often used in combination with Fructus Amomi, Rhizoma Atractylodis Macrocephalae, Poria, Rhizoma Pinelliae, Pericarpium Citri Reticulatae, etc.

In recent years the drug is used to treat cholecystitis, cholelithiasis, pancreatitis, appendicitis, intestinal obstruction, and other acute abdomen. In treating cholecystitis, cholelithiasis and pancreatitis, the drug can be used in combination with Radix Bupleuri, Radix Scutellariae, Radix et Rhizoma Rhei, etc. In treating appendicitis, the drug can be used in combination with Flos Lonicerae, Radix et Rhizoma Rhei and Cortex Moutan Radicis. In treating intestinal obstruction, the drug can be used in combination with Radix Euphorbiae Kansui, Semen Persicae, Radix Achyranthis Bidentatae, etc.

Dosage and Administration: Usually, 3–6 g of the drug is used in decoction. The crude drug is used to regulate flow of *Qi* and the roasted drug is used to arrest diarrhea. The drug should not be decocted for long.

Appendix: Radix Aristolochiae (青木香 *Qingmuxiang*)

This drug is also called *Tumuxiang* in Chinese. It consists of the root of the perennial twining herbage Aristolochia contorta Bge. (family Aristolochiaceae). The crude drug is cut into slices for use. This drug is pungent and bitter in taste and cold in nature with slight toxicity. It has the effect of inducing vomiting, removing toxin and subduing swelling, and can be used to treat food poisoning, painful swelling due to heat toxin, snake bite, etc. It can be both taken orally and applied externally. But overdosage is likely to cause vomiting. Usually, 3–6 g of the drug is used in decoction. Proper dosage of the drug powder can be used in external application.

Lindera Root (乌药 *Wuyao*)
Radix Linderae

This drug consists of the root of the evergreen shrub or arbor Lindera strychnifolia (Sieb. et Zucc.)Villar (family Lauraceae). The crude drug is dried in the sun and cut into slices for medication.

Nomenclature Used in Prescriptions: *Wuyao*, *Taiwuyao*

Properties and Channel Distribution: This drug is pungent in taste and warm in nature, and is distributed to the Spleen, Lung, Kidney and Urinary Bladder Channels.

Action and Indications:

1. Promoting flow of *Qi* to relieve pain: This drug can be used to treat stuffiness, distention and pain of the chest and abdomen, hernia, dysmenorrhea, etc. In treating pain of the abdomen due to cold in the middle warmer and stagnation of *Qi*, the drug can be used in combination with Lignum Aquilariae Resinatum, Rhizoma Zingiberis Recens, Radix Codonopsis Pilosulae, etc. In treating stuffy chest and poor appetite, the drug can be used in combination with Lignum Aquilariae Resinatum, Semen Arecae, etc. In treating hernia of small intestine due to accumulation of cold and stagnation of *Qi*, the drug can be used in combination with Fructus Foeniculi, Fructus Meliae Toosendan Radix Aucklandiae, etc. In treating abdominal distention due to stagnation of *Qi* and abdominal pain during menstruation, the drug can be used in combination with Radix Aucklandiae, Radix Angelicae Sinensis, etc.

2. Warming the kidney to disperse cold: In treating frequent

micturition due to cold of deficiency type, equal amount of the drug, Fructus Alpiniae Oxyphyllae and Rhizoma Dioscoreae can be ground into powder and made into pills with millet wine, and 10 g of the pills can be taken at a time with salt water, 2–3 times a day.

Dosage and Administration: Usually, 6–10 g of the drug is used in decoction.

Tangerine Peel (橘皮 *Jupi*) Pericarpium Citri Reticulatae

This drug consists of the ripe fruit and pericarp of the evergreen arbor Citrus reticulata Blanco (family Rutaceae). The crude drug is cut into slivers for medication.

Nomenclature Used in Prescriptions: *Jupi*, *Chenpi*, *Guangpi*, *Guangchenpi*, *Xinhuipi*

Properties and Channel Distribution: This drug is pungent and bitter in taste and warm in nature, and is distributed to the Spleen and Lung Channels.

Action and Indications:

1. Removing dampness and resolving phlegm: In treating cough with profuse sputum and stuffy chest due to stagnation of phlegm–dampness, the drug is often used in combination with Poria, Rhizoma Pinelliae, Radix Glycyrrhizae, etc.

2. Regulating flow of *Qi* and invigorating the spleen: In treating indigestion, abdominal distention, stuffy epigastrium, poor appetite, nausea, vomiting, etc.,the drug can be used in combination with Cortex Magnoliae Officinalis, Rhizoma Atractylodis Macrocephalae, Rhizoma Zingiberis Recens, etc.

Dosage and Administration: Usually, 3–10 g of the drug is used in decoction.

Notes: This drug is warm and dry in nature and should not be used for cases with deficiency of body fluid and excess heat syndrome.

Appendix:

1. Exocarpium Citri Grandis (橘红 *Juhong*): This drug consists of the red-coloured external layer of the pericarp of Citrus Reticulata, being rather drastic in nature and is similar in its action to Pericarpium Citri Reticulatae. It is especially effective in dispelling phlegm and removing dampness, and can be used to treat cough due to lung-cold and itchy throat with profuse sputum. Usually, 3–6 g of the drug is used in decoction.

2. Retinervus Citri Reticulatae Fructus (橘络 *Juluo*): This drug consists of the vascular bundles of the mesocarp of Citrus reticulata. It is sweet and bitter in taste and cold in nature, It has the effect of removing obstruction in the collaterals and resolving phlegm, and can be used to treat cough with pain in the chest and hypochondrium and accumulation of phlegm-heat in the channels and collaterals, so as to remove obstruction in the collaterals. Usually, 3–5 g of the drug is used in decoction.

3. Semen Citri Reticulatae (橘核 *Juhe*): This drug consists of the seed of Citrus Reticulata, It is bitter in taste and neutral in nature and is distributed to the Liver Channel. It has the effect of regulating flow of *Qi*, removing obstruction and relieving pain, and is used specially to treat hernia of the small intestine and swelling of testis. Usually, 6–12 g of the drug is used in decoction.

4. Folium Citri Sinensis (橘叶 *Juye*): This drug consists of the leaf of Citrus reticulata. It is bitter in taste and neutral in na-

ture, and is distributed to the Liver Channel. It has the effect of soothing the depressed liver and promoting flow of *Qi*, and can be used to treat pain of the chest and hypochondrium, swelling and pain of the breast, etc. due to depression of liver–*Qi*. Usually, 6–12 g of the drug is used in decoction.

Green Tangerine Orange Peel (青皮 *Qingpi*)
Pericarpium Citri Reticulatae Viride

This drug consists of the unripe fruit or green exocarp of the evergreen arbor Citrus reticulata Blanco (family Rutaceae). The pulp is removed and the drug is dried in the sun. The crude drug or the drug parched with vinegar is used for medication.

Nomenclature Used in Prescriptions: *Qingpi*, *Xiaoqingpi*, *Junqingpi*

Properties and Channel Distribution: This drug is bitter and pungent in taste and warm in nature, and is distributed to the Liver, Gall Bladder and Stomach Channels.

Action and Indications:

1. Soothing the liver and relieving stagnation of *Qi*: In treating distention and pain of the chest and hypochondrium due to stagnation of liver–*Qi*, the drug can be used in combination with Radix Bupleuri, Radix Curcumae, Rhizoma Cyperi, etc. In treating enlargement of the liver and spleen, the drug can be used in combination with Radix Bupleuri, Radix Curcumae, Rhizoma Cyperi, Carapax Trionycis, Radix Codonopsis Pilosulae, etc. In treating hypochondriac pain due to retention of phlegm, the drug can be used in combination with Semen Sinapis Albae. In treating acute mastitis, the drug can be used in combination with Herba

Taraxaci, Fructus Trichosanthis, Folium Citri Sinensis, etc. In treating nodule in the breast, swelling of the breast, stuffy chest, belching, hypochondriac pain, abdominal pain, etc. due to stagnation of *Qi*, 1.5 g of the drug powder can be taken as a dose, twice a day. In treating periumbilical colic due to cold, the drug can be used in combination with Radix Linderae, Fructus Foeniculi, Radix Aucklandiae, etc.

2. Removing food stagnancy: In treating stagnation of food with distention and pain of the epigastrium and abdomen, the drug can be used in combination with Fructus Crataegi, Fructus Hordei Germinatus, Semen Alpiniae Katsumadai, etc.

Dosage and Administration: Usually, 3–6 g of the drug is used in decoction. The drug parched with vinegar is used to soothe the liver.

Notes: This drug is drastic and is likely to damage *Qi*. It should, therefore, not be taken by those with deficiency of *Qi*.

Immature Bitter Orange (枳实 *Zhishi*)
Fructus Aurantii Immaturus

This drug consists of the immature fruit of the evergreen arbor Poncirus trifoliata (L.) Raf., Citrus aurantium L., or Citrus wilsonii Tanaka (family Rutaceae).The immature fruit collected around the Summer Solstice is called Fructus Aurantii Immaturus and the mature fruit collected in autumn is called Fructus Aurantii. The drug is cut into slices, dried in the sun and parched for medication.

Nomenclature Used in Prescriptions: *Xiaozhishi, Chaozhishi*

Properties and Channel Distribution: This drug is bitter in taste and slightly cold in nature, and is distributed to the Spleen, Stomach and Large Intestine Channels.

Action and Indications:

1. Removing stagnation of *Qi*: In treating abdominal pain, constipation, or diarrhea and dysentery with tenesmus due to accumulation of damp–heat in the intestine and stomach, the drug can be used in combination with Radix et Rhizoma Rhei, Rhizoma Coptidis, Rhizoma Atractylodis Macrocephalae, etc. In treating stasis of *Qi* and blood, abdominal pain and restlessness in women after childbirth, the drug can be ground into powder with Radix Paeoniae Alba (10 g each), and 6 g of the powder can be taken as a dose, twice a day.

2. Resolving phlegm and relieving stuffiness: In treating stuffy chest and hypochondrium due to retention of phlegm, the drug can be used in combination with Rhizoma Pinelliae, Poria, Pericarpium Citri Reticulatae, etc. In treating epigastric fullness and poor appetite or distention of the chest and abdomen and difficulty in defecation, the drug can be used in combination with Rhizoma Coptidis, Rhizoma Zingiberis, Cortex Magnoliae Officinalis, etc. In treating stuffy chest, abdominal distention and indigestion due to deficiency of the spleen, the drug is often used in combination with Rhizoma Atractylodis Macrocephalae.

Besides, in recent years it is used in combination with Radix Astragali seu Hedysari, Rhizoma Cimicifugae, etc. to treat gastroptosis, hysteroptosis, prolapse of rectum, etc.

Dosage and Administration: Usually, 3–6 g of the drug is used in decoction.

Notes: This drug should be used with care by those with deficiency of the spleen and stomach.

Appendix: Fructus Aurantii (枳壳 *Zhike*):

This drug consists of the mature fruit of Citrus aurantium L., etc. The fruit is deprived of the peel, cut into slices, dried in the sun and parched with bran for medication. Its properties and actions are the same as Fructus Aurantii Immaturus, yet with less powerful effect. It is used mainly to regulate *Qi*, comfort the middle warmer and relieve distention.

Toosendan Fruit (川楝子 *Chuanlianzi*) Fructus Meliae Toosendan

This drug consists of the fruit of the deciduous arbor Melia toosendan Sieb. et Zucc. (family Meliaceae) without the kernal. The crude drug or the drug parched with salt is used for medication.

Nomenclature Used in Prescriptions: *Chuanlianzi, Jinlingzi*

Properties and Channel Distribution: This drug is bitter in taste and cold in nature, and is distributed to the Liver, Stomach, Small Intestine and Urinary Bladder Channels.

Action and Indications:

1. Promoting flow of *Qi* and relieving pain

This drug is used to treat distention and pain of the chest and abdomen, painful hernia, etc. due to stagnation of liver–*Qi* and hyperactivity of fire in the liver and gall bladder. This drug is bitter in taste and cold and descending in nature with the effect of eliminating liver–heat. Therefore, it is often used to treat diseases due to heat. In treating distention and pain of the chest and abdomen, the drug is often used in combination with Rhizoma Corydalis to enhance the effect of relieving pain. In treating painful hernia with manifestation of cold, the drug can be used in combination with Radix Aucklandiae, Fructus Foeniculi, Fructus Euodiae, etc. to dispel cold, regulate flow of *Qi* and relieve pain.

2. Eliminating parasites

In treating abdominal pain due to enterositosis, the drug is often used with other drugs for destroying parasites such as Fructus Quisqualis, Semen Arecae, etc.

In addition, the drug can also be used to treat tinea capitis. The drug is baked till it turns brown, ground into powder, mixed with lard or sesame oil and applied to the local area. Before application, the affected part should be washed with warm salt water.

Dosage and Administration: Usually, 5–10 g of the drug is used in decoction. The crude drug is generally used and the drug parched with salt is used to treat hernia.

Notes: This drug is contraindicated for cold of deficiency type of the spleen and stomach.

Macrostem Onion (薤白 *Xiebai*)
Bulbus Allii Macrostemi

This drug consists of the underground bulb of the perennial herbage Allium macrostemon Bye., or A. chinense G. Don.(family Liliaceae). The drug is steamed for use.

Nomenclature Used in Prescriptions: *Xiebai, Xiebaitou*

Properties and Channel Distribution: This drug is pungent and bitter in taste and warm in nature, and is distributed to the Lung, Stomach and Large Intestine Channels.

Action and Indications:

1. Activating *Yang* and dispersing accumulation of pathogen

This drug can be used to treat accumulation of coldphlegm and stagnation of *Yang* in the chest, manifested by stuffy chest and epigastrium, cough with profuse sputum, stabbing pain in the chest and back, etc. This drug is pungent and bitter in taste and is characterized by its dispersing, descending, and warming functions. It can be used to disperse accumulation of cold and activating dispersing function of *Yang* in the chest, and is therefore a chief drug to remove obstruction of *Qi* in the chest. The drug is often used in combination with Fructus Trichosanthis and other drugs for regulating flow of *Qi* and activating blood circulation.

2. Sending down adverse flow of *Qi* to remove *Qi* stagnation

In treating diarrhea and dysentery with tenesmus due to stagnation of *Qi* in the intestine and stomach, the drug can be used in combination with Radix Bupleuri, Radix Paeoniae Alba, Fructus Aurantii Immaturus, etc.

In recent years it is used to treat angina pectoris seen in coronary heart disease. It is often used in combination with Radix Salviae Miltiorrhizae, Flos Carthami, Fructus Trichosanthis, etc. to activate blood circulation comfort the chest and relieve pain.

Dosage and Administration: Usually, 5–10 g of the drug is used in decoction.

Notes:

This drug is contraindicated for those with deficiency of *Qi* but without stagnation of *Qi*, anorexia due to deficiency of the stomach and intolerance to the taste of garlic.

Spikenard (甘松 *Gansong*)
Rhizoma Nardostachydis

This drug consists of the root and rhizome of the perennial low herbage Nardostachys chinensis Batal. (family Valerianaceae). The crude drug is cut into sections for use.

Nomenclature Used in Prescriptions: *Gansong, Gunsongxiang*

Properties and Channel Distribution: This drug is sweet in taste and warm in nature, and is distributed to the Spleen and Stomach Channels.

Action and Indications:

Promoting flow of *Qi*, relieving pain, inducing appetite and enlivening the spleen

In treating distention and pain of the epigastrium and abdomen, poor appetite, etc. due to stagnation of *Qi* as a result of invasion of cold into the spleen and stomach, the drug is often used in combination with Herba Agastachis, Fructus Hordei Germinatus, Fructus Amomi, etc.

Dosage and Administration: Usually, 3–10 g of the drug is used in decoction.

Finger Citron (佛手 *Foshou*)
Fructus Citri Sarcodactylis

This drug consists of the fruit of the evergreen arbor Citrus medica L. var. sarcodactylis (Noot.) Swingle (family Rutaceae). The crude drug is cut into slices and dried in the sun for medication.

Nomenclature Used in Prescriptions: *Foshoupian, Chenfoshou, Xianfoshou,Foshougan*

Properties and Channel Distribution: This drug is pungent, bitter and sour in taste and warm in nature, and is distributed to the Liver, Spleen, Stomach and Lung Channels.

Action and Indications:

1. Soothing the depressed liver to regulate flow of *Qi* and relieving pain

In treating distention and pain of the epigastrium and abdomen due to stagnation of *Qi* in the liver and stomach, the drug is often used in combination with drugs for regulating flow of *Qi* such as Radix Aucklandiae, Pericarpium Citri Reticulatae Viride, etc.

2. Invigorating the stomach and arresting vomiting

It is most effective for vomiting. In treating indigestion, poor appetite, belching, vomiting, etc., the drug can be used in combination with Fructus Amomi, Fructus Amomi Cardamomi, Rhizoma Pinelliae, etc.

Besides, the drug has the effect of relieving cough and resolving phlegm and can be used to treat cough with profuse sputum.

Dosage and Administration: Usually, 6–10 g of the drug is used in decoction.

Eagle Wood (沉香 *Chenxiang*)
Lignum Aquilariae Resinatum

This drug consists of the dark brown resinous wood of the evergreen arbor Aguilaria agallocha Roxb., or A. sinensis (Lour.)

Gilg (family Thymelaeaceae).The drug is ground into powder for medication.

Nowenclature Used in Prescriptions: *Chenxiang, Kui-Chenxiang*

Properties and Channel Distribution: This drug is pungent and bitter in taste and warm in nature, and is distributed to the Spleen, Stomach and Kidney Channels.

Action and Indications:

1. Promoting flow of *Qi* and relieving pain

In treating stuffiness and pain in the chest and hypochondrium due to stagnation of *Qi*, irregular menstruation and hypogastric pain, the drug can be used in combination with Rhizoma Cyperi, Fructus Amomi, etc. In treating stuffy chest with pain due to stagnation of *Qi* as a result of retention of phlegm, the drug can be used in combination with Radix Aucklandiae, Rhizoma Pinelliae, Poria, etc.

2. Sending down adverse flow of *Qi* to relieve asthma

In treating stuffy chest, asthma and dyspnea, the drug can be used in combination with Radix Linderae, Radix Aucklandiae and Semen Arecae. This drug is warm in nature and may both send down adverse flow of *Qi* and improve inspiration by invigorating kidney–*Qi*. Therefore, in treating asthma of deficiency type due to failure of the kidney in receiving *Qi* caused by cold of deficiency type, the drug can be used in combination with Radix Aconiti Praeparata and Rhizoma Zingiberis Recens, to warm the kidney and restore the kidney's function in receiving *Qi*.

3. Warming the middle warmer to arrest vomiting

In treating vomiting and hiccups due to stomachcold, the drug can be used in combination with Fructus Amomi Rotundus,

Flos Syzygii Aromatici, Calyx Kaki, etc.

Dosage and Administration: Usually, 1–3 g of the drug powder is taken following its infusion with boiling water. The drug should not be decocted.

Notes: Since this drug is pungent in taste and warm in nature and is likely to generate fire, it should not be taken by those with deficiency of *Yin* and hyperactivity of fire.

Sandlewood (檀香 *Tanxiang*)
Lignum Santali

This drug consists of the heartwood of the evergreen arbor Santalum album L. (family Santalaceae). After being cleaned, the drug is cut into slices or pieces for medication.

Nomenclature Used in Prescriptions: *Tanxiang, Saitanxiang*

Properties and Channel Distribution: This drug is pungent and warm in nature, and is distributed to the Spleen, Stomach and Lung Channels.

Action and Indications:

1. Promoting flow of *Qi* to relieve pain

In treating coldness and pain of the epigastrium and abdomen caused by stagnation of *Qi* and accumulation of cold and neurogenic gastritis, the drug can be used in combination with Lignum Aquilariae Resinatum, Radix Aucklandiae, Flos Syzygii Aromatici, Radix Linderae, etc. In treating gastralgia due to stasis of *Qi* and blood, angina pectoris, etc., the drug can be used in combination with Radix Salviae Miltiorrhizae.

2. Warming the stomach to arrest vomiting

In treating gastralgia due to cold and vomiting of gastric

juice, the drug can be used in combination with Rhizoma Acori Graminei, Flos Syzygii Aromatici, Radix Aucklandiae, etc.

Besides, in recent years the drug is used to treat coronary heart disease due to stasis of *Qi* and blood. and is always used in combination with Fructus Piperis Longi, Rhizoma Corydalis, Herba Asari, etc.

Dosage and Administration: Usually, 1–3 g of the drug is used in decoction.

Kaki Calyx (柿蒂 *Shidi*)
Calyx Kaki

This drug consists of the persistent calyx of the deciduous arbor Diospyros kaki L. f.(family Ebenaceae). The crude drug is dried in the sun for medication.

Nomenclature Used in Prescriptions: *Shidi*

Properties and Channel Distribution: This drug is bitter and puckery in taste and slightly warm in nature, and is distributed to the Stomach Channel.

Action and Indications:

Sending down adverse flow of *Qi* to arrest hiccups

In treating hiccups due to stomach–cold, the drug can be used in combination with Flos Syzygii Aromatici and Rhizoma Zingiberis Recens. In treating hiccups due to stomach–heat, the drug can be used in combination with Caulis Bambusae in Taeniam, Haematitum, etc.

Dosage and Administration: Usually, 6–10 g of the drug is used in decoction.

Litchi Seed (荔枝核 *Lizhihe*)
Semen Litchi

This drug consists of the ripe seed of the evergreen arbor Litchi chinensis Sonn (family Sapindaceae). The crude drug or the drug parched with salt water is used. The drug is broken into pieces before being used.

Nomenclature Used in Prescriptions: *Lizhihe*

Properties and Channel Distribution: This drug is sweet in taste and warm in nature, and is distributed to the Liver and Kidney Channels.

Action and Indications:

Promoting flow of *Qi* to relieve pain

This drug is used to treat enterocele, swelling of the testis, female stabbing pain in the hypogastrium due to stagnation of *Qi* and stasis of blood, etc. In treating hernia, the drug is often used in combination with Semen Citri Reticulatae, Fructus Foeniculi, Fructus Meliae Toosendan, etc. In treating female stabbing pain due to stagnation of *Qi* and stasis of blood, equal amount of the drug and Rhizoma Cyperi can be ground into powder and 6 g of the powder can be taken at a time with salt water or warm water.

Dosage and Administration: Usually, 6–10 g of the drug is used in decoction.

Notes: This drug is contraindicated for those without stagnation of *Qi* due to cold–dampness.

Rose (玫瑰花 *Meiguihua*)
Flos Rosae Rugosae

This drug consists of the flower of the deciduous shrub Rosa rugosa Thunb. (family Rosaceae). The drug is dried in the sun for medication.

Nomenclature Used in Prescriptions: *Meiguihua*

Properties and Channel Distribution: This drug is sweet and slightly bitter in taste and warm in nature, and is distributed to the Liver and Spleen Channels.

Action and Indications:

Promoting flow of *Qi*, activating blood circulation, soothing the liver and relieving pain

In treating distention and pain of the epigastrium and hypochondrium due to incoordination between the liver and stomach, the drug can be used in combination with Rhizoma Cyperi, Fructus Meliae Toosendan, etc.

Besides, the drug can also be used to treat irregular menstruation, distention and pain of the breast before menstruation, stasis of blood and pain due to trauma, etc., and in recent years it is included in the prescription for angina pectoris, because of its effect of regulating flow of *Qi* and activating blood circulation.

Dosage and Administration: Usually, 3–9 g of the drug is used in decoction.

9 Digestives

Drugs with the main functions in promoting digestion and removing stagnated food are called digestives.

This kind of drugs have the functions in promoting digestion and removing stagnated food. Some of the drugs also have the function in invigorating the spleen and stomach. The drugs are used to treat stagnation of undigested food, indigestion, distention of the epigastrium and abdomen, anorexia, belching, nausea, vomiting, abnormality in defecation, etc.

In using this kind of drugs, proper combination of drugs should be considered according to different conditions. For example, for treating those with stagnation of food accompanied by stagnation of *Qi*, drugs for promoting flow of *Qi* should also be used; for treating excessive heat resulted from retention of food, drugs bitter in taste and cold in nature for free bowel movement should also be used; for those with stagnation of food due to deficiency of the spleen and stomach with dysfunction in transportation and transformation accompanied by symptoms of deficiency of *Qi*, drugs for invigorating *Qi* and spleen should also be used.

Hawthorn Fruit (山楂 *Shanzha*)
Fructus Crataegi

This drug consists of the ripe fruit of the deciduous shrub Crataegus pinnatifida Bye. var. major N.E. Br. (family

Rosaceae). The kernal is removed and the crude, parched or carbonized drug is used in medication.

Nomenclature Used in Prescriptions: *Shenshanzha, Chaoshanzha, Jiaoshanzha, Shanzhatan*

Properties and Channel Distribution: This drug is sour and sweet in taste and slightly warm in nature, and is distributed to the Spleen, Stomach and Liver Channels.

Action and Indications:

1. Promoting digestion and removing stagnated food

In treating stagnation of food or greasy food, distention of chest and abdomen, infantile dyspepsia due to improper feeding, etc. the drug is often used in combination with Fructus Hordei Germinatus, Massa Fermentata Medicinalis, Semen Raphani, etc.

2. Activating blood circulation and removing blood stasis

In treating dysmenorrhea, postpartum abdominal pain, lochiorrhea, etc. due to stasis of blood, the drug is often used in combination with Radix Angelicae Sinensis, Rhizoma Ligustici Chuanxiong, Rhizoma Corydalis, Herba Leonuri, etc. In treating postpartum pain caused by uterine contraction, 30 g of the carbonized drug are prescribed. Take the decoction mixed with brown sugar and urine of a boy under 12 years old.

In addition, this drug also has the effect of activating blood circulation and promoting measles eruptions and can be used in combination with Pericarpium Citri Reticulatae to treat retarded eruption seen at the initial stage of measles with such manifestations as stasis of *Qi* and blood or indigestion. In recent years, the drug is used in combination with Semen Cassiae to treat hypertension. The drugs are infused in boiling water with sugar and the water is drunk everyday instead of tea. The drug can also be used to treat coronary heart disease, hyperlipemia and bacillary dysentery.

Dosage and Administration: Usually, 10–15 g of the drug is used in decoction. The parched drug is used for digestion, the carbonized for dysentery and blood stasis, and the crude for hypertension and measles eruptions.

Appendix: Semen Crataegi (山楂核 *Shanzhahe*)

This drug has the effect of softening hard mass and sending down adverse flow of *Qi* to relieve fullness in the chest. In treating enterocele and orchiocele, the drug is often used in combination with Semen Citri Reticulatae and Semen Litchi. In treating hiccups, the powder made of 30 g of it and 9 g of Fructus Amomi Rotundus is prescribed, 3 g is to be taken as one dose, twice a day.

Medicated Leaven (神曲 *Shenqu*)
Massa Fermentata Medicinalis

This drug consists of the mixture of fermented powders of wheat flour and other drugs (Herba Artemisiae Chinghao, Fructus Xanthii, Herba Polygoni Hydropiperis, Semen Armeniacae Amarum and sprout of Semen Phaseoli). The crude drug, the drug parched with bran or the carbonized drug is used in medication.

Nomenclature Used in Prescriptions: *Shengshenqu, Chaoshenqu, Jiaoshenqu, Liushenqu*

Properties and Channel Distribution: This drug is sweet and pungent in taste and warm in nature, and is distributed to the Spleen and Stomach Channels.

Action and Indications:

Promoting digestion and regulating the stomach

In treating indigestion due to stagnation of food or diarrhea, abdominal distention, etc. due to overeating, the drug is often used in combination with Fructus Crataegi, Fructus Hordei Germinatus, Semen Raphani, Endothelium Corneum Gigeriae Galli, etc.

Besides, the crude drug is also made into pills and taken together with pills with ingredients of metal or stone, which are hard to be digested and absorbed, such as "Magnetite and Cinnabar Pill", "Wan's Bezoar Sedative Bolus," etc., to assist digestion and absorption.

Dosage and Administration: Usually, 6–12 g of the drug is used in decoction. The parched drug is used to regulate the stomach and promote digestion, the carbonized drug, to arrest diarrhea and dysentery, and the crude drug, to be made into pills or paste.

Appendix: Massa Medicinalis (建曲 *Jianqu*)

This drug is also called *Fanzhiqu* in Chinese. It consists of the drugs in Massa Fermentata Medicinalis and other drugs without fermentation. Its actions are similar to that of Massa Fermentata Medicinalis and can be used to treat stagnation of food and stuffy chest due to invasion of wind–cold. The dosage is 6–12 g.

Germinated Barley (麦芽 *Maiya*)
Fructus Hordei Germinatus

This drug consists of the germinated fruit of the annual herbage Hordeum vulgare L. (family Gramineae). The crude or slightly carbonized drug is used in medication.

Nomenclature Used in Prescriptions: *Shengmaiya, Chaomaiya*

Properties and Channel Distribution: This drug is sweet in taste and neutral in nature, and is distributed to the Spleen, Stomach and Liver Channels.

Action and Indications:

1. Invigorating the stomach and promoting digestion

In treating indigestion with distention and stuffiness of the epigastrium and abdomen due to stagnation of food, the drug is often used in combination with Fructus Crataegi, Massa Fermentata Medicinalis, etc. In treating vomiting of milk in infants due to dyspepsia, the drug alone can be decocted and taken.

2. Comforting the liver and stopping milk secretion

In treating distention and stuffiness of the epigastrium and abdomen, belching, etc. due to stagnation of liver–*Qi*, the drug is often used in combination with Fructus Meliae Toosendan, Pericarpium Citri Reticulatae, etc. In treating distention and pain of the breast due to accumulation of milk, or for the purpose of stopping milk secretion, 60–120 g of the crude drug can be decocted and taken.

Dosage and Administration: Usually, 10–15 g or in large dosage 30–120 g, of the drug is used in decoction. The crude drug is used to comfort the liver or stop milk secretion and the slightly carbonized drug, to promote digestion.

Rice Sprout (谷芽 *Guya*)
Fructus Oryzae Germinatus

This drug consists of the dried germinant fruit of the annual herbage Oryza sativa L. (family Gramineae). The crude or slightly carbonized drug is used in medication.

Nomenclature Used in Prescriptions: *Shengguya, Chaoguya, Xiangdaoya, Chaodaoya*

Properties and Channel Distribution: This drug is sweet in taste and neutral in nature, and is distributed to the Spleen and Stomach Channels.

Action and Indications:

Invigorating the spleen, inducing appetite, removing stagnated food and regulating the middle warmer

In treating anorexia and indigestion due to deficiency of the spleen and stomach, the drug is often used in combination with Radix Codonopsis Pilosulae, Rhizoma Atractylod is Macrocephalae, Fructus Amomi, etc.

Dosage and Administration: Usually, 10–15 g of the drug is used in decoction. The crude drug is used to nourish the stomach and the slightly parched drug, to promote digestion.

Radish Seed (莱菔子 *Laifuzi*)
Semen Raphani

This drug consists of the ripe seed of the annual or biennial erect herbage Raphanus sativus L. (family Cruciferae). The drug is slightly parched and broken for medication.

Nomenclature Used in Prescriptions: *Laifuzi*

Properties and Channel Distribution: This drug is pungent and sweet in taste and neutral in nature, and is distributed to the Lung and Spleen Channels.

Action and Indications:

1. Removing stagnated food

In treating distention and stuffiness of the epigastrium and abdomen, belching with foul odour, abdominal pain with diarrhea, etc. due to stagnation of food, the drug is often used in combination with Fructus Crataegi, Fructus Hordei Germinatus, Massa Fermentata Medicinalis, etc. to enhance its effect of promoting digestion. For cases with dampness, Poria can be added, and for cases with heat, Fructus Forsythiae can be added.

2. Sending down adverse flow of *Qi* to resolve phlegm

In treating cough and asthma with phlegm, the drug is often used in combination with Fructus Perillae and Semen Sinapis Albae.

Dosage and Administration: Usually, 3–10 g of the drug is used in decoction.

Notes: Since this drug may exhaust anti-pathogenic factors, it should be used with care for those with deficiency of *Qi* and without stagnation of food or phlegm.

Chicken's Gizzard-membrane (鸡内金 *Jineijin*)
Endothelium Corneum Gigeriae Galli

This drug consists of the yellow lining membrance in the gizzard of Gallus gallus domesticus Brisson (family Phasianidae). The crude drug can be used. The drug may also be heated with hot sand and ground into powder for medication.

Nomenclature Used in Prescriptions: *Jineijin, Zhineijin*

Properties and Distributions: This drug is sweet and astringent to the taste and even in nature, and is distributed to the Spleen, Stomach and Urinary Bladder Channels.

Action and Indications:

1. Invigorating the stomach and promoting digestion

In treating indigestion, malnutrition in children, etc. due to stagnation of food, the drug may be used alone, or used in combination with Massa Fermentata Medicinalis, Fructus Hordei Germinatus and Fructus Crataegi.

2. Arresting polyuria

In treating enuresis and frequent micturition, the drug can be used in combination with Oötheca Mantidis, Radix Astragali seu Hedysari, Os Draconis, Concha Ostreae, etc. according to disease conditions.

3. Resolving stones

This drug can be used to treat lithiasis of the gall bladder, kidney and urinary bladder. In treating cholelithiasis, the drug is often used in combination with Herba Lysimachiae, Radix Curcumae, etc. In treating nephrolithiasis and cystolithiasis, the drug is often used in combination with Semen Juglandis, Spora Lygodii, etc.

Dosage and Administration: The dosage is 1.5–3 g to be taken in powder or pill form. The drug is usually not decocted because the active ingredients of the drug are not dissolved.

10 Anthelmintics

Drugs with the main function of expelling or destroying parasites are called anthelmintics.

Anthelmintics are mainly used for intestinal helminthic diseases such as ascariasis, ancylostomiasis, enterobiasis, teniasis, fasciolopsiasis, etc. The common clinical manifestations of helminthic diseases are frequent abdominal pain, abdominal distention, polyphagia or poor appetite or addephagia, and itching in the anus, ear and nose. Sallow complexion and emaciation may appear in chronic cases. Anthelmintics should be used to give radical treatment.

In using anthelmintics, proper combination of drugs should be considered in accordance with the patient's accompanying symptoms, constitution, etc. For example, for those with the accompanying symptom of constipation, purgatives should be used in combination with anthelmintics; for those with retention of food, drugs for removing food retention should be used; for those with deficiency of the spleen and stomach, drugs for invigorating the spleen should be used; for those with poor constitution, the method of reinforcement before reduction or that of reinforcement and reduction in combination can be used.

Due attention should be paid to those anthelmintics which have toxic effects.

Quisqualis Fruit (使君子 *Shijunzi*)
Fructus Quisqualis

This drug consists of the seed of the liana Quisgualis indica L. (family Combretaceae). The crude or parched kernel can be used, or the whole seed is crushed for medication.

Nomenclature Used in Prescriptions: *Shijunzi, Shijunrou*

Properties and Channel Distribution: The drug is sweet in taste and warm in nature, and is distributed to the Spleen and Stomach Channels.

Action and Indications:

This drug can be used to destroy parasites and remove food stagnancy and can be used in the treatment of ascariasis, enterobiasis, etc. It is especially suitable for children owing to its sweet and agreeable taste. For a mild case, therapeutic effect can be obtained by chewing the parched drug. For a severe case with many roundworms, the drug is often used in combination with Semen Arecae, Cortex Meliae, Fructus Mume, etc. In treating malnutrition of children, the drug is often used in combination with Semen Arecae, Rhizoma Picrorhizae, Radix Aucklandiae, etc.

Dosage and Administration: 6–12 g of the drug can be used in decoction. The drug can also be made into pill or powder. For adults, the parched drug is chewed, 10–20 pieces are taken for one dose. For children, the number of pieces to be taken is 1.5 multiplied by the age but the total number should not exceed 20 pieces.

Notes: Administration of large dosage may give rise to hiccups, dizziness, vomiting, nausea, etc. Hiccups may also be caused if the drug is taken with tea.

Chinaberry Bark (苦楝皮 *Kulianpi*)
Cortex Meliae

The drug consists of the bark of stem or root of the deciduous arbor Malia azedarach L. and M. toosendan S. et Z. (family Meliaceae). The crude or fresh drug is used.

Nomenclature Used in Precriptions: *Kuliangenpi, Kulianpi*

Properties and Channel Distibution: The drug is bitter in taste, cold in nature and with toxic effect. It is distributed to the Liver, Spleen and Stomach Channels.

Action and Indications:

This drug can be used to destroy parasites and remove food stagnation and is used in treating ascariasis, enterobiasis, ancylostomiasis, etc., which may cause abdominal pain. This drug is powerful in its effect to destroy parasites with satisfactory therapeutic effects. It may be used alone or in combination with other anthelmintics such as Semen Arecae, etc.

Dosage and Administration: Usually, 6–10 g or 15–30 g (fresh) can be used in decoction. Proper amount of the drug can be used in external treatment.

Notes: Owing to its cold nature and toxic effect, the drug should not be taken over a long period, and should be used with care by those with weak constitution. It is contraindicated for those with hepatitis.

Areca Seed (槟榔 *Binglang*)
Semen Arecae

This drug consists of the ripe seed of the evergreen arbor Areca catechu L. (family Palmae). The crude drug is used after being dried, pounded or cut into slices.

Nomenclature Used in Prescriptions: *Huabinglang, Binglangpian*

Properties and Channel Distribution: The drug is bitter and pungent in taste and warm in nature, and is distributed to the Stomach and Large Intestine Channels.

Action and Indications:

1. Destroying paracites and removing food stagnancy

The drug can be used in treating various intestinal parasitic diseases such as teniasis, ascariasis, enterobiasis, fasciolopsiasis, etc., with better therapeutic effect on teniasis. It can also be used in combination with other anthelmintics.

2. Descending the adverse flow of *Qi* and loosing the bowels

The drug can be used in treating stagnation of food and stasis of *Qi*, abdominal distention and pain, constipation, or tenasmus following diarrhea or dysentery, etc., and is often used in combination with Radix et Rhizoma Rhei, Radix Aucklandiae, etc.

3. Inducing diuresis to alleviate edema.

The drug can be used in treating flaccidity of lower limbs and is often used in combination with Fructus Perillae, Fructus Euodiae, Rhizoma Zingiberis Recens, etc.

In addition, the drug can also be used in treating malaria.

Dosage and Administration: The dosage is usually 6–10 g. When the drug is used alone, 30–120 g can be used. The drug is usually used in decoction.

Notes: It is not advisable for those with deficiency of the spleen and loose stool to use this drug.

Appendix: Pericarpium Arecae (大腹皮 *Dafupi*)

This drug consists of the dried pericarp of Areca catechu L. It is pungent in taste and slightly warm in nature and is distributed to the Spleen, Stomach, Large Intestine and Small Intestine Channels. This drug has the functions of descending adverse flow of *Qi*, comforting the middle warmer and inducing diuresis to alleviate edema, and can be used to treat stagnation of *Qi* due to obstruction by dampness, stuffy and distending epigastrium, difficulty in defecation, edema, flaccidity of the lower limbs, dysuria, etc. In recent years, it has also been used to treat ascites due to cirrhosis, nephrotic edema, etc. Usually, 6–12 g are used as a dose in decoction.

Pumpkin Seed (南瓜子 *Nanguazi*)
Semen Cucurbitae

This drug consists of the seed of the annual herbage Cucurbita moschata Duch. (family Cucurbitaceae). It is used in powder form but the fresh drug is more effective.

Nomenclature used in Prescriptions: *Nanguazi*

Properties and Channel Distribution: The drug is sweet in taste and warm in nature and is distributed to the Stomach and Large Intestine Channels.

Action and Indications:

This drug is used to destroy parasites and can be used in the treatment of teniasis. Usually, 60–120 g of the crude drug (with shell) is used. The drug is cleaned, ground into powder and is then taken with cold water. Two hours later, decoction of 60–120 g of Semen Arecae is to be taken. Half an hour after this, 15 g of Natrii Sulfas is to be taken with water to induce purgation, thus eliminating the parasites from the body.

Besides, the drug is also effective in treating schistosomiasis, ascariasis and enterobiasis.

Dosage and Administration: Usually, 60–120 g of the drug is to be chewed and swallowed as a dose.

Carpesium Fruit (鹤虱 *Heshi*)
Fructus Carpesii

This drug consists of the ripe fruit of the perennial herbage Carpesium abrotanoides L. (family Compositae) or the biennial herbage Daucus carota L. (family Umbelliferae). The fruit is dried in the sun and the crude or parched drug can be used in medication.

Nomenclature Used in Prescriptions: *Heshi*

Properties and Channel Distribution: This drug is bitter and pungent in taste and neutral in nature with mild toxic effect, and is distributed to the Large Intestine Channel.

Action and Indications:

This drug is used to destroy parasites and remove food stagnancy and can be used to treat abdominal pain and itching in the anus due to ascariasis, enterobiasis, teniasis, ancylostomiasis, etc. It is often used in combination with other anthelmintics.

Dosage and Administration: Usually, 3–10 g of the drug is used in decoction, When used in pill or powder form, it is often parched and when used in decoction, the crude drug is used.

Torreya Seed (榧子 *Feizi*)
Semen Torreyae

This drug consists of the ripe seed of the evergreen arbor Torreya grandis Fort. (family Taxaceae). The crude or parched drug is used with the shell removed for medication.

Nomenclature Used in Prescriptions: *Feizi, Feiziren, Feizirou*

Properties and Channel Distribution: This drug is sweet in taste and neutral in nature, and is distributed to the Lung, Stomach and Large Intestine Channels.

Action and Indications:

This drug is used to expel parasites and moisten the intestine, and can be used to treat the various kinds of abdominal pain due to ascariasis, filariasis, teniasis, ancylostomiasis, fasciolopsiasis, etc. It is often used in combination with Semen Arecae, fermentative mass of seed of Ulmus macrocarpa Hance, etc.

In addition, this drug has the function of moistening the intestine and relaxing the bowels and can be used to treat difficulty in defecation in patients with hemorrhoid.

Dosage and Administration: The dosage is 30–50 g. The parched kernel is chewed and swallowed or the drug can be made into pills or powder. The crude drug can also be used (with shell), or smashed and used in decoction. In treating ancylostomiasis, 34–40 pieces are prescribed as a dose to be taken before meals. No ceasation of drug taken until there is absence of eggs of worms in stools.

Fermentative Mass of Seed of Ulmus Macrocarpa Hance (芜荑 *Wuyi*)

This drug consists of the processed fruit of the deciduous arbor or bush Ulmus macrocarpa Hance (family Ulmaceae). The crude drug is used for medication.

Nomenclature Used in Prescriptions: *Chouwuyi, Baiwuyi*

Properties and Channel Distribution: This drug is pungent and bitter in taste and warm in nature, and is distributed to the Spleen and Stomach Channels.

Action and Indications:

This drug is used to destroy parasites and remove food stagnancy and can be used to treat abdominal pain caused by ascariasis, teniasis, etc., diarrhea due to malnutrition in children, etc. It is a chief drug for destroying parasites, and can be used alone or combined with other anthelmintics. For example, in treating malnutrition in children, abdominal pain due to presence of parasites or frequent diarrhea in those with emaciation and sallow complexion, the drug can be used in combination with Rhizoma Atractylodis Macrocephalae, Rhizoma Dioscoreae, Endothelium Corneum Gigeriae Galli, Radix Aucklandiae, etc.

Dosage and Administration: Usually, 3–10 g of the drug is used as a dose in decoction.

Omphalia (雷丸 *Leiwan*)
Omphalia

This drug consists of the sclerotium of Polyporus mylittae Cook. et Mass. (family Polyporaceae). The crude drug is cut into slices or ground into powder for medication.

Nomenclature Used in Prescriptions: *Leiwan*

Properties and Channel Distribution: This drug is bitter in taste and cold in nature with mild toxic effect, and is distributed to the Stomach and Large Intestine Channels.

Action and Indications:

This drug is used to destroy parasites and remove food stagnancy and can be used to treat teniasis, ancylostomiasis, ascariasis, etc. Experiments have shown that this drug may cause disintegration of tenia. The drug used alone is quite effective. It can also be used in combination with Semen Arecae, Semen Pharbitidis, Radix Aucklandiae etc. In treating malnutrition in children, it can be used in combination with Fructus Quisqualis, Rhizoma Picrorhizae, etc., and in treating cerebral cysticercosis, it can be used in combination with Rhizoma Pinelliae, Poria, etc.

Dosage and Administration: Usually, 3–6 g of the drug powder is taken as a dose. In treating teniasis, 12–18 g of the drug powder is taken with cold water after meals, 3 times a day for 3 days.

Notes: The drug is prepared into pill or powder, never given in decoction.

Agrimony Bud (鹤草芽 *Hecaoya*)
Gemma Agrimoniae

This drug consists of the winter bud of the perennial herbage Agrimonia Pilosa Ledeb. (family Rosaceae). The drug is dried in the sun and ground into powder for medication.

Nomenclature Used in Prescriptions: *Hecaoya*

Properties and Channel Distribution: This drug is puckery in taste and cool in nature, and is distributed to the Liver, Large Intestine and Small Intestine Channels.

Action and Indications:

This drug is used to destroy parasites and can be used to treat teniasis, with satisfactory result. It is the main drug for treating teniasis. The drug powder is taken in the morning at a drought before breakfast. Usually, the worms are eliminated 5–6 hours after the drug is taken.

Dosage and Administration: The drug is taken in powder form. The dosage for adults is 30–50 g , to be taken with warm water. For children, the dosage is determined according to the body weight, i. e. 0.7 0.8 g for each kilogram.

Brucea Fruit (鸦胆子 *Yadanzi*)
Fructus Bruceae

This drug consists of the ripe fruit of the evergreen bush or arbor Brucea javanica (L.) Merr. (family Simaroubaceae). The dried Kernel is used for medication.

Nomenclature Used in Prescriptions: *Yadanzi, Yadanyou*

Properties and Channel Distribution: This drug is bitter in taste and cold in nature, and is distributed to the Large Intestine and Liver Channels.

Action and Indications:

1. Destroying parasites to relieve dysentery

This drug can be used to treat dysentery with bloody stool due to noxious heat, dysentery with pus and blood, tenesmus, etc. This drug is the main drug for treating dysentery with bloody stool due to noxious heat and recurrent dysentery. The drug, when used alone, can be put into longan aril and taken. Fifteen pieces of the drug are prescribed as one dose, 3 times a day for 10–14 days. The drug is also used to treat acute and chronic amebic dysentery.

2. Destroying parasites to treat malaria

The drug can be used to treat malaria tertiana, malaria quartana and malignant malaria. The kernal of the drug is put into longan aril for oral administration, 10–15 pieces of the drug as a dose to be taken 3 times a day for 5–7 days.

3. Corroding verruca

The drug can be used to treat clavus and verruca vulgaris. The drug can be pounded and applied to the diseased area or the oil extracted from the drug can be applied to the diseased area, twice a day, Both methods will cause the falling off of the verruca.

Dosage and Administration: In treating dysentery, the drug is taken orally with 10–30 pieces each time for adults. In treating malaria, the drug is also taken orally with 10–15 pieces for adults and 1 piece for each year of age for children (the dosage should not exceed that for adults). The kernel is put into longan aril and then taken after meals, so as to avoid irritation of the stomach and intestine. Proper amount of the drug can also be used in external treatment.

Notes: The drug has mild toxic effect and may cause injury to the gastrointestinal tract, liver and kidney; it is therefore not advisable to use the drug with large dosage or over a long time. Those with bleeding in the stomach and intestine or with liver or kidney diseases should use the drug with care or avoid using the drug.

11 Hemostatics

Drugs with the main function of arresting various kinds of bleeding in the body are called hemostatics.

This kind of drugs are mainly used to treat various diseases characterized by bleeding, such as hemoptysis, epistaxis, hematemesis, hemafecia, hematuria, metrorrhagia and metrostaxis, purpura, traumatic bleeding, etc. The drugs can arrest bleeding timely and effectively to stop loss of blood. They are also of great significance in preventing massive loss of blood or collapse of *Qi* due to loss of blood.

Hemostatics have such different functions as arresting bleeding by means of cooling blood, astringing blood, removing blood stasis, warming the channels, etc. Bleeding is a symptom of certain diseases but the cause varies. Hemostatics are drugs only to treat the symptoms and they should not be used blindly in treating hemorrhagic diseases. Instead, proper combination of drugs should be considered according to the causes of bleeding in order to remove the original diseases. For example, when bleeding is due to blood−heat, hemostatics should be used in combination with drugs for clearing away heat and cooling blood; when bleeding is due to deficiency of *Yin* and hyperactivity of *Yang*, which results in adverse flow of blood with adverse flow of *Qi*, hemostatics should be used in combination with drugs for nourishing *Yin*, checking exuberance of *Yang* and sending down abnormal flow of *Qi*; when bleeding is due to deficiency of *Qi*, which results in failure to control blood, hemostatics should be used in combination with drugs for invigorating *Qi*. In this way, the symptoms and causes are treated at the same time and satisfactory result will be obtained.

In addition, attention should be paid to the presence of blood stasis. With the presence of blood stasis, hemastatics used alone may have the disadvantage of retaining the blood stasis. Therefore, at the initial stage of hemorrhagic diseases, it is advisable to used hemostatics with the function of removing blood stasis or to use hemostatics and drugs for promoting blood circulation in combination. For those with massive loss of blood and collapse, the method of invigorating *Qi* should be used first. This is known as "invigorating *Qi* in the case of collapse of blood".

Cat-tail Pollen (蒲黄 *Puhuang*)
Pollen Typhae

This drug consists of the pollen of the perennial herbage Typha angustifolia L. or other species of the same genus (family Typhaceae). The crude or carbonized drug is used for medication.

Nomenclature Used in Prescriptions: *Shengpuhuang, Chaopuhuang, Puhuangtan*

Properties and Channel Distribution: This drug is sweet in taste and neutral in nature, and is distributed to the Liver and Pericardium Channels.

Action and Indications:

1. Arresting blood (parched drug is used)

The drug can be used to treat hemoptysis, hematemesis, epistaxis, hematuria, hemafecia, metrorrhagia and metrostaxis, etc. The drug can be used alone (oral administration) or used in combination with other drugs. It may also be used alone in external treatment for traumatic bleeding.

2. Promoting blood circulation and removing blood stasis (crude drug is used)

The drug can be used to treat stasis of blood, gastralgia, abdominal pain, dysmenorrhea, postpartum abdominal pain due to stasis of blood, etc. The drug is often used in combination with Faeces Trogopterorum. In treating swelling, rigidity or heaviness of the tongue, the crude drug can be applied to the local area for several minutes.

In addition, the crude drug is often used to treat stranguria with blood to induce diuresis. It can be used in combination with Fructus Malvae Verticillatae, Radix Rehmanniae, etc. The drug is in recent years used to treat angina pectoris seen in coronary heart disease.

Dosage and Administration: Usually, 3–10 g of the drug is used in decoction (wrapped with cloth). Proper amount of the drug can also be used in external treatment.

Notes: Since the crude drug has the effect of contracting the uterus, it should be used with care by pregnant women. It can be used, however, in the treatment of bleeding due to improper uterine contraction after labour.

Agrimony (仙鹤草 *Xianhecao*)
Herba Agrimoniae

This drug consists of the whole plant of the perennial herbage Agrimonia Pilosa Ledeb. var. japonica (Miq.) Nakai (family

Rosaceae). The crude drug is cut and used for medication.

Nomenclature Used in Prescriptions: *Xianhecao*

Properties and Channel Distribution: This drug is bitter and puckery in taste and neutral in nature, and is distributed to the Heart, Spleen, Stomach and Large Intestine Channels.

Action and Indications:

1. Astringing blood to arrest bleeding

The drug can be used to treat various hemorrhagic diseases such as hemoptysis, hematemesis, epistaxis, hemafecia, hematuria, metrorrhagia and metrostaxis, etc. The drug is used extensively to treat various kinds of bleeding in various parts of the body, whether they are due to deficiency, excess, cold or heat. It can be used alone or combined with other drugs. For example, for bleeding due to blood–heat, this drug can be used in combination with drugs for cooling blood to arrest bleeding such as Radix Rehmanniae, Cortex Moutan Radicis, Cacumen Biotae, Radix Paeoniae Rubra, Nodus Nelumbinis Rhizomatis, etc.; for bleeding due to cold of deficiency type, the drug can be used in combination with Radix Codonopsis Pilosulae, Radix Astragali seu Hedysari, Rhizoma Rehmanniae Praeparata, Radix Angelicae Sinensis, Rhizoma Zingiberis Praeparata, Folium Artemisiae Argyi, Terra Flava Usta, etc.

2. Astringing blood to arrest diarrhea

This drug can be used to treat chronic diarrhea and dysentery. Usually, 30 g of the drug and 10 g of Flos Hibisci are used together. The drug can also be used in combination with other drugs in different cases.

3. Destroying parasites

This drug can be used to treat pruritus genitalium caused by trichomonal vaginitis. The thick decoction of 120 g of the drug can be used to wash the vagina, and then a cotton ball soaked with the decoction can be put into the vagina for 3 hours, treatment should be given once a day for a week.

In addition, the drug can also be used to treat patients with internal injury caused by overstrain. For those patients with listlessness but normal appetite, 30 g of the drug and 30 g of Chinese date are decocted and taken daily to invigorate *Qi* and blood and restore health. In treating carbuncle, sore, hemorrhoid, etc. a soft extract with honey made of the stalk and leaf of the plant can be given. This extract can be applied to the local area or taken orally.

Dosage and Administration: The usual dosage is 10–15 g and the large dosage is 30–60 g. Proper amount of the drug can also be used in external treatment.

Bletilla Tuber (白及 *Baiji*)
Rhizoma Bletillae

This drug consists of the tuber of the perennial herbage Bletilla striate (Thunb.) Reichb. f. (family Orchidaceae). The tuber is cut into slices for medication.

Nomenclature Used in Prescriptions: *Baiji*

Properties and Channel Distribution: The drug is bitter, sweet and puckery in taste and slightly cold in nature, and is distributed to the Lung, Liver and Stomach Channels.

Action and Indications:

1. Astringing blood to arrest bleeding

This drug can be used to treat bleeding of the lung or stomach. The drug powder can be used alone, e.g. for bleeding of the lung, or the drug can be used in combination with powder of Cyclina sinensis, Folium Eriobotryae, etc. In treating hemoptysis seen in pulmonary tuberculosis with cavitation, the drug can be used in combination with Colophonium, Rhizoma Anemarrhenae, Bulbus Lilii, etc. In treating bleeding of the stomach, ulcer and perforation of the stomach or duodenum, etc., the drug can be used in combination with Os Sepiellae seu Sepiae, etc. In treating bleeding due to unhealed trauma and sores, the drug powder alone or combined with Gypsum Fibrosum Usta can be applied to the local area. In treating scald or rhagas of the hand and foot, the drug can be mixed with sesame oil and then applied to the local area.

2. Subduing swelling and promoting tissue regeneration

In treating carbuncle and swelling, thc drug is often used in combination with Flos Lonicerae, Squama Manitis, Spina Gleditsiae, etc.

Dosage and Administration: The dosage is 3–10 g in decoction. When the drug is taken in powder form, the dosage is 1–3 g. Proper amount of the drug can also be used in external treatment.

Notes: The drug is antogonized by Radix Aconiti.

Lotus Node (藕节 *Oujie*)
Nodus Nelumbinis Rhizomatis

This drug consists of the node of perennial aquatic herbage Nelumbo nucifera Gaertn. (family Nymphaeaceae). The crude or carbonized drug is used for medication.

Nomenclature Used in Prescriptions: *Shengoujie, Oujietan*

Properties and Channel Distribution: The drug is sweet and puckery in taste and neutral in nature, and is distributed to the Liver. Lung, Urinary Bladder and Stomach Channels.

Action and Indications:

This drug is used to astringe blood to arrest bleeding and cool blood to remove blood stasis, and can be used to treat hemoptysis, hematemesis, epistaxis, hematuria, dysentery with blood, and metrorrhagia. It is especially effective for stasis of blood due to blood–heat. The fresh drug can be pounded and the extract is taken. The drug is often used in combination with other hemostatics such as Radix Rehmanniae, Cacumen Biotae, etc.

Dosage and Administration: Its usual dosage is 10–15 g. When fresh drug is used, 30–60 g are used in decoction. When the drug is used to cool blood and remove blood stasis, the crude drug is used, and when the drug is used to astringe blood to arrest bleeding, the carbonized drug is used.

Petiole of Windmill–palm (棕榈 *Zonglu*)
Petiolus Trachycarpi

This drug consists of the petiole of the evergreen arbor Trachycarpus Wagnerianus Becc. (family Palmae). It is also called *Zonglupi* in Chinese. The drug is cut into pieces and carbonized for medication.

Nomenclature Used in Prescriptions: *Zonglu,Zonglutan, Chenzonglu*

Properties and Channel Distribution: This drug is bitter and astringent in taste and neutral in nature, and is distributed to the

Lung, Liver and Large Intestine Channels.

Action and Indications:

This drug is used to astringe blood to arrest bleeding and can be used to treat hematemesis, epistaxis, hemafecia, metrorrhagia and metrostaxis, dysentery with blood and mucus, etc. without stasis of blood. Clinically, it is often used to treat metrorrhagia and metrostaxis. The drug may be used alone or combined with other drugs.

Dosage and Administration: Its usual dosage is 3–10 g, used in decoction.

Furnace Soil (灶心土 *Zaoxintu*)
Terra Flava Usta

This drug is the earth obtained from the kitchen range in which straw or wood is burnt over a long time. It is broken into small pieces for medication.

Nomenclature Used in Prescriptions: *Zaoxintu, Fulonggan*

Properties and Channel Distribution: This drug is pungent in taste and slightly warm in nature, and is distributed to the Spleen and Stomach Channels.

Action and Indications:

1. Astringing blood to arrest bleeding

This drug can be used to treat hematemesis, hemafecia, etc. due to cold of deficiency type, with such manifestations as dark blood, sallow complexion, cold limbs, pale tongue and thready pulse. The drug can be used in combination with Rhizoma Atractylodis Macrocephalae, Radix Rehmanniae, Radix Aconiti Praeparata, etc., with the effect of warming the middle warmer and astringing blood so as to arrest bleeding.

2. Warming the middle warmer to arrest vomiting

This drug can be used to treat vomiting due to cold of deficiency type, pernicious vomiting, etc. It can be used in combination with Pericarpium Citri Reticulatae, Rhizoma Zingiberis Recens, etc.

Besides, it can also be used to treat diarrhea due to deficiency of the spleen, with the effect of warming the spleen to arrest diarrhea.

Dosage and Administration: Usually, 15–30 g of the drug is wrapped with cloth and decocted before other drugs. Alternatively, 60–120 g of the drug can be decocted and drunk instead of drinking water.

Notoginseng (三七 *Sanqi*)
Radix Notoginseng

This drug consists of the root of the perennial herbage Panax pseudo–ginseng Wall. var. notoginseng (Burkill) Hoo & Tseng (family Araliaceae). The drug is ground into powder for medication.

Nomenclature Used in Prescriptions: *Sanqifen*

Properties and Channel Distribution: This drug is sweet and slightly bitter in taste and warm in nature, and is distributed in the Liver and Stomach Channels.

Action and Indications:

1. Arresting bleeding and removing blood stasis

This drug can be used to treat hematemesis, epistaxis, dysentery with blood, hemafecia, metrorrhagia, massive loss of blood after labour, etc. This drug is the major drug for arresting blood and has the characteristic of arresting bleeding without retaining blood stasis. It has special therapeutic effect whether it is taken orally or used in external treatment, and is especially effective for those with bleeding accompanied by blood stasis. The drug powder can be used alone, to be taken with rice water or warm water (1.5–3 g as a dose). The drug can also be used in combination with Ophicalcitum. The drug powder can also be applied to the wound in treating bleeding due to trauma.

2. Subduing swelling and relieving pain

The drug can be used to treat traumatic injury, pain due to stasis of blood, carbuncle, sore, etc. The drug powder can be mixed with vinegar and applied to the affected area.

In addition, the drug has been used in recent years to treat angina pectoris seen in coronary heart disease with certain effect.

Dosage and Administration: Its dosage is usually 1.5–3 g. The drug is often made into pills or powder. The drug powder can also be used in decoction. Proper amount of the drug can also be used in external treatment.

Notes: This drug is warm in nature and therefore in treating bleeding accompanied by dry mouth due to deficiency of *Yin*, the drug is often used in combination with drugs for nourishing *Yin* and cooling blood.

Rubia Root (茜草根 *Qiancaogen*)
Radix Rubiae

This drug consists of the root of the perennial trailing herbage Rubia cordifolia L. (family Rubiaceae). The drug is dried in the sun and cut into sections for use. The crude or carbonized drug can be used for medication.

Nomenclature Used in Prescriptions: *Qiancaogen, Qiancaotan*

Properties and Channel Distribution: This drug is bitter in taste and cold in nature, and is distributed to the Liver Channel.

Action and Indications:

1. Arresting bleeding and removing blood stasis

This drug can be used to treat hematemesis, epistaxis, hemafecia, metrorrhagia and metrostaxis, etc. which are due to heat. It can be used in combination with Radix Rehmanniae, Cacumen Biotae, Colla Corii Asini, etc. In treating dysentery with bloody stool, the drug can be used in combination with Radix Scutellariae, Rhizoma Coptidis, etc.; in treating metrorrhagia and metrostaxis due to cold of deficiency type, the drug can be used in combination with Os Sepiellae seu Sepiae, Concha Ostreae, Radix Astragali seu Hedysari, etc. to astringe blood and build up strength; in treating allergic purpura, the drug can be used in combination with Radix Arnebiae seu Lithospermi, Radix Salviae Miltiorrhizae, etc.

2. Cooling blood and promoting blood circulation

This drug can be used in combination with Radix Salviae Miltiorrhizae to treat stasis of blood due to blood-heat, dysmenorrhea, amenia, etc., or in combination with Flos Carthami, Radix Paeoniae Rubra, etc. to treat traumatic injury.

Dosage and Administration: Usually, 6–10 g of the drug is used in decoction.

Ophicalcite (花蕊石 *Huaruishi*)
Ophicalcitum

This drug consists of the marble containing green serpentine, i. e. Ophicalcite. The marble is calcined and ground into fine powder with water for medication.

Nomenclature Used in Prescriptions: *Huaruishi*

Properties and Channel Distribution: This drug is sour and astringent in taste and neutral in nature, and is distributed to the Liver Channel.

Action and Indications:

This drug is used to arrest bleeding and remove blood stasis, and can be used to treat hematemesis, epistaxis, postpartum fainting, retention of placenta, etc. This drug can be used to treat all kinds of internal bleeding with blood stasis. The drug can be used alone (6 g as a dose), taken with urine of a boy under 12 and wine or vinegar, or the drug can be used in combination with Radix Notoginseng, Crinis Carbonisatus, etc. In treating traumatic bleeding, the drug can be ground into fine powder and applied to the affected part.

Dosage and Administration: Usually, 3–10 g of the drug is used in decoction, and the drug is to be decocted longer than other drugs. Pills or powder are preferred. It can also be used in external treatment.

Carbonized Hair (血余炭 *Xueyutan*)
Crinis Carbonisatus

This drug is the carbonized human hair, which is ground into small pieces or fine powder for medication.

Nomenclature Used in Prescriptions: *Xueyutan, Fatan*

Properties and Channel Distribution: This drug is bitter in taste and neutral in nature, and is distributed to the Liver and Kidney Channels.

Action and Indications:

This drug is used to arrest bleeding and remove blood stasis, and can be used to treat hematemesis, epistaxis, hematuria, stranguria with blood, dysentery with bloody stool, hemafecia, metrorrhagia and metrostaxis, etc. The drug is often used in combination with other hemostatics. In treating traumatic bleeding or persistent ulcer, a soft extract made of its powder is applied to the affected part.

Besides, this drug also has the effect of inducing diuresis.

Dosage and Administration: Its usual dosage is 3–10 g, used in decoction. Proper amount of the drug can also be used in external treatment.

Field Thistle (小蓟 *Xiaoji*)
Herba Cephalanoploris

This drug consists of the whole plant of the perennial herbage Cephalanoplos Segetum (Bge.) Kitam. (family Compositae). The drug is cut into sections. The crude or parched drug is used.

Nomenclature Used in Prescriptions: *Xiaoji, Xiaojitan*

Properties and Channel Distribution: This drug is sweet in taste and cool in nature, and is distributed to the Heart, Small Intestine and Urinary Bladder Channels.

Action and Indications:

This drug is used to cool blood to arrest blood and remove blood stasis, and can be used to treat hematemesis, epistaxis, hematuria, stranguria with blood, hemafecia, metrorrhagia and metrostaxis, etc. due to heat in the blood system. Since this drug has the effect of inducing diuresis, it is effective for stranguria with blood. It is often used in combination with Radix Rehmanniae, Fructus Gardeniae, Nodus Nelumbinis Rhizomatis, Talcum, Pollen Typhae, etc. In treating hematemesis, it is often used in combination with Herba seu Radix Cirsii Japonici, Cacumen Biotae, Rhizoma Imperatae, Fructus Gardeniae, Radix Rubiae, etc.

Dosage and Administration: Usually, 10–15 g of the drug or 30–60 g of the fresh drug is used in decoction.

Appendix: Herba seu Radix Cirsii Japonici (大蓟 *Daji*)

This drug consists of the root, stem and leaf of the perennial herbage Cirsium japonicum DC. (family Compositae). The properties, actions and dosage of this drug are the same as those of Herba Cephalanoploris. Besides, this drug has the effect of subduing swelling and therefore can be used to treat carbuncles and pyogenic infections. This drug can be both taken orally and applied externally. The fresh drug is more effective.

Biota Tops (侧柏叶 *Cebaiye*)
Cacumen Biotae

This drug consists of the leafy twigs of the evergreen arbor Biota orientalis (L.) Endl. (family Cupressaceae). The crude or carbonized drug is used for medication.

Nomenclature Used in Prescriptions: *Shengcebai, cebaiye*

Properties and Channel Distribution: This drug is bitter and puckery in taste and slightly cold in nature, and is distributed to the Lung, Liver and Large Intestine Channels.

Action and Indications:

1. Cooling blood and arrest bleeding

This drug can be used to treat hemoptysis, hematemesis, epistaxis, hematuria, hemafecia, metrorrhagia and metrostaxis, etc. which are due to heat in the blood system. This is a drug for astringing and cooling blood and arresting bleeding. It can be used alone or in combination with other drugs for cooling blood and arresting bleeding, such as Radix Rehmanniae, Folium Nelumbinis, etc. In treating bleeding due to cold of deficiency type, the drug can be used in combination with Folium Artemisiae Argri, Rhizoma Zingiberis Praeparata, etc.

2. Promoting the growth of hair and blackening hair

This drug can be used to treat deficiency of blood due to blood−heat, baldness after disease, or premature greying of hair seen in young or middle−aged persons. It is often used in combination with Radix Polygoni Multiflori, Fructus Ligustri Lucidi, Radix Rehmanniae, etc.

Besides, this drug can also be used to relieve cough and dispel phlegm and can be used to treat cough and asthma with much sputum, It can also be used to treat abnormal leukorrhea due to damp–heat owing to its effect of eliminating dampness. In external treatment, the drug can be used to treat seborrheic dermatitis. A solution of 60 g of the fresh drug mixed in 60% alcohol (or spirit) for 7 days can be applied to the affected area.

Dosage and Administration: Usually, 6–10 g of the drug is used in decoction.

Imperata Rhizome (白茅根 *Baimaogen*)
Rhizoma Imperatae

This drug consists of the rhizome of the perennial herbage Imperata cylindrica (L.) Beauv. var, major (Nees) C. E. Hubb. (family Graminae). The drug is cut into sections and the crude or freesh drug can be used in medication.

Nomenclature Used in Prescriptions: *Baimaogen, Maogen, Xianmaogen*

Properties and Channel Distribution: This drug is sweet in taste and cold in nature, and is distributed to the Heart, Lung, Stomach and Urinary Bladder Channels.

Action and Indications:

1. Cooling blood and arresting bleeding

This drug can be used to treat bleeding due to blood–heat, such as hematemesis, epistaxis, hematuria, etc. It can used alone or in combination with Radix Rehmanniae, Fructus Gardeniae Praeparatae, Nodus Nelumbinis Rhizomatis, etc.

2. Clearing away heat to induce diuresis

This drug can be used to treat pain seen in stranguria due to heat, edema, dysuria, etc. It can be used alone or in combination with Semen Plantaginis, etc. When decocted with Semen Phaseoli, it can be used to treat jaundice.

3. Clearing away heat to promote the production of body fluid

This drug can be used to treat febrile diseases, thirst due to heat in the stomach, vomiting of foul food, cough due to heat in the lung, or cough with yellow sputum. Since the drug is sweat in taste and cold in nature and therefore has the effect of clearing away heat in the heart, lung and stomach, it is most suitable for those with febrile diseases accompanied by deficiency of body fluid. The drug can be used in combination with Rhizoma Phragmitis, Gypsum Fibrosum, etc. In treating measles at its initial stage with retarded eruptions, the drug can be used alone or in combination with Rhizoma Phragmitis or other drugs for promoting eruption.

Dosage and Administration: Usually, 10–30 g of the drug or 30–60 g of the fresh drug is used in decoction. The fresh drug is more effective.

Sanguisorba Root (地榆 *Diyu*)
Radix Sanguisorbae

This drug consists of the rhizome and root of the perennial herbage Sanguisorba officinalis L. (family Rosaceae). The drug is cut into slices and the crude or carbonized drug is used for medication.

Nomenclature Used in Prescriptions: *Shengdiyu, Diyutan*

Properties and Channel Distribution: This drug is bitter, sour and puckery in taste and slightly cold in nature, and is distributed to the Liver, Stomach and Large Intestine Channels.

Action and Indications:

1. Cooling blood to arrest bleeding

This drug can be used to treat hematemesis, epistaxis, hematuria, metrorrhagia and metrostaxis, etc. It is often used in combination with Radix Rubiae, Nodus Nelumbinis Rhizomatis, etc. In treating hemafecia, hemorrhoid with bleeding, dysentery with blood, etc., the drug is often used in combination with Fructus Sophorae, Radix Rehmanniae, Spica Schizonepetae, Radix Ledebouriellae, etc. In treating gastric or duodenal ulcer, hematemesis and hemafecia, it can be used in combination with Rhizoma Bletillae, etc.

2. Subduing swelling and relieving pain

This drug can be used to treat scald and burns. Since this drug has the effect of astringing blood and purging fire, it is an important drug for scald and burns. The crude drug is ground into powder, mixed with sesame oil and applied to the local area. This can reduce exudate, relieve pain and speed up healing. Alternatively, 30 g of the drug, 30 g of crude Radix et Rhizoma Rhei and 1.5 g of Borneolum Syntheticum are ground into powder, mixed with sesame oil and applied to the local area. In treating carbuncle and sores, the drug can be used in combination with Flos Lonicerae, Herba Taraxaci, etc.

Dosage and Administration: Usually, 10–30 g of the drug is used in decoction. The drug can also be used in external treatment. In treating burns and swelling, the crude drug can be used. In arresting bleeding, the carbonized drug can be used.

Sophora Fruit (槐角 *Huaijiao*)
Fructus Sophorae

This drug consists of the fruit of the deciduous arbor Sophora japonica L. (family Leguminosae). The crude or carbonized drug is used for medication.

Nomenclature Used in Prescriptions: *Huaijiao, Huaishi, Huaijiaotan*

Properties and Channel Distribution: This drug is bitter in taste and cold in nature, and is distributed to the Liver and Large Intestine Channels.

Action and Indications:

1. Cooling blood to arrest bleeding

This drug can be used to treat hemafecia, hemorrhoid with bleeding, dysentery with blood, etc. This drug is especially effective for lower bleeding, particularly bleeding from the intestine. It is often used in combination with Radix Sanguisorbae and Radix Scutellariae. In treating downward flow of damp–heat, yellowish vaginal discharge and metrostaxis, the drug can be used in combination with crude Cacumen Biotae, crude Radix Sanguisorbae, Herba Houttuyniae, Flos Lonicerae, Radix Glycyrrhizae, etc.

2. Clearing away heat in the liver and brightening the eye

This drug can be used to treat the liver–heat, dizziness and conjunctival congestion. It is often used in combination with Rhizoma Coptidis.

Dosage and Administration: Usually, 6–12 g of the drug is used in decoction. In clearing away heat, cooling blood or brightening the eye, the crude drug is used. In arresting blood, the carbonized drug can be used.

Appendix: Flos Sophorae Immaturus and Flos Sophorae (槐米,槐花 *Huaimi, Huaihua*)

The former refers to the flower–bud of the plant and the latter, the flower. Both are bitter in taste and slightly cold in nature. They have better effect of cooling blood to arrest bleeding than Fructus Sophorae, and can be used to treat hemafecia, hemorrhoid with blood, hematemesis, epistaxis, etc. Since the crude drugs have the effect of bringing down blood pressure, they are often used to treat hypertension. The dosage is the same as that of Fructus Sophorae.

Boehmeriu Root (苎麻根 *Zhumagen*) Radix Boehmeriae

This drug consists of the root of the perennial herbage Boehmeria nivea (L.) Gaud, (family Urticaceae). The drug is cut into slices and sections and the crude drug is used for medication.

Nomenclature Used in Prescriptions: *Zhumagen*

Properties and Channel Distribution: This drug is sweat in taste and cold in nature, and is distributed to the Liver and Heart Channels.

Action and Indications:

1. Arresting bleeding to prevent abortion

This drug can be used to treat threatened abortion, vaginal bleeding during pregnancy, etc. It is a special drug for preventing abortion and is used frequently. It can be used in combination with Radix Rehmanniae, Radix Angelicae Sinensis, Colla Corii Asini, etc.

2. Clearing away heat and removing toxins

This drug can be used to treat boils at its initial stage, hemorrhoid with swelling and pain, prolapse of rectum, etc. The fresh drug can be washed, pounded into paste and applied to the local area twice a day. This method can also be used to treat snake bite and insect sting.

3. Inducing diuresis

This drug can be used to treat stranguria with hematuria, in combination with Talcum Herba Dianthi, Herba Polygoni Avicularis, etc.

Dosage and Administration: Usually, 6–12 g of the drug is used in decoction. Proper amount of the drug can also be used in external treatment.

Argyi Leaf (艾叶 *Aiye*)
Folium Artemisiae Argyi

This drug consists of the leaf of the perennial herbage Artemisia Argyi Levl. et Vant. (family Compositae). The crude or carbonized drug is used for medication.

Nomenclature Used in Prescriptions: *Shengaiye, Aiyetan, Airong*

Properties and Channel Distribution: This drug is pungent and bitter in taste and warm in nature, and is distributed to the Liver, Spleen and Kidney Channels.

Action and Indications:

1. Warming the channels to arrest bleeding

This drug can be used to treat metrorrhagia and metrostaxis, threatened abortion, irregular menstruation, etc., which are of cold of deficiency type. It is often used in combination with Colla

Corii Asini, Radix Rehmanniae, etc. In treating hematemesis and epistaxis due to blood–heat, the crude drug can be used in combination with crude Cacumen Biotae, crude Radix Rehmanniae, crude Folium Nelumbinis, etc.

2. Dispersing cold and removing dampness

This drug can be used to treat abnormal leukorrhea due to cold uterus, irregular menstruation, abdominal pain, infertility, etc. It is often used in combination with Rhizoma Cyperi, Fructus Euodiae, Cortex Cinnamomi, etc.

In addition, this drug can also be used to treat itching of the skin seen in eczema. The drug can be decocted with Cortex Dictamni Radicis and Fructus Kochiae and the decoction can be used to wash the local area. In treating retention of placenta due to cold, the parched drug can be applied to the hypogastrium while still hot. The drug can also be made into wool, put on the acupoints and ignited. This can send heat into the tendons and bones so as to treat arthralgia due to cold. The drug is therefore the main material used in applying warming moxibustion.

Dosage and Administration: Usually, 3–10 g of the drug is used in decoction. The drug can also be used in external treatment. In dispersing cold and dampness and regulating the flow of *Qi* and blood, the crude drug is used. In warming the uterus so as to arrest bleeding, the carbonized drug is used.

12 Drugs for Promoting the Circulation of Blood and Removing Blood Stasis

This is a kind of drugs with the main functions of removing obstruction from the blood vessels, promoting blood circulation and dispersing blood stasis, in which those with strong power of promoting blood circulation and removing blood stasis are also called drastic drugs for removing blood stasis.

This kind of drugs are mostly pungent in taste and warm in nature. Pungency can remove blood stasis and warmth can promote blood circulation, and therefore disperse stasis, subdue swelling and relieve pain. This kind of drugs are often used in the treatment of pain caused by stasis of *Qi* and blood, traumatic injury, masses in the abdomen, carbuncle, phlegmon, painful swelling, amenorrhea, dysmenorrhea, etc.

There are various causes of stasis of blood, and therefore the causes should be found out by differentiation of syndromes and proper combination of drugs worked out. Since *Qi* and blood are closely related to each other, i.e. free flow of *Qi* leads to free flow of blood and stasis of *Qi* results in stasis of blood and vice versa, this kind of drugs are often used in combination with drugs for regulating the flow of *Qi*.

Since this kind of drugs has the function of promoting blood circulation, it is not advisable to use them to treat menorrhagia and deficiency of blood without blood stasis. Besides, since drugs for promoting menstrual flow have the function of promoting the contraction of the uterus, they should not be given to pregnant women so as to avoid miscarriages.

Chuanxiong Rhizome (川芎 *Chuanxiong*)
Rhizoma Ligustici Chuanxiong

This drug consists of the rhizome of the perennial herbage Ligusticum chuanxiong Hort. (family Umbelliferae). The crude drug is cut into pieces for medication.

Nomenclature Used in Prescriptions: *Chuanxiong, Fuxiong*

Properties and Channel Distribution: This drug is pungent in taste and warm in nature, and is distributed to the Liver, Gall Bladder and Pericardium Channels.

Action and Indications:

1. Activating blood circulation and flow of *Qi*

In treating angina pectoris seen in coronary heart disease, the drug can be used in combination with Flos Carthami, Radix Salviae Miltiorrhizae, etc. In treating stasis of *Qi* and blood, irregular menstruation, amenorrhea, dysmenorrhea, difficult labour, retention of placenta, etc., the drug is often used in combination with Radix Angelicae Sinensis, Radix Paeoniae Alba, Radix Rehmanniae, etc. In treating blood stasis and swelling due to traumatic injury, pain in the hypochondrium due to stasis of *Qi*, carboncle and sores, etc., the drug is often used in combination with Semen Persicae, Flos Carthami, Resina Boswelliae Carterii, Resina Commiphorae Myrrhae, etc.

2. Dispelling wind to relieve pain

This drug can be used to treat headache. The drug has quite satisfactory effect of dispelling wind to relieve pain and the drug effect may reach the vertex, and therefore it is a good drug for headache. In treating common cold and headache due to wind-cold, the drug can be used in combination with Herba Schizonepetae, Radix Angelicae Dahuricae, Radix Ledebouriellae, etc.; in treating the same disease due to wind-heat, the drug can be used in combination with Flos Chrysanthemi, Herba Menthae, etc.; if the disease is due to wind-dampness, the drug can be used in combination with Rhizoma seu Radix Notopterygii, Rhizoma Ligustici, Radix Ledebouriellae, etc. In treating headache due to stasis of blood or deficiency of blood, the drug can be used in combination with drugs for activating blood circulation or drugs for nourishing blood. In treating arthralgia due to wind-dampness, the drug can be used in combination with Rhizoma seu Radix Notopterygii, Radix Angelicae Pubescentis, Radix Ledebouriellae, etc.

Dosage and Administration: Usually, 3-6 g of the drug is used in decoction.

Notes: Since this drug is pungent in taste and warm in nature with ascending and dispersing properties, it should not be used in the cases of hyperactivity of fire due to deficiency of *Yin*, red tongue and dry mouth, headache due to liver-*Yang*, menorrhagia, and hemorrhagic diseases.

Red Sage Root (丹参 *Danshen*)
Radix Salviae Miltiorrhizae

This drug consists of the root of the perennial herbage Salvia miltiorrhiza Bge. (family Labiatae). The crude drug is cut into slices for medication.

Nomenclature Used in Prescriptions: *Danshen, Zidanshen, Xuedanshen*

Properties and Channel Distribution: This drug is bitter in taste and slightly cold in nature, and is distributed to the Heart and Liver Channels.

Action and Indications:

1. Activating blood circulation to remove blood stasis

This drug can be used to treat stasis of blood due to blood–heat, irregular menstruation, dysmenorrhea, amenorrhea, abdominal masses, lochiorrhea, etc. The drug may be given alone in powder form with millet wine, 6 g as one dose, 3 times a day. Or, it may be used in combination with other drugs for activating blood circulation and tonifying blood. In treating angina pectoris seen in coronary heart disease, it can be used in combination with Rhizoma Ligustici Chuanxiong, Flos Carthami, etc. In treating hypochondriac pain due to depression of the liver, it can be used in combination with Folium Isatidis, Herba Taraxaci, Carapax Trionycis, Concha Ostreae, Radix Paeoniae Rubra, Pericarpium Citri Reticulatae Viride, etc. In treating gastralgia due to stasis of *Qi* and blood, it can be used in combination with Lignum Santali Albi, etc.

2. Relieving restlessness and calming the mind

This drug can be used to treat restlessness and insomnia due to damage of the nutrient system seen in febrile diseases, and is often used in combination with Radix Rehmanniae, Radix Scrophulariae, Herba Lophatheri, etc. In treating neurathenia manifested by long–lasting insomnia, headache, dizziness, listlessness, etc., 50 g of the drug (ground into powder) can be put into 500 ml. of 95% alcohol with addition of 500 ml. of boiled water. The mixture is filtered 1–2 days later and 10 ml. of the extract is to be taken every night before sleep. In severe cases, the extract may be taken both in the morning and at night.

3. Subduing swelling to relieve pain

This drug can be used to treat carbuncle, sore and painful swelling, and is often used in combination with Flos Lonicerae, Fructus Forsythiae, Resina Olibani, Resina Commiphorae Myrrhae, etc., which have the effect of activating blood circulation and removing toxins. In treating arthritis of heat type manifested by pain in the joints and muscles, 30 g of the drug can be decocted and taken.

In recent years, it is used to treat chronic hepatitis, early cirrhosis with hepatomegaly, mild thromboangitis obliterans, ectopic pregnancy, etc.

Dosage and Administration: Its usually dosage is 10–15 g. In treating angitis, 30–60 g of the drug can be decocted. Large dosage should not be used for those with bleeding.

Peach Kernel (桃仁 *Taoren*)
Semen Persicae

This drug consists of the ripe kernel of the deciduous arbor Prunus Persica (L.) Batsch. (family Rosaceae). The kernel is dried, cooked and pounded into pieces (with the shell removed) for medication.

Nomenclature Used in Prescriptions: *Taoren, Taorenni*

Properties and Channel Distribution: This drug is bitter and

sweat in taste and neutral in nature, and is distributed to the Heart, Liver and Large Intestine Channels.

Action and Indications:

1. Removing blood stasis and promoting blood circulation

This drug can be used to treat amenorrhea, dysmenorrhea, abdominal masses, etc., which are due to stasis of blood. The drug is often used in combination with Flos Carthami, Rhizoma Ligustici Chuanxiong, Radix Angelicae Sinensis, Radix Rehmanniae Praeparata, Radix Paeoniae Alba, etc. In treating traumatic injury manifested by painful swelling due to stasis of blood, the drug is often used in combination with drugs for activating blood circulation and subduing swelling such as Flos Carthami, Squama Manitis (bake–stirred with hot sand), wine–fried Radix et Rhizoma Rhei, etc. In treating pulmonary abscess, the drug is often used in combination with Rhizoma Phragmitis. Semen Benincasae, Semen Coicis, etc. In treating periappendicular abscess, the drug is often used in combination with Radix et Rhizoma Rhci, Cortex Moutan Radicis, etc.

2. Moistening the intestine and ralaxing the bowels

This drug can be used to treat constipation due to dry intestine, and is often used in combination with Semen Armeniacae Amarum, Fructus Cannabis, etc.

Besides, the drug can also be used in combination with Semen Armeniacae Amarum to treat cough due to abnormal rising of *Qi*. In recent years it is also used to treat pulmonary abscess, acute appendicitis, etc.

Dosage and Administration: Usually, 6–10 g of the drug is used in decoction.

Notes: This drug is contraindicated for those with

amenorrhea due to exhaustion of blood and for pregnant women.

Safflower (红花 *Honghua*)
Flos Carthami

This drug consists of the flower of the annual herbage Carthamus tinctorius L. (family Compositae). The crude drug is used for medication.

Nomenclature Used in Prescriptions: *Honghua, Nanhonghua, Caohonghua*

Properties and Channel Distibution: This drug is pungent in taste and warm in nature, and is distributed to the Heart and Liver Channels.

Action and Indications:

1. Activating blood circulation and restoring menstrual flow

This drug can be used to treat amenorrhea, dysmenorrhea, abdominal masses, etc.,which are due to stasis of blood, and is often used in combination with Semen Persicae, Radix Angelicae Sinensis, Rhizoma Ligustici Chuanxiong, etc.

2. Removing blood stasis to relieve pain

This drug can be used to treat angina pectoris seen in coronary heart disease, and is often used in combination with Rhizoma Ligustici Chuanxiong, Radix Salviae Miltiorrhizae, etc. In treating hypochondriac pain due to stasis of blood, carbuncle, and hematemesis with blood stasis, the drug can be used in combination with Semen Persicae, Resina Boswelliae Carterii, Resina Commiphorae Myrrhae, etc. In treating ecchymoma, cyanosis and painful swelling due to traumatic injury, contusion and sprain, the drug can be mixed with spirit and applied to the local area. In treating thromboangitis obliterans manifested by dark red or bluish purple foot, which is due to stasis of *Qi* and blood, the drug is often used in combination with Radix Angelicae Sinensis, Semen Persicae, Radix Paeoniae Rubra, Resina Boswelliae Carterii, Resina Commiphorae Myrrhae, etc.

Dosage and Administration: Usually, 3–10 g, or 10–15 g, of the drug is used in decoction.

Notes: This drug should be used with care by pregnant women and should not be used by those with bleeding.

Appendix: Stigma Croci (藏红花 *Zanghonghua*)

This drug consists of the dried flower of the perennial herbage Crocus sativus L. (family Iridaceae). It is sweat in taste and cold in nature, and is distributed to the Heart and Liver Channels. Its effect is the same as, but better than, that of Flos Carthami. Besides, it also has the effect of removing heat from blood and removing toxins and therefore can be used to treat eruptions accompanied by fever seen in epidemic febrile disease at the stage when heat enters the nutrient system. Its dosage is 1–3 g, used in decoction.

Motherwort Herb (益母草 *Yimucao*)
Herba Leonuri

This drug consists of the whole plant of the annual or biennial herbage Leonurus heterophyllus Sweet (family Labiatae). The crude drug can be used, or the drug is made into soft extract for medication.

Nomenclature Used in Prescriptions: *Yimucao, Kuncao*

Properties and Channel Distribution: This drug is pungent and slightly bitter in taste and slightly cold in nature, and is distributed to the Liver, Heart and Kidney Channels.

Action and Indications:

1. Activating blood circulation to remove blood stasis

This drug can be used to treat irregular menstruation, dysmenorrhea, postpartum abdominal pain, lochiorrhea, metrorrhagia and metrostaxis, etc., which are due to stasis of blood. The drug can be used alone, to be made into soft extract with sugar, or used in combination with Rhizoma Angelicae Sinensis, Radix Paeoniae Rubra, etc.

2. Inducing diuresis to subdue edema

This drug can be used to treat edema and dysuria. It can be used alone, or in combination with Rhizoma Imperatae, Poria, Cortex Mori Radicis, etc.

3. Clearing away heat and removing toxins

This drug can be used as one of the ingredients to treat sores and itchy rashes.

In recent years it is also used to treat chronic nephritic edema, hypertension and coronary heart disease.

Dosage and Administration: Usually, 12–30 g of the drug is used in decoction. In treating nephritis, the drug is used in decoction, with 60–120 g of the dried drug or 120–240 g of the fresh drug.

Appendix: Semen Leonuri (茺蔚子 *Chongweizi*)

This drug consists of the seed of Herba Leonuri. The crude drug is used. It is sweat in taste and slightly cold in nature. It has the functions of activating blood circulation to remove blood stasis and cooling the liver to improve vision. It is often used to treat conjunctival congestion with swelling and pain due to liver–heat, hyphemia, or nebula, and is often used in combination with Semen Celosiae, Semen Cassiae, etc. Its dosage is 3–10 g. It is contraindicated for those with deficiency of blood in the liver and dilatation of the pupil.

Bugleweed (泽兰 *Zelan*)
Herba Lycopi

This drug consists of the stem and leaf, or just the leaf, of the perennial herbage Lycopus Lucidus Turcz., or Iycopus lucidus Turcz. var. hirtus Regel (family Labiatae). The crude drug is used for medication.

Nomenclature Used in Prescriptions: *Zelan, Zelanye*

Properties and Channel Distribution: This drug is bitter and pungent in taste and slightly warm in nature, and is distributed to the Liver, Spleen and Kidney Channels.

Action and Indications:

1. Activating blood circulation to remove blood stasis

This drug can be used to treat amenorrhea, dysmenorrhea, irregular menstruation, abdominal masses, postpartum abdominal pain, etc., which are due to stasis of blood. It can be used in combination with Radix Angelicae Sinensis, Radix Paeoniae, Radix Glycyrrhizae, etc. In treating stasis of blood and swelling due to traumatic injury, the fresh drug can be pounded into paste and applied to the local area.

2. Inducing diuresis to subdue edema

This drug can be used to treat postpartum dribbling urination, abdominal pain, edema of the body and face, ascites due to cirrhosis, etc. It can be used in combination with other drugs for inducing diuresis to subdue edema.

Dosage and Administration: Its usual dosage is 6–12 g, to be used in decoction.

Burreed Tuber (三棱 *Sanleng*)
Rhizoma Sparganii

This drug consists of the tuber of the perennial herbage Sparganium stoloniferum Buch—Ham. (family Sparganiaceae). The drug is parched with vinegar or bran for medication.

Nomenclature Used in Prescriptions: *Sanleng, Jingsanleng, Cusanleng*

Properties and Channel Distribution: This drug is bitter in taste and neutral in nature, and is distributed to the Liver and Spleen Channels.

Action and Indications:

1. Removing blood stasis and promoting flow of *Qi*

This drug can be used to treat amenorrhea, abdominal masses, postpartum abdominal pain, etc., which are due to stasis of blood. It is often used in combination with Rhizoma Zedoariae, Rhizoma Ligustici Chuanxiong, etc. In treating enlargement of the liver and spleen, it is often used in combination with Rhizoma Zedoariae, Pericarpium Citri Reticulatae Viride, Fructus Hordei Germinatus, etc.

2. Removing food stagnancy to relieve pain

This drug can be used to treat abdominal pain due to food stagnancy, and is often used in combination with Rhizoma Zedoariae, Pericarpium Citri Reticulatae Viride, Fructus Hordei Germinatus, etc.

Dosage and Administration: Usually, 3–10 g of the drug is used in decoction. When parched with vinegar, the drug's effect of relieving pain and removing blood stasis is enhanced.

Notes:

The drug is contraindicated for wowen with menorrhagia and pregnant wowen.

Zodoary (莪术 *Ezhu*)
Rhizoma Zedoariae

This drug consists of the rhizome of the perennial herbage Curcuma Kwangsiensis S. G. Lee et C. F. Liang (family Zingiberaceae). The drug is steamed, cut into slices and parched with vinegar for medication.

Nomenclature Used in Prescriptions: *Ezhu, Pengezhu, Cuezhu*

Properties and Channel Distribution: This drug is bitter and pungent in taste and warm in nature, and is distributed to the Liver and Spleen Channels.

Action and Indications:

1 Promoting flow of *Qi* and removing blood stasis

This drug can be used to treat amenorrhea, abdominal masses, etc. which are due to stasis of blood. It is often used in combination with Rhizoma Sparganii, Rhizoma Ligustici Chuanxiong, etc. In treating the enlargement of the liver and spleen, it is often used in combination with Rhizoma Sparganii, Flos Carthami, Radix Paeoniae Rubra, Rhizoma Cyperi, etc. In treating traumatic injury, the fresh rhizome of the drug can be pounded into paste, mixed with wine, parched and then applied to the local area while the drug is still hot.

2. Removing food stagnancy to relieve pain

This drug can be used to treat stagnation of food, distention and pain of the chest and abdomen, vomiting with sour fluid, etc. It is often used in combination with Rhizoma Sparganii, Pericarpium Citri Reticulatae Viride, Fructus Setariae Germinatus, etc.

Besides, the drug is also used to treat cancerous tumour nowadays. In treating carcinoma of uterine cervix, 10–30 ml. of the liquid medicine made from the drug can be injected into the local area daily, and this treatment should last for about 3 months (a course of treatment). At the same time, the decoction made from 10 g of Rhizoma Zedoariae and 10 g of Rhizoma Sparganii (both parched with vinegar) can be taken orally twice a day (before breakfast and after supper). As another treatment, the volatile oil ointment made from the drug can be applied to the local area. The above methods of treatment are also effective for carcinoma of vulva and skin.

Dosage and Administration: Usually, 3–10 g of the drug is used in decoction.

Notes: This drug is contraindicated for women with menorrhagia and pregnant women.

Curcuma Root (郁金 *Yujin*)
Radix Curcumae

This drug consists of the tuberous root of the perennial herbage Curcuma aromatica salisb. and C. zedoaria (Berg) Rosc. or C. longa L. or C. kwangsiensis S. Lee et C. F. Liang. (family Zingiberaceae). The drug is boiled, dried and cut into slices for medication.

Nomenclature Used in Prescriptions: *Yujin, Guangyujin, Huangyujin, Chuanyujin, Heiyujin*

Properties and Channel Distribution: This drug is pungent and bitter in taste and cold in nature, and is distributed to the Heart, Lung, Liver and Gall Bladder Channels.

Action and Indications:

1. Promoting flow of *Qi* and removing blood stasis

This drug can be used to treat distention and pain of the chest, epigastrium and abdomen, dysmenorrhea, etc. due to stasis of *Qi* and blood. It can be used in combination with Radix Bupleuri, Rhizoma Cyperi, Radix Angelicae Sinensis, Radix Paeoniae Alba, etc.

2. Clearing away heat from the heart to relieve depression

In treating damp–warm disease, mental confusion due to phlegm and unconsciousness, the drug is often used in combination with Rhizoma Acori Graminei, Fructus Gardeniae, Talcum, etc. In treating epilepsy and mania as a result of mental confusion due to phlegm–heat, the drug is often used in combination with Alumen, or with Rhizoma Cyperi, Scolopendra, etc.

3. Cooling blood to arrest bleeding

This disease can be used to treat hematemesis, epistaxis, hematuria, retrograde menstruation, etc. due to accumulation of blood–heat. It is often used in combination with other drugs for cooling blood to arrest bleeding such as Radix Rehmanniae, Cortex Moutan Radicis, Fructus Gardeniae, etc.

In addition, since this drug has cholagogic effect, it is often used in combination with Herba Lysimachiae, Herba Artemisiae Scopariae, Fructus Gardeniae, etc. to treat cholecystolith and jaundice. The drug is also commonly used to treat hepatalgia caused by cirrhosis, chronic hepatitis, hematuria seen in renal tuberculosis, and " encephalitis B" and " epidemic encephalitis" which are manifested by coma, schizophrenia and mania.

Dosage and Administration: Usually, 3–10 g of the drug is used in decoction.

Notes: The drug should not be used together with Flos Caryophylli.

Turmeria (色姜黄 *Sejianghuang*)
Rhizoma Curcumae Longae

This drug consists of the rhizome of the perennial herbage Curcuma longa L. (family Zingiberaceae). It is also called *Sejianghuang, Yingjianghuang* or *Zijianghuang* in Chinese. The bark is removed and the drug is cut into thin slices or pounded and made into powder for medication.

Nomenclature Used in Prescriptions: *Jianghuang, Sejianghuang*

Properties and Channel Distribution: This drug is pungent and bitter in taste and cold in nature, and is distributed to the Liver, Gall Bladder, Spleen and Stomach Channels.

Action and Indications:

1. Cooling blood to arrest bleeding

This drug can be used to treat preceded menstrual cycle due to blood–heat, and can be used in combination with Radix Scutellariae, Rhizoma Corydalis, Rhizoma Rehmanniae Praeparatae, etc.

2. Removing blood stasis, subduing swelling, promoting flow

of *Qi* to relieve pain

This drug can be used to treat stasis of blood and painful swelling due to traumatic injury, and can be used in combination with Semen Persicae, Lignum Sappan, Resina Olibani, etc. In treating pain in the chest, hypochondrium, epigastrium and abdomen due to stasis of *Qi* and blood, the drug is often used in combination with Radix Angelicae Sinensis, Radix Paeoniae Alba, Rhizoma Ligustici Chuanxiong, Rhizoma Zedoariae, etc. In treating sore throat due to obstruction by wind–heat, the drug is often used in combination with Bombyx Batryticatus, Periostracum Cicadae, Radix et Rhizoma Rhei, etc. In treating pyogenic infection and ulceration of skin, the drug is often used in combination with Radix Trichosanthis, Cortex Phellodendri, Radix et Rhizoma Rhei, etc., which are made into powder and applied to the local area.

Dosage and Administration: Usually, 3–10 g of the drug is used in decoction. Proper amount of the drug is used in external treatment.

Corydalis Tuber (延胡索 *Yanhusuo*)
Rhizoma Corydalis

This drug consists of the small round tuber of the perennial herbage Corydalis *Yanhusuo* W. T. Wang (family Papaveraceae). The drug is parched with vinegar and then pounded or ground into powder for medication.

Nomenclature Used in Prescriptions: *Yanhusuo, Xuanhu, Yuanhu, Cuyanhu*

Properties and Channel Distribution: This drug is pungent and bitter in taste and warm in nature, and is distributed to the Liver, Spleen and Heart Channels.

Action and Indications:

Activating blood circulation, removing blood stasis and promote flow of *Qi* to relieve pain

In treating pain in the epigastrium, hypochondrium and stomach due to stasis of *Qi* and blood, this drug is often used in combination with Fructus Meliae Toosendan. In treating dysmenorrhea, abdominal masses, postpartum abdominal pain, etc. due to stasis of blood, the drug is often used in combination with Radix Angelicae Sinensis, Radix Paeoniae Alba, Rhizoma Sparganii, Rhizoma Zedoariae, etc. In treating painful hernia, the drug is often used in combination with Fructus Meliae Toosendan, Fructus Foeniculi, etc. In treating pain all over the body due to stasis of *Qi* and blood, pain and swelling due to traumatic injury, etc., the drug can be used in combination with Radix Angelicae Sinensis, Ramulus Cinnamomi, etc.

In recent years, this drug has often been used in combination with drugs for activating blood circulation and promoting flow of *Qi* in the treatment of angina pectoris seen in coronary heart disease, arrhythmia, etc.

Dosage and Administration: Usually, 3–10 g of the drug is used in decoction. Or, 1.5–3 g of the drug powder can be taken orally with water or with the drug decoction. The drug parched with vinegar is more effective.

Trogopterus Dung (五灵脂 *Wulingzhi*)
Faeces Trogopterorum

This drug consists of the faeces of the mammalian vertebrate Trogopterus Xanthipes Milne–Edwards (family Petauristidae). The faeces is dried and parched with vinegar or carbonized for medication.

Nomenclature Used in Prescriptions: *Wulingzhi, Culingzhi, Lingzhitan*

Properties and Channel Distribution: This drug is sweat in taste and warm in nature, and is distributed to the Liver Channel.

Action and Indications:

1. Removing obstruction from blood vessel and dispersing blood stasis to relieve pain

This drug can be used to treat cardiac, abdominal, hypochondriac and costal pains due to stasis of *Qi* and blood, hernia, amenorrhea, dysmenorrhea, postpartum blood stasis, after–pains, etc. Like Resina Olibani and Resina Commiphorae Myrrhae, this drug has strong power of relieving pain, and therefore is quite effective against any pain due to stasis of *Qi* and blood. The drug can be used alone (the drug powder can be taken with wine) or in combination with Pollen Typhae.

2. Removing blood stasis to arrest bleeding

This drug can be used in combination with Radix Rehmanniae, Rhizoma Rehmanniae Praeparata, Colla Corii Asini, Radix Salviae Miltiorrhizae, etc. to treat metrorrhagia and metrostaxis.

Besides, the drug is in recent years used to treat angina

pectoris seen in coronary heart disease, bleeding and pain due to gastric and duodenal ulceration, etc.

Dosage and Administration: Usually, 3–10 g of the drug is used in decoction. In activating blood circulation, the drug parched with vinegar is used; in arresting bleeding, carbonized drug is used.

Notes: This drug should be used with care by pregnant women.

Frankincense (乳香 *Ruxiang*)
Resina Olibani

This drug consists of the gum–resin obtained from the low shrub Boswellia carterii Birdw. (family Burseraceae). The drug is often parched for medication.

Nomenclature Used in Prescriptions: *Zhiruxiang, Mingruxiang*

Properties and Channel Distribution: This drug is pungent and bitter in taste and warm in nature, and is distributed to the Heart, Liver and Spleen Channels.

Action and Indications:

1. Activating blood circulation to relieve pain

In treating traumatic injury, stasis of blood, painful swelling or muscular constricture, this drug is often used in combination with Resina Commiphorae Myrrhae, Resina Draconis, Flos Carthami, etc. The drug can also be used to treat angina pectoris due to stasis of blood in the heart, and gastralgia, abdominal pain, dysmenorrhea, postpartum abdominal pain, etc. due to stasis of blood. This drug has strong power of relieving pain, and therefore is quite effective against pain due to stasis of blood seen in internal medicine, gynecology, surgery, traumatology, etc. It is a main drug used in surgery and traumatology and is often used in combination with drugs for activating blood circulation and removing blood stasis such as Resina Commiphorae Myrrhae.

2. Subduing swelling and promoting tissue regeneration

This drug can be used to treat carbuncle, phlegmon, painful swelling or ulceration which does not heal over a long time. It may be taken orally and is often used in combination with Resina Commiphorae Myrrhae, Realgar, Moschus, etc. For external application, the powder made of it and Resina Commiphorae Myrrhae is applied to the affected area, which is then covered with plaster.

3. Relieving rigidity of muscles and joints

This drug can be used to treat muscular constricture seen in arthralgia, and is often used in combination with drugs for dispelling wind and removing dampness such as Rhizoma seu Radix Notopterygii, Radix Angelicae Sinensis, etc.

Dosage and Administration: Usually, 3–10 g of the drug is used in decoction. Proper amount of the drug can be used in external treatment.

Notes: This drug is bitter in taste and its decoction is turbid. It is therefore likely to cause vomiting in those with deficiency of the stomach and large dosage is not advisable, especially for those with deficiency of the stomach. It is contraindicated for those without blood stasis and for pregnant women.

Appendix: Resina Myrrhae (没药 *Moyao*)

This drug consists of the gum–resin obtained from the stem of the arbor Commiphora myrrha Engl. (family Burseraceae) and other plants of the same genus. The processing method of the drug is the same as that of Resina Olibani. This drug is bitter in taste and neutral in nature and its channel distribution and actions are the same as those of Resina Olibani. Experience has proved that Resina Olibani is good at activating blood circulation and relieving rigidity of muscles and joints, while Resina Myrrhae is more effective in dispersing blood stasis. In treating arthralgia, the former is used rather than the latter. In treating pain due to stasis of *Qi* and blood, the two drugs are used in combination to produce better effect.

This drug also has the effect of subduing swelling and promoting tissue regeneration. It can be used in external treatment and is always used in combination with Resina Olibani.

Its dosage is 3–10 g, to be used in decoction. Proper amount of the drug can be used in external treatment. Attention should be paid to combining this drug with Resina Olibani.

Sappan Wood (苏木 *Sumu*)
Lignum Sappan

This drug consists of the heart–wood of deciduous shrub or arbor Caesalpinla sappan L. (family Leguminosae). The drug is cut into thin slices or small pieces for medication.

Nomenclature Used in Prescriptions: *Sumu, Sufangmu*

Properties and Channel Distribution: This drug is sweat, salty and pungent in taste and neutral in nature, and is distributed to the Heart, Liver and Spleen Channels.

Action and Indications:

This drug is used to activate blood circulation, remove blood stasis, and subdue swelling to relieve pain. In treating stasis of blood and painful swelling due to traumatic injury, the drug is often used in combination with Resina Olibani, Resina Commiphorae Myrrhae, Resina Draconis, Flos Carthami, etc. In treating abdominal pain in women due to amenorrhea caused by stasis of blood, postpartum stasis of blood, etc., the drug is often used in combination with Radix Paeoniae Rubra, the tip of Radix Angelicae Sinensis, Semen Persicae, Flos Carthami, Rhizoma Ligustici Chuanxiong, etc.

Dosage and Administration: Usually, 3–10 g of the drug is used in decoction. Proper amount of the drug can be used in external treatment.

Notes: The drug is contraindicated in pregnant women.

Dalbergia Wood (降真香 *Jiangzhenxiang*)
Lignum Dalbergiae Odoriferae

This drug consists of the heartwood of the arbor Dalbergia odorifera T. Chen (family Leguminosae). It is cut into slices for medication.

Nomenclature Used in Prescriptions: *Jiangxiang, Jiangzhenxiang, Zijiangxiang*

Properties and Channel Distribution: This drug is pungent in taste and warm in nature, and is distributed to the Heart and Liver Channels.

Action and Indications:

This drug is used to remove blood stasis, arrest bleeding and relieve pain. In treating stasis of blood and painful swelling due to traumatic injury or internal and external hemorrhage, etc., the drug can be ground into powder and applied to the local area or used in combination with drugs for activating blood circulation and regulating flow of *Qi* such as Resina Boswelliae Carterii, Resina Commiphorae Myrrhae, Radix Notoginseng, etc. In treating angina pectoris seen in coronary heart disease, it is often used in combination with Rhizoma Ligustici Chuanxiong, Flos Carthami, Radix Paeoniae Rubra, etc.

Besides, this drug can be used in combination with Herba Agastachis, Radix Aucklandiae, etc. to treat vomiting and abdominal pain due to intake of contaminated food.

Dosage and Administration: Its dosage is 3–6 g. In treating angina pectoris, 12 g can be used. The drug is usually decocted.

Notes: This drug is contraindicated for those with hyperactivity of fire due to deficiency of *Yin* and bleeding due to blood–heat but without blood stasis.

Achyranthes Root (牛膝 *Niuxi*)
Radix Achyranthis Bidentatae

This drug consists of the root of the perennial herbage Achyranthes bidentata Blume and C. officinalis Kuan (family Amaranthaceae). The drug is cut into small sections for medication.

Nomenclature Used in Prescriptions: *Niuxi, Huainiuxi, Chuanniuxi*

Properties and Channel Distribution: This drug is bitter and sour in taste and neutral in nature, and is distributed to the Liver and Kidney Channels.

Action and Indications:

1. Activating blood circulation to restore menstrual flow

This drug can be used to treat amenorrhea, dysmenorrhea, retarded menstrual cycle, abdominal masses, difficult labour, etc. which are due to stasis of blood. It is often used in combination with Radix Angelicae Sinensis, Semen Persicae, Radix Paeoniae Rubra, Cortex Moutan Radicis, etc. When combined with Fructus Malvae Verticillatae, the drug can be used to treat retention of placenta.

2. Relaxing tendons and muscles to treat arthralgia

This drug can be used to treat aching pain of the low back and knee joints and arthralgia of the lower limbs due to wind–dampness. If the diseases are due to damp–heat, the drug is often used in combination with Rhizoma Atractylodis, Cortex Phellodendri in treatment; if the diseases are due to cold, the drug is often used in combination with Radix Angelicae Pubescentis, Fructus Chaenomelis, etc.; if the diseases are due to deficiency of the kidney, the drug is often used in combination with Cortex Eucommiae, Radix Dipsaci, etc.

3. Ensuring proper downward flow of blood

In treating pain and swelling of the gum, hematemesis, hemoptysis, epistaxis, etc. caused by hyperactivity of fire due to deficiency of *Yin*, the drug is often used in combination with drugs for nourishing *Yin* and purging fire such as Rhizoma Rehmanniae Praeparatae, Radix Ophiopogonis, Gypsum Fibrosum, Rhizoma Anemarrhenae, etc. In treating hypertension due to hyperactivity of the liver yang and headache due to spasm of the cerebral blood vessels, the drug can be used in combination with Ochra, Os Draconis, Concha Ostreae, Radix Scrophulariae, etc.

4. Inducing diuresis to treat stranguria

This drug can be used to treat stranguria due to heat and hematuria, and is often used in combination with Herba Dianthi, Talcum, Medulla Tetrapanacis, etc.

Dosage and Administration: Its dosage is 6—12 g, or up to 30 g, to be used in decoction. This drug is of two kinds, Radix Cyathulae and Radix Achyranthis Bidentatae. The former is usually used to activate blood circulation, restore menstrual flow and relax muscles and tendons to treat arthralgia while the latter, to tonify the liver and kidney and strengthen tendons and bones.

Pangolin Scales (穿山甲 *Chuanshanjia*) Squama Manitis

This drug consists of the scale of the vertebrate Manis Pentadactyla L. (family Manidae). The scale is heated with hot sand till it becomes loose and turns brown for medication.

Nomenclature Used in Prescriptions: *Chuanshanjia, Zhishanjia, Paojiapian, Shanjiazhu*

Properties and Channel Distribution: This drug is salty in taste and slightly cold in nature, and is distributed to the Liver and Stomach Channels.

Action and Indications:

1. Subduing swelling and evacuating pus

This drug can be used to treat initial swelling or pus without diabrosis, etc. This drug is characterized by ever moving and therefore the drug effect may run along the channels to reach the diseased area. In treating initial swelling, the drug can subdue swelling and in treating pus, the drug can cause diabrosis and evacuation of pus. The drug is often used in combination with Spina Gleditsiae, Flos Lonicerae, Resina Boswelliae Carterii, Resina Commiphorae Myrrhae, etc.

2. Restoring menstrual flow and promoting milk secretion

In treating galactostasis, the drug powder can be taken with millet wine (6 g as a dose, twice a day), or the drug can be used in combination with Semen Vaccariae, Herba Dianthi, etc. In treating amenorrhea due to stasis of blood, the drug can be used in combination with drugs for removing blood stasis and restoring menstrual flow, such as Radix Angelicae Sinensis, Radix Paeoniae Rubra, Flos Carthami, Radix et Rhizoma Rhei, etc.

In addition, the drug can also be used to treat arthralgia due to wind–dampness and contracture of limbs, and is often used in combination with Radix Angelicae Sinensis, Rhizoma Ligustici Chuanxiong, Rhizoma seu Radix Notopterygii, Radix Ledebouriellae, etc.

Dosage and Administration: Usually, 3–10 g of the drug is used in decoction. The drug can also be ground into powder and taken orally (1–1.5 g as a dose). The drug powder taken orally is better in effect.

Notes: The drug is contraindicated in pregnant women.

Thorn of Chinese Honeylocust
(皂角刺 *Zaojiaoci*)
Spina Gleditsiae

This drug consists of the thorn on the stem of the deciduous arbor Gleditsia sinensis Lan. (family Leguminosae). The crude drug is cut into slices for medication.

Nomenclature Used in Prescriptions: *Zaojiaoci, Zaoci, Zaozhen*

Properties and Channel Distribution: This drug is pungent in taste and warm in nature, and is distributed to the Liver and Stomach Channels.

Action and Indications:

1. Subduing swelling and evacuating pus

This drug can be used to treat carbuncle, phlegmon, sores, acute mastitis, scrofula, subcutaneous nodule, etc., and is often used in combination with Squama Manitis, Flos Lonicerae, crude Radix Glycyrrhizae, etc.

2. Calming wind and destroying parasite

In treating leprosy, the drug can be used in combination with oil of Semen Hydnocarpi, Radix et Rhizoma Rhei, etc. In treating skin tinea, thick decoction of the drug and vinegar is prepared and applied to the local area.

Dosage and Administration: Usually, 3–10 g of the drug is used in decoction. Proper amount of the drug can be used in external treatment.

Spatholobus Stem (鸡血藤 *Jixueteng*)
Caulis Spatholobi

This drug consists of the stem of the climbing shrubs Spatholobus suberectus Dunn, Millettia dielsiana Harms, etc. (family Leguminosae). The crude drug can be cut into slices or decocted into gelatin for medication.

Nomenclature Used in Prescriptions: *Jixueteng*

Properties and Channel Distribution: This drug is bitter and

slightly sweat in taste and warm in nature, and is distributed to the Liver and Kidney Channels.

Action and Indications:

This drug is used to promote blood circulation, tonify the blood, and relax muscles and joints. In treating arthralgia due to wind–dampness, aching pain of the waist and knee and numbness of the tendon and bone, the drug is often used in combination with drugs for invigorating *Qi*, nourishing blood and dispelling wind–dampness such as Fructus Mori, Rhizoma Atractylodis Macrocephalae, Radix Angelicae Sinensis, Radix Cyathulae, Radix Stephaniae Tetrandrae, Caulis Piperis Futokadsurae, etc. In treating irregular menstruation, amenorrhea, abdominal pain, etc. due to deficiency of blood, the drug is often used in combination with Radix Angelicae Sinensis, Rhizoma Ligustici Chuanxiong, Radix Paeoniae Alba, Radix Rehmanniae, etc.

Dosage and Administration: Usually, 10–15 g, or in large dosage up to 60 g, of the drug can be used in decoction. The drug can also be put into wine and the wine is drunk. When the drug is taken in gelatin form, the dosage is 6–10 g. The gelatin should be melted and or dissolved in warm water before taken.

Vaccaria Seed (王不留行 *Wangbuliuxing*)
Semen Vaccariae

This drug consists of the ripe seed of the annual or bienniel herbage Vaccaria segetalis (Neck) Garcke (family Caryophyllaceae).The crude drug is used.

Nomenclature Used in Prescriptions: *Wangbuliuxing, Buliuxing*

Properties and Channel Distribution: This drug is sweat and bitter in taste and neutral in nature, and is distributed to the Liver and Stomach Channels.

Action and Indications:

1. Promoting milk secretion and subduing swelling

In treating galactostasis, the drug is often used in combination with Squama Manitis, Herba Dianthi, etc. In treating acute mastitis at its initial stage without formation of pus, the drug can be used in combination with Herba Taraxaci, Radix Angelicae Dahuricae, etc.

2. Activating blood circulation to restore menstrual flow

In treating amenorrhea due to stasis of blood, the drug can be used in combination with Radix Angelicae Sinensis, Rhizoma Ligustici Chuanxiong, Semen Persicae, Flos Carthami, etc.

Besides, the drug can also be used to treat testitis. For example, in treating mumps complicated by testitis, the drug can be used in combination with Fructus Meliae Toosendan, Radix Isatidis, Radix Scutellariae, Radix Rehmanniae, Cortex Moutan Radicis, etc.

Dosage and Administration: Usually, 6–10 g of the drug is used in decoction.

Notes: This drug should be used with care by pregnant women.

Pyrite (自然铜 *Zirantong*)
Pyritum

This drug is the iron disulphide obtained from a natural brassy yellow mineral, Pyrite, crystallizing in the cubic system.

The mineral is calcined thoroughly and quenched with vinega and this is repeated two or three times. Then the mineral is put under the ground to rid it of fire-toxins. Finally the mineral is ground into fine powder with water for medication.

Nomenclature Used in Prescriptions: *Zirantong, Duanzirantong*

Properties and Channel Distribution: This drug is pungent in taste and neutral in nature, and is distributed to the Liver Channel.

Action and Indications:

This drug is used to disperse blood stasis to relieve pain and to set broken bones and tendons. It can be used to treat fractures and pains with blood stasis. Since this drug has the effect of promoting blood circulation to remove blood stasis and setting broken bones and tendons, it is a main drug used in setting bones in traumatology. It can be used in combination with Resina Boswelliae Carterii, Resina Commiphorae Myrrhae, Radix Angelicae Sinensis, Rhizoma seu Radix Notopterygii, etc. In treating sudden sprain in the lumbar region, feeling of pain in the chest when breathing and lumbago, 30 g of the drug and 30 g of Eupolyphaga seu Steleophaga can be ground into powder and taken with warm water (2 g as a dose, twice a day).

Dosage and Administration: Its dosage is 1-3 g. The drug is usually taken in pill or powder form and is not to be decocted.

Leech (水蛭 *Shuizhi*)
Hirudo

This drug consists of the dried body of annelid Whitmania

pigra (Whitman), Whitmania acranulate (Whitman), Hirudo nipponica Whitman, etc. (family Hirudinidae). It is cut into sections and roasted with talcum for medication.

Nomenclature Used in Prescriptions: *Shuizhi*

Properties and Channel Distribution: This drug is salty and bitter in taste and neutral in nature with toxic effect, and is distributed to the Liver Channel.

Action and Indications:

This drug is used to disperse blood retention and remove blood stasis. In treating amenorrhea due to stasis of blood, abdominal masses, blood retention etc., it is often used in combination with Tabanus Bivittatus, Semen Persicae, Radix et Rhizoma Rhei, etc. In treating traumatic injury with blood stasis, swelling and pain, cardiac and abdominal distention and pain and constipation, the drug is ground into fine powder together with Radix et Rhizoma Rhei and Semen Pharbitidis and taken with warm wine.

Besides, this drug is also of cértain effect in the treatment of thrombocytosis. In this case it is not to be decocted for long.

Dosage and Administration: Usually, 3–6 g of the drug is used in decoction. When taken in pill or powder form, 1–1.5 g of the drug is used.

Notes: This drug is contraindicated in pregnant women.

Gradfly (虻虫 *Mengchong*)
Tabanus

This drug consists of the female insect Tabanus bivittatus Mats. (family Tabanidae). The crude or parched drug is used.

Nomenclature Used in Prescriptions: *Mengchong*

Properties and Channel Distribution: This drug is bitter in taste and slightly cold in nature with slight toxic effect, and is distributed to the Liver Channel.

Action and Indications:

This drug is used to remove blood stasis. In treating amenorrhea due to stasis of blood, abdominal masses and unsmooth flow of blood, it is often used in combination with Hirudo, Semen Persicae, and Radix et Rhizoma Rhei. In treating traumatic injury with blood stasis and painful swelling, the drug can be ground into powder together with Cortex Moutan Radicis and taken with wine.

Dosage and Administration: Usually, 1.5–3 g of the drug is used in decoction. When taken in powder form, 0.3–0.6 g of the drug is used.

Notes: This drug is contraindicated in pregnant women.

Ground Beetle (䗪虫 *Zhechong*)
Eupolyphaga seu Steleophaga

This drug consists of the dried female insect Eupolyphaga sinensis Walker (family Corydiidae).

Nomenclature Used in Prescriptions: *Zhechong, Dibiechong, Tuyuan*

Properties and Channel Distribution: This drug is salty in taste and cold in nature with slight toxic effect, and is distributed to the Liver Channel.

Action and Indications:

1. Removing blood stasis

In treating amenorrhea due to stasis of blood, irregular menstruation and postpartum stasis of blood, the drug is often used in combination with drugs for removing blood stasis such as Radix et Rhizoma Rhei, Semen Persicae, etc. In treating acute abdominal pain due to ectopic pregnancy and abdominal masses, the drug can be used in combination with Squama Manitis Preaparata, mashed Semen Persicae, Sargassum, the whole plant of Angelica Sinensis, Rhizoma Corydalis, Resina Commiphorae Myrrhae, Concha Ostreaeusta, etc. In treating hepatomegaly due to chronic hepatitis, early cirrhosis, and dull pain in the hepatic region, the drug can be used in combination with Radix Codonopsis Pilosulae, Placenta Hominis, Rhizoma Curcumae Longae, Radix Curcumae, Radix Notoginseng, Endothelium Corneum Gigeriae Galli, etc. which are ground into powder and taken before meals. In treating swollen and rigid tongue, five ground beetles and 15 g of table salt are decocted and the decoction is taken while still hot, and this treatment should stop when the patient is able to spit out saliva and the symptom is relieved. In treating swollen tongue, the live ground beetles and fresh Herba Menthae are pounded to take the liquid, which is then soaked with gauze and the gauze is put beneath the tongue where there is swelling.

2. Setting broken bones and tendons

This drug can be used to treat fractures. Twenty ground beetles, 6 g of Pyritum (quenched with vinegar), 6 g of Os Draconis, 6 g of Resina Boswelliae Carterii, 6 g of Resina Commiphorae Myrrhae and 0.3 g of Moschus are ground into fine powder and this powder is taken with millet wine. (1.5 g as a dose. three times a day).

Dosage and Administration: Usually, 5–10 g of the drug is used in decoction. When taken in pill or powder form, 1–2 g can be used.

Notes: This drug is contraindicated in pregnant women.

13 Antitussives, Antiasthmatics and Expectorants

Drugs with the main functions of relieving cough and asthma are called antitussives and antiasthmatics, while drugs with the main function of resolving and expelling phlegm are called expectorants. Since antitussives and antiasthmatics can also be used to resolve phlegm and expectorants also have the function of relieving cough, these drugs are generally referred to as antitussives, antiasthmatics and expectorants.

Cough and phlegm are closely related to each other in pathogenesis. Generally speaking, cough may be accompanied by presence of phlegm, which, in turn, usually causes cough. In treatment, therefore, antitussives and antiasthmatics are often used in combination with expectorants, and vice versa. Antitussives and antiasthmatics are mainly used to treat cough, asthma, phthisical cough, long-lasting cough, etc. Expectorants are mainly used to treat cough with profuse sputum, asthma due to retention of phlegm, difficulty in expectoration, and other diseases caused by phlegm, such as epilepsy, convulsion, scrofula, multiple abscess, etc.

Diseases either due to internal damage or exogenous invasion may lead to profuse sputum and cough. Therefore, it is necessary in treatment not only to use proper antitussives, antiasthmatics and expectorants according to the disease condition, but also to work out necessary combination of drugs according to various etiological factors and with due consideration of the exterior and interior, deficiency and excess, and heat and cold of the disease, if satisfactory therapeutic effect is to be obtained. For example, in treating cough due to invasion by exogenous factors, drugs for relieving exterior syndrome should be used in combination; in treating cough due to consumption, tonics should be used in combination; in treating heat-phlegm and dry-phlegm, the method of clearing away heat and moistening should also be used; and in treating cold-phlegm and damp-phlegm, warming and drying methods should also be used. On the other hand, undesirable results will be given rise to if astringing method is used for cough due to exogenous invasion, consuming and dispersing methods are used for cough due to consumption, warming and drying methods are used for heat-phlegm and dry-phlegm, or the methods of clearing away heat and moistening are used for cold-phlegm and damp-phlegm.

For cough with blood, it is not advisable to use potent expectorants. Otherwise, it is likely to cause bleeding.

According to the main properties of the antitussives and expectorants, they are subdivided into three kinds, namely, drugs for relieving cough and asthma, drugs for clearing away heat and resolving heat-phlegm, and drugs for warming and resolving phlegm due to cold.

13.1 Drugs for Relieving Cough and Asthma

This kind of drugs has the main function of relieving cough or asthma, and may have the effect of promoting the dispersing function of the lung to remove phlegm, moistening the lung to relieve cough, sending down adverse flow of *Qi* to relieve asthma, etc. They are used to treat cough and asthma due to dysfunction of the lung–*Qi*.

Cough may be manifested by dry cough, cough with thin or thick sputum. Cough may by caused by exogenous invasion or consumption, cold or heat, deficiency or excess. Therefore, this kind of drugs should be used in combination with other drugs according to differentiation of syndromes and should not be used alone.

For example, in treating measles at its initial stage or diseases with eruptions due to exogenous evils, it is not advisable to use antitussives warm in nature and with astringing effect, although there presents cough, because eruptions may be suppressed and the case becomes deteriorated.

Bitter Apricot Kernel (杏仁 *Xingren*)
Semen Armeniacae Amarum

This drug consists of the kernel of the deciduous arbor Prunus armeniaca L. (family Rosaceae). The drug is dried in the sun and the crude or parched drug (broken into pieces) is used for medication.

Nomenclature Used in Prescriptions: *Kuxingren, Xingrenni*

Properties and Channel Distribution: This drug is bitter and pungent in taste and warm in nature with slight toxic effect, and is distributed to the Lung and Large Intestine Channels.

Action and Indications:

1. Relieving cough and asthma

In treating common cold due to wind–cold with cough and

asthma, this drug can be used in combination with Folium Perillae, Rhizoma Pinelliae, Poria, etc. In treating cough due to wind-heat, the drug is often used in combination with Folium Mori, Flos Chrysanthemi, Radix Platycodi, ect. In treating cough due to dryness in the lung, the drug is often used in combination with Radix Adenophorae Strictae, etc. In treating long-lasting cough with asthma, the drug can be used in combination with Cortex Mori Radicis, Radix Asteris, Fructus Schisandrae, etc.

2. Moistening the intestine and relaxing the bowels

This drug can be used to treat constipation in the elderly or in women after childbirth, and is often used in combination with Fructus Cannabis, Semen Persicae, etc.

Dosage and Administration: Usually, 6-10 grams of the drug is used in decoction.

Appendix: Sweet Apricot Seed (甜杏仁 *Tianxingren*)

This drug consists of the kernel of Prunus amygdalus Batsch (family Rosaceae). It is sweat in taste and neutral in nature without toxic effect. It has the functions of moistening and nourishing the lung and send down adverse flow of *Qi* to relieve cough. It is specially used to treat prolonged cough due to consumption, stuffy chest, constipation, etc. Its dosage is the same as that of Semen Armeniacae Amarum.

Stemona Root (百部 *Baibu*)
Radix Stemonae

This drug consists of the tuberous root of the perennial herbage Stemona japonica (Bl.) Miq. Stemona sessilifolia (Miq.) Franch. et Sav., or Stemona tuberosa Lour., etc. (family

Stemonaceae). The drug is cut into sections and the crude or honey– fried drug is used.

Nomenclature Used in Prescriptions: *Baibu, Zhibaibu*

Properties and Channel Distribution: This drug is sweat and bitter in taste and slightly warm in nature, and is distributed to the Lung Channel.

Action and Indications:

1. Moistening the lung to relieve cough

This drug can be used to treat cough due to exopathogens or cough which occurs after common cold. This drug is warm rather than dry in nature and can be used to treat both initial or longlasting cough, being much effective for the latter. It is often used in combination with Radix Asteris, Radix Platycodi, Herba Schizonepetae, etc. In treating long–lasting cough due to deficiency of the lung, the drug can be used in combination with Radix Adenophorae Strictae, Radix Astragali seu Hedysari, Bulbus Lilii, etc. In treating cough with bloody sputum due to impairment of the lung caused by overstrain (tuberculosis of the lung with cavitation), the drug can be used in combination with Rhizoma Bletiilae, Bulbus Fritillariae Thunbergii, Radix Notoginseng, etc. In recent years, this drug is made into syrup to be used to treat whooping cough in children.

2. Destroying louse and parasites

The infusion of the drug can be applied externally to treat head louse, body louse, pubic louse and clothes louse (not effective against louse eggs). When sprayed, the drug can destroy bedbug. When taken orally, the drug can be used to treat enterobiasis; and the disease can also be treated by washing the anus with the decoction of the drug.

Dosage and Administration: Usually, 6–10 g of the drug is used in decoction. Proper amount of the drug can also be used in external treatment.

Root and Rhizome of Tatarian Aster (紫菀 *Ziwan*) Radix Asteris

This drug consists of the root and rhizome of the perennial herbage Aster tataricus L.f. (family Compositae). The crude or honey–fried drug is used for medication.

Nomenclature Used in Prescriptions: *Ziwan, Zhiziwan*

Properties and Channel Distribution: This drug is pungent and bitter in taste and slightly warm in nature, and is distributed to the Lung Channel.

Action and Indications

This drug is used to moisten the lung, bring down adverse rising of *Qi*, resolve phlegm and relieve cough. Since this drug is moist rather than dry in nature, it is a main drug for resolving phlegm and relieving cough, whether the cough is due to lung–heat or lung–cold. In treating pulmonary tuberculosis with consumptive fever due to deficiency of *Yin* and cough with blood, the drug can be used in combination with Rhizoma Anemarrhenae, Bulbus Fritillariae,Colla Corii Asini, etc. In treating long–lasting cough, the drug can be used in combination with Flos Farfarae, Radix Stemonae, etc. In treating cough and asthma without fever due to deficiency of lung–*Qi*, the drug can be used in combination with Radix Codonopsis Pilosulae, Radix Astragali seu Hedysari, Rhizoma Zingiberis, etc. In treating cough with profuse sputum due to exogenous wind–cold, the drug can be used in combination with Herba Schizonepetae, Rhizoma Cynanchi Stauntonii, Pericarpium Citri Reticulatae, etc.

Dosage and Administration: Usually, 6–10 g of the drug is used in decoction. In treating cough due to exopathogen, the crude drug is used; in treating long–lasting cough and asthma, the honey–fried drug is used.

Coltsfoot Flower (款冬花 *Kuandonghua*)
Flos Farfarae

This drug consists of the flower–bud of the perennial herbage Tussilago farfara L. (family Compositae). The crude or honey–fried drug is used.

Nomenclature Used in Prescriptions: *Kuandonghua, Zhikuandong*

Properties and Channel Distribution: This drug is pungent and sweat in taste and warm in nature, and is distributed to the Lung Channel.

Action and Indications:

This drug is used to moisten the lung, relieve cough, resolve phlegm and bring down adverse rise of *Qi*. This is an effective drug for moistening the lung, resolving phlegm and relieving cough and can be used to treat cough, whether it is due to exogenous invasion or internal damage, cold or heat, deficiency or excess. In treating cough and asthma which are induced by cold, the drug can be used in combination with Herba Ephedrae, Semen Armeniacae Amarum, Fructus Perillae, etc. In treating cough with blood, the drug and Bulbus Lilii can be ground into powder and made into pills with honey. In treating severe cough, the drug can be used in combination with Semen Armeniacae Amarum, Bulbus Fritillariae Cirhosae, Fructus Schisandrae, etc.

Dosage and Administration: Usually, 6–10 g of the drug is used in decoction. The crud drug is used for cough due to exogenous invasion and the prepared, for long–lasting cough of deficiency type.

Mulberry Bark (桑白皮 *Sangbaipi*)
Cortex Mori Radicis

This drug consists of the root–bark of the deciduous arbor Morus alba L. (family Moraceae). The bark is deprived of its cork and cut into stripes, and the crude or fried drug is used.

Nomenclature Used in Prescriptions: *Shengsangpi, Zhisangpi*

Properties and Channel Distribution: This drug is sweat in taste and cold in nature, and is distributed to the Lung Channel.

Action and Indications:

1. Purging fire accumulated in the lung and relieving asthma

This drug can be used to treat cough and asthma due to lungheat. This drug is specially used to purge lung–fire and relieve asthma, and can be used in combination with Cortex Lycii Radicis, Semen Oryzae Sativae, Radix Glycyrrhizae, etc.

2. Inducing diuresis to subdue edema

This drug can be used to treat dropsy and edema due to dysuria and is often used in combination with Pericarpium Arecae, Extra Poriae, Exocarpium Zigiberis Recens, etc.

Besides, the drug is also used to treat hypertension, owing to its effect of lowering blood pressure.

Dosage and Administration: Usually, 6–12 g of the drug is used in decoction. In inducing diuresis, the crude drug is used; in relieving cough and asthma, the fried drug is used.

Notes: This drug should not be used to treat cough due to lung–cold or wind–cold.

Ioquat Leaf (枇杷叶 *Pipaye*)
Folium Eriobotryae

This drug consists of the leaf of the evergreen arbor Eriobotrya japonica (Thunb.) Lindl. (family Rosaceae). The down is removed and the leaf is cleaned and cut into stripes. The crude or honey–fried drug is used.

Nomenclature Used in Prescriptions: *Shengpaye, Zhipaye*

Properties and Channel Distribution: This drug is bitter in taste and neutral in nature, and is distributed to the Lung and Stomach Channels.

Action and Indications:

1. Resolving phlegm and relieving cough

This drug can be used to treat cough and asthma due to lungheat, bitter taste, dry throat, etc. This drug is bitter in taste, neutral or slightly cool in nature, and is characterized by its descending function. Therefore, it can be used to purify and descend lung–*Qi* so as to resolve phlegm and relieve cough. It can be used in combination with Radix Adenophorae Strictae, Cortex Mori Radicis, Fructus Gardeniae, etc. In treating whooping cough, the drug can be used in combination with Radix Stemonae, Bulbus Allii, etc.

2. Sending down adverse ascending of *Qi* to stop vomiting

In treating nausea and vomiting due to adverse ascending of stomach–*Qi*, the drug can be used in combination with Rhizoma Pinelliae, Poria, etc. In treating vomiting due to stomach–heat, the drug can be used in combination with Caulis Bambusae in Taeniam, Exocarpium Citri Grandis, and Rhizoma Zingiberis Recens.

Dosage and Administration: Usually, 6–12 g of the drug is used in decoction. In relieving cough, the fried drug is used; in stopping vomiting, the crude drug is used.

Aristolochia Fruit (马兜铃 *Madouling*)
Fructus Aristolochiae

This drug consists of the fruit of the perennial trailing or creeping herbage Aristolochia debilis Sieb. et Zucc. or Aristolochia contorta Bge. (family Aristolochiaceae). The crude or honey–fried drug is used for medication.

Nomenclature Used in Prescriptions: *Madouling, Zhidouling*

Properties and Channel Distribution: This drug is bitter and slightly pungent in taste and cold in nature, and is distributed to the Lung and Large Intestine Channels.

Action and Indications:

This drug is used to clear away heat in the lung, descend adverse flow of *Qi*, and relieve cough and asthma. In treating cough and asthma due to hyperactivity of fire as a result of deficiency of the lung, the drug can be used in combination with Colla Corii Asini, Semen Armeniacae Amarum, Semen Oryzae Glutinosae, etc. In treating measles in its final stage accompanied by fever and dry cough, the drug can be used in combination with Bulbus

Fritillariae Thunbergi, Fructus Arctii, Radix Ophiopogonis, etc.

In addition, this drug can also be used to treat hemorrhoid with blood and swelling and pain around the anus, using the decoction of the drug to wash the local area. This drug has slow and persistent effect of lowering blood pressure and can be used to treat hypertension manifested by dizziness and flushed face due to hyperactivity of liver–*Yang*. It can be used in combination with Spica Prunellae, Ramulus Uncariae cum Uncis, Radix Scutellariae, etc.

Dosage and Administration: Usually, 3–10 g of the drug is used in decoction. Proper amount of the drug can be used in external treatment. In relieving cough, the fried drug is used, and when the drug is applied externally the crude drug is used.

Notes: The drug is contraindicated for those with cough and asthma due to cold of deficiency type or those with colds accompanied by cough. It is also not advisable to use the drug for cough with sputum due to lung–heat in pregnant women during the period of pernicious vomiting or in those with deficiency of stomach–*Qi*, because the drug can cause vomiting even when a small dosage is used.

Iepidium Seed (葶苈子 *Tinglizi*)
Semen Lepidii seu Descurainiae

This drug consists of the ripe seed of the annual or biennial herbage Lepidium apetalum Willd. or Descurainia sophia (L.) webb. (family Cruciferae). The crude or slightly parched drug is broken into pieces for medication.

Nomenclature Used in Prescriptions: *Tinglizi, Kutingli,*

Tiantingli

Properties and Channel Distribution: This drug is pungent and bitter in taste and cold in nature, and is distributed to the Lung, Urinary Bladder and Large Intestine Channels.

Action and Indications:

1. Purging heat accumulated in the lung and relieving asthma

This drug can be used to treat retention of phlegm, stuffy chest, asthma, insomnia and general edema. It can be used in combination with Fructus Ziziphi Jujubae in decoction. In recent years, the drug has been proved effective for exudative pleurisy and thoracic hydrops.

2. Sending down adverse flow of *Qi* and inducing diuresis

This drug can be used to remove obstruction by the lung *Qi* to induce diuresis and subdue swelling, It can be used to treat abdominal distention, dry mouth and lips, etc. due to retention of fluid in the intestine, and can be used in combination with Radix Stephaniae Tetrandrae, Semen Zanthoxyli, etc. which are made into pills. In treating thoracic hydrops, constipation and scanty urine, the drug can be used in combination with Semen Armeniacae Amarum, Radix et Rhizoma Rhei, etc., which are made into bolus with honey.

Dosage and Administration: Usually, 3–10 g of the drug is used in decoction.

Notes: The drug is contraindicated for those with cough and asthma due to deficiency of the lung and edema due to deficiency of the spleen.

Perilla Fruit (紫苏子 *Zisuzi*)
Fructus Perillae

This drug consists of the seed of the annual herbage Perilla frutescens (L.) Britt. var. crispa (Thunb.) Hand–Mazz. (family Labiatae). The drug is slightly Parched and broken into pieces for medication.

Nomenclature Used in Prescriptions: *Suzi, Zisuzi, Chaosuzi*

Properties and Channel Distribution: This drug is pungent in taste and warm in nature, and is distributed to the Lung and Large Intestine Channels.

Action and Indications:

This drug is used to send down adverse flow of *Qi*, resolve phlegm and relieve cough and asthma. It can be used to treat accumulation of phlegm, stuffy chest, adverse flow of *Qi*, and cough and asthma, and is often used in combination with Radix Peucedani, Cortex Magnoliae Officinalis, Rhizoma Pinelliae, Pericarpium Citri Reticulatae, etc. It can also be used in combination with Semen Sinapis Albae and Semen Raphani.

Besides, since this drug can moisten the intestine and treat constipation due to dryness in the intestine, it is often administered with such drugs as Fructus Cannabis, Semen Armeniacae Amarum, Fructus Aurantii, etc. to moisten the intestine and send down the adverse frow of *Qi*.

Dosage and Administration: Usually, 6–10 g of the drug is used in decoction.

Notes: This drug is contraindicated for those with loose stools due to deficiency of the spleen.

Gingko Nut (白果 *Baiguo*)
Semen Ginkgo

This drug consists of the ripe seed of the deciduous arbor Ginkgo biloba L. (family Ginkgoaceae). The drug is pounded into pieces and the crude or roasted drug is used for medication.

Nomenclature Used in Prescriptions: *Baiguoren, Baiguorou, Chaobaiguo*

Properties and Channel Distribution: This drug is sweet, bitter and puckery in taste and neutral in nature with slight toxic effect, and is distributed to the Lung Channel.

Action and Indications:

1. Astringing the lung to relieve asthma

This drug can be used to treat profuse sputum, shortness of breath, cough and asthma which are due to internal accumulation of phlegm–heat. It is often used in combination with Herba Ephedrae, Semen Armeniacae Amarum, Radix Scutellariae, etc.

2. Treating leukorrhea and eliminating turbidity

In treating leukorrhea with yellow and sticky discharge due to damp–heat, the drug is often used in combination with Cortex Phellodendri, Rhizoma Dioscoreae,etc. In treating chronic stranguria with turbid urine without pain, parched Semen Ginkgo and parched Rhizoma Dioscoreae are ground into fine powder and 10 g of the powder is to be taken at a time, 3 times a day.

Besides, the drug also has the effect of arresting polyuria. The roasted drug can be chewed as a treatment for polyuria.

Dosage and Administration: Usually, 6–10 g of the drug or

5–10 pieces of the drug is used in decoction. The crude drug is used in decoction. The drug can also be taken in powder form or by chewing.

Notes: Overdosage of the drug should be avoided because the crude drug has toxic effect and taking the drug too much may also cause poisoning, The drug should not be used by those suffering from common cold and cough.

Datura Flower (洋金花 *Yangjinhua*) Flos Daturae

This drug consists of the flower of the annual herbage Datura metel L. or Datura innoxia Mill. (family Solanaceae). The crude drug is dried for medication.

Nomenclature Used in Prescriptions: *Yangjinhua*

Properties and Channel Distribution: This drug is pungent in taste and warm in nature with powerful toxic side effect. It is distributed to the Lung Channel.

Action and Indications:

1. Relieving asthma

In treating asthma and cough without or with little sputum, the drug can be made into powder for oral administration or made into cigarette (with an equal amount of tobacco) for smoking.

2. Relieving pain

In treating gastralgia and abdominal pain, 0.3 g of the drug can be used in decoction. In treating arthralgia due to wind, cold and dampness, the decoction of 10 g of the drug can be used to wash the local area.

3. Relieving spasm

In treating spasm seen in epilepsy or chronic infantile convulsion, the drug can be used in combination with Rhizoma Gastrodiae, Scorpio, etc.

According to modern research on anesthesia by traditional Chinese drugs, this drug is used as the main drug used in anesthesia, which is made into injection together with Radix Aconiti, Radix Aconiti Kusnezoffii, Radix Stephaniae Tetrandrae, etc.

Dosage and Administration: When used for oral administration, 0.3 g of the drug is used in decoction. When used for smoking, 0.6–1 g of the drug is used. Proper amount of the drug can also be used in external treatment.

Notes: This drug is contraindicated for those with cough due to invasion by exopathogen, glaucoma and hypertension. Also, since this drug has powerful toxic effect, special attention should be paid to dosage to avoid poisoning.

13.2 Drugs for Clearing Away Heat and Resolving Heat–phlegm

This kind of drugs are mostly cold in nature with the function of clearing away heat and resolving heat–phlegm. They can be used to treat cough with sticky and foul sputum, difficulty in expectoration, epilepsy, convulsion, scrofula, multiple abscess, etc., and are often used in combination with drugs for clearing away heat.

Generally, drugs in this kind are mostly mild in their actions, except Lapis Chloriti or Lapis Micae Aureus, which is rather drastic. This kind of drugs should not be used by those with cold–phlegm and deficiency of the spleen and stomach.

Platycodon Root (桔梗 *Jiegeng*)
Radix Platycodi

This drug consists of the root of the perennial herbage platycodaon grandiflorum (Jacg.) A. DC. (family Campanulaceae).The crude drug is cut into slices for medication.

Nomenclature Used in Prescriptions: *Jiegeng, Kujiegeng, Baijiegeng*

Properties and Channel Distribution: This drug is pungent and bitter in taste and neutral in nature, and is distributed to the Lung Channel.

Action and Indications:

1. Promoting the lung's dispersing function and dispelling phlegm

This drug has both the ascending and discending functions and can be used effectively to dissipate and elevate the lung-*Qi* and comfort the chest and diaphragm. It also has desirable function of dispelling phlegm. It can be used to treat cough with profuse sputum, whether the disease is due to cold or heat in the lung. In treating cough with sticky sputum difficult to be expectorated due to heat in the lung, the drug can be used in combination with Folium Mori, Semen Armeniacae Amarum, Folium Eriobotryae, Herba Menthae, Radix Glycyrrhizae, etc. In treating cough with thin sputum and running nose due to wind-cold, the drug can be used in combination with Folium Perillae, Semen Armeniacae Amarum, Rhizoma Pinelliae, Pericarpium Citri Reticulatae, Rhizoma Cynanchi Stauntonii, Radix Glycyrrhizae, etc. In treating sore throat due to failure of the lung's dispersing function, the drug can be used in combination with Radix Glycyrrhizae, or, in addition Calyx seu Fructus Physalis, Caulis Lonicerae, etc.

2. Evacuating pus to subdue swelling

In treating pulmonary abscess, the drug can be used in combination with Herba Houttuyniae, Semen Coicis, Semen Benincasae, etc.

Dosage and Administration: Usually, 6–10 g of the drug is used in decoction.

Peucedanum Root (前胡 *Qianhu*)
Radix Peucedani

This drug consists of the root of the perennial herbage Peucedanum Praeruptorum Dunn or Peucedanum decursivum (Miq.) Maxim. (family Umbelliferae), The crude drug is used.

Nomenclature Used in Prescriptions: *Qianhu, Nenqianhu*

Properties and Channel Distribution: This drug is bitter and pungent in taste and slightly cold in nature, and is distributed to the Lung Channel.

Action and Indications: Sending down adverse flow of *Qi* to eliminate phlegm

In treating cough with yellow and sticky sputum and stuffy chest due to heat in the lung, the drug can be used in combination with Semen Armeniacae Amarum, Cortex Mori Radicis, etc. In treating cough with shortness of breath due to accumulation of lung–*Qi*, or vomiting and poor appetite, the drug can be used in combination with Rhizoma Pinelliae, Pericarpium Citri Reticulatae, Fructus Perillae, etc.

Dosage and Administration: Usually, 6–10 g of the drug is used in decoction.

Sichuan Fritillary Bulb (川贝母 *Chuanbeimu*)
Bulbus Fritillariae Cirhosae

This drug consists of the bulb of the perennial herbage Fritillaria cirrhosa D. Don. var. cirrhosa Franch. and F. cirrhosa D. Don. or F. delavayi Franch., or F. roylei Hook., or F. przewalskii Maxim. (family Liliaceae). The drug is pounded into pieces for medication.

Nomenclature Used in Prescriptions: *Chuanbeimu, Chuanbei*

Properties and Channel Distribution: This drug is bitter and sweet in taste and slightly cold in nature, and is distributed to the Heart and Lung Channels.

Action and Indications:

1. Moistening the lung to resolve phlegm

In treating cough with little sputum due to deficiency of *Yin* and excessive heat in the lung, honeted bolus made of Bulbus Fritillariae Thunbergii and Rhizoma Anemarrhenae is administered. In treating cough with sticky sputum due to dryness of the lung, the drug is often used in combination with Radix Asteris, Flos Farfarae, etc.

2. Purging away heat and dissolving lumps and masses

In treating scrofula and subcutaneous nodules, the drug is often used in combination with Radix Scrophulariae, Concha Ostreae, etc. In treating painful swelling at the initial stage of acute mastitis, the drug is often used in combination with Herba Taraxaci, Fructus Forsythiae, Radix Trichosanthis, etc.

Dosage and Administration: Usually, 3–10 g of the drug is used in decoction.

Notes: The drug should not be used in combination with Radix Aconiti.

Appendix: Bulbus Fritillariae Thunbergii (浙贝母 *Zhebeimu*)

This drug is also called *Xiangbei* and *Dabei* in Chinese. It consists of the bulb of the perennial herbage F. thunbergii Miq. (family Liliaceae). The drug is cut into thick slices for use. It is bitter in taste and cold in nature, and has the actions of promoting the lung's dispersing function, resolving phlegm, relieving cough, clearing away heat and dissolving lumps and masses. Owing to its function of dispersion and purgation, it is often used to treat cough due to invasion of exogenous wind and accumulation of phlegm–heat in the lung, sores, carbuncle, swelling, scrofula, subcutaneous nodule, etc. Usually, 6–12 g of the drug is used in decoction. The drug should not be used in combination with Radix Aconiti.

Trichosanthes Fruit (栝楼 *Gualou*)
Fructus Trichosanthis

This drug consists of the fruit of the perennial liana climber Trichosanthes kirilowii Maxim. (family Cucurbitaceae). When the whole fruit is used, the drug is called the whole Fructus Trichosanthis; When the peel is used, the drug is called Pericarpium Trichosanthis; when the seed is used, the drug is called Semen Trichosanthis, which is parched and broken into pieces for use; when the oil is removed from the seed, the drug is called frost of Semen Trichosanthis.

Nomenclature Used in Prescriptions: *Guangualou, Gualoupi, Gualouren, Gualoushuang*

Properties and Channel Distribution: This drug is sweet in taste and cold in nature, and is distributed to the Lung, Stomach and Large Intestine Channels.

Action and Indications:

1. Clearing away heat and resolving phlegm

In treating cough due to accumulation of lung–*Qi* and phlegmheat Pericarpium Trichosanthis is often used in combination with drugs for promoting the lung's dispersing function and resolving phlegm such as Bulbus Fritillariae Thunbergii, Semen Armeniacae Amarum, Radix Platycodi, etc. In treating accumulation of phlegm due to retention of fluid, stuffy chest and shortness of breath, the drug can be used in combination with Rhizoma Pinelliae, Fructus Aurantii Immaturus, etc. In treating dyspnea in children, 15 g of the drug can be used in decoction.

2. Comforting the chest and dispersing accumulation of *Qi*

In treating obstruction of *Qi* in the chest and chest pain, the drug is often used in combination with Bulbus Allii Macrostemi, etc. In treating stuffy chest or chest pain due to accumulation of phlegm and heat, the drug can be decocted together with Rhizoma Pinelliae, Rhizoma Coptidis, etc.

3. Subduing swelling

In treating pulmonary abscess and cough with pus and blood, the drug is often used in combination with Flos Lonicerae, Herba Houttuyniae, Rhizoma Phragmitis, etc. In treating acute mastitis with redness, swelling and burning pain, the drug is often used in combination with Herba Taraxaci, Flos Lonicerae, Fructus Forsythiae, etc.

4. Moistening the intestine to relax the bowel

In treating constipation due to dryness of the intestine, a decoction of 30 g of the drug and 6 g of Radix Glycyrrhizae is taken with honey added to the decoction. In treating constipation due to indigestion, honeyed bolus made of equal dosage of Semen Trichosanthis, Massa Fermentata Medicinalis, Fructus Crataegi, and Rhizoma Pinelliae is administered.

In recent years it is used to treat angina pectoris seen in coronary heart disease and mammary cancer.

Dosage and Administration: Usually, 12–30 g of the whole drug, 6–12 g of Pericarpium Trichosanthis, 3–10 g of Semen Trichosanthis and 3–10 grams of frost of Semen Trichosanthis are used in decoction. The whole drug is often used to treat obstruction of *Qi* in the chest, swelling and constipation; Pericarpium Trichosanthis is often used to clear away heat, resolve phlegm, send down adverse flow of *Qi* and comfort the chest; Semen Trichosanthis is used to moisten the lung to dispel phlegm or moisten the intestine to relax the bowel; frost of Semen Trichosanthis is similar in its effect to Semen Trichosanthis, but the effect of moistening the intestine is much milder.

Notes: This drug is antagonized by Radix Aconiti

Bamboo Shavings (竹茹 *Zhuru*)
Caulis Bambusae in Taeniam

This drug consists of the culm shavings of the perennial evergreen bamboo–like arbor or shrub Phyllostachys nigra (Lodd.) Munro var henonis (Mitf.) Stapf ex Rendle (family Gramineae). The crude of slightly parched (with ginger juice) drug is used.

Nomenclature Used in Prescriptions: *Danzhuru, Jiangzhuru*

Properties and Channel Distribution: This drug is sweet in taste and slightly cold in nature, and is distributed to the Lung, Stomach and Gall Bladder Channels.

Action and Indications:

1. Clearing away heat and resolving phlegm

In treating restlessness, insomnia, etc. due to deficiency of the gall bladder and accumulation of phlegm–heat, the drug is often used in combination with Fructus Aurantii Immaturus, Rhizoma Pinelliae, Poria, etc. In treating wind–stroke manifested by mental confusion due to phlegm and rigid tongue, the drug is often used in combination with Arisaema cum Bile, Rhizoma Acori Graminei, Poria, Rhizoma Pinelliae, etc. In treating cough due to heat–phlegm, the drug is often used in combination with Radix Scutellariae, Fructus Trichosanthis, etc.

2. Clearing away heat and arresting vomiting

In treating vomiting due to damp–heat, the drug can be used in combination with Rhizoma Coptidis, Rhizoma Pinelliae, etc. In treating vomiting or hiccup due to heat of deficiency type in the stomach, the drug can be used in combination with Exocarpium Citri Grandis, Radix Codonopsis Pilosulae, Radix Glycyrrhizae, Rhizoma Zingiberis Recens, and Fructus Ziziphi Jujubae.

Dosage and Administration: Usually, 6–12 g of the drug is used in decoction. The crude drug is used to dispel phlegm and the parched drug (with ginger juice) is used to arrest vomiting.

Appendix: Succus Bambosae (竹沥 *Zhuli*)

This drug is also called *Zhuyou, Zhulishui* and *Zhuligao* in Chinese. It consists of the juice excreted from the baked fresh bamboo stem. This drug is slippery, and is sweet in taste and cold in nature. It can be used to clear away fire from the Heart, Lung and Stomach Channels so as to dispel phlegm, relieve restlessness and arrest convulsion. It can be used in combination with ginger juice or other drugs to treat wind–stroke manifested by aphasia, epilepsy, convulsion, etc. due to obstruction by phlegm, or cough and asthma due to accumulation of phlegm–heat in the lung, or numbness and contracture of the limbs due to retention of phlegm in the channels. However, since this drug is cold in nature and is likely to damage the stomach and intestine, it is contraindicated for those with cold–dampness or loose stools. The common dosage is 30–60 g.

Tabasheer (天竺黄 *Tianzhuhuang*)
Concretio Silicea Bambusae

This drug consists of the concrete mass in the hollow stem of the perennial evergreen plant Bambusa textilis Mcclure, etc. (family Gramineae). The drug is broken into pieces for use.

Nomenclature Used in Prescriptions: *Tianzhuhuang, Zhuhuang*

Properties and Channel Distribution: This drug is sweet in taste and cold in nature, and is distributed to the Heart, Stomach and Liver Channels.

Action and Indications:

1. Clearing away heat and eliminating phlegm

In treating shortness of breath, cough and asthma in children due to accumulation of phlegm–heat, the drug can be used in combination with Rhizoma Coptidis, Bombyx Batryticatus,

Cinnabaris, etc.

2. Cooling the heart to arrest convulsion

In treating infantile convulsion, fever with soporous state, and clonic convulsion due to accumulation of phlegm, the drug is often used in combination with Arisaema cum Bile, Cinnabaris, etc. In treating infantile convulsion and night crying, the drug can be used in combination with Periostracum Cicadae, Bombyx Batryticatus, Radix Curcumae, etc.

Dosage and Administration: Usually, 3–10 g of the drug is used in decoction, or 0.6–1 g of the drug powder is taken as a dose.

Costazia Bone (海浮石 *Haifushi*)
Os Costaziae

This drug consists either of the rock formed from the volcano lava or of the bone of Costazia aculeata Canuet Bassler or Costazia costazii Audouin, etc. (family Poripidae). The drug is dried and broken into pieces for medication.

Nomenclature Used in Prescriptions: *Haifushi, Fuhaishi*

Properties and Channel Distribution: This drug is salty in taste and cold in nature, and is distributed to the Lung Channel.

Action and Indications:

1. Clearing away heat and resolving phlegm

In treating cough and asthma due to phlegm–heat, and accumulation of stubborn phlegm, the drug can be used in combination with Arisaema cum Bile, Bulbus Fritillariae Thunbergii, etc. In treating pulmonary tuberculosis manifested by hemoptysis and cough with yellow sputum, 60 g of Os Costaziae, 180 g of

Rhizoma Bletillae and 60 g of Radix Notoginseng are ground into powder, and 3 g of the powder is to be taken at a time, 2–3 times a day.

2. Softening and resolving hard mass

In treating scrofula and tuberculosis, the drug used alone may not be quite effective, and therefore it is often used together with other drugs.

3. Resolving stones and treating stranguria

In treating stranguria with urolithiasis, stranguria caused by the passage of urinary stone, stranguria complicated by hematuria, dysuria, etc., 3 g of the drug powder is taken at a time with decoction of Radix Glycyrrhizae, 3 times a day.

Dosage and Administration: Usually, 6–10 g of the drug is used in decoction. The drug can also be made into pills or powder.

Clam Shell (海蛤壳 *Haigeqiao*)
Concha Meretricis

This drug consists of the shell of Cyclina sinensis (Gmelin), or Meretrix meretrix L. (family Veneridae). The drug is ground into pieces and the crude or calcined drug is used for medication.

Nomenclature Used in Prescriptions: *Haigeqiao, Haigefen, Duangeqiao*

Properties and Channel Distribution: This drug is salty in taste and cold in nature, and is distributed to the Lung and Kidney Channels.

Action and Indications:

1. Clearing away heat from the lung and resolving phlegm

In treating cough due to phlegm–fire or stuffy chest due to accumulation of phlegm, the drug can be used in combination with Indigo Naturalis, Radix Asparagi, Radix Scutellariae, etc. In treating chest pain due to accumulation of phlegm–heat, equal amount of the powder of the drug and Semen Trichosanthis are made into pills and taken.

2. Softening and resolving hard mass

In treating goiter and scrofula, the drug can be used in combination with Thallus Laminariae seu Echloniae, Sargassum, etc.

3. Inducing diuresis to relieve edema

In treating edema due to damp–heat and dysuria, the drug can be used in combination with Caulis Akebiae, Talcum, Polyporus Umbellatus, etc. In treating tympanites, ascites and dysuria, the drug can be used in combination with Radix Stephaniae Tetrandrae, Semen Lepidii seu Descurainiae, Semen Pruni, etc.

Besides, the drug can also be used to relieve hyperacidity and pain and therefore can be used to treat gastralgia with acid regurgitation. When mixed with vegetable oil, the drug can be applied externally to treat scald and eczema, etc.

Dosage and Administration: Usually, 10–15 g of the drug is used in decoction. The drug powder should be wrapped in a piece of cloth before being decocted with other drugs. The drug can also be made into pills or powder. The crude drug is used for oral administration and the calcined drug is used to relieve hyperacidity or in external treatment.

Sargassum Seaweed (海藻 *Haizao*)
Sargassum

This drug consists of the dried seaweed of the marine perennial plant Sargassum fusiforme (Harv.) Setch., or Sargassum pallidum (Turn.) C. Ag. (family Sargassaceae). The drug is cut into sections for medication.

Nomenclature Used in Prescriptions: *Haizao, Danhaizao*

Properties and Channel Distribution: This drug is bitter and salty in taste and cold in nature, and is distributed to the Liver, Stomach and Kidney Channels.

Action and Indications:

Resolving phlegm and hard mass

In treating scrofula, tuberculosis and goiter, the drug is often used in combination with Thallus Laminariae seu Eckloniae, Concha Meretricis, Bombyx Batryticatus, etc. In treating swelling and pain of the testis, the decoction of the drug is taken.

In addition, the drug can also be used to treat dropsy due to beriberi and edema, owing to its effect of inducing diuresis and relieving edema.

Dosage and Administration: Usually, 15–30 g of the drug is used in decoction.

Notes: The drug should not be used in combination with Radix Glycyrrhizae

Laminaria or Ecklonia (昆布 *Kunbu*)
Thallus Laminariae or Thallus Eckloniae

This drug consists of the thallus of the marine plants Ecklonia kurome Okam. and Undaria pinnatifida (Harv.) Suring (family Alariaceae), or Laminaria japonica Aresch (family Laminariaceae). The drug is cut into slivers or small pieces for medication.

Nomenclature Used in Prescriptions: *Kunbu, Dankunbu*

Properties and Channel Distribution: This drug is salty in taste and cold in nature, and is distributed to the Liver, Stomach and Kidney Channels.

Action and Indications:

Resolving phlegm and hard mass

In treating goiter and scrofula, the drug is often used in combination with Sargassum, etc. This effect of this drug is the same as but more powerful than that of Sargassum and the two drugs combined may have better therapeutic effect. They are both the main drugs for treating goiter and scrofula. In treating enlargement of the liver and spleen, the drug is often used in combination with Rhizoma Sparganii, Rhizoma Zedoariae, Carapax Trionycis, etc.

Besides, the drug can also be used to treat edema and beriberi, owing to its effect of inducing diuresis and relieving edema. It can also be used to treat orchioscheocele. In recent years it has been used to treat endemic goiter, adenoma, tuberculosis of lymph node, and cirrhosis.

Chlorite–schist or Mica–schist (礞石 *Mengshi*)

This drug consists of the metamorphic rock of Chlorite–schist or Mica–schist. The rock is calcined together with nitre till it turns golden in colour. Then it is refined with water to remove toxins and dried for medication.

Nomenclature Used in Prescriptions: *Mengshi, Jinmengshi*

Properties and Channel Distribution: This drug is sweet and salty in taste and neutral in nature, and is distributed to the Lung and Liver Channels.

Action and Indications:

Sending down adverse flow of *Qi*, promoting expectoration of phlegm, checking hyperfunction of the liver and relieving convulsion

In treating dyspnea due to internal accumulation of stubborn phlegm, constipation, or epilepsy, mania, dysphoria, etc. due to accumulation of phlegm, the drug is often used in combination with Lignum Aquilariae Resinatum, Radix et Rhizoma Rhei, etc. In treating acute infantile convulsion due to phlegm–heat, 1.5–3 g of the drug powder can be taken at a time with decoction of Herba Menthae mixed with honey.

Dosage and Administration: Usually, 6–10 g of the drug is used in decoction. When taken in pill or powder form, 1.5–3 g of the drug is used at a time.

13.3 Drugs for Warming and Resolving Phlegm due to Cold

This kind of drugs are mostly warm and dry in nature and have the function of warming and resolving phlegm due to cold or eliminating dampness to resolve phlegm. They can be used to treat those with thin and cold phlegm, cold or damp phlegm easy to be expectorated, cough and asthma due to this kind of phlegm, aching pain of the limbs, multiple abscess due to accumulation of cold phlegm occurring in the deep layer of tissues, etc. To improve the therapeutic effect. this kind of drugs should be used together with drugs for warming and dispersing cold-dampness. They should be used with care by those with dry cough due to deficiency of *Yin* or with the history of hemoptysis and hematemesis.

Pinellia Tuber (半夏 *Banxia*)
Rhizoma Pinelliae

This drug consists of the tuber of the perennial herbage Pinellia ternata (Thunb.) Breit. (family Araceae). The crude or processed drug is used. The drug is divided, according to the processing method, into Rhizoma Pinelliae prepared with alum, Rhizoma Pinelliae prepared with Radix Glycyrrhizae and lime and Rhizoma Pinelliae Prepared with alum and ginger.

Nomenclature Used in Prescriptions: *Qingbanxia, Jiangbanxia, Fabanxia, Shengbanxia*

Properties and Channel Distribution: This drug is pungent in taste and warm in nature with slight toxic effect, and is distributed to the Spleen and Stomach Channels.

Action and Indications:

1. Eliminating dampness and resolving phlegm

In treating cough with profuse thin sputum due to damp–phlegm or dizziness due to phlegm, the drug is often used in combination with Pericarpium Citri Reticulatae, Poria, etc. In treating vomiting due to wind–phlegm, headache and blurred vision, stuffy chest and poor appetite, the drug can be used in combination with Rhizoma Arisaematis, etc.

2. Sending down adverse flow of *Qi* to arrest vomiting

In treating vomiting due to cold in the stomach or retention of phlegm, 15 g of Rhizoma Pinelliae and 10 g of Rhizoma Zingiberis Recens are prescribed. In treating vomiting due to deficiency of the stomach, 12 g of Rhizoma Pinelliae and 15 g of Radix Codonopsis Pilosulae can be decocted, with addition of 30 g of honey. In treating stuffy chest and vomiting due to phlegm–heat, the drug is often used in combination with Rhizoma Coptidis and Rhizoma Zingiberis.

3. Disintegrating masses

This drug has the effect of disintegrating masses and resolving phlegm. In treating stuffy chest due to accumulation of phlegmheat, the drug can be used in combination with Rhizoma Coptidis, Semen Trichosanthis, etc. In treating stagnation of *Qi*, accumulation of phlegm and globus hystericus, the drug can be used in combination with Cortex Magnoliae Officinalis, Folium Perillae, Poria, etc. In treating goiter and subcutaneous nodule, the drug can be used in combination with drugs for softening and disintegrating hard masses such as Thallus Laminariae seu Eckloniae, Sargassum, Bulbus Fritillariae Thunbergii, etc. In treating carbuncle, phlegmon and swelling, the drug powder is mixed with egg white and applied to the local area.

Dosage and Administration: Usually, 3–10 g of the drug is used in decoction. It is customary to use Rhizoma Pinelliae Prepared with alum to resolve damp–phlegm, Rhizoma Pinelliae prepared with ginger and alum to arrest vomiting, Rhizoma Pinelliae prepared with Radix Glycyrrhizae and lime to eliminate dampness and regulate the stomach, and crude Rhizoma Pinelliae to treat carboncle, phlegmon and swelling.

Notes: This drug is antagonized by Radix Aconiti. Since it is warm and dry in nature, it should be used with care or should not be used by those with dry cough due to deficiency of *Yin*, blood disorders, heat–phlegm, etc.

Arisaema Tuber (天南星 *Tiannanxing*)
Rhizoma Arisaematis

This drug consists of the tuber of the perennial herbage Arisaema consanguineum Schott, Arisaema amurense Maxim., or Arisaema heterophyllum Bl. (family Araceae). The crude drug or the drug prepared by soaking it in the alum solution, decocting it together with ginger, cutting it into slices and then drying it, can both be used.

Nomenclature Used in Prescriptions: *Shengnanxing*, *Zhinanxing*

Properties and Channel Distribution: This drug is bitter and pungent in taste and warm in nature with toxic effect. It is distributed to the Lung, Liver and Spleen Channels.

Action and Indications:

1. Eliminating dampness and resolving phlegm

In treating cough due to stubborn phlegm and damp phlegm, stuffy chest, etc., the drug is often used in combination with Rhizoma Pinelliae, Poria, Fructus Aurantii Immaturus, etc., or the drug, Rhizoma Atractylodis Macrocephalae, and Rhizoma Pinelliae can be made into pills. In treating profuse yellow sticky sputum due to lung– heat, the drug can be used in combination with Rhizoma Pinelliae, Radix Scutellariae, etc. In treating cough with thin sputum, the drug, Rhizoma Pinelliae, Cortex Cinnamomi can be made into pills, to be taken with decoction of Rhizoma Zingiberis Recens.

2. Dispelling wind and relieving spasm

In treating excessive sputum, severe numbness of hands and feet, hemiplegia, deviation of mouth and eye which are due to retention of wind–phlegm in the channels, the drug can be used in combination with Rhizoma Pinelliae, Rhizoma Typhonii, Radix Aconiti, etc. In treating tetanus manifested by spasm of limbs, lockjaw, neck rigidity, etc., equal amount of the drug and Radix Ledebouriellae can be ground into powder, to be used for oral administration or in external treatment.

3. Removing toxins and treating skin and external diseases

In treating boils, carbuncles, scrofula and tuberculosis, the drug can be soaked in vinegar and the concentrated solution is applied to the local area. In treating snake bite, the fresh drug is pounded and applied to the bite, or the dry drug and Realgar are ground into powder, mixed with alcohol and applied to the bite.

Besides, the drug is in recent years used to treat carcinoma of uterine cervix.Pharmacological research has proved that the drug has antineoplastic action.

Dosage and Administration: Usually, 3–10 g of the drug is used in decoction. In external treatment, proper amount of the crude drug can be used.

Notes: This drug should be used with care by pregnant women.

Appendix: Arisaema cum Bile (胆南星 *Dannanxing*)

This drug is the mixture of powdered Arisaema Tuber and bile of ox, which is made into small pieces or cylinder–like pieces. It is more bitter in taste but cool in nature. It has the effect of calming wind, resolving phlegm and relieving convulsion and can be used to treat coma, convulsion, epilepsy, etc. due to invasion of heat–phlegm to the seven orifices. Usually, 3–6 g of the drug is used in decoction.

Giant Typhonium Tuber (白附子 *Baifuzi*)
Rhizoma Typhonii

This drug consists of the tuber of the perennial herbage Typhonium giganteum Engl. (family Araceae). The crude or prepared drug is used for medication.

Nomenclature Used in Prescriptions: *Baifuzi, Zhibaifuzi*

Properties and Channel Distribution: This drug is pungent and sweet in taste and hot in nature with toxic effect. It is distributed to the Liver and Spleen Channels.

Action and Indications:

1. Removing phlegm and relieving pain

In treating dizziness due to wind–phlegm and headache due to phlegm syndrome, the drug can be decocted together with Rhizoma Arisaematis and Rhizoma Pinelliae.

2. Dispelling wind to relieve spasm

In treating wind-stroke manifested by deviation of mouth and eye, the drug is often used in combination with Scorpio and Bombyx Batryticatus. In treating convulsion and vomiting due to excessive phlegm, the drug can be used in combination with Rhizoma Arisaematis, Scorpio, Bombyx Batryticatus, etc. In treating tetanus manifested by lock jaw and spasm, the drug can be used in combination with Rhizoma Arisaematis, Radix Ledebouriellae, Rhizoma Gastrodiae, etc.

3. Removing toxin and disintegrating mass

In treating snake bite, the drug alone can be applied to the bite, or the drug can be used with other drugs for removing snake poisons, to be taken orally or applied externally. In treating scrofula and subcutaneous nodules, the fresh drug can be pounded and applied to the local area.

Dosage and Administration: Usually, 3–5 g of the drug is used in decoction. Proper amount of the drug is used in external treatment.

Notes: The drug is contraindicated for pregnant women. The crude drug is usually not used for oral administration.

White Mustard Seed (白芥子 *Baijiezi*) Semen Sinapis Albae

This drug consists of the ripe seed of the Brassica alba (L.) Boiss., or B. juncea (L.) Czern. et Coss. (family Cruciferae). The former is called *Baijiezi* and the latter is called huangjiezi in Chinese. The crude or parched drug is used for medication.

Nomenclature Used in Prescriptions: *Baijiezi, Chaojiezi*

Properties and Channel Distribution: This drug is pungent in taste and warm in nature, and is distributed to the Lung and Stomach Channels.

Action and Indications:

1. Eliminating phlegm and promoting flow of *Qi*

In treating cough and asthma with profuse thin sputum, distention in the chest and hypochondrium, etc. due to accumulation of cold phlegm in the lung, the drug is often used in combination with Fructus Perillae, Semen Raphani, etc. In treating reversed flow of *Qi* due to retention of phlegm, cough and asthma with chest pain, hydrops in the chest and hypochondrium, etc., the drug is often used in combination with Radix Euphorbiae Kansui and Radix Euphorbiae Pekinensis. In treating pain in the limbs and joints due to stasis of *Qi* and retention of phlegm, 10 g of Semen Sinapis Albae, 10 g of Resina Commiphorae Myrrhae, 10 g of ortex Cinnamomi, 10 g of Radix Aucklandiae, and 3 g of Semen Momordicae are ground into powder and 3 g of the powder is to be taken at a time with warm wine, twice a day.

2. Disintegrating mass and subduing swelling

In treating scrofula, subcutaneous nodules, swelling caused by accumulation of cold, etc., equal amount of the drug and Bulbus Allii Fistulos can be pounded into mash and applied to the local area once a day. The powdered drug mixed with vinegar can be used to treat pyogenic infections.

Besides, the drug has been used in recent years to treat exudative pleurisy to remove hydrops in the thoracic cavity.

Dosage and Administration: Usually, 3–10 g of the drug is used in decoction. Proper amount of the drug can be used in external treatment.

Notes: Since the drug has the effect of forming blister on the skin, it should not be used by those with dermal allergy.

Swallowwort Rhizome (白前 *Baiqian*) Rhizoma Cynanchi Stauntonii

This drug consists of the rhizome and root of the perennial herbage Cynanchum stauntoni (Decne.) Schltr. ex Levl., or Cynanchum glaucescens (Decne.) Hand-Mazz. (family Asclepiadaceae). The drug is cut into sections and the crude drug or the honey-fried drug is used for medication.

Nomenclature Used in Prescriptions: *Baiqian, Zhibaiqian*

Properties and Channel Distribution: This drug is bitter and pungent in taste and slightly warm in nature, and is distributed to the Lung Channel.

Action and Indications:

Promoting the lung's dispersing function, sending down adverse flow of *Qi*, dispelling phlegm and relieving cough

This drug is a main drug for cough due to disorder of the lung because it can effectively send down adverse flow of *Qi*, thus eliminating phlegm and therefore relieve cough. In treating cough with profuse sputum due to obstruction of the lung-*Qi*, stuffy chest, shortness of breath, etc., the drug can be used in combination with Herba Ephedrae, Flos Farfarae, Semen Armeniacae Amarum, Radix Glycyrrhizae, etc. In treating cough and asthma with yellow and sticky sputum difficult to be expectorated due to lung-heat, the drug can be used in combination with Cortex Mori Radicis, Radix Rehmanniae, Cortex Lycii Radicis, etc. In treating cough due to exogenous wind-cold, the drug is often used in combination with Herba Schizonepetae, Radix Platycodi, Pericarpium Citri Reticulatae, etc.

Dosage and Administration: Usually, 6–10 g of the drug is used in decoction. The honey–fried drug can be used to treat long–lasting cough with sticky sputum difficult to be expectorated.

Inula Flower (旋复花 *Xuanfuhua*)
Flos Inulae

This drug consists of the capitulum of the perennial herbage Inula britannica L. var. chinensis (Rupr.) Reg., or Inula britannica L. (family Compositae). The crude or honey–fried drug is used.

Nomenclature Used in Prescriptions: *Xuanfuhua*

Properties and Channel Distribution: This drug is bitter, pungent and salty in taste and slightly warm in nature, and is distributed to the Lung, Stomach and Large Intestine Channels.

Action and Indications:

1. Removing obstruction and dissolving phlegm

In treating stuffy chest, shortness of breath, etc. due to retention of phlegm, the drug can be used in combination with Radix Platycodi, Cortex Mori Radicis, Semen Arecae, etc. In treating cough and asthma with sputum due to febrile diseases, the drug is often used in combination with Herba Schizonepetae, Herba Asari, Radix Peucedani, etc.

2. Sending down adverse flow of *Qi* and arrest belching

In treating stuffy chest and belching due to deficiency of *Qi* in the spleen and stomach or adverse ascending of phlegm–dampness, the drug is often used in combination with Haematitum , Rhizoma Pinelliae, etc.

Dosage and Administration: Usually, 6–12 g of the drug is used in decoction (wrapped with cloth).

14 Tranquilizers

Drugs with the main function of calming the mind are called tranquilizers.

Tranquilizers are divided, according to their properties, into two kinds: drugs consisting of heavy minerals, metals or shells for tranquilization and drugs consisting of plants for tranquilization by nourishing the heart and liver.

The first kind of the drugs have tranquilizing effect and are often used to treat excess syndromes due to flaring-up of *Yang-Qi* and manifested by irritability. However, though this kind of drugs can calm down the floating *Yang*, they can't eliminate other factors causing the flaring-up of *Yang*. They should, therefore, be used in combination with other drugs. The second kind of the drugs are mostly used to treat deficiency syndromes due to deficiency of blood in the heart and liver manifested by restlessness. In this case they are often used in combination with drugs for nourishing *Yin* and blood.

Although the first kind of drugs are often used in excess syndromes and the second kind, deficiency syndromes, they are sometimes used in combination in treating syndromes of both excess and deficiency so as to enhance the therapeutic effect.

14.1 Drugs with Heavy Materials for Tranquilization

This kind of drugs has tranquilizing effect and are used to

treat flaring–up of *Yang–Qi*, palpitation, insomnia, epilepsy induced by terror, mania, irritability, etc. If the diseases are due to hyperactivity of pathogenic heat, they should be used in combination with drugs for clearing away heat and purging fire; if the diseases are due to ascending of liver–*Yang*, they should be used in combination with drugs for calming the liver and suppressing *Yang* hyperactivity.

Cinnabar (朱砂 *Zhusha*)
Cinnabaris

This drug consists of the natural mineral Cinnabar. The mineral is refined into powder with water for medication.

Nomenclature Used in Prescriptions: *Zhusha, Feizhusha, Dansha, Chensha*

Properties and Channel Distribution: This drug is sweet in taste and cold in nature, and is distributed to the Heart Channel.

Action and Indications

1. Relieving palpitation and calming the mind

In treating restlessness, vexation and insomnia due to deficiency of blood in the heart and hyperactivity of the heart–fire, the drug is often used in combination with Rhizoma Coptidis, Radix Rehmanniae or Succinum, etc. In treating epilepsy, the drug can be used in combination with Rhizoma Arisaematis, Succinum, Alumen, etc.

2. Removing toxin and treating skin and external diseases

In treating sores and pyogenic infections, the drug and Realgar, etc. can be ground into powder and applied to the local area. In treating ulcer of the mouth or nose, sore throat, etc., the drug and Borneolum, Syntheticum, Borax, etc. can be ground into powder and applied to the local area by insufflation.

Besides, the drug has antiseptic effect and its powder can be used as pill coating.

Dosage and Administration: Its dosage is 0.3–1 g. The drug is made into pills or powder and should not be decocted. The drug powder can be taken following its infusion with water. Proper amount of the drug can be used in external treatment. The crude drug is always used.

Notes: The drug should not be calcined with fire because when the drug is calcined, mercury will separate out and this is likely to cause poisoning. When used for oral administration the drug should not be taken continually for a long time and overdosage is also not advicable, so as to avoid mercury poisoning. The drug should be used with care for those with abnormal function of the liver and kidney to avoid aggravating the disease.

Dragon's Bone (龙骨 *Longgu*)
Os Draconis

This drug consists of the fossil bone of ancient large mammals, such as Stegodon orientalis and Rhinocerus sinensis, etc. The bone is broken into pieces and the crude or calcined drug is used.

Nomenclature Used in Prescriptions: *Shenglonggu*, *Duanlonggu*

Properties and Channel Distribution: This drug is sweet and puckery in taste and neutral in nature, and is distributed to the

Heart and Liver Channels.

Action and Indications:

1. Relieving palpitation and calming the mind

In treating mental disorder, palpitation, poor memory, insomnia, etc., equal amount of the drug, Plastrum Testudinis, Rhizoma Acori Graminei and Radix Polygalae are ground into powder and made into pills with water, and 3 g of the pills are taken at a time, three times a day.

2. Calming the liver and suppressing *Yang* hyperactivity

In treating dizziness, blurred vision, vexation, mania due to terror, etc. which are caused by deficiency of liver–*Yin* and floating of *Yang* of deficiency type, the drug is often used in combination with Concha Ostreae, Radix Paeoniae Alba, Radix Cynanchi Atrati, Flos Chrysanthemi, Ramulus Uncariae cum Uncis, Radix Scrophulariae, etc.

3. Inducing astringency and arresting discharge

In treating seminal emission, abnormal leukorrhea, spontaneous sweating, night sweating, menorrhagia, etc., the drug is often used in combination with Concha Ostreae, Rhizoma Dioscoreae, Os Sepiellae seu Sepiae, Poria, etc.

4. Promoting tissue regeneration and healing sores

In treating sores and ulceration which do not heal over a long time, umbilical sore with watery discharge, bleeding from incised wound, etc., equal amount of the drug and Alumen are ground into fine powder and applied to the local area.

Dosage and Administration: The dosage is 10–30 g. When used in decoction, the drug should be decocted longer than other drugs. Proper amount of the drug can be used in external treatment. The crude drug is used to soothe the mind and liver and the calcined drug is used to induce astringency and arrest discharge.

Amber (琥珀 *Hupo*)
Succinum

This drug consists of the fossil formed from the resin of ancient maple or pine. The resin is ground into powder for medication.

Nomenclature Used in Prescriptions: *Hupo, Xuepo, Laohupo*

Properties and Channel Distribution: This drug is sweet in taste and neutral in nature, and is distributed to the Heart, Liver and Urinary Bladder Channels.

Action and Indications:

1. Relieving palpitation and calming the mind

In treating palpitation due to terror, severe palpitation, poor memory, dream-disturbed sleep, insomnia, epilepsy, etc., the drug can be used in combination with Cinnabaris, Rhizoma Arisaematis, Poria, Radix Polygalae, Rhizoma Acori Graminei, etc.

2. Inducing diuresis and treating stranguria

In treating retention of urine, stranguria with blood, stranguria due to heat, stranguria from urolithiasis, etc., the drug is often used in combination with other drugs for inducing diuresis and removing blood stasis.

3. Activating blood circulation and removing blood stasis

In treating amenorrhea due to stasis of *Qi* and blood, the drug can be used in combination with Radix Angelicae Sinensis, Rhizoma Zedoariae, etc.

In addition, the drug can also be used to treat sores,

ulceration and pyogenic infection to activate blood circulation and subdue swelling. It can be used as a drug for inducing astringency in external treatment. In recent years the powder of it and Radix Notoginseng is used to treat coronary heart disease. The drug powder can also be taken orally to treat scrotal and labial hematoma or uterine passive congestion.

Dosage and Administration: The dosage is 1.5–3 g. The drug should not be decocted. The drug is usually in powder or pill form.

Magnetite (磁石 *Cishi*)
Magnetitum

This drug consists of the magnetic iron ore Magnetite. It is broken into pieces or quenched with vinegar and ground into powder for medication.

Nomenclature Used in Prescriptions: *Cishi, Lingcishi, Huocishi, Duancishi*

Properties and Channel Distribution: This drug is pungent and salty in taste, slightly cold in nature, and distributed to the Liver and Kidney Channels.

Action and Indications:

1. Suppressing *Yang* hyperactivity to calm the mind

In treating dizziness, headache, palpitation, insomnia, vexation, epilepsy, etc.due to deficiency of *Yin* and hyperactivity of *Yang*, the drug is often used in combination with Cinnabaris.

2. Improving the functions of eye and ear

In treating tinnitus, deafness, poor vision, etc. due to deficiency of the liver and kidney, the drug can be used in combination with Rhizoma Rehmanniae Praeparatae, Fructus Corni, Fructus Schisandrae, etc.

3. Helping inspiration to relieve asthma

In treating senile asthma due to deficiency of kidney–*Qi*, the drug can be used in combination with Rhizoma Rehmanniae Praeparatae, Fructus Corni, Rhizoma Dioscoreae, etc.

Dosage and Administration: Usually, 10–30 g of the drug is used in decoction. When used in decoction, the crude drug is to be used or the drug should be broken and decocted longer than other drugs. When made into pill or powder for oral administration, the drug should be thoroughly calcined; otherwise it may cause stomachache.

Notes: Since the drug may impair digestion, the pill or powder should not be over–taken or taken over a long time.

14.2 Drugs for Tranquilization by Nourishing the Heart

This kind of drugs have the functions of nourishing the heart and liver and replenishing *Yin* to nourish the blood. They are often used to treat palpitation or severe palpitation, insomnia, dream-disturbed sleep, mental disorder, restlessness, etc. due to deficiency of blood in the heart and liver, disturbed mind, and abnormal activity of the seven emotional factors. They are often used in combination with drugs for nourishing blood and *Yin* to enhance the therapeutic effect.

Wild or Spiny Jujuba Seed (酸枣仁 *Suanzaoren*)
Semen Ziziphi Spinosae

This drug consists of the kernel of the deciduous shrub or arbor Ziziphus jujuba Mill. (family Rhamnaceae). The crude or parched kernel is used for medication.

Nomenclature Used in Prescriptions: *Suanzaoren, Chaozaoren*

Properties and Channel Distribution: This drug is sweet and sour in taste and neutral in nature, and is distributed to the Heart, Liver, Gall Bladder and Spleen Channels.

Action and Indications:

1. Nourishing the heart to calm the mind

In treating dysphoria with smothery sensation, insomnia, palpitation due to terror or severe palpitation due to deficiency of blood, which fails to nourish the heart and liver, the drug is often used in combination with Rhizoma Anemarrhenae, Poria, Rhizoma Ligustici Chuanxiong and Radix Glycyrrhizae. In treating neurasthenia, poor memory, dream-disturbed sleep, poor appetite and listlessness due to deficiency of heart and spleen *Qi*, the drug can be used in combination with Radix Codonopsis Pilosulae, Poria, Radix Polygalae, Rhizoma Acori Graminei, etc.

2: Nourishing *Yin* to arrest sweating

In treating profuse sweating due to deficiency of *Yin*, the drug can be used in combination with Radix Ginseng and Poria, which are ground into powder and taken with rice water, or the drug can be used in combination with Radix Rehmanniae, Radix Paeoniae Alba, Radix Ophiopogonis, Fructus Schisandrae, Arillus Longan, etc.

Dosage and Administration: Usually, 10–15 g of the drug can be used in decoction. The drug can also be ground into powder and taken before sleep, 1.5–3 g as a dose.

Arborvitae Seed (柏子仁 *Baiziren*)
Semen Biotae

This drug consists of the seed of the evergreen arbor Biota orientalis (L.) End l. (family Cupressaceae). The shell is removed and the crude drug or the drug with the oil removed is used.

Nomenclature Used in Prescriptions: *Baiziren, Cebairen, Baizishuang*

Properties and Channel Distribution: This drug is sweet in taste and neutral in nature, and is distributed to the Heart and Spleen Channels.

Action and Indications:

1. Nourishing the heart to calm the mind

In treating restlessness, insomnia, dream–disturbed sleep, palpitation or severe palpitation, poor memory, etc. due to deficiency of heart blood, the drug can be used in combination with Rhizoma Rehmanniae Praeparatae, Radix Angelicae Sinensis, Poria, Rhizoma Acori Graminei, etc. If the above diseases are accompanied by night sweating, Radix Ginseng, Fructus Schisandrae and Concha Ostreae can also be used.

2. Invigorating the spleen and moistening the intestine

In treating senile or postpartum constipation due to deficiency of *Yin*, the drug is often used in combination with Semen Pini, Semen Pruni, etc.

Dosage and Administration: Usually, 6–10 g of the drug is used in decoction. The drug with the oil removed is used for those with loose stool.

Polygala Root (远志 *Yuanzhi*)
Radix Polygalae

This drug consists of the root of the perennial herbage Polygala tenuifolia Willd., or P. sibirica L. (family Polygalaceae). The crude or prepared drug is used for medication.

Nomenclature Used in Prescriptions: *Yuanzhi, Yuanzhirou, Chaoyuanzhi*

Properties and Channel Distribution: This drug is bitter and pungent in taste and warm in nature, and is distributed to the Heart, Kidney and Lung Channels.

Action and Indications:

1. Nourishing the heart to calm the mind

In treating palpitation due to terror, restlessness, poor memory, etc., the drug is often used in combination with Radix Codonopsis Pilosulae, Poria, Rhizoma Acori Graminei, Semen Ziziphi Spinosae, etc.

2. Dispelling phlegm to induce resuscitation

In treating mental disorder, confusion of the mind, palpitation due to terror, etc. which are caused by obstruction of the heart by phlegm, the drug is often used in combination with Radix Curcumae, Rhizoma Acori Graminei, Alumen, etc. to reinforce the effect of dispelling phlegm to induce resuscitation. In treating cough with profuse sputum or with sticky sputum difficult to be expectorated, the drug can be used in combination with Pericarpium Citri Reticulatae and Radix Glycyrrhizae.

Besides, the drug can also be used to treat carbuncle, phlegmon, pyogenic infections and swelling and pain of the breast. The drug powder is taken orally with wine or applied externally to the local area.

Dosage and Administration: Usually, 3–6 g of the drug is used in decoction. Proper amount of the drug is used in external treatment.

Notes: Since this drug is warm and dry in nature, it should be used with care by those with phlegm–heat, ulceration or gastritis.

Albizia Bark (合欢皮 *Hehuanpi*)
Cortex Albiziae

This drug consists of the bark of the deciduous arbor Albizzia julibrissin Durazz. (family Leguminosae). The crude drug is cut into slices for medication

Nomenclature Used in Prescriptions: *Hehuanpi*

Preperties and Channel Distribution: This drug is sweet in taste and neutral in nature, and is distributed to the Heart and Spleen Channels.

Action and Indications:

1. Calming the mind and relieving depression

In treating vexation, depression, anger, poor memory, insomnia, etc., the drug may be used alone or combined with Radix Paeoniae Alba, Semen Biotae, Dens Draconis, Succinum, etc.

2. Activating blood circulation to subdue swelling

In treating pulmonary abscess and cough with turbid sputum, the drug can be used alone or decocted together with Radix Ampelopsis, In treating traumatic injury with stasis of blood, swelling and pain, the drug can be used in combination with Radix Angelicae Sinensis, Radix Paeoniae Rubra, Rhizoma Ligustici Chuanxiong, Semen Persicae, etc.

3. Promoting tissue regeneration and reunion of fractured bones

In treating fractures, the drug and Semen Sinapis Albae can be ground into powder and taken orally with millet wine or applied externally to the local area.

Dosage and Administration: Usually, 10–15 g of the drug is used in decoction.

Appendix: Flos Albiziae (合欢花 *Hehuanhua*)

This drug consists of the flower of Albizzia julibrissin Durazz. It has similar functions to those of Cortex Albiziae but is especially effective in regulating flow of *Qi*, relieving depression, and normalizing the function of the stomach and spleen. Its dosage is 6–12 g.

15 Drugs for Calming the Liver and Subduing Wind

Drugs with the function of calming the liver–wind or checking exuberance of *Yang* for tranquilization are under this category.

This kind of drugs have the functions of clearing away heat in the liver, checking exuberance of *Yang*, relieving convulsion, etc. respectively and are often used to treat coma, convulsion and spasm or even opisthotonus due to high fever, or dizziness, burning pain in the brain, flushed face due to hyperactivity of the liver–*Yang* and up–stirring of the liver–wind, or sudden syncope, deviation of the mouth and eyes, hemiplegia, etc. due to internal stirring of liver wind. The drugs consisting of insects can also be used to treat intractable rheumatic arthralgia, numbness of the muscles, etc.

In using this kind of drugs, due attention should be paid to the combination of drugs according to the causes of diseases. For example, if the diseases are caused by high fever, drugs for clearing away heat and purging fire should be used; if the diseases are caused by wind–phlegm, drugs for resolving phlegm should be used; if the diseases are caused by failure of the kidney to nourish the liver, drugs for nourishing the kidney–*Yin* should be used; if the diseases are caused by deficiency of blood, drugs for enriching blood and nourishing the liver should be used. The wind syndromes are characterized by rapid change. The fire and wind may stir up each other and the ascending of fire and *Qi* may result in ascending of phlegm, giving rise to coma, etc. In such a case, it is important to first eliminate phlegm to induce resuscitation, and when consciousness is restored, the disease is then treated according to differentiation of syndromes. Also, since epilepsy induced by terror and convulsion are often accompanied by palpitation, insomnia, etc., this kind of drugs are often used in combination with drugs for calming the mind.

This kind of drugs have different properties and therefore should be used according to diseased conditions. Drugs of cold or cool nature should not be used for chronic convulsion due to deficiency of the spleen; drugs of warm and dry nature should be used with care for those with deficiency of *Yin* and blood.

Antelope's Horn (羚羊角 *Lingyangjiao*) Cornu Saigae Tataricae

This drug consists of the horn of Saiga tatarica L. (family Bovidae). The horn is cut into pieces, filed into powder or ground with water to take the liquid for oral administration.

Nomenclature Used in Prescriptions: *Lingyangpian, Lingyangfen*

Properties and Channel Distribution: This drug is salty in taste and cold in nature, and is distributed to the Liver, Heart and Lung Channels.

Action and Indications:

1. Cooling the liver and calming the wind

In treating up-stirring of the liver wind due to hyperactivity of heat in febrile diseases and manifested by contracture of the limbs or even opisthotonus, the drug can be used in combination with Ramulus Uncariae cum Uncis, Flos Chrysanthemi, Bulbus Fritillariae Thunbergii, Scorpio, Scolopendra, etc.

2. Clearing away heat in the liver and improving vision

In treating headache and conjunctival congestion due to hyperactivity of the liver–fire, the drug can be used in combination with Radix Gentianae, Fructus Gardeniae, Radix Scutellariae, etc.

Besides, the drug also has the effect of removing blood stasis and toxin, and can be used to treat skin eruption with redness, swelling, itching and pain due to toxic heat, and measles with retarded appearance of eruption due to invasion of toxic heat into the interior. The drug is ground with water to take the liquid for oral administration.

Dosage and Administration: The dosage is 3–6 g. When used in decoction, the drug should be decocted separately from other drugs. The drug can also be ground with water to take the liquid or filed into powder, and 0.6–1.5 g of the drug is to be used at a time.

Abalone Shell (石决明 *Shijueming*)
Concha Haliotidis

This drug consists of the shell of Haliotis diversicolor Reeve, or Haliotis gigantea discus Reeve, etc. (family Haliotidae). The crude or calcined drug is used.

Nomenclature Used in Prescriptions: *Shijueming, Shengshijue, Duanshijue*

Properties and Channel Distribution: This drug is salty in taste and cold in nature, and is distributed to the Liver and Lung Channels.

Action and Indications:

1. Calming the liver and suppressing *Yang* hyperactivity

In treating dizziness, vexation, insomnia and ascending of liver–*Yang* due to deficiency of *Yin*, the drug is often used in combination with Concha Ostreae, Radix Paeoniae Alba, Radix Rehmanniae, Fructus Ligustri Lucidi, Flos Chrysanthemi, Radix Achyranthis Bidentatae, etc.

2. Removing nebula to improve visual acuity

In treating nebula, optic atrophy, night blindness and conjunctival congestion with swelling and pain due to liver–heat, the drug can be used in combination with Flos Chrysanthemi, Flos Eriocauli, Periostracum Serpentis, etc. Another method of treatment of optic atrophy is putting the drug powder into the sheep liver, binding the liver with thread, cooking the liver in a clay pot and eating the liver every day (10 g of the drug at a time).

Dosage and Administration: Usually, 10–30 g of the drug is used in decoction and the drug should be decocted longer than other drugs.

Notes: This drug should be used with care by those with deficiency of the spleen–*Yang* due to invasion of cold, indigestion and achlorhydria.

Oyster Shell (牡蛎 *Muli*)
Concha Ostreae

This drug consists of the shell of Ostrea gigas Thunb. and O.

talienwhanensis crosse or O. ri–vularis Gould, etc. (family Ostreidae). The shell is broken into pieces and the crude or calcined drug is used.

Nomenclature Used in Prescriptions: *Shengmuli, Duanmuli*

Properties and Channel Distribution: This drug is salty and puckery in taste and slightly cold in nature, and is distributed to the Liver and Kidney Channels.

Action and Indications:

1. Calming the liver and suppressing *Yang* hyperactivity

In treating headache, dizziness, tinnitus, numbness of the limbs, etc. due to deficiency of *Yin* and hyperactivity of *yang*, the drug is often used in combination with Os Draconis, Ochra, Plastrum Testudinis, Radix Paeoniae Alba, etc.

2. Inducing tranquilization to calm the mind

In treating palpitation, fear, terror, vexation, insomnia, etc. due to deficiency of the liver–*Yin*, the drug is often used in combination with drugs for calming the mind such as Os Draconis, Semen Ziziphi Spinosae, Radix Polygalae, Caulis Polygoni Multiflori, etc.

3. Inducing astringency and arresting discharge

In treating afternoon fever, night sweating and spontaneous sweating seen in tuberculosis, 30 g of the drug can be decocted and taken orally. In treating seminal emission and spermatorrhea, the drug can be used in combination with Stamen Nelumbinis, Semen Euryales, etc. In treating metrorrhagia, metrostaxis and leukorrhea, the drug can be used in combination with Colla Corii Asini, Halloysitum Rubrum, Radix Dipsaci, etc.

4. Softening and resolving hard mass

In treating scrofula, subcutaneous nodules, etc. due to accumulation of phlegm–fire, the drug is often used in combination with Radix Scrophulariae, Bulbus Fritillariae Thunbergii, etc.

Besides, the drug has in recent years been used to relieve hyperacidity and is effective in treating acid regurgitation seen in gastropathy.

Dosage and Administration: Usually, 15–30 g of the drug is used in decoction, to be decocted longer than other drugs. The crude drug is used to suppress *Yang* hyperactivity and softening hard mass and the calcined drug is used to induce astringency and relieve hyperacidity.

Pearl (珍珠 *Zhenzhu*)
Margarita

This drug consists of the pearl formed in Pteria martensii Dunker. (family Pteriidae), and Hyriopsis cumingii Lea, Cristaria plicata Leach, or Anodonta woodiana Lea, etc. (family Unionidae). Before taken, the drug is wrapped in a piece of silk cloth, and cooked with bean curd for 4 hours. After that it is taken out and refined into powder with water for medication.

Nomenclature Used in Prescriptions: *Zhenzhufen, Lianzhufen*

Properties and Channel Distribution: This drug is sweet and salty in taste and cold in nature, and is distributed to the Heart and Liver Channels.

Action and Indications:

1. Calming the heart to relieve convulsion

In treating palpitation, epilepsy, acute convulsion due to heat, etc., the drug can be used in combination with Cinnabaris, Succinum, Arisaema cum Bile, Concretio Silicea Bambusae, etc.

2. Clearing away heat in the liver to remove nebula

In treating conjunctival congestion and painful nebula due to deficiency of the liver and presence of heat, eye drops can be prepared from the drug, Calamina, Borneolum Syntheticum, etc.

3. Promoting tissue regeneration and healing sores

In treating ulcers and sores that do not heal, the drug can be used in combination with Borneolum Syntheticum, elephant's thick skin, Resina Draconis, etc. In treating erosion of throat and ulcerative gingivitis, 9 g of the drug and 3 g of Calculus Bovis can be ground into powder and applied to the local area.

Dosage and Administration: The dosage is 0.3–1 g. Only the pill form is available. No decoction is made from it. Proper amount of the drug can be used in external treatment.

Appendix: Concha Margaritifera (珍珠母 *Zhenzhumu*)

This drug consists of the shell of Hyriopsis cumingii (Lea) or Pteria martensisi Dunker, etc. It is sweet and salty in taste and cold in nature. It can be used to calm the liver, suppress *Yang* hyperactivity, clear away heat in the liver and improve vision. Its main indications are headache, dizziness tinnitus, nebula, epilepsy induced by terror, etc. The dosage is 15–30 g.

Red Ochre (代赭石 *Daizheshi*)
Ochra Haematitum

This drug consists of the red coloured iron ore Hematite. The crude drug is broken into pieces for use, or calcined, treated with vinegar and then broken into pieces for medication.

Nomenclature Used in Prescriptions: *Shengzheshi, Duanzheshi*

Properties and Channel Distribution: This drug is bitter and

sweet in taste and cold in nature, and is distributed to the Liver and Heart Channels.

Action and Indications:

1. Calming the liver and purging away heat

In treating headache and dizziness due to hyperactivity of the liver–*Yang*, the drug can be used in combination with Concha Haliotidis, Spica Prunellae, Radix Achyranthis Bidentatae, etc.

2. Relieving vomiting and sending down adverse flow of *Qi*

In treating vomiting, belching, fullness sensation in the chest and abdomen, salivation, etc. due to adverse ascending of *Qi*, the drug is often used in combination with Flos Inulae, Rhizoma Pinelliae, etc. In treating vomiting and hiccup due to ascending of the liver–fire, the drug can be used in combination with Indigo Naturalis, Radix Gentianae, Fructus Evodiac, etc.

3. Cooling blood to arrest bleeding

In treating hematemesis and epistaxis due to blood–heat, the drug can be used in combination with Radix Paeoniae Alba, Caulis Bambusac in Tacniam, Fructus Arctii, etc. In treating metrorrhagia and metrostaxis, the calcined drug is ground into powder and 10 g of the powder is taken as a dose, 3 times a day. The powder can also be applied to the local area to treat bleeding due to trauma.

Dosage and Administration

Usually, 10–30 g of the drug is used in decoction. The crude drug is usually used to calm the liver, relieve vomiting and cool blood and the calcined drug, to astringe blood to arrest bleeding.

Gastrodia Tuber (天麻 *Tianma*)
Rhizoma Gastrodiae

This drug consists of the tuber of the perennial parasitic herbage Gastrodia elata Bl. (family Orchidaceae). The skin of the tuber is removed and the tuber is soaked thoroughly in hot water, cut into slices and dried in the sun for medication.

Nomenclature Used in Prescriptions: *Tianma, Mingtianma, Tianmapian*

Properties and Channel Distribution: This drug is sweet in taste and neutral in nature and is distributed to the liver Channel.

Action and Indications:

1. Calming the wind to relieve convulsion

In treating convulsion due to tetanus, the drug is often used in combination with Rhizoma Arisaematis, Radix Ledebouriellae, etc. In treating dizziness due to internal accumulation of phlegm-dampness, the drug is often used in combination with Rhizoma Pinelliae, Rhizoma Atractylodis Macrocephalae, etc. In treating migraine, aching all over the head and blurred vision, equal amount of the drug and Rhizoma Ligustici Chuanxiong are made into water-paste pills and 3 g of the pills are taken as a dose, 3 times a day.

2. Removing obstruction in the channels to relieve pain

In treating joint pain and numbness due to wind, cold and dampness, the drug can be used in combination with Radix Achyranthis Bidentatae, Scorpio, etc. In treating flaccidity and numbness of the limbs due to deficiency of the liver and kidney, the drug can be used in combination with Cortex Eucommiae, Radix Achyranthis Bidentatae, Radix Rehmanniae, Radix

Angelicae Sinensis, etc.

Dosage and Administration: Usually, 3–6 g of the drug is used in decoction.

Hooked Uncaria (钩藤 *Gouteng*)
Ramulus Uncariae cum Uncis

This drug consists of the hooked stem of evergreen liana Uncaria rhynchophylla (Mig.) Jacks. (family Rubiaceae). The crude drug is dried in the sun for medication.

Nomenclature Used in Prescriptions: *Gouteng, Shuangouteng, Nengouteng*

Properties and Channel Distribution: This drug is sweet in taste and slightly cold in nature, and is distributed to the Liver and Heart Channels.

Action and Indications:

1. Calming the wind to relieve convulsion

In treating epilepsy and convulsion due to formation of wind caused by liver–heat, tetanus, etc., the drug is often used in combination with Rhizoma Gastrodiae, Flos Chrysanthemi, Periostracum Cicadae, Cornu Saigae Tataricae, etc.

2. Calming the liver and clearing away heat

In treating headache due to liver–heat, headache due to wind-heat, dizziness, etc., the drug is often used in combination with Folium Mori, Flos Chrysanthemi, Herba Menthae, etc.

Besides, the drug also has satisfactory effect of lowering blood pressure, and can be used effectively to treat hypertension due to hyperactivity of the liver–heat.

Dosage and Administration: Usually, 10–15 g of the drug is used in decoction.

Notes: This drug should not be decocted for long since when decocted for over 20 minutes the drug's effect of lowering blood pressure is reduced.

Tribulus Fruit (白蒺藜 *Baijili*)
Fructus Tribuli

This drug consists of the fruit of the annual or perennial herbage Tribulus terrestris L. (family Zygophyllaceae). The fruit is dried in the sun, parched with salt water till it turns yellow and then the thorn is removed for medication.

Nomenclature Used in Prescriptions: *Baijili, Cijili*

Properties and Channel Distribution: This drug is bitter and pungent in taste and neutral in nature, and is distributed to the Liver and Lung Channels.

Action and Indications:

1. Dispelling wind and soothing the liver

In treating dizziness and headache due to wind, the drug can be used in combination with drugs for dispersing wind-heat such as Folium Mori, Flos Chrysanthemi, Fructus Viticis, Ramulus Uncariae cum Uncis, etc. In treating conjunctival conjestion with delacrimation, the drug can be used in combination with Flos Chrysanthemi, Semen Cassiae, Semen Celosiae, etc. In treating rubella with itching sensation, the drug is always used in combination with Periostracum Cicadae, Herba Schizonepetae, etc. In treating discomfort in the chest and hypochondrium and galactostasis due to depression of the liver-*Qi*, the drug can be used in combination with drugs for soothing the liver such as

Pericarpium Citri Reticulatae Viride, Folium Citri Sinensis, Radix Curcumae, etc.

2. Promoting flow of *Qi* and activating blood circulation

In treating distention and pain in the hypogastrium, the drug can be used in combination with Radix Linderae, Radix Paeoniae Alba, Fructus Meliae Toosendan, Rhizoma Cyperi, etc.

Dosage and Administration: Usually, 6–10 g of the drug is used in decoction.

Batryticated Silkworm (僵蚕 *Jiangcan*) Bombyx Batryticatus

This drug consists of the larva of the silkworm Bombyx mori L. (family Bombycidae), dead and stiffened due to the infection of Beauveria bassiana. The crude drug or the drug parched with wheat bran is used for medication.

Nomenclature Used in Prescriptions: *Jiangcan, Baijiangcan, Zhijiangcan, Zhitianchong*

Properties and Channel Distribution: This drug is salty and pungent in taste and neutral in nature, and is distributed to the Liver and Lung Channels.

Action and Indications:

1. Resolving phlegm and relieving convulsion

In treating acute infantile convulsion, phlegm–dyspnea and spasm, the drug can be used in combination with Scorpio, Arisaema cum Bile, Rhizoma Gastrodiae, etc. In treating fever with headache and cough accompanied by epilepsy and convulsion, the drug can be used in combination with Periostracum Cicadae, Ramulus Uncariae cum Uncis, Flos Chrysanthemi, etc.

2. Dispelling wind and clearing away heat

In treating headache due to wind–heat, lachrymation, sore throat due to wind–heat, etc., the drug can be used in combination with Folium Mori, Herba Schizonepetae, Herba Menthae, Herba Equiseti Hiemalis, etc. In treating cutaneous pruritus, the drug can be used alone (ground into powder) but generally it is used with other drugs.

3. Subduing swelling and resolving mass

In treating scrofula and subcutaneous nodules, the drug can be used alone (in powder form). In treating acute mastitis at the initial stage, the drug powder is mixed with vinegar and applied to the local area.

Dosage and Administration: Usually, 3–10 g of the drug is used in decoction. The prepared drug is generally used but the crude drug is used to disperse wind–heat.

Scorpion (全蝎 *Quanxie*)
Scorpio

This drug consists of the whole body of Buthus martensi Karsch (family Buthidae). The whole body or the distal part of the body is used for medication.

Nomenclature Used in Prescriptions: *Quanxie, Xiewei, Quanchong*

Properties and Channel Distribution: This drug is sweet and pungent in taste and neutral in nature, and is distributed to the Liver Channel.

Action and Indications:

1. Calming the wind to relieve convulsion

This drug has satisfactory effect of calming the wind to relieve convulsion. In treating spasm and convulsion caused by damp–warm syndrome, tetanus, epilepsy, acute infantile convulsion, etc., and excess syndrome of opisthotonus, equal amount of the drug, Bombyx Batryticatus and Scolopendra can be ground into powder and 1–1.5 g of the powder is to be taken as a dose, once or twice a day. In treating deviation of mouth and eye due to wind–stroke, the drug is often used in combination with Bombyx Batryticatus, Rhizoma Typhonii, etc.

2. Removing Stagmation of *Qi* of channels and collaterals to relieve pain

In treating arthralgia due to wind–dampness, 3 g of the drug and 0.06 g of Moschus can be ground into powder and 1.5 g of the powder is taken with warm wine as a dose, or 1.5 g of the powder of Scorpio is taken with warm wine at a time. In treating chronic arthritis, the drug can be used in combination with Radix Aconiti Praeparata, Resina Boswelliae Carterii, Squama Manitis, etc.

3. Removing toxin and resolving mass

In treating sores, ulceration, Pyogenic infection, scrofula, tuberculosis, mumps, etc., the drug can be used in combination with Fructus Gardeniae, Radix Angelicae Dahuricae, etc. Mumps can also be treated by eating two fried scorpions.

Dosage and Administration: Usually, 1.5–5 g of the whole scorpion or 3–8 pieces of the distal part of the scorpion are used in decoction. When it is ground into powder, the dosage is to be reduced.

Notes: Overdosage is forbidden because this drug has toxic effect. The drug should be used with care by those with wind syndrome due to deficiency of the blood.

Centipede (蜈蚣 *Wugong*)
Scolopendra

This drug consists of the whole body of Scolopendra subspinipes mutilans L. Koch. (family Scolopendridae). The whole body is dried in the sun or by the fire and then cut into pieces or ground into powder for medication.

Nomenclature Used in Prescriptions: *Wugong, Jintouwugong*

Properties and Channel Distribution: This drug is pungent in taste and warm in nature with toxic effect, and is distributed to the Liver Channel.

Action and Indications:

1. Calming the wind to relieve convulsion

In treating contracture of the limbs, lockjaw and opisthotonus due to liver–wind, or infantile convulsion, epilepsy, tetanus, facial paralysis, etc., the drug is often used in combination with drugs for calming the wind such as Bombyx Batryticatus, Scorpio, etc.

2. Removing toxin and resolving mass

In treating sores, ulceration, pyogenic infection, scrofula, tuberculosis, etc., the drug can be used in combination with other drugs for removing toxin.

3. Removing Stagnation of *Qi* of channels and collaterals to relieve pain

In treating intractable spasm and pain of the head, arthralgia due to wind–dampness, etc., the drug is always used in combination with Scorpio, or with Bombyx Batryticatus, Rhizoma

Gastrodiae, Rhizoma Ligustici Chuanxiong, etc., usually with good therapeutic effect.

Dosage and Administration: Usually, 2–5 g of the drug or 1–3 centipedes are used in decoction. When the drug powder is taken orally, 0.6–1 g is used. Proper amount of the drug is used in external treatment.

Notes: The drug in contraindicated for pregnant women or those with convulsion due to deficiency of blood.

Earthworm (地龙 *Dilong*)
Lumbricus

This drug consists of the dried whole body of annelid Pheretima asiatica Michalsen and Allolobophora caliginosa trapezoides (Duges) (family Megascolecidae). The crude or baked drug is used.

Nomenclature Used in Prescriptions: *Dilong, Gandilong, Dilongrou, Xiandilong*

Properties and Channel Distribution: This drug is salty in taste and cold in nature, and is distributed to the Liver, Kidney and Lung Channels.

Action and Indications:

1. Clearing away heat to relieve convulsion

In treating vexation due to high fever, convulsion and spasm, the drug can be used in combination with Ramulus Uncariae cum Uncis, Scorpio, Gypsum Fibrosum, etc., or 10 g of the drug and 3 g of Cinnabaris are ground into powder and half of the powder is to be taken at a time. In treating encephalitis B with persistent high fever and coma, the six live earthworms and 18 g of

Melanterite are pounded and applied to the patient's fontanel (with the hair shaved), and the same treatment can be given 5 hours later if fever still persists.

2. Removing obstruction in the collaterals and treating arthralgia

In treating arthralgia with redness, swelling and burning pain due to wind, dampness and heat, the drug is often used in combination with Caulis Trachelospermi, Caulis Lonicerae, Cortex Erythrinae, etc. In treating arthralgia due to wind-cold, the drug can be used in combination with Radix Aconiti, Radix Aconiti Lateralis Praeparata, Ramulus Cinnamomi, etc. In treating limb pain due to obstruction of channels by damp-phlegm and blood stasis, or hemiplegia, the drug can be used in combination with Radix Aconiti and Rhizoma Arisaematis, or Semen Persicae, Flos Carthami, Radix Angelicae Sinensis, etc.

3. Clearing away heat in the lung to relieve asthma

In treating cough and asthma due to burning of the lung by fire and whooping cough in children, the decoction of 100 earthworms is concentrated into soft extract with sugar and one spoonful of the extract is to be taken at a time with water, or 3 g of the drug powder is to be taken as a dose, twice a day.

4. Inducing diuresis to treat stranguria

In treating anuresis due to accumulation of heat and painful stranguria from urolithiasis, the drug powder can be taken, or the drug can be used in combination with other drugs for inducing diuresis.

Dosage and Administration: Usually, 6-10 g of the drug is used in decoction. When live earthworm is used, the dosage is 10-20 g. When the drug is used in pill or powder form, the dosage is 1–3 g. Proper amount of the drug is used in external treatment.

Dogbane Leaf (罗布麻 *Luobuma*) Folium Apocyni Veneti

This drug consists of the leaf of the perennial herbage Apocynum venetum L. (family Apocynaceae). The drug is dried and cut into pieces for medication.

Nomenclature Used in Prescriptions: *Luobuma*

Properties and Channel Distribution: This drug is slightly bitter in taste and cool in nature, and is distributed to the Liver Channel.

Action and Indications:

1. Calming the liver and tranquilizing the mind

It has been proved by experiments that this drug has the effect of lowering blood pressure. In treating hypertension due to hyperactivity of liver–*Yang* or Liver–heat manifested by headache, dizziness, vexation, insomnia, etc., the drug can be put into boiling water and the water is drunk instead of tea, or the drug can be used in combination with Spica Prunellae, Ramulus Uncariae cum Uncis, Flos Chrysanthemi Indici, etc.

2. Clearing away heat and inducing diuresis

In treating dysuria, edema, etc. due to heat, the drug can be used in combination with drugs for inducing diuresis such as Semen Plantaginis, Rhizoma Alismatis, etc.

Dosage and Administration: The dosage is 6–15 g, to be decocted or put into boiling water.

16 Drugs for Inducing Resuscitation

Drugs with the main functions of restoring consciousness, inducing resuscitation and refreshing the mind are called drugs for inducing resuscitation.

This kind of drugs are mostly of aromatic odour and are characterized by ever moving. They have the functions of restoring consciousness, inducing resuscitation and refreshing the mind and are used mainly to treat sudden syncope seen in wind–stroke, syncope due to disorder of *Qi*, phlegm syncope, epilepsy, etc., or excess syndrome of loss of consciousness due to febrile diseases. Some of the drugs may be used to remove nasal obstruction.

Coma may be seen not only in excess syndrome of stroke but also in prostration syndrome. The former is manifested by lockjaw, clenching of the fist, lustrous complexion and forceful pulse while the latter, on the contrary, is manifested by opening of the mouth, relaxing of the hands, dim complexion, forceless pulse, etc. The former is the internal obstruction due to excess of pathogenic factors and therefore should be treated with aromatic drugs for inducing resuscitation to remove the obstruction; the latter, on the other hand, is the external collapse due to deficiency of *Qi* and therefore should be treated by invigorating the primordial *Qi*, recuperating depleted *Yang* and rescuing the patient from collapse, but should not be treated with aromatic drugs to induce resuscitation so as to avoid exhausting the primordial *Qi* and aggravating the case. In addition, the excess syndrome of stroke may be due to cold or heat. In the former case, the disease is manifested by blueish complexion, cold body, white tongue coating and slow pulse; in the latter case, the disease is manifested by flushed face, fever, yellow tongue coating and rapid pulse. In the former case, the disease should be treated by combining this kind of drugs with drugs for dispelling cold, while in the latter case, with drugs for clearing away heat.

This kind of drugs is only to be used temporarily and should not be used over a long time. Otherwise, the primordial *Qi* may be consumed. Only very few drugs of this kind are used in decoction, and others are only used in pill or powder form.

Cow–bezoare (牛黄 *Niuhuang*)
Calculus Bovis

This drug consists of the stone in the gall bladder, biliary duct or hepatic duct of Bos taurus domesticus Gmelin, or Bubalus bubalis L. (family Bovidae). The stone is ground into powder for use.

Nomenclature Used in Prescriptions: *Nuhuang,Xihuang*

Properties and Channel Distribution: This drug is bitter in taste and cool in nature, and is distributed to the Heart and Liver Channels.

Action and Indications:

1. Eliminating phlegm to induce resuscitation

In treating coma, delirium and restlessness seen in febrile disease, acute infantile convulsion, and unconsciousness and accumulation of phlegm-heat seen in wind-stroke, the drug is often used in combination with Cinnabaris, Fructus Gardeniae, Rhizoma Coptidis, etc.

2. Calming the wind to relieve convulsion

In treating convulsion and spasm due to hyperactivity of heat, the drug is often used in combination with Cinnabaris, Moschus, the tip of Scorpio, etc.

3. Clearing away heat and removing toxin

This drug is a main drug for antisepsis and removing toxin. In treating breast carcinoma, scrofula, subcutaneous noduels, pulmonary abscess, acute appendicitis, etc., the drug can be used in combination with Moschus, Resina Boswelliae Carterii, Resina Commiphorae Myrrhae, etc. In treating sore throat, diphtheria, aphthous stomatitis, etc. due to flaring-up of fire, the drug is often used in combination with Moschus, Borneolum Syntheticum, Cinnabaris, etc. In treating carbuncle, ulceration, Pyogenic infection, and infantile sores and boils due to fetal toxicosis, the drug is often used in combination with Flos Lonicerae, Radix Glycyrrhizae and Rhizoma Paridis

Dosage and Administration: The dosage is usually 0.15-0.3 g. The drug is used in pill or powder form and should not be decocted. Proper amount of the drug can be used in external treatment.

Musk (麝香 *Shexiang*)
Moschus

This drug consists of the dried secretion obtained from the musk gland of the musk deer Moschus Moschiferus L. (family

Cervidae). The drug is ground into powder for medication.

Nomenclature Used in Prescriptions: *Shexiang, Cunxiang, Yuancun, Danmenzi*

Properties and Channel Distribution: This drug is pungent in taste and warm in nature, and is distributed to the twelve regular channels.

Action and Indications:

1. Inducing resuscitation

In treating coma and convulsion seen in febrile diseases and excess syndromes of stroke such as phlegm–syncope, syncope due to disorder of *Qi* and sudden syncope, the drug is often used in combination with Cornu Rhinoceri, Borneolum Syntheticum, Calculus Bovis, Cinnabaris, etc.

2. Activating blood circulation and subduing swelling

In treating traumatic injury with stasis of blood and pain all over the body, the drug is often used in combination with Resina Draconis, Resina Boswelliae Carterii, Catechu, etc. In treating sore throat, the drug is often used in combination with Calculus Bovis, Realgar, Borneolum Syntheticum, etc. In treating carbuncle, phlegmon and pyogenic infection, the drug is often used in combination with drugs for removing toxin.

3. Removing obstruction from channels and collaterals

In treating mass in the abdomen and amenorrhea, the drug can be used in combination with Rhizoma Sparganii, Rhizoma Zedoariae and Cortex Cinnamomi.

4. Inducing labour

In treating retention of dead fetus and retention of placenta, 0.15 g of the drug and 1.5 g of Cortex Cinnamomi are ground into powder and half of the powder is to be taken at a time.

Dosage and Administration: The dosage is 0.1–0.15 g. The drug is used in pill or powder form and should not be decocted. Proper amount of the drug can be used in external treatment.

Notes: The drug is contraindicated for pregnant women.

Borneol (冰片 *Bingpian*)
Borneolum Syntheticum

This drug consists of the processed crystalline organic compound from the resin of the evergreen arbor Dryobalanops aromatica Gaertn. f. (family Dipterocarpaceae). The drug may also be produced chemically with turpentine oil as the main raw material and is called jipian in Chinese. Another kind of the drug is produced from Blumea balsamifera DC. (family Compositae). The drug is ground into powder for medication.

Nomenclature Used in Prescriptions: *Bingpian, Meipian*

Properties and Channel Distribution: This drug is pungent and bitter in taste and slightly cold in nature, and is distributed to the Heart and Liver Channels.

Action and Indications:

1. Inducing resuscitation

In treating coma with feeble breathing seen in any kind of fulminating disease of grievous bodily injury, the drug can be used in combination with Cinnabaris, Realgar, Natrii Sulfas, etc. In treating dizziness, vomiting, diarrhea and unconsciousness due to pathogenic summer–heat, cholera morbus and eruptive disease, the drug is often used in combination with Calculus Bovis, Realgar, Natrii Sulfas, etc.

2. Dispersing heat to relieve pain and subduing swelling

In treating sore throat and aphthous stomatitis, the drug is often used in combination with Borax, etc. In treating furunculosis, the drug is often used in combination with Cinnabaris, Calomelas, Semen Ricini, etc. In treating acute conjunctivitis, the drug is often used in combination with Calamina, Rhizoma Coptidis, etc.

Besides, the drug can also be used in combination with Resina Liquidambaris Orientalis to treat angina pectoris seen in coronary heart disease, with certain effect.

Dosage and Administration: The dosage is 0.15–0.3 g. The drug is used in pill or powder form and should not be decocted. Proper amount of the drug can be used in external treatment.

Notes: This drug should be used with care by pregnant women.

Storax (苏合香 *Suhexiang*)
Resina Liquidambaris Orientalis

This drug consists of the yellow and thick balsam obtained from the deciduous arbor Liguidambar orientalis Mill. (family Hamamelidaceae). The balsam is made into pills for medication.

Nomenclature Used in Prescriptions: *Suhexiang*

Properties and Channel Distribution: This drug is pungent in taste and warm in nature, and is distributed to the Heart and Spleen Channels.

Action and Indications:

Inducing resuscitation and eliminating phlegm

In treating sudden syncope, lockjaw and coma due to wind–stroke or syncope due to disorder of *Qi*, sudden syncope due to accumulation of phlegm and obstruction of *Qi*, distention and pain in the chest and abdomen, epidemic disease, malignant malaria, etc., the drug can be used in combination with Benzoinum, Moschus, Borneolum, Syntheticum, Flos Syzygii Aromatici, Lignum Santali, etc.

In recent years, the drug has been used in combination with Lignum Santali, Borneolum Syntheticum, Resina Boswelliae Carterii, etc. to treat angina pectoris from coronary heart disease with good effect of relieving pain. The pill made from this drug and Borneolum Syntheticum has similar effect.

Dosage and Administration: The dosage is 0.3–1 g. The drug is often used in pill form and shouid not be decocted.

Grassleaved Sweetflag Rhizome (菖蒲 *Changpu*) Rhizoma Acori Graminei

This drug consists of the rhizome of the perennial herbage Acorus gramineus Soland. (family Araceae) and the perennial herbage Anemone altaica Fisch. (family Ranunculaceae). The drug is dried and cut into sections for medication.

Nomenclature Used in Prescriptions: *Shichangpu, Jiujiechangpu*

Properties and Channel Distribution: This drug is pungent and bitter in taste and warm in nature, and is distributed to the Heart, Spleen and Stomach Channels.

Action and Indications:

1. Inducing resusciation and eliminating phlegm

In treating coma and delirium due to mental confusion caused by turbid phlegm, the drug can be used in combination with Radix Curcumae, Rhizoma Pinelliae, Caulis Bambusae in

Taeniam, Succus Bambusae, Succus Zingiberis, etc.

2. Refreshing the mind and invigorating the brain

In treating insomnia due to fright, epilepsy, poor memory, etc., the drug is often used in combination with Radix Polygalae, Dens Draconis, Cinnabaris, Poria, etc.

3. Removing dampness to induce appetite and digestion

In treating poor appetite due to profuse sputum, the drug can be used in combination with Radix Curcumae, Rhizoma Pinelliae, Herba Eupatorii, etc. In treating dysentery with no desire to eat, the drug can be used in combination with Rhizoma Coptidis; Semen Caesalpiniae, poria, etc.

Besides, the drug may be used alone or in combination with other drugs to treat deafness and tinnitus.

Dosage and Administration: Usually, 3–6 g of the drug is used in decoction.

17 Tonics

Drugs which can be used to invigorate the body's *Qi*, blood, *Yin* and *Yang* so as to treat various diseases of deficiency type, are called tonics.

Diseases of deficiency type are divided into the following: deficiency of *Qi*, deficiency of *Yang*, deficiency of blood and deficiency of *Yin*, Tonics are divided, according to the property and indication, into tonics for invigorating, *Qi*, tonics for reinforcing yang, tonics for nourishing blood and tonics for repleniching *Yin*. *Qi*, blood, *Yin* and *yang* are mutually interdependent and interacting. Deficiency of *Yang* is often accompanied by deficiency of *Qi*, deficiency of *Qi* is likely to lead to deficiency of *Yang*, and deficiency of *Qi* and deficiency of *Yang* are the manifestation of deficiency of the body's physiological function. Deficiency of *Yin* is always accompanied by deficiency of blood, deficiency of blood often results in deficiency of *Yin*, and deficiency of blood and deficiency of *Yin* are the manifestation of exhaustion of the body fluid. Therefore, the methods of invigorating *Qi*, reinforcing *Yang*, nourishing blood and replenishing *Yin* should be used according to the disease conditions. In treating deficiency of both *Qi* and blood, or both *Yin* and *Yang*, the four kinds of tonics may be used in combination and the method of invigorating both *Qi* and blood or of replenishing both *Yin* and *Yang* can be used.

Tonics should not be used for those diseases where the pathogenic factors of excess type are not eliminated so as to avoid retaining the pathogenic factors. If the pathogenic factors are not eliminated but the anti–pathogenic factors are weak, tonics can be used with drugs for eliminating pathogenic factors so as to reinforce the body's resistance, i.e. to reinforce the anti–pathogenic factors so as to eliminate pathogenic ones.

17.1 Tonics for Invigorating *Qi*

This kind of tonics have strengthening effect and can be used to improve the body's physiological function and physical activity. They are mainly used to treat diseases due to deficiency of *Qi*, especially due to deficiency of *Qi* in the spleen and lung. The spleen provides the material basis of the acquired constitution and is the source of production and transformation. Deficiency of the *Qi* of the spleen, therefore, may lead to listlessness, poor appetite, distention in the chest and abdomen and diarrhea. The spleen dorminates the *Qi* in the body, and deficiency of the spleen–*Qi* will give rise to shortness of breath, low voice, and spontaneous sweating. The above manifestations can all be treated with this kind of drugs.

In using tonics for invigorating *Qi*, a choice should be made among the various drugs according to different kinds of diseases due to deficiency of *Qi*. If deficiency of *Qi* is accompanied by deficiency of *Yin* or *Yang*, tonics for replenishing *Yin* or reinforcing *yang* should also be used. Since there is a close relation between *Qi* and blood and affluent *Qi* may lead to formation of blood, tonics for invigorating *Qi* are often used to treat diseases due to deficiency of blood.

This kind of drugs are mostly sweet in taste and taking the drug for a long time may give rise to distention of the chest and poor appetite. Therefore, drugs for regulating flow of *Qi* such as Radix Aucklandiae, Fructus Aurantii, etc. can be added when necessary.

Ginseng (人参 *Renshen*)
Radix Ginseng

This drug consists of the root of the perennial herbage Panax ginseng C. A. Meg. (family Araliaceae). The wild ginseng is called *Yeshanshen* in Chinese and the cultivated ginseng, *Yuanshen* or *Yangshen*. This drug may have different forms and names owing to different growing areas and methods of preparation. The drug is cut into slices or ground into powder for medication.

Nomenclature Used in Prescriptions: *Renshen, Jilinshen, Liaodongshen, Hongshen, Dalishen, Baishen, Biezhishen, Renshenxu*

Properties and Channel Distribution: This drug is sweet and slightly bitter in taste and slightly warm in nature, and is distributed to the Spleen, Lung and Heart Channels.

Action and Indications:

1. Invigorating *Qi* to rescue the patient from collapse

In treating extreme deficiency manifested by shortness of breath, listlessness and weak pulse almost imperceptible seen after serious or long–lasting diseases or loss of too much blood, this drug can be used to greatly invigorate the primordial *Qi* and rescue the patient from collapse. The drug may be used alone and decocted into concentrated decoction. If the collapse is accompanied by cold limbs and spontaneous sweating which indicate exhaustion of *Yang*, Radix Aconiti Praeparata can be added.

2. Invigorating the spleen and reenforcing the lung

This drug is the main drug for treating consumptive disease and internal injury. In treating listlessness, myasthenia of limbs, shortness of breath and poor appetite due to deficiency of *Qi* of the spleen and stomach, distention of the epigastrium, diarrhea, or deficiency of *Qi* and weak physique due to various causes, the drug is often used in combination with Rhizoma Atractylodis Macrocephalae, Radix Glycyrrhizae, etc. In treating deficiency of both *Qi* and blood, the drug can be used in combination with Rhizoma Rehmanniae Praeparatae, Radix Angelicae Sinensis, etc. In treating loose stool and diarrhea due to deficiency of the spleen and dampness, the drug can be used in combination with drugs for invigorating the spleen and removing dampness such as Rhizoma Dioscoreae, Semen Dolichoris, Semen Nelumbinis, etc. In treating long–lasting diarrhea and prolapse of rectum due to sinking of *Qi* of the middle warmer, the drug can be used in combination with drugs for invigorating *Qi* and elevating *Yang* such as Radix Astragali seu Hedysari, Rhizoma Cimicifugae, Radix Bupleuri, etc. In treating asthma due to deficiency of the lung and kidney, the drug is often used in combination with Juglandis Regiae, Fructus Schisandrae, Gecko, etc.

3. Promoting production of body fluid to quench thirst

In treating exhaustion of *Qi* and body fluid by heat in febrile diseases, shortness of breath, thirst, or heart failure with weak and thready pulse due to exhaustion of body fluid, the drug is often used in combination with Radix Ophiopogonis and Fructus Schisandrae. In recent years, the drug is made into pulseactivating injection used in the first aid of infectious–toxic shock, with certain effect. In treating diabetes with thirst and polyuria, the drug is often used in combination with Radix Rehmanniae Praeparata, Radix Trichosanthis, etc.

4. Calming the mind and improving mental activity

In treating palpitation, poor memory, listlessness, etc. due to deficiency of the heart and spleen, the drug is often used in combination with Radix Astragali seu Hedysari, Rhizoma Atractylodis Maerocephalae, Arillus Longan, Semen Ziziphi Spinosae, etc. In treating palpitation, insomnia, listlessness, etc. due to break–down of the normal physiological corrdination between the heart and kidney, the drug can be used in combination with Poria, Radix Polygalae, Semen Ziziphi Spinosae, Os Draconis, Concha Ostreae, etc. In treating spontaneous sweating, the drug is often used in combination with Fructus Schisandrae, Radix Paeoniae Alba, Fructus Tritici Levis, etc.

In addition, the drug can be used in combination with drugs for enriching blood or drugs for warming and invigorating kidney–*Yang* to treat deficiency of blood and impotence. Small dosage of the drug can also be used in combination with drugs for relieving exterior syndromes or drugs for purgation to treat those patients with weak physique and exogenous invasion or with interior excess and weak physique who can hardly endure the method of purgation and elimination of pathogens, to build up the body' s resistance and reinforce the anti–pathogenic factors so as to eliminate pathogenic ones.

Dosage and Administration: The usual dosage is 3–10 g and the large dosage is 15–30 g. The drug should be decocted alone with gentle fire and then the decoction can be mixed with decoction of other drugs. The drug can also be ground into powder and 1–2 g of the powder is taken at a time, 2–3 times a day.

When used as a tonic, small dosage is used; when used in first aid, large dosage is used. The ginseng growing in Jilin Province is slow in effect and therefore large dosage can be used; the ginseng growing in Korea is powerful in effect and therefore small dosage should be used. When the drug is taken by those with weak physique, the drug can be taken once in 5–7 days.

Notes: The drug is contraindicated for those with excess syndromes or febrile diseases with strong body resistance. The drug is antagonized by Rhizoma et Radix Veratri and Fructus Gleditsiae Sinenses. Tea and turnip should be avoided when the drug is taken so as not to reduce the drug effect.

Pilose Asiabell Root (党参 *Dangshen*)
Radix Codonopsis Pilosulae

This drug consists of the root of the perennial herbage Codonopsis pilosula (Franch.) Nannf. (family Campanulaceae). The wild drug is called yetaishen in Chinese while the cultivated drug, ludangshen. The crude drug is cut into slices for medication.

Nomenclature Used in Prescriptions: *Dangshen, Taishen, Ludangshen, Yetaishen, Fangdang*

Properties and Channel Distribution: This drug is sweet in taste and neutral in nature, and is distributed to the Spleen and Lung Channels.

Action and Indications:

1. Invigorating *Qi* in the middle warmer

This drug is effective in invigorating the spleen, nourishing the stomach and promoting flow of *Qi* in the middle warmer, and is often used clinically. In treating poor appetite and loose stool due to deficiency of the spleen and stomach, cough due to deficiency of the lung, shortness of breath, listlessness, and deficiency of *Qi* and weak physique due to various causes, the drug is often used in combination with Rhizoma Atractylodis Macrocephalae, Poria and Radix Glycyrrhizae Praeparata. This drug is similar in the effect of invigorating *Qi* to Radix Ginseng and is often used instead of the latter in the prescription for invigorating *Qi* and spleen. The drug' s effect of invigorating *Qi*, however, is not so powerful as that of Radix Ginseng, and therefore can not be used instead of the latter in the serious cases of collapse.

2. Nourishing blood and promoting production of body fluid

In treating dizziness due to deficiency of blood, sallow complexion or edema, the drug can be used in combination with Rhizoma Rehmanniae Praeparatae, Radix Angelicae Sinensis, Radix Paeoniae Alba, Caulis Spatholobi, etc. In treating shortness of breath and thirst due to consumption of *Qi* and body fluid by heat, the drug is often used in combination with Radix Ophiopogonis, Fructus Schisandrae, etc.

Besides, the drug can also be used to treat edema from nephritis to reduce the excretion of urinary protein.

Dosage and Administration: The usual dosage is 10–15 g and the large dosage is up to 30 g.

Notes: The drug is contraindicated for those with abdominal distention and excess of pathogens.

Pseudostellaria Root (太子参 *Taizishen*) Radix Pseudostellariae

This drug consists of the tuberous root of the perennial herbage Pseudostellaria heterophyll (Mig) Pax ex pax et Hoffm. (family Caryophyllaceae). The crude drug is used for medication.

Nomenclature Used in Prescriptions: *Haiershen, Taizishen, Tongzishen*

Properties and Channel Distribution: This drug is sweet and slightly bitter in taste and neutral in nature, and is distributed to the Spleen and Lung Channels.

Action and Indications:

Invigorating the spleen, tonifying the lung, invigorating *Qi* and promoting production of body fluid

In treating deficiency of *Qi* manifested by week physique, listlessness, poor appetite, dry mouth, dryness in the lung due to deficiency of *Yin*, cough with little sputum, emaciation of children after disease, spontaneous sweating, etc., the drug is often used in combination with other drugs for invigorating *Qi* and promoting production of body fluid to enhance the therapeutic effect. In treating deficiency of the spleen–*Qi* and stomach–*Yin*, the drug can be used in combination with Radix Codonopsis Pilosulae, Rhizoma polygonati Odorati and Rhizoma Dioscoreae. In treating deficiency of *Qi* and *Yin*, spontaneous sweating and thirst, the drug can be used in combination with Fructus Schisandrae and Radix Astragali seu Hedysari. In treating spontaneous sweating in children, the drug can be used in combination with Fructus Tritici Levis. For deficiency of *Yin*, dryness in the lung and cough with little sputum, the drug can be used in combination with Radix Adenophorae Strictae and Radix Ophiopogonis.

The drug has similar action to Radix Ginseng in invigorating *Qi*, promoting production of body fluid and invigorating the spleen and lung, but it is milder in effect than the latter and is considered to be a mild tonic among drugs of invigorating *Qi*.

Dosage and Administration: Usually, 10–30 g of the drug is used in decoction.

Astragalus Root (黄芪 *Huangqi*)
Radix Astragali seu Hedysari

This drug consists of the root of the perennial herbage Astragalus membranaceus (Fisch.) Bunge. and A. mongholicus Bunge. (family Leguminosae). The drug is cut into slices and the crude or honey–fried drug is used for medication.

Nomenclature Used in prescriptions: *Shenghuangqi, Zhihuangqi*

Properties and Channel Distribution: This drug is sweet in taste and warm in nature, and is distributed to the Spleen and Lung Channels.

Action and Indications:

1. Invigorating *Qi* and strengthening *Yang*

In treating deficiency of *Qi* manifested by weak physiques, listlessness, lassitude, poor appetite, etc., the drug is often used in combination with Radix Ginseng to enhance the effect of invigorating *Qi*. If the above condition is accompanied by deficiency of *Yang*, Radix Aconiti Praeparata can be added; if the above condition is accompanied by deficiency of blood, Radix Angelicae Sinensis can be added. In treating fever due to deficiency of blood or collapse due to loss of too much blood, large dosage of the drug can be used in combination with Radix Angelicae Sinensis to invigorate *Qi* and promote production of blood. The drug can also be used to treat deficiency of *Qi*, stasis of blood, numbness of limbs, hemiplegia as a sequela of wind–stroke, weak pulse, etc. In treating blood–arthralgia, the drug is often used in combination with Ramulus Cinnamomi, Radix Paeoniae Alba, etc. In the case of arthralgia of shoulder and arm, Radix Ledebouriellae and Rhizoma Curcumae Longae can be added;. in the case of hemiplegia, large dosage of the drug can be used in combination with Semen Persicae, Flos Carthami, Rhizoma Ligustici Chuanxiong, Lumbricus, etc. In treating sinking of *Qi* in the middle warmer manifested by visceroptosis, hysteroptosis, long–lasting diarrhea with prolapse of rectum, etc., the drug is often used in combination with Radix Ginseng, Rhizoma Cimicifugae, Radix Bupleuri, etc.

2. Consolidating superficial resistance to arrest sweating

In treating spontaneous sweating, night sweating, etc. due to weak physique and exterior deficiency, the drug is often used in combination with Rhizoma Atractylodis Macrocephalae and Radix Ledebouriellae, or with Concha Ostreae, Fructus Tritici Levis, Radix Ephedrae, etc.

3. Promoting pus discharge and tissue regeneration

In treating carbuncle and ulceration due to deficiency of *Qi* and blood, the drug is often used in combination with Radix Angelicae Sinensis, Rhizoma Ligustici Chuanxiong, Squama Manitis, Spina Gleditsiae, etc. In treating smallpox with retarded appearance of eruption due to weak body physique, the drug can be used with drugs for promoting eruption. In treating ulceration with thin pus, the drug is often used in combination with Radix Codonopsis Pilosulae and Cortex Cinnamomi. In treating diabetes complicated by carbuncle and boils, 180 g of the drug and 30 g of crude Radix Glycyrrhizae are ground into powder and 9 g of the powder is to be taken as a dose, 2–3 times a day, or the two drugs can be decocted and taken.

4. Inducing diuresis and relieving edema

In treating edema of the face and limbs, dysuria, palpitation, shortness of breath, etc. due to deficiency of *Yang* of the heart and kidney, the drug is often used in combination with Rhizoma Atractylodis Macrocephalae, Radix Stephaniae Tetrandrae, etc. In treating chronic nephritis manifested by presence of urinary protein and edema of the face and body, large dosage of the drug (15–30 g) can be used in decoction.

Besides, the drug can be used in combination with Rhizoma Dioscoreae, Radix Rehmanniae, Radix Trichosanthis, Fructus Schisandrae, etc. to treat diabetes.

Dosage and Administration: The usual dosage is 10–15 g and the large dosage is 30–60 g. The drug is used in decoction. The honey–fried drug has strong effect of invigorating *Qi*, and the crude drug is usually used to arrest sweating, induce diuresis and promote pus discharge and tissue regeneration.

Notes: Since the drug is warm in nature and fire may be generated by it, it is contraindicated for those with internal heat of excess type, hyperactivity of liver–*Yang*, ascending of *Qi* and fire, stasis of *Qi* due to damp–heat, carbuncle and phlegmon at the initial stage or after diabrosis but with hyperactivity of heat–toxin, or exterior excess and hyperactivity of pathogens.

Bighead Atractylodes Rhizoma (白术 *Baizhu*)
Rhizoma Atractylodis Macrocephalae

This drug consists of the rhizome of the perennial herbage Atractylodes macrocephala Koidz. (family Compositae). The crude drug, the parched drug, the drug parched till it is scorched or the drug parched with earth can be used for medication.

Nomenclature Used in Prescriptions: *Shengbaizhu, Chaobaizhu, Jiaobaizhu, Tubaizhu*

Properties and Channel Distribution: This drug is sweet and bitter in taste and warm in nature, and is distributed to the Spleen and Stomach Channels.

Action and Indications:

1. Invigorating the spleen and strengthening *Qi*

This drug can be used to treat poor appetite, abdominal distention of deficiency type, listlessness, loose stool, etc. due to deficiency of *Qi* of the spleen and stomach and abnormality of transportation and transformation. The drug is the main drug for invigorating the spleen-*Qi* and is often used in combination with Radix Ginseng, poria, Radix Glycyrrhizae Praeparata, etc. In the case of severe cold syndrome of deficiency type, the drug can be used in combination with Radix Codonopsis Pilosulae and Rhizoma Zingiberis.

2. Removing dampness and inducing diuresis

In treating failure of the spleen in transportation and retention of water within the body manifested by edema of the limbs, sallow complexion, poor appetite, loose stool, listlessness, cold limbs, thin and white tongue coating and deep pulse, the drug is often used in combination with drugs for removing dampness and inducing diuresis. In mild cases, the drug can be used in combination with Poria, Rhizoma Alismatis, Ramulus Cinnamomi, etc. to enhance the effect of inducing diuresis. In the case of marked deficiency and cold of the spleen and kidney, the drug is to be used in combination with Radix Aconiti Praeparata, Rhizoma Zingiberis or Rhizoma Zingiberis Recens. In the case of retention of phlegm due to retention of water within the body, which results in distention of the chest and hypochondrium and dizziness, the drug can be used in combination with Poria, Ramulus Cinnamomi and Radix Glycyrrhizae.

3. Consolidating superficial resistance to arrest sweating

In treating spontaneous sweating due to weak superficial resistance and especially poor appetite and spontaneous sweating in children due to weak physique after disease, the drug is indispensable, and can be used in combination with Rhizoma Dioscoreae, Fructus Tritici Levis, Radix Ephedrae, etc. In treating spontaneous sweating due to deficiency of *Yang* and susceptibility to cold, the drug can be used in combination with Radix Astragali seu Hedysari and Radix Ledebouriellae.

In addition, the drug can be used in combination with Radix Scutellariae to treat threatened abortion due to heat–syndrome in pregnancy. The drug can also be used to treat rheumatic arthralgia to dispel wind–dampness and relieve pain.

Dosage and Administration: Usually, 3–10 g of the drug is used in decoction. The parched drug or the drug parched till it is scorched can be used to invigorate the spleen and regulate the stomach. The drug parched with earth is used to invigorate the spleen to arrest diarrhea. The crude drug is used to induce diuresis to relieve edema, consolidate superficial resistance to arrest sweating and treat arthralgia due to wind–dampness.

Notes: This drug is dry in nature and is likely to consume *Yin*. Therefore, it is contraindicated for those with internal heat due to deficiency of *Yin*, deficiency of body fluid and diabetes.

Chinese Yam (山药 *Shanyao*)
Rhizoma Dioscoreae

This drug consists of the rhizome of the perennial trailing herbage Dioscorea opposita Thunb. (family Dioscoreaceae). The drug is cut into slices and dried in the sun. The crude or parched drug is used for medication.

Nomenclature Used in Prescriptions: *Huaishanyao, Shengshanyao, Chaoshanyao*

Properties and Channel Distribution: This drug is sweet in taste and neutral in nature, and is distributed to the Spleen, Lung and Kidney Channels.

Action and Indications:

1. Invigorating the spleen to arrest diarrhea

In treating poor appetite and listlessness due to deficiency of the spleen and stomach, or diarrhea, loose stool, etc. due to deficiency of the spleen the drug is often used in combination with Radix Codonopsis Pilosulae, Rhizoma Atractylodis Macrocephalae, Poria, etc. In treating deficiency of the spleen and stomach of children manifested by indigestion, emaciation, loose stool, etc., the drug can be used in combination with Herba Agastachis, Rhizoma Pinelliae, Fructus Oryzae Germinatus,

Massa Fermentata Medicinalis, etc.

2. Nourishing the lung and replenishing *Yin*

In treating cough and asthma due to deficiency of the lung, cough due to consumptive disease, etc., the drug can be used in combination with Radix Codonopsis Pilosulae, Bulbus Fritillariae Cirrhosae, etc. The drug alone can also be decocted and the decoction can be drunk instead of tea.

3. Tonifying the kidney to control nocturnal emission

In treating nocturnal emission, abnormal leukorrhea or frequent micturition, etc. due to deficiency of the kidney, the drug can be used in combination with Semen Nelumbinis, Semen Euryales, Rhizoma Atractylodis Macrocephalae, etc. In treating deficiency and consumption of the kidney−*Yin*, the drug is often used in combination with Radix Rehmanniae Praeparata, Fructus Corni, etc.

4. Nourishing *Yin* and promoting production of body fluid

The drug can be used to treat diabetes, exhaustion of body fluid due to deficiency of *Yin*, dysphoria with smothery sensation and thirst. In treating mild diabetes, 150 g of the drug can be decocted daily and the decoction can be drunk over a long time instead of tea, or the drug can be used in combination with Radix Astragali seu Hedysari, Radix Puerariae, Radix Trichosanthis, Rhizoma Anemarrhenae, etc. In treating thirst due to exhaustion of body fluid, the drug can be used in combination with Radix Ophiopogonis, Rhizoma Polygonati Odorati, etc.

Dosage and Administration: The usual dosage is 10−30 g and the large dosage is 60−120 g. The drug is usually decocted. When parched and ground into powder, 6−10 g of the drug is used as a dose. The crude drug is used to nourish *Yin* and the parched drug is used to invigorate the spleen to arrest diarrhea or to be made into pills or powder.

Notes: The drug is contraindicated for those with deficiency of the spleen with hyperactivity of dampness and stuffy chest and fullness of abdomen.

Hyacinth Bean (扁豆 *Biandou*)
Semen Dolichoris

This drug consists of the seed of the annial trailing herbage Dolichos lablab L. (family Leguminosae). The crude or parched drug is pounded into pieces for medication.

Nomenclature Used in Prescriptions: *Baibiandou, Shengbiandou, Chaobiandou*

Properties and Channel Distribution: This drug is sweet in taste and slightly warm in nature, and is distributed to the Spleen and Stomach Channels.

Action and Indications:

1. Invigorating the spleen to arrest diarrhea

In treating diarrhea or abnormal leukorrhea due to deficiency of the spleen, the drug is often used in combination with drugs for invigorating the spleen such as Rhizoma Atractylodis Macrocephalae, Rhizoma Dioscoreae, etc. The drug can also be parched and ground into powder to treat abnormal leukorrhea with reddish discharge, 6 g of the powder being used as a dose.

2. Removing summer–heat and resolving dampness

In treating vomiting, diarrhea and abdominal pain caused by summer–heat and dampness, equal amount of the drug and Herba Agastachis can be ground into powder and 6 g of the powder is to be taken with water as a dose. In preventing and treating summer–heat diseases, the drug can be used in combination with Herba Agastachis, Cortex Magnoliae Officinalis and Radix Glycyrrhizae.

Dosage and Administration: Usually, 10–15 g of the drug is used in decoction. The crude drug is used to remove summer–heat, resolve dampness and remove toxin and the parched drug is used to invigorate the spleen and regulate the stomach.

Appendix:

1. Testa Dolichoris (扁豆衣 *Biandouyi*).

This drug consists of the skin of the dried seed of Dolichos lablab. Its actions are the same as but milder than those of Semen Dolichoris. It is often used to treat vomiting and diarrhea due to summer–heat and dampness. The dosage is 6–10 g.

2. Flos Dolichoris (扁豆花 *Biandouhua*)

This drug consists of the flower of Dolichos lablab. It can be used to remove summer–heat and resolve dampness, and is often used to treat common cold, vomiting and diarrhea in summer, summer–heat, dysentery, metrorrhagia, metrostaxis, abnormal leukorrhea, etc. The dried flower can be used to treat diarrhea and dysentery with pus and blood.Its dosage is the same as Testa Dolichoris.

Liquorice (甘草 *Gancao*)
Radix Glycyrrhizae

This drug consists of the root and rhizome of the perennial herbage Glycyrrhiza uralensis Fisch. (family Leguminosae). The drug is cut into slices and dried in the sun. The crude or honeyfried drug is used for medication.

Nomenclature Used in Prescriptions: *Gancao, shenggancao, Fengancao, Zhigancao, Gancaoshao*

Properties and Channel Distribution: This drug is sweet in taste and neutral in nature, and is distributed to the Spleen, Stomach, Heart and Lung Channels.

Action and Indications

1. Invigorating the spleen and replenishing *Qi*

In treating the various diseases due to deficiency of *Qi* in the spleen and stomach, the drug is often used in combination with Radix Codonopsis Pilosulae, Rhizoma Atractylodis Macrocephalae, etc. In treating listlessness due to internal injury caused by overstrain and deficiency of primordial *Qi*, the drug is often used in combination with Radix Codonopsis Pilosulae, Radix Astragali seu Hedysari, etc. In treating palpitation, spontaneous sweating, knotted or intermittent pulse, etc., the parched drug is often used in combination with Radix Rehmanniae, Radix Ophiopogonis, Radix Codonopsis Pilosulae, Ramulus Cinnamomi, etc.

2. Dispelling phlegm and relieving cough

The drug can be used to treat cough and asthma. In treating cough due to invasion of wind–cold into the lung, the drug can be used in combination with Herba Ephedrae and Semen Armeniacae Amarum. In treating cough due to wind–heat, the drug can be used in combination with Radix Platycodi, Fructus Arctii, Radix Peucedani, Folium Mori, etc. In treating cough due to wind–cold, the drug can be used in combination with Herba Ephedrae, Folium Perillae, Semen Armeniacae Amarum, etc. In treating cough due to heat–phlegm, the drug can be used in combination with Fructus Trichosanthis, Bulbus Fritillariae

Thunbergii, Radix Scutellariae and Cortex Mori Radicis. In treating cough due to cold—phlegm, the drug can be used in combination with Rhizoma Zingiberis, Herba Asari and Fructus Schisandrae.

3. Relieving spasm and pain

This drug can be used to treat gastralgia, abdominal pain, spasm and pain of muscles, etc. In treating sharp pain of the epigastric region which is not relieved after taking other drugs, 120 g of the drug and 30 g of Rhizoma Atractylodis Macrocephalae can be decocted and the decoction taken frequently. In treating gastric or duodenal ulcer, the drug alone can be made into soft extract or ground into powder with calcined Concha Arcae and taken. In treating pain of the epigastrium or the gastrocnemius muscle of the leg, the drug is often used in combination with Radix Paeoniae Alba.

4. Clearing away heat and removing toxin

This drug can be used to treat skin and external diseases, pyogenic infections, sore throat, and pesticide or food poisoning. In treating pyogenic infections, the drug is often used in combination with Flos Lonicerae, Fructus Forsythiae, etc. In treating sore throat, the drug is often used in combination with Radix Platycodi or Caulis Lonicerae, etc. In treating pesticide or food poisoning, the drug is often taken together with decoction of Semen Phaseoli Radiatus or decocted with Radix Ledebouriellae.

5. Regulating drug properties

This drug is often used in various kinds of prescriptions to reduce or modify drastic properties or toxic effect of the drugs.

Besides, this drug also has the effect of inducing diuresis and the tip of Radix Glycyrrhizae is traditionally used as an adjuvant drug in the treatment of stranguria due to heat and dysuria.

Dosage and Administration: The dosage is 3–6 g. When used as a principal drug, 10–30 g of the drug can be used. The drug is usually decocted. The crude drug has the effect of removing obstruction and the prepared drug has tonifying effect. The former is used to clear away heat and the latter is used for tonifying purpose.

Notes: Edema may be caused if the drug is taken over a long time or large dosage is used. The drug is contraindicated for those with hyperactivity of dampness, stuffy chest, abdominal distention and vomiting. It is antagonized by Radix Euphorbiae Pekinensis, Flos Genkwa and Radix Euphorbiae Kansui.

Chinese–date (大枣 *Dazao*)
Fructus Ziziphi Jujubae

This drug consists of the ripe fruit of the deciduous shrub or arbor Ziziphus jujuba Mill. var. inermis (Bge.) Rehd. (family Rhamnaceae). The crude drug is used after being dried in the sun.

Nomenclature Used in Prescriptions: *Dazao, Hongzao*

Properties and Channel Distribution: This drug is sweet in taste and slightly warm in nature, and is distributed to the Spleen, Stomach, Heart and Liver Channels.

Action and Indications:

1. Tonifying the spleen and regulating the nutrient system

This drug can be used to treat poor appetite and listlessness due to deficiency of the spleen and stomach, diarrhea due to deficiency of the spleen, incoordination between the nutrient and defensive systems, etc. In tonifying the spleen and stomach, the drug is often used in combination with Radix Codonopsis Pilosulae and Rhizoma Atractylodis Macrocephalae and in coordinating the nutrient and defensive systems, the drug is always used in combination with Rhizoma Zingiberis Recens.

2. Nourishing the heart and calming the mind

In treating restlessness of deficiency type and insomnia, the drug is often used in combination with Semen Ziziphi Spinosae, Radix Polygalae, etc. In treating hysteria, the drug is often used in combination with Radix Glycyrrhizae, Fructus Tritici Levis, etc.

3. Modifying drug properties

The drug is used in prescriptions containing drastic or pungent drugs to modify the drug properties so as to avoid damage to the spleen and stomach.

Besides, this drug has been used in recent years to treat thrombocytopenia and allergic purpura and large dosage of the drug is often taken continually, with certain therapeutic effect.

Dosage and Administration: The dosage is usually 3–12 pieces and the large dosage may be 30–60 g. The drug is usually decocted after being cut. The drug is often used in prescriptions to modify drug properties.

Notes: Since the drug can generate dampness, it is contraindicated for those with abdominal distention, painful dental caries, etc. due to accumulation of dampness.

Malt Extract (饴糖 *Yitang*)
Saccharum Granorum

This drug is prepared by mixing cooked polished glutinous rice powder, polished nonglutinous rice powder or flour with malt and then boiling the mixture down with gentle fire. The drug is often used when it is soft.

Nomenclature Used in Prescriptions: *Yitang*

Properties and Channel Distribution: This drug is sweet in taste and slightly warm in nature, and is distributed to the Spleen, Stomach and Lung Channels.

Action and Indications:

1. Tonifying the spleen and relieving pain

In treating deficiency of *Qi* in the middle warmer, damage of the spleen due to overstrain, abdominal pain alleviated by warmth and pressing due to cold of deficiency type, etc., the drug is often used in combination with Ramulus Cinnamomi, Radix Paeoniae, etc. In treating patients with serious deficiency of *Qi*, the drug can be used in combination with Radix Ginseng and Radix Astragali seu Hedysari. In treating patients with deficiency of blood, the drug can be used in combination with Radix Angelicae Sinensis. In treating patients affected seriously by cold, the drug can be used in combination with Rhizoma Zingiberis and Pericarpium Zanthoxyli.

2. Moistening the lung to relieve cough

In treating cough without sputum due to deficiency of the lung, the drug is often used in combination with Mel, Radix Stemonae, etc.

Dosage and Administration: The dosage is 30–60 g. The drug is usually melted in decoction and is not to be decocted.

Notes: This drug is sweet in taste and frequent administration of the drug may lead to distention. Therefore, it is contraindicated for those with abdominal distention and vomiting due to damp–heat or cough due to phlegm–heat.

Honey (蜂蜜 *Fengmi*)
Mel

This drug consists of the honey made by the insects Apis cerana Fabricius, etc. (family Apidae). The crude honey is filtered or heated to remove water for medication.

Nomenclature Used in Prescriptions: *Fengmi, Shengmi, Baimi, Huangmi, Lianmi*

Properties and Channel Distribution: This drug is sweet in taste and neutral in nature, and is distributed to the Lung, Spleen and Large Intestine Channels.

Action and Indications:

1. Tonifying the middle warmer and relieving spasm

This drug can be used to treat listlessness, poor appetite and pain in the epigastrium due to deficiency of the spleen and stomach. In treating duodenal ulceration, decoction of 60 g of Mel, 10 g of Radix Paeoniae, 10 g of Radix Glycyrrhizae and 6 g of Pericarpium Citri Reticulatae can be taken. This drug has tonifying effect and can be used to regulate drug properties, and therefore tonics are often made into bolus or soft extract with honey. Some tonics are fried with honey to enhance the tonifying effect.

2. Moistening the intestine to relax the bowel

In treating constipation due to dry intestine, 2 spoonfuls of honey (or with an addition of 1 spoonful of sesame oil) can be taken with water once a day before meals or the drug can be made into suppository and inserted into the anus.

3. Moistening the lung to relieve cough

This drug can be used to treat chronic cough due to deficiency of the lung and unproductive cough due to dryness of the lung. In treating unproductive cough with dry throat, one spoonful of the drug can be taken with water twice a day. When used to moisten the lung to relieve cough, many drugs for relieving cough and resolving phlegm are fried with honey.

Besides, this drug can be applied externally to treat sores, swelling and scald because it functions to remove toxin. The drug can be used to remove toxicity of drugs such as Radix Aconiti, Radix Aconiti Praeparata, etc.

Dosage and Administration: The dosage is 15–30 g. The drug is not to be decocted but is put into decoction. Proper amount of the drug can be used in external treatment. The crude drug is used to moisten the intestine, rclax the bowel and remove toxin; the heated drug is used to relieve cough and pain.

Notes: This drug is slippery in nature and therefore should not be used by those with accumulation of damp–heat, stuffy chest and loose stool due to deficiency of the spleen.

17.2 Tonics for Reinforcing *Yang*

This kind of drugs are mainly used to treat diseases caused by deficiency of *Yang*, which includes deficiency of the heart–*Yang*, spleen–*Yang*, kidney–*Yang*, etc. Since the kidney–*Yang* is the primordial *Yang*, deficiency of *Yang* often refers to deficiency of the kidney–*Yang* and to reinforce *Yang* is to tonify the kidney. Therefore, tonics for reinforcing *Yang* are in fact drugs for warming and tonifying the kidney–*Yang*.

Deficiency of the kidney–*Yang* is manifested by the decline of general body functions, impotence, seminal emission, etc. Tonics for reinforcing *Yang* have the functions of warming and tonifying the kidney–*Yang*, replenishing vital essence and marrow, strengthening muscles and bones, etc. They are, therefore, used to treat listlessness, aversion to cold, cold limbs, lassitude in loin and knee, impotence, seminal emission, frequent micturition, enuresis, etc. due to deficiency of the kidney–*Yang*. Also, some of the tonics for reinforcing *Yang* can be used to treat diarrhea and asthma of deficiency type, since failure of the kidney–fire to warm the spleen and stomach may lead to dysfunction of the two organs, causing diarrhea, and deficiency of the kidney–*Qi* often cause asthma.

Since tonics for reinforcing *Yang* are mostly warm and dry in nature, they should not be used by those with deficiency of *Yin* and hyperactivity of fire, so as to avoid assisting fire and consuming *Yin*.

Pilose Antler (鹿茸 *Lurong*)
Cornu Cervi Pantotrichum

This drug consists of the hairy young horn of the male deers Cervus nippon Temminck or Cervus elaphus L. (family Cervidae). The former is called "*Hualurong*" in Chinese and the latter, "*Malurong*". The horn is cut into slices or ground into powder for medication.

Nomenclature Used in Prescriptions: *Lurong, Lurongpian, Lurongfen*

Properties and Channel Distribution: This drug is sweet and salty in taste and warm in nature, and is distributed to the Liver and Kidney Channels.

Action and Indications:

Tonifying kidney–*Yang*, replenishing vital essence and blood and strengthening muscles and bones

In treating aversion to cold, listlessness, impotence, seminal emission, enuresis, frequent micturition, infertility, etc. due to deficiency of kidney–*Yang*, the drug can be used alone or in combination with Rhizoma Rehmanniae Praeparatae, Fructus Corni, Radix Morindae Officinalis, Fructus Psoraleae, Herba Epimedii, etc. In treating metrorrhagia and metrostaxis due to cold of deficiency type, the drug can be used in combination with Colla Corii Asini, Os Sepiellae seu Sepiae, etc. In treating lassitude in loin and knee, listlessness, dizziness, tinnitus, etc. due to deficiency of vital essence and blood, the drug is often used in combination with drugs for tonifying the kidney and nourishing blood. In treating infantile metopism, poor development of bones and muscles, retardation in walking and tooth eruption, etc. due to deficiency of the liver and kidney, the drug can be used in combination with Rhizoma Rehmanniae Praeparatae, Fructus Corni, Rhizoma Dioscoreae, etc.

In addition, the drug can also be used to treat cellulitis of *Yin* nature with thin pus, which does not heal due to deficiency of *Qi* and blood. In recent years, the drug is used to treat deficiency of the heart, palpitation, aching loin, and neurasthenia with symptoms of deficiency of the kidney.

Dosage and Administration: Usually, 0.5–1 g of the drug powder is taken. The drug can also be made into pills.

Notes: In taking this drug, it is advisable to use small dosage at first and then increase the dosage gradually. If large dosage is used at the beginning, dizziness and conjunctival congestion may be caused as a result of floating of *Yang* and stirring–up of wind. The drug is contraindicated for those with deficiency of *Yin* and hyperactivity of *Yang*, or with heat in the blood system.

Appendix:

1. Cornu Cervi (鹿角 *Lujiao*)

This drug consists of the ossified horn of the male deer Cervus nippon Temminck or other male deers. The drug is called *Lujiaopian* or *Lujiaoxie* in prescriptions. It is salty in taste and warm in nature, and is distributed to the Kidney Channel. The horn is parched till it turns brown for use. It can be used instead of Cornu Cervi Pantotrichum to tonify the kidney–*Yang* and strengthen muscles and bones, but its effect is less powerful than the latter. The crude drug can be used to activate blood circulation and subdue swelling and is often used to treat skin diseases or pyogenic infections. It can be both taken orally or ground into powder with vinegar and applied externally. The drug is effective especially for diseases caused by deficiency of *Qi* and cold of deficiency type. Usually, 6–10 g of the drug is used in decoction.

2. Colla Cornus Cervi (鹿角胶 *Lujiaojiao*)

This drug consists of the gelatin made from Cornu Cervi. It is sweet and salty in taste and warm in nature, and is distributed to the Liver and Kidney Channels. With less effect than Cornu Cervi Pantotrichum, the drug can be used to warm and tonify the liver and kidney and replenish vital essence and blood. In addition, it has the effect of arresting bleeding. It is used to treat deficiency of vital essence and blood, consumptive diseases, internal injury due to overstrain, epistaxis, metrorrhagia, metrostaxis, deficiency and cold of the uterus, cellulitis of *Yin* nature invading the deep interior of the body, etc. Usually, 6–10 g of the drug is melted in water, millet wine or drug decoction and taken.

3. Cornu Cervi Degelatinatum (鹿角霜 *Lujiaoshuang*)

This drug consists of the residue after Colla Cornus Cervi is prepared, gathered and removed. It is salty in taste and warm in nature. Its effect is similar to but less powerful than Cornu Cervi. It can be used to treat deficiency of kidney–*Yang* and blood, coldness of vital essence, metrorrhagia with metrostaxis, vomiting and anorexia due to deficiency of spleen–*Yang*, etc. When used in external treatment, the drug has the effect of astringing blood. Usually, 6–10 g of the drug is used in decoction.

Morinda Root (巴戟天 *Bajitian*)
Radix Morindae Officinalis

This drug consists of the root of the perennial twining or climbing liana Morinda officinalis How (family Rubiaceae). The drug is cut into sections and parched with salt water for medication.

Nomenclature Used in Prescriptions: *Baji, Bajitian, Bajirou*

Properties and Channel Distribution: This drug is pungent and sweet in taste and slightly warm in nature, and is distributed to the Kidney Channel.

Action and Indications:

1. Tonifying kidney–*Yang*

In treating impotence due to deficiency of kidney–*Yang*, infertility and irregular menstruation due to coldness of the uterus, deficiency and coldness of the lower warmer, coldness and pain of the hypogastrium, incontinence of urine, frequent urination, etc., the drug is often used in combination with drugs for tonifying the kidney and astringency.

2. Strengthening muscles and bones and dispelling cold

In treating rheumatic pain of the loin and knee or myophagism and myasthenia, the drug is often used in combination with Cortex Eucommiae, Radix Achyranthis Bidentatae, Radix Dipsaci, Fructus Corni, etc.

Dosage and Administration: Usually, 6–10 g of the drug is used in decoction.

Notes: The drug is contraindicated for those with deficiency of *Yin* and hyperactivity of fire, dry mouth and lips, and dysuria.

Desertliving Cistanche (肉苁蓉 *Roucongrong*)
Herba Cistanchis

This drug consists of the fleshy stem of the annial parasitic herbage Cistanche salsa (C.A. Mey.) G. Beck (family Orobanchaceae). The drug is dried and cut into slices for medication.

Nomenclature Used in Prescriptions: *Dancongrong*, *Tiancongrong*

Properties and Channel Distribution: This drug is sweet and salty in taste and warm in nature, and is distributed to the Kidney and Large Intestine Channels.

Action and Indications:

1. Tonifying kidney–*Yang*

In treating impotence due to deficiency of the kidney, coldness and pain of the low back and knee, female infertility, etc., the drug is often used in combination with Fructus Psoraleae, Semen Cuscutae, Fructus Cnidii, Radix Morindae Officinalis, Semen Astragali Complanati, Fructus Corni, etc.

2. Moistening the intestine to relax the bowel

In treating constipation in the elderly or patients with weak physiques, the drug is often used in combination with Fructus Cannabis, Lignum Aquilariae Resinatum, etc. If the disease is due to deficiency of blood and body fluid, the drug can be used in combination with Radix Rehmanniae and Radix Angelicae Sinensis.

Dosage and Administration: Usually, 10–18 g of the drug is used in decoction. The large dosage may be 30 g.

Notes: The drug is contraindicated for those with hyperactivity of kidney–fire, loose stool due to deficiency of the spleen and constipation due to heat of excess type.

Curculigo Rhizome (仙茅 *Xianmao*)
Rhizoma Curculiginis

This drug consists of the rhizome of the perennial herbage Curculigo orchioides Gaertn (family Amaryllidaceae). The crude drug is used after being dried in the sun.

Nomenclature Used in Prescriptions: *Xianmao*

Properties and Channel Distribution: This drug is pungent in taste and heat in nature with slight toxic effect, and is distributed to the Kidney Channel.

Action and Indications:

1. Warming the kidney and reinforcing *Yang*

In treating impotence, seminal emission and premature ejaculation due to deficiency of kidney–*Yang*, the drug is often used in combination with Rhizoma Rehmanniae Praeparatae, Herba Epimedii, Fructus Lycii, etc.

2. Dispelling cold and dampness and strengthening muscles and bones

In treating lassitude in the low back and knee due to deficiency of the kidney and arthralgia due to cold and dampness, the drug is often used in combination with drugs for treating arthralgia and relieving pain.

Besides, the drug has been used in recent years in combination with Herba Epimedii to treat hypertension in women during climacterium.

Dosage and Administration: Usually, 3–10 g of the drug is used in decoction.

Notes: This drug should not be taken for a long time as a tonic. It is contraindicated for those with deficiency of *Yin* and hyperactivity of fire, or with hyperactivity of *Yang*.

Epimedium (淫羊藿 *Yinyanghuo*)
Herba Epimedii

This drug consists of the stem and leaf of the perennial herbage Epimedium grandiglorum Morr. and Epimedium brevicornum Maxim. or E. sagittatum (S. et Z.) Maxim. (family Berberidaceae). The drug is died in shade or in the sun, cut into slivers and fried with fat from sheep for medication.

Nomenclature Used in Prescriptions: *Yinyanghuo,Xianlingpi*

Properties and Channel Distribution: This drug is pungent and sweet in taste and warm in nature, and is distributed to the Liver and Kidney Channels.

Action and Indications:

1. Tonifying kidney–*Yang*

In treating impotence, lassitude in the low back and knee, incontinence of urine, female infertility, etc. due to deficiency of kidney–*Yang*, 30 g of the drug can be put into 0.5 kg of rice wine and 5 ml. of the wine is drunk at a time, 3 times a day. The drug can also be used in combination with other drugs for tonifying the kidney.

2. Dispelling wind and removing dampness

In treating arthralgia due to wind, cold and dampness, paralysis of the lower limbs, spasm of muscles, numbness of hand and foot, etc., the drug can be used in combination with drugs for treating arthralgia and relieving pain such as Ramulus Loranthi, Radix Gentianae Macrophyllae, etc.

In addition, the drug can also be used in combination with drugs for reinforcing *Yang* and replenishing *Yin* such as Rhizoma Curculiginis, Radix Morindae Officinalis, Cortex Phellodendri, Rhizoma Anemarrhenae, etc. to treat hypertention in women during clmacterium with symptoms of deficiency of both *Yin* and *Yang*.

Dosage and Administration: Usually, 6–10 g of the drug is used in decoction.

Notes: This drug is rather drastic and may damage *Yin* and assist fire, and therefore should not be taken by those with deficiency of *Yin* and hyperactivity of fire, or with sufficient *Yang*.

Eucommia Bark (杜仲 *Duzhong*)
Cortex Eucommiae

This drug consists of the bark of the deciduous arbor Eucommia ulmoides Oliv. (family Eucommiaceae). The drug is dried in the sun, cut into pieces, fried with salt water and then cut into slivers for medication.

Nomenclature Used in Prescriptions: *Duzhong, Duzhongtan*

Properties and Channel Distribution: This drug is sweet in taste and warm in nature, and is distributed to the Liver and Kidney Channels.

Action and Indications:

1. Tonifying the liver and kidney and strengthening muscles and bones

In treating lassitude in the low back and knee, weakness of muscles and bones, impotence, frequent micturition, etc. due to deficiency of the liver and kidney, the drug is often used in combination with drugs for tonifying the liver and kidney such as Radix Dipsaci, Radix Achyranthis Bidentatae, Rhizoma Rehmanniae Praeparatae, Fructus Corni, etc. In treating low back pain due to cold and dampness, the drug can be used in combination with Ramulus Cinnamomi, Radix Angelicae Pubescentis, Radix Gentianae Macrophyllae, etc. In treating low back pain during menstruation, the drug can be used in combination with Radix Angelicae Sinensis, Rhizoma Ligustici Chuanxiong, Radix Paeoniae Alba, etc.

2. Curing metrorrhagia and preventing abortion

In treating metrorrhagia, threatened abortion, viginal bleeding during pregnancy, etc., carbonized Cortex Eucommiae is often used in combination with other drugs for curing metrorrhagia such as Radix Dipsaci.

In addition, this drug has the effect of reducing blood pressure and can be used in combination with Ramulus Loranthi, Radix Achyranthis Bidentatae, Spica Prunellae, etc. to treat hypertension with symptoms of deficiency of the kidney.

Dosage and Administration: Usually, 10–15 g of the drug is used in decoction. Large dosage is 30–60 g.

Notes: The drug is contraindicated for those with deficiency of *Yin* and hyperactivity of fire.

Dipsacus Root (续断 *Xuduan*)
Radix Dipsaci

This drug consists of the root of the perennial herbage Dipsacus asper Wall. or Dipsacus japonicus Miq. (family Dipsacaceae). The crude drug is cut into slices for medication.

Nomenclature Used in Prescriptions: *Xuduan, Chuanduan, Chuanduanrou*

Properties and Channel Distribution: This drug is bitter, sweet and pungent in taste and slightly warm in nature, and is distributed to the Liver and Kidney Channels.

Action and Indications:

1. Tonifying the liver and kidney and activating channel function to relieve pain

In treating soreness and pain of the loin and leg and weakness of the foot and knee due to deficiency of the liver and kidney and sluggishness of blood circulation, arthralgia due to wind, coldness and dampness, muscular spasm, etc., the drug is often used in combination with Cortex Eucommiae, Radix Achyranthis Bidentatae, Fructus Chaenomelis, etc.

2. Promoting reunion of fractured bones

In treating traumatic injury, contusion, sprain, and closed fracture, the drug is often used in combination with Resina Boswelliae Carterii, Resina Commiphorae Myrrhae, Pyritum, Eupolyphaga seu steleophaga, Rhizoma Drynariae, etc.

3. Preventing metrorrhagia and abortion

In treating metrorrhgia, metrostaxis, leukorrhea, threatened abortion, viginal bleeding during pregnancy, etc., the drug is often used in combination with Radix Angelicae Sinensis, Radix Rehmanniae Praeparata, Colla Corii Asini, Folium Artemisiae Argyi, etc.

Dosage and Administration: Usually, 10–15 g of the drug is used in decoction.

Cibot Rhizome (狗脊 *Gouji*)
Rhizoma Cibotii

This drug consists of the rhizome of the perennial herbage Cibotium barometz (L.) J. Sm. (family Dicksoniaceae). The root and hairy part are removed and the drug is cut into slices after being heated in hot sand.

Nomenclature Used in Prescriptions: *Gouji, Jinmaogouji*

Properties and Channel Distribution: This drug is bitter and sweet in taste and warm in nature, and is distributed to the Liver and Kidney Channels.

Action and Indications:

1. Tonifying the liver and kidney and strengthening loin and

back

In treating deficiency of the liver and kidney manifested by low back pain, stiffness of the spine, difficulty in turning the body, pain of the knee, weakness of the muscles and bones, incontinence of urine, abnormal leukorrhea, etc., the drug is often used in combination with Cortex Eucommiae, Ramulus Loranthi, Semen Cuscutae, Radix Achyranthis Bidentatae, Radix Rehmanniae Praeparata, Fructus Corni, Colla Cornus Cervi, etc.

2. Dispelling wind–dampness to treat arthralgia

In treating arthralgia due to wind–dampness, numbness of the limbs, lassitude of the loin and knee, weakness in walking, etc., the drug is often used in combination with drugs for tonifying *Qi* and blood and treating arthralgia.

Dosage and Administration: Usually, 3–10 g of the drug is used in decoction.

Drynaria Rhizome (骨碎补 *Gusuibu*)
Rhizoma Drynariae

This drug consists of the rhizome of perennial pteriodophyte Drynaria fortunei (Kunze) J. Sm. (family Polypodiaceae). The drug is heated in hot sand to remove hairy part and pounded into pieces for medication.

Nomenclature Used in Prescriptions: *Gusuibu*

Properties and Channel Distribution: This drug is bitter in taste and warm in nature, and is distributed to the Liver and Kidney Channels.

Action and Indications:

1. Tonifying the kidney, strengthening tooth and relieving

pain

In treating low back pain, debility, tinnitus, deafness, toothache, etc. due to deficiency of the kidney, the drug is often used in combination with Radix Rehmanniae Praeparata, Fructus Corni, Fructus Psoraleae, etc.

2. Activating blood circulation, promoting reunion of fractured bones and treating injury

In treating fracture, the drug can be used in combination with Radix Dipsaci, Resina Boswelliae Carterii, Resina Commiphorae Myrrhae, etc. The drug can be ground into powder and applied to the local area.

Besides, the drug can also be used to treat long-lasting diarrhea due to deficiency of the kidney.

Dosage and Administration: Usually, 3–10 g of the drug is used in decoction. Proper amount of the drug can be used in external treatment.

Psoralea Fruit (补骨脂 *Buguzhi*)
Fructus Psoraleae

This drug consists of the fruit of the annual herbage Psoralea corylifolia L. (family Leguminosae). The drug is dried in the sun and parched with salt water for medication.

Nomenclature Used in Prescriptions: *Buguzhi, Poguzhi*

Properties and Channel Distribution: This drug is pungent and bitter in taste and warm in nature, and is distributed to the Kidney and Spleen Channels.

Action and Indications:

1. Tonifying kidney–*Yang*, arresting seminal emission and

reducing urination

In treating impotence, seminal emission, frequent micturition, enuresis, coldness and pain of low back and knee, etc. due to deficiency of kidney–*Yang*, the drug is often used in combination with Semen Cuscutae, Radix Dipsaci, Rhizoma Dioscoreae, Herba Epimedii, etc.

2. Warming the spleen to arrest diarrhea

In treating deficiency of spleen and kidney *Yang* manifested by diarrhea before dawn with borborygmus and abdominal pain which are alleviated after diarrhea, the drug is often used in combination with Semen Myristicae.

Besides, the drug is used in combination with Juglandis Regiae, Mel, etc. to treat cough and asthma due to cold of deficiency type.

Dosage and Administration: Usually, 3–10 g of the drug is used in decoction.

Notes: The drug is contraindicated for those with deficiency of *Yin* and presence of fire, or with constipation.

Bitter Cardamon (益智仁 *Yizhiren*)
Fructus Alpiniae Oxyphyllae

This drug consists of the ripe fruit of the perennial herbage Alpinia oxyphylla Miq. (family Zingiberaceae). The shell is removed and the kernel is parched with salt water for use.

Nomenclature Used in Prescriptions: *Yizhiren*

Properties and Channel Distribution: This drug is pungent in taste, warm in nature, and distributed to the Spleen and Kidney Channels.

Action and Indications:

1. Tonifying kidney, arresting seminal emission and reducing urination

In treating seminal emission, enuresis, frequent micturition, cloudy urine, etc. due to deficiency of the kidney, the drug is often used in combination with Semen Cuscutae, Oötheca Mantidis, Rhizoma Dioscoreae, Radix Linderae, etc.

2. Warming the spleen to arrest diarrhea and arresting salivation

In treating deficiency of spleen–*Yang* manifested by coldness and pain of the abdomen, vomiting, diarrhea, anorexia or salivation, the drug is often used in combination with Radix Codonopsis Pilosulae, Rhizoma Atractylodis Macrocephalae, Rhizoma Zingiberis, Fructus Amomi, etc.

Dosage and Administration: Usually, 3–10 g of the drug is used in decoction.

Notes: The drug is contraindicated for those with deficiency of *Yin* and hyperactivity of fire, or with diseases due to damp–heat.

Cordyceps (冬虫夏草 *Dongchongxiacao*)
Cordyceps

This drug consists of the whole mass of the stroma of the fungus Cordyceps sinensis (Berk.) Sacc. (family Clavicipitaceae) and the larva of its host Hepialus varians Staudinger. The crude drug is dried for medication.

Nomenclature Used in Prescriptions: *Dongchongcao*, *Dongchongxiacao*

Properties and Channel Distribution: This drug is sweet in taste and warm in nature, and is distributed to the Kidney and Lung Channels.

Action and Indications:

Nourishing the lung and kidney, arresting bleeding and resolving phlegm

In treating cough with sputum and blood due to overstrain, impotence, seminal emission, consumptive diseases which do not recover, etc., the drug alone can be taken for a long time. In treating phthisical cough with blood and chest pain, the drug is often used in combination with Bulbus Fritillariae Cirrhosae,Radix Ophiopogonis, Colla Corii Asini, Radix Adenophorae Strictae, etc. In treating impotence, seminal emission, and lassitude of the loin and leg, the drug can be used in combination with Cortex Eucommiae, Herba Epimedii, Herba Cistanchis, etc.

Dosage and Administration: Usually, 6–10 g of the drug is used in decoction, or 1.5–3 g of the drug powder is taken as a dose.

Gecko (蛤蚧 *Gejie*)
Gecko

This drug consists of the dried body of Gekko gecko (L.) (family Geckonidae), deprived of the viscera. The drug is cleaned after the head and claw are removed and then is ground into powder for medication.

Nomenclature Used in Prescriptions: *Gejie*, *Gejiewei*

Properties and Channel Distribution: This drug is salty in taste and neutral in nature with slight toxic effect, and is distributed to the Lung, Kidney and Heart Channels.

Action and Indications:

Nourishing the lung and kidney and helping inspiration to relieve asthma

In treating long–lasting asthma or cough with bloody sputum due to overstrain, which are both caused by deficiency of the lung and kidney and failure of the kidney in receiving air, the drug is often used in combination with Radix Ginseng, Semen Juglandis, Radix Stemonae, Radix Asteris, Fructus Schisandrae, Bulbus Fritillariae Cirrhosae, etc. In treating impotence, seminal emission, frequent micturition, etc. due to deficiency of the kidney, the drug can be ground into powder and taken, or used in combination with Radix Ginseng, Fructus Schisandrae, Semen Juglandis, Radix Morindae Officinalis, etc.

Dosage and Administration: Usually, 1–1.5 g of the drug powder is used as a dose. The drug can also be made into pills or put into wine and taken.

Notes: The drug is contraindicated for those with asthma caused by wind–cold or heat of excess type. It is not to be decocted.

Walnut Kernel (胡桃肉 *Hutaorou*)
Semen Juglandis

This drug consists of the kernel of the deciduous arbor Juglans regia L. (family Juglandaceae). The crude or parched drug is used for medication.

Nomenclature Used in Prescriptions: *Hutaorou*, *Hetaorou*, *Hutaoren*

Properties and Channel Distribution: This drug is sweet in taste and warm in nature, and is distributed to the Kidney, Lung and Large Intestine Channels.

Action and Indications:

1. Tonifying the kidney to treat low back pain

In treating low back pain due to deficiency of the kidney, the drug is often used in combination with drugs for tonifying the kidney such as Fructus Psoraleae, Cortex Eucommiae, etc.

2. Astringing the lung to relieve asthma

In treating asthma due to deficiency of the lung and kidney, the drug is often used in combination with Radix Ginseng, Gecko, Radix Asteris, Flos Farfarae, etc.

In addition, the drug alone or used in combination with Herba Cistanchis, Fructus Cannabis, Radix Angelicae Sinensis, etc., is effective for constipation in the elderly after diseases due to dryness of the intestine. In recent years, the drug has been used in combination with Herba Lysimachiae, Endothelium Corneum Gigeriae Galli, Talcum, Spora Lygodii, etc. to treat low back pain from nephrolithiasis.

Dosage and Administration: Usually, 10–30 g of the drug is used in decoction. The drug can also be baked and chewed, with 3–5 pieces at a time.

Notes: Strong tea should not be drunk during drug administration.

Human Placenta (紫河车 *Ziheche*)
Placenta Hominis

This drug consists of the placenta of healthy parturient. It is ground into powder for medication.

Nomenclature Used in Prescriptions: *Taipanfen*, *Ziheche*

Properties and Channel Distribution: This drug is sweet and salty in taste and warm in nature, and is distributed to the Lung, Liver and Kidney Channels.

Action and Indications:

1. Tonifying the kidney and replenishing vital essence

In treating deficiency of the liver and kidney, internal injury due to overstrain, impotence, seminal emission, afternoon fever, spontaneous sweating, etc., the drug can be ground into powder and taken, or used in combination with Rhizoma Rehmanniae Praeparatae, Plastrum Testudinis, etc.

2. Tonifying *Qi* and blood

In treating deficiency of *Qi* and blood manifested by emaciation, listlessness, sallow complexion, and hypogalactia after childbirth, the drug can be ground into powder and taken, or used in combination with other drugs for tonifying *Qi* and blood such as Radix Ginseng, Rhizoma Rehmanniae Praeparatae, etc.

3. Tonifying the lung to relieve cough

In treating cough, asthma and hemoptysis due to deficiency of lung–*Yin* or kidney–*Yin*, the drug can be ground into powder and taken, or used in combination with Bulbus Fritillariae Cirhosae, Radix Stemonae, Radix Asparagi, Fructus Schisandrae, etc.

Dosage and Administration: The dosage is 1.5–3 g. The drug can also be made into pills, powder or tablets.

Dodder Seed (菟丝子 *Tusizi*)
Semen Cuscutae

This drug consists of the seed of the annual parasitic trailing plant Cuscuta chinensis Lam. or Cuscuta japonica Choisy (family Convolvulaceae). The drug is infused in wine or pounded into mash and made into cakes for medication.

Nomenclature Used in Prescriptions: *Tusizi*, *Tusibing*

Properties and Channel Distribution: This drug is sweet and pungent in taste and neutral in nature, is distributed into the Liver and Kidney Channels.

Action and Indications:

1. Tonifying the kidney and replenishing vital essence

In treating impotence, seminal emission, tinnitus, lassitude of low back and knee, frequent urination, etc. due to deficiency of the kidney, the drug is often used in combination with Fructus Lycii, Fructus Rubi, Fructus Schisandrae or Fructus Psoraleae, Cortex Eucommiae, etc. In the case of deficiency of kidney−*Yin*, the drug can be used in combination with Radix Rehmanniae Praeparata, Rhizoma Dioscoreae, etc.

2. Nourishing the liver to improve vision

In treating poor eyesight, blurred vision, dizziness, etc. due to deficiency of the liver and kidney, the drug can be used in combination with Radix Rehmanniae Praeparata, Fructus Lycii, Fructus Mori, Fructus Ligustri Lucidi, etc.

3. Invigorating the spleen to arrest diarrhea

In treating anorexia and loose stool due to deficiency of the spleen and kidney, the drug can be used in combination with

Rhizoma Dioscoreae, Semen Nelumbinis, Radix Codonopsis Pilosulae, Poria, etc.

In addition, the drug can be used in combination with drugs for tonifying the kidney and regulating menstruation to treat threatened abortion, irregular menstruation due to deficiency of the kidney.

Dosage and Administration: Usually, 10–15 g of the drug is used in decoction.

Notes: The drug is contraindicated for those with deficiency of *Yin* and hyperactivity of fire, or with constipation.

Flatstem Milkvetch Seed (沙苑子 *Shayuanzi*)
Semen Astragali Complanati

This drug consists of the ripe seed of the annual herbage Astragalus complanatus R. Br. (family Leguminosae). The crude drug or the drug parched with salt water is used.

Nomenclature Used in Prescriptions: *Shayuanzi, Tongjili*

Properties and Channel Distribution: This drug is sweet in taste and warm in nature, and is distributed to the Kidney and Liver Channels.

Action and Indications:

1. Tonifying the kidney to arrest seminal emission

In treating lassitudc of low back and knee, seminal emission, premature ejaculation, incontinence of urine, etc. due to deficiency of the kidney, the drug is often used in combination with Rhizoma Dioscoreac, Stamen Nelumbinis, air–bladdle glue of fish, etc.

2. Nourishing the liver to improve vision

In treating blurred vision and dizziness due to deficiency of the liver and kidney, the drug can be ground into powder and taken, or used in combination with Radix Rehmanhiae Praeparata, Fructus Lycii, Fructus Ligustri Lucidi, etc.

Dosage and Administration: Usually, 10–15 g of the drug is used in decoction.

Notes: The drug is contraindicated for those with deficiency of *Yin* and hyperactivity of fire, or with dysuria.

17.3 Tonics for Nourishing Blood

This kind of drugs are mainly used to treat diseases due to deficiency of blood, which are usually manifested by lusterless complexion, pale lip and nail, dizziness, palpitation, irregular menstruation, etc. In application, if diseases are due to deficiency of blood accompanied by deficiency of *Qi*, tonics for nourishing blood should be used in combination with drugs for invigorating *Qi*; if diseases are due to deficiency of blood accompanied by deficiency of *Yin*, drugs for replenishing *Yin* should also be used; if the diseases are due to deficiency of the spleen and stomach, drugs for invigorating thc spleen and stomach should also be used.

This kind of drugs are mostly thick and sticky in nature and should therefore not be taken by those with distention of the middle warmer due to accumulation of dampness, anorexia and loose stool.

Prepared Rehmannia Root (熟地 *Shudi*)
Radix Rehmanniae Praeparata

This drug consists of the tuberous root of the perennial

herbage Rehmannia glutinosa Libosch. (family Scrophulariaceae). The drug is steamed and cut into slices for medication.

Nomenclature Used in Prescriptions: *Shudi*, *Shudihuang*

Properties and Channel Distribution: This drug is sweet in taste and slightly warm in nature, and is distributed to the Heart, Liver and Kidney Channels.

Action and Indications:

1. Nourishing blood to regulate menstruation

In treating dizziness, palpitation, metrorrhagia, metrostaxis, irregular menstruation, etc. due to deficiency of blood in the heart and liver, the drug can be used in combination with Radix Angelicae Sinensis, Rhizoma Dioscoreae, Rhizoma Ligustici Chuanxiong. etc.

2. Nourishing the kidney to replenish *Yin*

In treating hectic fever, afternoon fever, spontaneous sweating, seminal emission, lassitude of the low back and knee, diabetes, etc. due to deficiency of the kidney–*Yin*, the drug is often used in combination with Fructus Corni, Rhizoma Dioscoreae or Rhizoma Anemarrhenae, Plastrum Testudinis, etc.

Dosage and Administration: Usually, 15–30 g of the drug is used in decoction. The large dosage is 30–60 g.

Notes: This drug is thick and sticky in nature and is likely to generate dampness and disturb thc normal function of the stimach. Therefore, it is contraindicated for those with deficiency of the spleen and presence of dampness, or with profuse sputum and stasis of *Qi*.

Fleece-flower Root (何首乌 *Heshouwu*)
Radix Polygoni Multiflori

This drug consists of the tuberous root of the perennial twining herbage Polygonum multiflorum Thunb.(family Polygonaceae). The crude or prepared drug is used after being cut into slices.

Nomenclature Used in Prescriptions: *Zhishouwu*, *Shengshouwu*

Properties and Channel Distribution: This drug is bitter, sweet and puckery in taste and slightly warm in nature, and is distributed to the Liver and Kidney Channels.

Action and Indications:

1. Tonifying the liver and kidney and replenishing vital essence and blood (prepared)

In treating deficiency of the liver and kidney and deficiency of blood and *Yin*, manifested by palpitation, insomnia, dizziness, tinnitus, lassitude of the low back and knee, metrorrhagia, leukorrhea, seminal emission, etc., the drug is often used in combination with Semen Ziziphi Spinosae, Radix Paeoniae Alba, Radix Rehmanniae Praeparata, Radix Angelicae Sinensis, Os Draconis, etc. In treating deficiency of blood and exhaustion of vital essence manifested by premature greying of hair, baldness, etc., the drug can be used in combination with Radix Rehmanniae Praeparata, Cacumen Biotae,Fructus Ligustri Lucidi, etc., or with Radix Rehmanniae Praeparata, Radix Angelicae Sinensis, Rhizoma seu Radix Notopterygii, etc.

2. Relaxing the bowel, treating external diseases and preventing attack of malaria (crude)

In treating constipation due to deficiency of blood and body fluid, the drug alone can be decocted and taken, and fresh drug is more effective. In treating scrofula, carbuncles and sores due to deficiency of *Yin*, the drug can be used with other drugs according to disease conditions. In treating rubella due to deficiency of blood, the drug can be used in combination with Radix Rehmanniae, Radix Angelicae Sinensis, Periostracum Cicadae, Fructus Tribuli, etc. In treating itching sores and tinea, the drug can be decocted with Folium Artemisiae Argyi and the decoction is applied to the local area. In treating long-lasting malaria due to deficiency of *Qi* and blood, the drug can be used in combination with Radix Codonopsis Pilosulae, Radix Angelicae Sinensis, etc.

Besides, the drug alone (prepared) taken for a long time is effective for disturbance in spermatogenesis and spermateliosis.

Dosage and Administration: Usually, 10–15 g of the drug is used in decoction. The prepared drug is used to replenish blood and vital essence and the crude drug, to relax the bowel and treat external diseases.

Appendix: Caulis Polygoni Multiflori (夜交藤 *Yejiaoteng*)

This drug consists of the vine of Radix Polygoni Multiflori, and is also called *Shouwuteng* in Chinese. It is sweet in taste and neutral in nature, and is distributed to the Heart and Liver Channels. It has the functions of nourishing the heart to calm the mind and relieving itching, and can be used to treat insomnia, profuse sweating and soreness and pain due to deficiency of blood. Its decoction can also be applied externally to treat cutaneous pruritus. Usually, 15–30 g of the drug is used in decoction. Proper amount of the drug can be decocted and used in external treatment.

Chinese Angelica Root (当归 *Danggui*)
Radix Angelicae Sinensis

This drug consists of the root of the perennial herbage Angelica sinensis (Oliv.) Diels (family Umbelliferae). The crude drug or the drug parched with wine is used for medication.

Nomenclature Used in Prescriptions: *Danggui*, *Quandanggui*, *Dangguishen*, *Dangguiwei*, *Jiudanggui*

Properties and Channel Distribution: This drug is sweet, pungent and bitter in taste and warm in nature, and is distributed to the Liver, Heart and Spleen Channels.

Action and Indications:

1. Nourishing blood to regulate menstruation

In treating irregular menstruation, amenorrhea, dysmenorrhea, etc. due to deficiency of blood in the heart and liver, the drug is often used in combination with Rhizoma Ligustici Chuanxiong, Radix Paeoniac Alba, Radix Rehmanniae, etc. If the above diseases are due to stasis of blood, drugs for activating blood circulation and promoting flow of *Qi* can be used.

2. Activating blood circulation to relieve pain

In treating traumatic injury, carbuncle, phlegmon, sores, arthralgia due to wind–dampness, stasis of blood and pain after childbirth, etc., the drug is often used in combination with Resina Boswelliae Carterii, Resina Commiphorae Myrrhae or Semen Persicae, Flos Carthami, Squama Manitis, etc.

3. Moistening the intestine to relax the bowel

In treating constipation due to deficiency of blood and dryness of the intestine, the drug is often used in combination with Fructus Cannabis, Radix Polygoni Multiflori, Herba Cistanchis, etc.

Dosage and Administration: Usually, 6–15 g of the drug is used in decoction. The drug proper is used to nourish blood, the tip of the drug is used to activate blood circulation, and the whole drug is used to regulate blood circulation. The crude drug is used to nourish blood and moisten the intestine and the drug parched with wine is used to restore menstrual flow and activate blood circulation.

Notes: The drug is contraindicated for those with distention of the middle warmer due to hyperactivity of dampness, or with diarrhea.

White Peony Root (白芍药 *Baishaoyao*) Radix Paeoniae Alba

This drug consists of the root of the perennial herbage Paeonia lactiflora Pall. (family Ranunculaceae). The drug is dried in the sun and cut into slices. The crude drug, parched drug or the drug parched with wine is used for medication.

Nomenclature Used in Prescriptions: *Baishao, Shengbaishao, Jiushao, Chaohangshao*

Properties and Channel Distribution: This drug is bitter and sour in taste and slightly cold in nature, and is distributed to the Liver and Spleen Channels.

Action and Indications:

1. Tonifying blood and astringing *Yin*

In treating irregular menstruation, dysmenorrhea,

metrorrhagia, metrostaxis, etc. due to deficiency of blood, the drug is often used in combination with Radix Angelicae Sinensis, Rhizoma Ligustici Chuanxiong, Radix Rehmanniae Praeparata, etc. In treating exterior syndrome of deficiency with spontaneous sweating and aversion to wind due to invasion of wind–cold, the drug can be used in combination with Ramulus Cinnamomi to regulate the nutrient and defensive systems. The drug can also be used to treat night sweating.

2. Nourishing the liver and relieving pain

In treating pain of the chest, hypochondrium, stomach, abdomen, etc. due to dysfunction of liver–*Qi*, the drug is often used in combination with drugs for relieving depressed liver such as Radix Bupleuri, Rhizoma Cyperi, etc. In treating pain of the epigastrium and abdomen and spasm and pain of the limbs, the drug is often used in combination with Radix Glycyrrhizae. In treating diarrhea and dysentery with abdominal pain, the drug is often used in combination with Rhizoma Coptidis, Radix Scutellariae, Radix Aucklandiae, etc.

3. Nourishing *Yin* and soothing the liver

In treating headache, dizziness, etc. due to deficiency of liver–*Yin* and hyperactivity of liver–*Yang*, the drug is often used in combination with Radix Rehmanniae. Concha Haliotidis, Ramulus Uncariae cum Uncis, Flos Chrysanthemi, etc.

Dosage and Administration: Usually, 6–12 g of the drug is used in decoction. The crude drug is used to astringe *Yin*, soothe the liver and treat dysentery. The parched drug is used to nourish the liver, regulate the spleen and relieve pain. When the drug is parched with wine, its cold nature is reduced.

Donkey–hide Gelatin (阿胶 *Ejiao*)
Colla Corii Asini

This drug consists of the gelatin prepared from the hide of the ass Equus asinus L. (family Equidae) with the hair removed. The drug is broken into pieces or parched with powder of Concha Meretricis seu Cyclinae and Pollen Typhae Powder into small beads for medication.

Nomenclature Used in Prescriptions: *Shengejiao*, *Ejiaozhu*

Properties and Channel Distribution: This drug is sweet in taste and neutral in nature, and is distributed to the Liver, Lung and Kidney Channels.

Action and Indications:

1. Tonifying blood and arrest bleeding

In treating hematemesis, hemoptysis, etc. due to deficiency of blood, the drug is often used in combination with Radix Rehmannia, Radix Ophiopogonis, etc. In treating metrorrhagia and metrostaxis after childbirth, the drug is often used in combination with Folium Artemisiae Argyi, Radix Angelicae Sinensis, Radix Paeoniae Alba, etc.

2. Nourishing *Yin* and removing dryness

In treating vexation and insomnia due to deficiency of *Yin*, the drug is often used in combination with Rhizoma Coptidis, yolk, Radix Scutellariac, Radix Paeoniae Alba, Radix Rehmannia, etc. In treating dry cough due to deficiency of the lung and presence of heat, the drug is often used in combination with Semen Armeniacae Amarum, Fructus Aristolochiae, Fructus Arctii, etc. In treating convulsion and spasm due to deficiency of blood, which fails to nourish the muscles, the drug can be used in combination with Plastrum Testudinis, Concha Ostreae, yolk, etc.

Dosage and Administration: The dosage is 6–15 g. The crude drug (melted and taken with water) can be used to nourish *Yin* and remove dryness; the drug parched with Pollen Typhae is used to arrest bleeding; the drug parched with powder of Concha Meretricis seu Cyclinae is used to clear away heat in the lung.

Notes: The crude drug is contraindicated for those with deficiency of the spleen and stomach and indigestion.

Longan Aril (龙眼肉 *Longyanrou*)
Arillus Longan

This drug consists of the ripe fruit of the evergreen arbor Euphoria longan (Lour.) Steud. (family Sapindaceae). The kernel is removed and the drug is dried in the sun for medication.

Nomenclature Used in Prescriptions: *Guiyuanrou, Longyanrou, Yuanrou*

Properties and Channel Distribution: This drug is sweet to the taste, even in nature, and distributed to the Heart and Spleen Channels.

Action and Indications:

Nourishing blood and calming the mind

In treating insomnia, poor memory, palpitation, etc. due to deficiency of heart blood, the drug is often used in combination with Semen Ziziphi Spinosae, Radix Polygalae, Poria, etc.

Dosage and Administration: Usually, 6–12 g of the drug is used in decoction.

17.4 Tonics for Replenishing *Yin*

Drugs which have the functions of nourishing *Yin*, promoting the production of body fluid, removing dryness, etc. and are used to treat diseases due to deficiency of *Yin* and body fluid, are called tonics for replenishing *Yin* or tonics for nourishing *Yin*. Deficiency of lung–*Yin* is manifested by dry cough, hemoptysis, fever of deficiency type, and polydipsia; deficiency of stomach–*Yin* is manifested red tongue with desire for drinks, or even vomiting; deficiency of liver–*Yin* is manifested by poor vision, night blindness, dizziness, tinnitus, dry nail, and insomnia; and deficiency of kidney–*Yin* is manifested by afternoon fever, night sweating, etc. Tonics for replenishing *Yin* may be used selectively for the above diseases.

Glehnia Root (北沙参 *Beishashen*)
Radix Glehniae

This drug consists of the root of the perennial herbage Glehnia littoralis F. Schmidt ex Miq. (family Umbelliferae). The crude drug is cut into sections or slices for medication.

Nomenclature Used in Prescriptions: *Beishashen*

Properties and Channel Distribution: This drug is sweet and slightly bitter in taste and slightly cold in nature, and is distributed to the Lung and Stomach Channels.

Action and Indications:

1. Moistening the lung to relieve cough

This drug has the effect of clearing away heat in the lung and replenishing lung–*Yin*, and is often used in combination with

Radix Ophiopogonis, Rhizoma Polygonati Odorati, Radix Trichosanthis, etc. to treat dry cough with little sputum or long–lasting cough with hoarse voice.

2. Nourishing the stomach and promoting the production of body fluid

In treating dry throat and thirst due to exhaustion of body fluid by febrile disease, the drug is often used in combination with Radix Ophiopogonis, Rhizoma Polygonati Odorati, etc.

Dosage and Administration: Usually, 10–15 g of the drug is used in decoction.

Ophiopogon Root (麦门冬 *Maimendong*)
Radix Ophiopogonis

This drug consists of the tuberous root of the perennial herbage Ophiopogon japonicus Ker–Gawl. or Liriope spicata Lour. (family Liliaceae). The crude drug is used after been dried in the sun.

Nomenclature Used in Prescriptions: *Maimendong*, *Maidong*, *Cundong*

Properties and Channel Distribution: This drug is sweet and slightly bitter in taste and slightly cold in nature, and is distributed to the Lung, Heart and Stomach Channels.

Action and Indications:

Moistening the lung, clearing away heat from the lung, nourishing the stomach and promoting production of body fluid

In treating cough from consumptive disease, dry mouth and throat, and dry cough with thick sputum due to exhaustion of *Yin* in the lung and stomach, the drug is often used in combination with Rhizoma Pinelliae, Radix Codonopsis Pilosulae, etc., or equal amount of the drug and Radix Asparagi are made into soft extract with honey and one or two spoonful of the extract is taken before meals, three times a day. In treating thirst due to exhaustion of body fluid, the drug is often used in combination with Radix Adenophorae Strictae, Radix Rehmanniae, etc. In treating vexation and insomnia due to invasion of heat from febrile disease into the heart, the drug is often used in combination with Cornu Rhinoceri, Radix Rehmanniae, Radix Salviae Miltiorrhizae, etc. In treating constipation due to dryness of the intestine as a result of deficiency of body fluid, the drug is often used in combination with Radix Rehmanniae and Radix Scrophulariae.

Dosage and Administration: Usually, 6–12 g of the drug is used in decoction.

Notes: The drug is contraindicated for those with diarrhea due to cold of deficiency type, or with cough caused by exopathogens.

Lucid Asparagus Root (天门冬 *Tianmendong*)
Radix Asparagi

This drug consists of the tuberous root of the perennial climbing herbage Asparagus cochinchinensis (Lour.) Merr. (family Liliaceae). The crude drug is cut into sections for medication.

Nomenclature Used in Prescriptions: *Tianmendong*, *Tiandong*

Properties and Channel Distribution: This drug is sweet and slightly bitter in taste and cold in nature, and is distributed to the Lung and Kidney Channels.

Action and Indications:

Moistening the lung, nourishing the kidney, clearing away heat and resolving phlegm

In treating dry cough with sticky sputum difficult to be expectorated, hemoptysis, etc. due to lung–heat, the drug is often used in combination with Radix Ophiopogonis. In treating thirst due to deficiency of *Yin* and body fluid, the drug is often used in combination with Radix Rehmanniae Pracparata, Radix Ginseng, etc. In treating constipation due to dryness of the intestine, the drug can be used in combination with Radix Rehmanniae, Radix Angelicae Sinensis, Fructus Cannabis, Radix Scrophulariae, etc.

Dosage and Administration: Usually, 6–12 g of the drug is used in decoction.

Dendrobium (石斛 *Shihu*)
Herba Dendrobii

This drug consists of the stem of the perennial herbage Dendrobium nobile Lindll. (family Orchidaceae) and other plants of the same genus. The crude or fresh drug is cut into sections for medication.

Nomenclature Used in Prescriptions: *Jinshihu, Chuangshihu, Huoshihu, Xianshihu*

Properties and Channel Distribution: This drug is sweet in taste and cold in nature, and is distributed to the Lung, Stomach and Kidney Channels.

Action and Indications:

Nourishing the stomach, promoting production of body fluid, replenishing *Yin* and clearing away heat

In treating dry mouth and polydipsia due to exhaustion of body fluid by febrile diseases, the drug is often used in combination with fresh Radix Rehmanniae, fresh Radix Ophiopogonis, Radix Trichosanthis, Rhizoma Polygonati Odorati, etc. In treating gastralgia and retching, the drug is often used in combination with Herba Agastachis, Cortex Moutan Radicis, Exocarpium Citri Grandis, etc. In treating fever due to deficiency of *Yin*, the drug is often used in combination with Radix Ophiopogonis, Radix Rehmanniae, Radix Scrophulariae, etc.

Dosage and Administration: Usually, 6–12 g of the drug, or 15–30 g of the fresh drug is used in decoction. The fresh drug is much more effective than the dry drug in clearing away heat and promoting the production of body fluid, and therefore is used to treat deep red tongue and polydipsia due to exhaustion of body fluid by febrile diseases. The dry drug decocted for a long time can be used to treat dry tongue due to deficiency of *Yin*.

Notes: This drug is likely to retain pathogens and assist dampness and should therefore not be taken by those with damp–warm syndrome and should not be taken too early by those with damp–heat disease without dryness formation.

Fragrant Solomonseal Rhizome (玉竹 *Yuzhu*)
Rhizoma Polygonati Odorati

This drug consists of the rhizome of the perennial herbage Polygonatum odoratum (Mill.) Druce (family Liliaceae). The drug is dried in the sun, cut into slices and steamed for medication.

Nomenclature Used in Prescriptions: *Yuzhu, Weirui*

Properties and Channel Distribution: This drug is sweet in taste and slightly cold in nature, and is distributed to the Lung and Stomach Channels.

Action and Indications:

Nouring *Yin*, removing dryness, promoting production of body fluid and relieving cough

In treating cough with thick sputum and dry throat due to dryness of the lung, the drug is often used in combination with Radix Adenophorae Strictae, Radix Ophiopogonis, etc. In treating exhaustion of body fluid and thirst due to dry–heat of the lung and stomach, or polydipsia due to hyperactivity of stomach–heat, the drug is often used in combination with Radix Adenophorae Strictae, Radix Ophiopogonis, Radix Glycyrrhizae, etc. In treating common cold, headache, fever, cough, dry mouth, sore throat, etc. due to deficiency of *Yin*, the drug is often used in combination with Radix Cynanchi Atrati, Radix Platycodi, Herba Menthae, Bulbus Allii Fistulosi, etc.

Dosage and Administration: The dosage is 10–30 g.

Siberian Solomonseal Rhizome (黄精 *Huangjing*) Rhizoma Polygonati

This drug consists of the rhizome of the perennial herbage Polygonatum sibiricum Redoute or Polygonatum cyrtonema Hua (family Liliaceae), and various other plants of the same genus. The drug is cut into sections and steamed with millet wine for medication.

Nomenclature Used in Prescriptions: *Huangjing*

Properties and Channel Distribution: This drug is sweet in taste and neutral in nature, and is distributed to the Spleen, Lung and Kidney Channels.

Action and Indications:

1. Replenishing *Yin* and moistening the lung

In treating dry cough without sputum due to deficiency of lung–*Yin*, the drug alone can be made into soft extract and taken, or used in combination with drugs for clearing away heat from the lung and nourishing and moistening the lung such as Radix Adenophorae Strictae, Rhizoma Anemarrhenae, Bulbus Fritillariae Cirrhosae, etc. In treating lassitude of the low back and knee and premature greying of the hair due to deficiency of the kidney–essence, the drug can be used in combination with Radix Asparagi, Cacumen Biotae, Rhizoma Atractylodis, Cortex Lycii Radicis, etc., which are ground into powder and made into pills with honey.

2. Invigorating *Qi* in the middle warmer

In treating listlessness and anorexia due to deficiency of the spleen and stomach, debility after disease, etc., the drug is often used in combination with Radix Codonopsis Pilosulae and Radix Astragali seu Hedysari. In treating exhaustion of vital essence due to deficiency of *Qi*, the drug can be used in combination with Radix Rehmanniae Praeparata and Fructus Lycii.

Dosage and Administration: Usually, 10–30 g of the drug is used in decoction.

Lily Bulb (百合 *Baihe*)
Bulbus Lilii

This drug consists of the fleshy bulb of the perennial herbage Lilium brownii F.E. Brown var. colchesteri Wils. or Lilium pumilum DC. (family Liliaceae). The crude or honey–fried drug is used.

Nomenclature Used in Prescriptions: *Shengbaihe, Zhibaihe*

Properties and Channel Distribution: This drug is sweet in taste and slightly cold in nature, and is distributed to the Heart and Lung Channels.

Action and Indications:

1. Moistening the lung to relieve cough

In treating cough with bloody sputum due to dryness of the lung, the drug can be made into soft extract with Flos Farfarae, or used in combination with Radix Rehmanniae, Radix Ophiopogonis, Bulbus Fritillariae Cirrhosae, Radix Scrophulariae, etc.

2. Clearing away heat from the heart to calm the mind

In treating restlessness of deficiency type, palpitation, insomnia, dream–disturbed sleep, etc. at the late stage of febrile disease when heat is not completely cleared away, the drug is often used in combination with Rhizoma Anemarrhenae or Radix Rehmanniae.

Dosage and Administration: Usually, 10–30 g of the drug is used in decoction. The crude drug is used to clear away heat in the lung and the honey–fried drug, to moisten the lung.

Wolfberry Fruit (枸杞子 *Gouqizi*)
Fructus Lycii

This drug consists of the fruit of the perennial deciduous shrub Lycium chinese Mill. or Lycium barbarum L. (family Solanaceae). The crude drug is used for medication.

Nomenclature Used in Prescriptions: *Gouqi, Gangouqi, Gouqizi*

Properties and Channel Distribution: This drug is sweet in taste and neutral in nature, and is distributed to the Liver and Kidney Channels.

Action and Indications:

1. Nourishing the liver and kidney

In treating lassitude of the low back and knee due to deficiency of the kidney–essence, the drug can be used in combination with Rhizoma Polygonati.

2. Nourishing the liver to improve vision

In treating dizziness, blurred vision and poor eyesight due to deficiency of *Yin* of the liver and kidney, the drug is often used in combination with Flos Chrysanthemi, Radix Rehmanniae Praeparata, etc.

Dosage and Administration: Usually, 10–15 g of the drug is used in decoction.

Glossy Privet Fruit (女贞子 *Nüzhenzi*)
Fructus Ligustri Lucidi

This drug consists of the fruit of the evergreen shrub or arbor Ligustrum lucidum Ait. (family Oleaceae). The drug is steamed with millet wine and dried in the sun for medication.

Nomenclature Used in Prescriptions: *Nüzhenzi, Nüzhenshi*

Properties and Channel Distribution: This drug is sweet and bitter in taste and cool in nature, and is distributed to the Liver and Kidney Channels.

Actions and Indications:

Nourishing the liver and kidney, blackening hair and improving vision

In treating hectic fever, consumptive fever, lassitude of the low back and knee, premature greying of hair, etc. due to deficiency of *Yin* of the liver and kidney, the drug is often used in combination with Herba Ecliptae. In treating poor vision due to deficiency of *Yin* of the liver and kidney, the drug is often used in combination with Radix Rehmanniae, Fructus Lycii, Flos Chrysanthemi, Semen Astragali Complanati, etc.

Dosage and Administration: Usually, 10–15 g of the drug is used in decoction.

Mulberry (桑椹子 *Sangshenzi*)
Fructus Mori

This drug consists of the ripe fruit of the deciduous arbor Morus alba L. (family Moraceae). The crude drug is used, or the drug can be made into soft extract with honey for medication.

Nomenclature Used in Prescriptions: *Sangshenzi, Hesangshen, Sangshengao*

Properties and Channel Distribution: This drug is sweet and sour in taste and cold in nature, and is distributed to the Heart, Liver and Kidney Channels.

Action and Indications:

Replenishing *Yin* and blood

In treating dizziness, insomnia, etc. due to deficiency of *Yin* and blood, equal amount of the drug, Fructus Ligustri Lucidi and Herba Ecliptae are ground into powder and made into pills with honey. In treating thirst or diabetes due to deficiency of body fluid, the drug is often used in combination with Radix Rehmanniae, Radix Ophiopogonis, Radix Trichosanthis, etc. In treating constipation due to dryness of the intestine as a result of deficiency of *Yin* and blood, the drug alone can be made into soft extract or decocted with Radix Rehmanniae with addition of little honey for oral administration.

Dosage and Administration: Usually, 10–15 g of the drug is used in decoction, or 15–30 g of the soft extract made from the drug is taken with water.

Eclipta (旱莲草 *Hanliancao*)
Herba Ecliptae

This drug consists of the whole plant of the annual herbage Eclipta alba (L.) Hassk. (family Compositae). The crude drug is cut into sections for medication.

Nomenclature Used in Prescriptions: *Hanliancao, Mohanlian*

Properties and Channel Distribution: This drug is sweet and sour in taste and cold in nature, and is distributed to the Liver and Kidney Channels.

Action and Indications:

Nourishing the liver and kidney, cooling blood and arresting bleeding

In treating dizziness, blurred vision, premature greying of

hair, etc. due to deficiency of *Yin* of the liver and kidney, the drug is often used in combination with Fructus Ligustri Lucidi, Fructus Mori, etc. In treating the various blood disorders due to deficiency of *Yin* and blood–heat, such as hemoptysis, epistaxis, hemafecia, hematuria, metrorrhagia, metrostaxis, etc., the drug alone can be used with effect, or in combination with drugs for replenishing *Yin*, cooling blood and arresting bleeding.

Besides, the fresh drug can be pounded and applied to the local area to treat bleeding due to trauma.

Dosage and Administration: Usually, 6–15 g of the drug is used in decoction. Proper amount of the drug can also be used in external treatment.

Tortoise Plastron (龟板 *Guiban*)
Plastrum Testudinis

This drug consists of the plastron of Chinemys reevesii (Gray) (family Testudinidae). The crude or vigenar–fried drug is used.

Nomenclature Used in Prescriptions: *Shengguiban, Zhiguiban*

Properties and Channel Distribution: This drug is salty and sweet in taste and neutral in nature, and is distributed to the Kidney and Liver Channels.

Action and Indications:

1. Replenishing *Yin* and checking exuberance of *Yang*

In treating hectic fever, consumptive fever and night sweating due to deficiency of *Yin* and hyperactivity of fire, the drug is often used in combination with Cortex Phellodendri, Rhizoma Anemarrhenae, Radix Rehmanniae Praeparata, etc. In treating dizziness and blurred vision due to deficiency of *Yin* and hyperactivity of *Yang*, the drug is often used in combination with Radix Asparagi, Radix Scrophulariae, Os Draconis, Concha Ostreae, etc. In treating spasm of muscles and contracture of hand and foot due to exhaustion of *Yin* by heat from febrile diseases, the drug is often used in combination with Radix Paeoniae Alba, Radix Ophiopogonis, Radix Rehmanniae. etc.

2. Tonifying the kidney to strengthen the bone

In treating lassitude of the low back and feet, stiffness of muscles and bones, infantile metopism, etc. due to deficiency of kidney–*Yin*, the drug is often used in combination with Os Tigris, Radix Rehmanniae Praeparata, Radix Paeoniae Alba, etc.

3. Restoring normal menstruation and arresting metrorrhagia

In treating menorrhagia, metrorrhagia, metrostaxis, leukorrhea, etc. due to deficiency of *Yin* and heat in the blood, the drug is often used in combination with Radix Paeoniae Alba, Cortex Phellodendri, Cortex Ailanthi, Rhizoma Cyperi, etc.

Dosage and Administration: Usually, 10–30 g of the drug is used in decoction. The crude drug is decocted to replenish *Yin* and the fried drug is used when the drug is made into pills or powder. The drug should be boiled first before other drugs are thown in.

Notes: The drug is contraindicated for those with cold of deficiency type of the spleen and stomach, or with exopathogens which are not eliminated.

Fresh–water Turtle Shell (鳖甲 *Biejia*)
Carapax Trionycis

This drug consists of the carapace of Amyda sinensis (Weigmann).

The crude or vinegar–fried drug is used.

Nomenclature Used in Prescriptions: *Shengbiejia, Zhibiejia*

Properties and Channel Distribution: This drug is salty in taste and cold in nature, and is distributed to the Liver and Spleen Channels.

Action and Indications:

1. Replenishing *Yin* and reducing fever

In treating consumptive fever, hectic fever and night sweating due to deficiency of *Yin*, the drug is often used in combination with Radix Gentianae Macrophyllae, Cortex Lycii Radicis, Rhizoma Anemarrhenae, etc. In treating exhaustion of *Yin*–fluid at the late stage of seasonal febrile disease with fever at night and chills in the morning, the drug is often used in combination with Herba Artemisiae Chinghao, Cortex Moutan Radicis, Radix Rehmanniae, etc. In treating exhaustion of *Yin* by pathogenic heat, which affects the lower warmer, dry tongue and dark teeth, and involuntary movement of fingers, this drug can be used in combination with Radix Rehmanniae, Colla Corii Asini, Radix Paeoniae Alba, Concha Ostreae, etc. to replenish *Yin* and check exuberance of *Yang*.

2. Softening and resolving hard masses

In treating enlargement of the liver and spleen, abdominal blood clots, etc., the drug is often used in combination with

Rhizoma Cyperi, Pericarpium Citri Retculatae Viride, Rhizoma Sparganii, Rhizoma Zedoariae, etc.

Dosage and Administration: Usually, 10–30 g of the drug is used in decoction. The crude drug is decocted to replenish *Yin*, and the fried drug is used to soften hard masses or to be made into pills or powder. The drug should be decocted longer than other drugs.

18 Astringents

Drugs with the main functions of inducing astringency and arresting discharge are called astringents.

This kind of drugs are mostly sour and puckery in taste and have the functions in inducing astringency and arresting discharge. They can be used to treat the various kinds of involuntary discharge, including spontaneous sweating, night sweating, long–lasting cough with asthma of deficiency type, seminal emission, spermatorrhea, frequent micturition, enuresis, long–lasting diarrhea with prolapse of rectum, metrorrhagia and metrostaxis, long–lasting abnormal leukorrhea, etc.

It is the purpose of using astringents to induce astringency to prevent decline of anti–pathogenic factors and appearance of complications caused by involuntary discharge. The drugs are used to treat only the symptoms, not the root cause of diseases. Since the cause of involuntary discharge is deficiency of anti–pathogenic factors, astringents should be used in combination with appropriate tonics, to treat both the principal and secondary aspects of diseases.

Astringents have the functions in arresting sweating, relieving cough, controlling seminal emission, reducing urination, arresting diarrhea, bleeding, and leukorrhea, etc. They should not be used too early by those with pathogens of excess type which have not been eliminated, or at the initial stage of diarrhea, dysentery and cough, so as not to retain the pathogens.

Schisandra Fruit (五味子 *Wuweizi*)
Fructus Schisandrae

This drug consists of the ripe fruit of the perennial deciduous liana Schisandra chinensis (Turcz.) Baill. (family Magnoliaceae). The drug is pounded for medication.

Nomenclature Used in Prescriptions: *Wuweizi, Beiwuwei*

Properties and Channel Distribution: This drug is sour in taste and warm in nature, and is distributed to the Lung, Heart and Kidney Channels.

Action and Indications:

1. Astringing the lung to relieve cough

In treating cough and asthma due to deficiency of the lung, the drug can be used in combination with Radix Codonopsis Pilosulae, Radix Ophiopogonis, Semen Armeniacae Amarum, etc.

2. Consolidating superficial resistance to arrest sweating

In treating night sweating due to deficiency of *Yin* or spontaneous sweating due to deficiency of *Yang*, the drug is often used in combination with Concha Ostreae, Rhizoma Atractylodis Macrocephalae, Radix Ephedrae, etc.

3. Controlling nocturnal emission and arresting diarrhea

In treating nocturnal emission due to deficiency of the kidney, the drug is often used in combination with Oötheca Mantidis, Radix Aconiti Praeparata, Os Draconis, etc. In treating diarrhea before dawn due to cold of deficiency type of the spleen and kidney, the drug is often used in combination with Semen Myristicae, Fructus Euodiae, etc.

4. Promoting production of body fluid to quench thirst

In treating dry mouth and thirst due to deficiency of body fluid, the drug is often used in combination with Radix Codonopsis Pilosulae, Radix Ophiopogonis, etc.

5. Relieving mental stress

In treating restlessness of deficiency type, palpitation, insomnia, or dream–disturbed sleep due to deficiency of blood in the heart and kidney, the drug can be used in combination with Radix Rehmanniae, Radix Ophiopogonis, Radix Salviae Miltiorrhizae, Semen Ziziphi Spinosae, etc.

Besides, this drug ground into powder is effective in lowering transaminase level in those suffering from chronic hepatitis.

Dosage and Administration: Usually, 3–10 g of the drug is used in decoction. Relatively small dosage (1.5–3 g) is to be used to astringe the lung and relieve cough, and relatively large dosage (6–10 g) is to be used to replenish *Yin*.

Notes: The drug is contraindicated for those with exopathogenic factors which are not eliminated, or with cough at the initial stage of measles.

Black Plum (乌梅 *Wumei*)
Fructus Mume

This drug consists of the unripe green fruit of the deciduous arbor Prunus mume (sieb.)Sieb. et Zucc. (family Rosaceae). The crude or carbonized drug is used for medication.

Nomenclature Used in Prescriptions: *Wumeirou*, *Wumeitan*

Properties and Channel Distribution: This drug is sour and puckery in taste and neutral in nature, and is distributed to the

Spleen, Lung and Large Intestine Channels.

Action and Indications:

1. Astringing the lung to relieve cough

In treating long–lasting cough due to deficiency of the lung, the drug can be used in combination with Pericarpium Papaveris, Semen Armeniacae Amarum, Colla Corii Asini, etc.

2. Astringing the intestine to arrest diarrhea

In treating long–lasting diarrhea or dysentery, the drug can be used in combination with Semen Myristicae, Radix Codonopsis Pilosulae, Radix Aucklandiae etc.

3. Promoting production of body fluid to quench thirst

In treating diabetes due to heat of deficiency type, the drug can be used in combination with Radix Ophiopogonis, Radix Trichosanthis, Radix Puerariae, etc.

4. Regulating the stomach and relieving colic caused by ascariasis

In treating abdominal pain, vomiting, etc caused by intestinal ascariasis, the drug is often used in combination with Rhizoma Coptidis, Cortex Phellodendri, Rhizoma Zingiberis, Pericarpium Zanthoxyli, etc. In treating biliary ascariasis, 30 g of the drug and 30 g of Herba Artemisiae Scopariae can be decocted and half of the decoction is to be taken as a dose. This decoction should be taken every 2 hours successively for 4 times.

5. Arresting bleeding of the lower part of the body

In treating hemafecia, hematuria, metrorrhagia, metrostaxis, etc., the drug powder can be made into pills as large as the seeds of Chinese parasol tree (mixed with vinegar) and 30 pills are to be taken as a dose, 3 times a day. Or, the drug can be decocted with other drugs.

Besides, in treating lockjaw, the drug can be used to rub the local area; in treating protrusion of vegetations after diabrosis of carbuncle or phlegmon, the carbonized drug can be ground into powder and applied to the local area; in treating callosity and clavus, the drug and Calomelas can be ground into powder and the powder is mixed with vinegar and applied to the local area.

Dosage and Administration: The usual dosage is 3–10 g and large dosage may be up to 30 g. The drug is usually decocted. Proper amount of the drug can be used in external treatment. To arrest bleeding, the carbonized drug is used.

Chinese Gall (五倍子 *Wubeizi*)
Galla Chinensis

This drug consists of the gall produced by the insects Melaphis chinensis (Bell), or Melaphis paitan Tsai et Tang on the leaf of the deciduous shrub or arbor Rhus chinensis, R. punjabensis, R. punjabensis sincia (family Anacardiaceae). The crude or calcined drug is used.

Nomenclature Used in Prescriptions: *Webeizi*

Properties and Channel Distribution: This drug is sour and salty in taste and cold in nature, and is distributed to the Liver, Stomach and Large Intestine Channels.

Action and Indications:

1. Astringing the lung and purging fire

In treating long–lasting cough due to deficiency of the lung, the drug is often used in combination with drugs for astringing the lung, such as Fructus Schisandrae, Pericarpium Papaveris, etc.

2. Astringing the intestine to arrest diarrhea

In treating long–lasting diarrhea or dysentery, prolapse of rectum, etc., the drug alone can be used, or used in combination with Fructus Chebulae, Fructus Schisandrae, etc.

3. Controlling seminal emission and reducing urination

In treating seminal emission and enuresis, the drug can be used in combination with Poria.

4. Arresting sweating and promoting production of body fluid

In treating night sweating, the drug powder mixed with water can be applied to the umbilicus, covered with gauze, and the drug is to be applied at night and removed the next morning. In treating diabetes, the drug alone can be taken.

5. Inducing astringency to arrest bleeding

In treating metrorrhagia, metrostaxis, hemafecia, etc., the drug is often used in combination with drugs for arresting bleeding such as Fructus Mume, Folium Artemisiae Argyi, etc.

Besides, the drug powder applied to the local area or the drug decoction used to fumigate and wash the local area, is effective for sores, tinea, pyogenic infection, ulceration of the skin, prolapse of rectum, hysteroptosis, etc.

Dosage and Administration: Usually, 3–6 g of the drug is used in decoction. The drug is often made into pills or powder. Proper amount of the drug is used in external treatment.

Ephedra Root (麻黄根 *Mahuanggen*)
Radix Ephedrae

This drug consists of the root of the perennial herbaceous

shrub Ephedra sinica Stapf, or E. eguisetina Bunge (family Ephedraceae). The drug is cut into sections for use.

Nomenclature Used in Prescriptions: *Mahuanggen*

Properties and Channel Distribution: This drug is sweet in taste and neutral in nature, and is distributed to the Lung Channel.

Action and Indications:

Arresting sweating

This drug can be used to treat spontaneous sweating and night sweating and can be used in combination with other drugs according to different disease conditions. In treating spontaneous sweating due to deficiency of the superficial defence, the drug can be used in combination with drugs for invigorating *Qi* such as Radix Astragali seu Hedysari, Rhizoma Atractylodis Macrocephalae, etc. In treating spontaneous sweating due to deficiency of *Yang*, the drug can be used in combination with drugs for invigorating *Yang* such as Radix Ginseng, Radix Aconiti Praeparata, etc. In treating night sweating due to deficiency of *Yin*, the drug can be used in combination with drugs for replenishing *Yin* and inducing astringency such as Radix Rehmanniae Praeparata, Fructus Corni, Os Draconis, Concha Ostreae, etc. In treating sweating due to debility after childbirth, the drug can be used in combination with drugs for nourishing blood and consolidating superficial resistance such as Radix Angelicae Sinensis, Radix Astragali seu Hedysari, etc.

Dosage and Administration: Usually, 3–10 g of the drug is used in decoction. The drug powder can be used in external treatment.

Notes: The drug is contraindicated for those affected by exopathogen.

Light Wheat (浮小麦 *Fuxiaomai*)
Fructus Tritici Levis

This drug consists of the dry blighted caryopsis of the annual herbage Tritcum aestivum L. (family Gramineae). The crude or parched drug is used for medication.

Nomenclature Used in Prescriptions: *Fuxiaomai*

Properties and Channel Distribution: This drug is sweet in taste and cool in nature, and is distributed to the Heart Channel.

Action and Indications: Invigorating *Qi*, clearing away heat and arresting sweating

In treating night sweating, the drug can be decocted and taken, or the drug powder can be taken with rice water. In treating spontaneous sweating, the drug can be used in combination with Radix Astragali seu Hedysari, Concha Ostreae, Radix Ephedrae, etc. In treating hectic fever and fever of deficiency type, 30 g of the drug and 10 g of Cortex Lycii Radicis can be decocted and taken.

Dosage and Administration: Usually, 15–30 g of the drug is used in decoction. The drug is to be parched when made into powder for oral administration.

Appendix: Triticum aestivum L. (小麦 *Xiaomai*)

This drug consists of the ripe wheat. It is sweet in taste and cool in nature, and is distributed to the Heart Channel. It can be used to nourish the heart to relieve restlessness and is indicated in female hysteria, grief, etc. The drug is often used in combination with Radix Glycyrrhizae and Fructus Ziziphi Jujubae. Usually,

30–60 g of the drug is used in decoction.

Ailanthus Bark (椿皮 *Chunpi*)
Cortex Ailanthi

This drug consists of the root–bark of the deciduous arbor Toona sinensis (A. Juss.) Roem, or Ailanthus altissima (Mill.) Swingle (family Simaroubaceae). The crude or parched dried is used for medication.

Nomenclature Used in Prescriptions: *Chunshupi, Chushupi*

Properties and Channel Distribution: This drug is bitter and puckery in taste and cold in nature, and is distributed to the Stomach and Large Intestine Channels.

Action and Indications:

1. Eliminating dampness and clearing away heat

In treating abnormal leukorrhea with bloody discharge, the drug is often used in combination with Cortex Phellodendri, Rhizoma Alpiniae Officinarum, Radix Paeoniae Alba, Radix Angelicae Sinensis, etc. In treating abnormal leukorrhea due to damp–heat, the drug can be used in combination with Radix Paeoniae, Cortex Phellodendri, Rhizoma Dryopteris Crassirhizomae, etc.

2. Astringing the intestine to arrest diarrhea

In treating long–lasting diarrhea and dysentery, the drug can be used in combination with Fructus Chebulae, Radix Aucklandiae, Flos Syzygii Aromatici, etc.

3. Arresting lower bleeding

In treating menorrhea with dark discharge, etc. due to deficiency of *Yin* and hyperactivity of fire, the drug can be used in combination with Plastrum Testudinis, Cortex Phellodendri, etc. In treating hemafecia, the drug powder can be used.

Besides, in treating scabies humida, tinea, etc., the drug decoction can be used to wash the local area, to eliminate dampness and clear away heat.

Dosage and Administration: Usually, 3–10 g of the drug is used in decoction.

Chebula Fruit (诃子 *Hezi*)
Fructus Chebulae

This drug consists of the ripe fruit of the deciduous arbor Terminalia chebula Retz. (family Combretacae). The crude or roasted drug is used.

Nomenclature Used in Prescriptions: *Hezi, Hezipi, Hezirou, Weihezi*

Properties and Channel Distribution: This drug is sour and bitter in taste and neutral in nature, and is distributed to the Lung and Large Intestine Channels.

Action and Indications:

1. Astringing the intestine to arrest diarrhea

In treating long–lasting diarrhea and dysentery, the drug can be used in combination with Rhizoma Coptidis, Radix Aucklandiae, etc., or in combination with Pericarpium Papaveris, Rhizoma Zingiberis, etc.

2. Astringing the lung to relieve cough

In treating cough and asthma due to deficiency of the lung, or aphonia due to long–lasting cough, decoction of the drug, Radix Platycodi (9 g) and Radix Glycyrrhizae (6 g) can be taken.

Dosage and Administration: The dosage is 3–10 g. The crude drug is used to astringe the lung and purge fire and the roasted drug, to astringe the intestines and arrest diarrhea.

Nutmeg (肉豆蔻 *Roudoukou*)
Semen Myristicae

This drug consists of the ripe seed of the arbor Myristica fragrans Houtt. (family Myristicaceae). The seed is covered with flour and roasted to get rid of the oil for medication.

Nomenclature Used in Prescriptions: *Roudoukou, Rouguo, Yuguo, Weirouguo*

Properties and Channel Distribution: This drug is pungent in taste and warm in nature, and is distributed to the Spleen, Stomach and Large Intestine Channels.

Action and Indications

1. Astringing the intestine to arrest diarrhea

In treating long–lasting cough, prolapse of rectum, etc. due to deficiency of spleen–*Yang*, the drug can be used in combination with Fructus Chebulae, Pericarpium Papaveris, Radix Codonopsis Pilosulae, Rhizoma Atractylodis Macrocephalae, Cortex Cinnamomi, etc. In treating diarrhea before dawn due to cold of deficiency type of the spleen and kidney, the drug can be used in combination with Fructus Psoraleae, Fructus Euodiae and Fructus Schisandrae.

2. Warming the middle warmer to promote flow of *Qi*

In treating distention of the epigastrium and stomach, poor appetite, vomiting, etc. due to deficiency of spleen–*Yang*, the drug can be used in combination with Radix Aucklandiae,

Rhizoma Pinelliae Praeparata, etc.

Dosage and Administration: Usually, 3–10 g of the drug is used in decoction.

Red Halloysite (赤石脂 *Chishizhi*)
Halloysitum Rubrum

This drug consists of the hydrated soil–like mineral Halloysite (Monoclinic system). The mineral is ground into powder with water or calcined and ground into powder with water for medication.

Nomenclature Used in Prescriptions: *Chishizhi*

Properties and Channel Distribution: This drug is sweet, sour and puckery in taste and warm in nature, and is distributed to the Kidney and Large Intestine Channels.

Action and Indications:

1. Astringing the intestine to arrest diarrhea

In treating long–lasting diarrhea, dysentery, hemafecia, etc., the drug can be used in combination with Rhizoma Zingiberis, Semen Oryzae Sativae, or Radix Codonopsis Pilosulae, Rhizoma Atractylodis Macrocephalae, Os Draconis, etc.

2. Arresting bleeding

In treating hemafecia, menorrhea, metrorrhagia, metrostaxis and abnormal leukorrhea due to cold of deficiency type, the drug can be used in combination with Cacumen Biotae and Os Sepiellae seu Sepiae, which are calcined and ground into powder for oral administration.

3. Promoting tissue regeneration and healing of wounds

In treating carbuncles, sores or ulceration with wounds that do not heal, the drug is often used in combination with elephant's thick skin, Os Draconis, Resina Draconis, etc.

Dosage and Administration: Usually, 10–20 g of the drug is used in decoction.

Limonite (禹余粮 *Yuyuliang*) Limonitum

This drug consists of a kind of iron ore (Monoclinic system). The ore is broken into pieces and calcined for medication.

Nomenclature Used in Prescriptions: *Yuyuliang, Yuliangshi*

Properties and Channel Distribution: This drug is sweet and puckery in taste and neutral in nature, and is distributed to the Stomach and Large Intestine Channels.

Action and Indications:

1. Astringing the intestine to arrest diarrhea

In treating long–lasting diarrhea and dysentery, the drug is often used in combination with Halloysitum Rubrum.

2. Arresting bleeding

In treating hemafecia, dysentery with blood, metrorrhagia, metrostaxis, abnormal leukorrhea, etc., equal amount of the drug, Halloysitum Rubrum, Os Sepiellae seu Sepiae, ignited yellow earth, Concha Ostreae Usta and Cortex Cinnamomi can be ground into powder and 6 g of the powder is to be taken as a dose with millet wine, twice a day.

Dosage and Administration: Usually, 10–24 g of the drug is used in decoction.

Poppy Capsule (罂粟壳 *Yingsuke*)
Pericarpium Papaveris

This drug consists of the dried capsule of the annual or biennial herbage Papaver somniferum L. (family Papaveraceae). The vinegar–fried or honey–fried drug is used for medication.

Nomenclature Used in Prescriptions: *Yingsuke, Yumike, Zhimike*

Properties and Channel Distribution: This drug is sour and puckery in taste and neutral in nature, and is distributed to the Lung, Large Intestine and Kidney Channels.

Action and Indications:

1. Astringing the lung to relieve cough

In treating long–lasting cough of deficiency type, the drug can be used in combination with Fructus Mume.

2. Astringing the intestine to arrest diarrhea

In treating frequent diarrhea, the drug can be used in combination with Fructus Ziziphi Jujubae. In treating long–lasting dysentery, dysentery with blood, etc., the drug can be used in combination with Radix Aucklandiae, Rhizoma Coptidis, Rhizoma Zingiberis Recens, etc.

3. Relieving pain

In treating stomach pain and pain of bones and muscles, the drug alone can be used, or used in combination with other drugs.

Dosage and Administration: Usually, 3–10 g of the drug is used in decoction. The honey–fried drug is used to relieve cough and the vinegar–fried drug, to arrest diarrhea and relieve pain.

Notes: The drug is contraindicated for the onset of cough, diarrhea or dysentery. Since this drug has toxic effect, overdosage or persistent administration are not advisable.

Lotus Seed (莲子 *Lianzi*)
Semen Nelumbinis

This drug consists of the seed of the perennial aquatic herbage Nelumbo nucifera Gaertn. (family Nymphaeaceae). The plumule is removed and the drug is broken into pieces for use.

Nomenclature Used in Prescriptions: *Lianzi, Lianzirou*

Properties and Channel Distribution: This drug is sweet and puckery in taste and neutral in nature, and is distributed to the Spleen, Kidney and Heart Channels.

Action and Indications:

1. Invigorating the spleen to arrest diarrhea

In treating diarrhea due to deficiency of the spleen, the drug is often used in combination with Poria, Rhizoma Atractylodis Macrocephalae, Rhizoma Dioscoreae, Fructus Amomi, etc.

2. Nourishing the heart to calm the mind

In treating palpitation and insomnia due to breakdown of the normal physiological coordination between the heart and kidney, the drug can be used in combination with Semen Ziziphi Spinosae, Radix Polygalae, Poria, etc.

3. Tonifying the kidney to control seminal emission

In treating seminal emission, metrorrhagia, metrostaxis, abnormal leukorrhea, etc. due to deficiency of the kidney, the drug can be used in combination with Semen Astragali Complanati, Semen Euryales, Os Draconis, Concha Ostreae, Stamen Nelumbinis, etc.

Dosage and Administration: Usually, 10—15 g of the drug is used in decoction.

Appendix:

1. Stamen Nelumbinis (莲须 *Lianxu*)

This drug consists of the stamen of Nelumbo nucifera. It is sweet and puckery in taste and neutral in nature, and is distributed to the Heart and Kidney Channels. It has the effect of clearing away heat from the heart, strengthening the kidney, controlling seminal emission and arresting bleeding, and can be used to treat nocturnal emission, spermatorrhea, frequent micturition, enuresis, hematemesis, metrorrhagia, metrostaxis, etc. The dosage is 3—6 g.

2. Receptaculum Nelumbinis (莲房 *Lianfang*)

This drug consists of the receptacle of Nelumbo nucifera. It is bitter and puckery in taste and warm in nature, and is distributed to the Heart and Liver Channels and the blood system. It has the effect of removing blood stasis and arresting bleeding, and can be used to treat all kinds of bleeding, hematuria, metrorrhagia, etc. The drug is usually carbonized and its dosage is 6—10 g.

3. Plumula Nelumbinis (莲子心 *Lianzixin*)

This drug consists of the green and tender plumule in the seed of Nelumbo nucifera. It is bitter in taste and cold in nature, It has the effect of clearing away heat from the heart to calm the mind, and can be used in combination with Radix Scrophulariae, leaves bud of Herba Lophatheri, Fructus Forsythiae, etc. to treat coma and delirium due to invasion of pathogenic factors into the pericardium seen in epidemic febrile disease, or used in combination with drugs for calming the mind and controlling seminal emission to treat vexation, insomnia, seminal emission, etc. Its dosage is 1.5–3 g.

4. Folium Nelumbinis (荷叶 *Heye*)

This drug consists of the leaf of Nelumbo nucifera. It is bitter and puckery in taste and neutral in nature. It has the effect of clearing away summer–heat, removing dampness, sending up lucid *Yang*, enlivening the spleen, removing blood stasis and arresting bleeding, and can be used to treat febrile disease, diarrhea due to deficiency of the spleen and all kinds of blood disorders. Usually, 10–15 g of the drug or 1/4 of a fresh leaf is used in decoction. The fresh drug is used to clear away heat or summer–heat, the dry drug is used to send up lucid *Yang* and enliven the spleen, and the dry or carbonized drug is used to remove blood stasis and arrest bleeding.

Gordon Euryale Seed (芡实 *Qianshi*)
Semen Euryales

This drug consists of the seed of the annual aquatic herbage Euryale ferox Salisb. (family Nymphaeaceae). The drug is broken into pieces for medication.

Nomenclature Used in Prescriptions: *Qianshi, Qianshimi*

Properties and Channel Distribution: This drug is sweet and puckery in taste and neutral in nature, and is distributed to the Spleen and Kidney Channels.

Action and Indications:

1. Invigorating the spleen to arrest diarrhea

In treating long–lasting diarrhea due to deficiency of the spleen, the drug is often used in combination with Radix

Codonopsis Pilosulae, Rhizoma Atractylodis Macrocephalae, Rhizoma Dioscoreae, Poria, etc.

2. Tonifying the kidney to arrest seminal emission

In treating nocturnal emission, incontinence of urine, etc. due to deficiency of the kidney, the drug is often used in combination with Fructus Rosae Laevigatae.

3. Removing dampness to arrest abnorma leukorrhea

In treating abnormal leukorrhea due to damp–heat, the drug is often used in combination with Rhizoma Dioscoreae, Cortex Phellodendri, Semen Ginkgo, Semen Plantaginis, etc. In treating abnormal leukorrhea, equal amount of the drug and Poria can be ground into powder and made into pills with honey, and 10 g of the pills is to be taken with salt water as a dose

Dosage and Administration: Usually, 10–15 g of the drug is used in decoction.

Dogwood Fruit (山茱萸 *Shanzhuyu*)
Fructus Corni

This drug consists of the ripe sarcocarp of the deciduous arbor Cornus officinalis Sieb. et Zucc. (family Cornaceae). The drug is dried in the sun for medication.

Nomenclature Used in Prescriptions: *Shanzhuyu, Shanyurou*

Properties and Channel Distribution: This drug is sour and puckery in taste and slightly warm in nature, and is distributed to the Liver and Kidney Channels.

Action and Indications:

1. Tonifying the liver and kidney, controlling seminal emission and reducing urination

In treating impotence, seminal emission, lassitude of the low back, dizziness, tinnitus, deafness, frequent micturition, etc. due to deficiency of the liver and kidney, the drug is often used in combination with Fructus Psoraleae, Radix Angelicae Sinensis, etc.

2. Controlling menstruation and arresting bleeding

In treating menorrhea, metrostaxis, etc. due to weak physiques, the drug is often used in combination with Os Sepiellae seu Sepiae, Petiolus Trachycarpi Carbonisetus, Radix Rubiae, etc.

3. Arresting sweating and preventing collapse

In treating collapse after profuse sweating or after longlasting diseases, the drug can be used in combination with Radix Codonopsis Pilosulae, Os Draconis, Concha Ostreae, etc.

Dosage and Administration: Usually, 6–10 g of the drug is used in decoction. The large dosage may be up to 30 g.

Notes: The drug is contraindicated for those with hyperactivity of kidney–*Yang*, damp–heat or dysuria.

Cherokee Rose hip (金樱子 *Jinyingzi*) Fructus Rosae Laevigatae

This drug consists of the ripe fruit of the evergreen climbing shrub Rosa laevigate Michx. (family Rosaceae). The crude drug is used after the thorn and kernel are removed.

Nomenclature Used in Prescriptions: *Jinyingzi*

Properties and Channel Distribution: This drug is sour and puckery in taste and neutral in nature, and is distributed to the Kidney, Urinary Bladder and Large Intestine Channels.

Action and Indications:

1. Controlling seminal emission and reducing urination

In treating seminal emission, enuresis, abnormal leukorrhea, etc. due to deficiency of the kidney, the drug alone can be used, or equal amount of the drug and Semen Euryales can be ground into powder and made into pills and 6 g of the pills is to be taken as a dose with rice water.

2. Astringing the intestine to arrest diarrhea

In treating long–lasting diarrhea due to deficiency of the spleen, the drug is often used in combination with Rhizoma Dioscoreae, Semen Euryales, Rhizoma Atractylodis Macrocephalae, Poria, Fructus Schisandrae, etc.

Dosage and Administration: Usually, 6–15 g of the drug is used in decoction. The drug can also be made into pills or soft extract.

Mantis Egg–case(桑螵蛸 *Sangpiaoxiao*) Oötheca Mantidis

This drug consists of the egg–case of the insect Statilia maculata Thunb. (family Mantidae). The drug is dried in the sun for medication.

Nomenclature Used in Prescriptions: *Sanpiaoxiao*

Properties and Channel Distribution: This drug is sweet and salty in taste and neutral in nature, and is distributed to the Liver and Kidney Channels.

Action and Indications:

Tonifying the kidney–*Yang*, controlling seminal emission and reducing urination

The drug can be used to treat enuresis, frequent micturition, seminal emission, premature ejaculation, etc. due to deficiency of kidney–*Yang*. In treating enuresis and frequent micturition, the drug is often used in combination with Radix Codonopsis Pilosulae, Os Draconis, Concha Ostreae, etc. In treating seminal emission and premature ejaculation, the drug is often used in combination with Fructus Schisandrae, Os Draconis Ustum, etc.

Dosage and Administration: Usually, 3–10 g of the drug is used in decoction. The drug can also be made into pills or powder.

Raspberry (覆盆子 *Fupenzi*)
Fructus Rubi

This drug consists of the unripe fruit of the deciduous thrub Rubus chingii Hu (family Rosaceae). The drug is mixed with wine, steamed and then dried in the sun for medication.

Nomenclature Used in Prescriptions: *Fupenzi*

Properties and Channel Distribution: This drug is sweet and sour in taste and slightly warm in nature, and is distributed to the Liver and Kidney Channels.

Action and Indications

1. Tonifying the kidney and reducing urination

In treating frequent micturition, enuresis, etc., the drug is often used in combination with Oötheca Mantidis, Fructus Alpiniae Oxyphyllae, Semen Cuscutae, Fructus Corni, etc.

2. Tonifying the kidney and controlling seminal emission

In treating seminal emission, impotence, etc., the drug is often used in combination with Fructus Lycii, Semen Cuscutae,

Fructus Schisandrae, Semen Plantaginis, etc.

Dosage and Administration: Usually, 6–12 g of the drug is used in decoction.

Cuttle–bone(乌贼骨 *Wuzeigu*)
Os Sepiella seu Sepiae

This drug consists of the internal shell of the mollusc Sepiella maindroni de Rochebrune. or Sepia esculenta Hoyle (family Sepiidae). The drug is fried till it turns brown for medication.

Nomenclature Used in Prescriptions: *Wuzeigu, Haipiaoxiao*

Properties and Channel Distribution: This drug is salty and puckery in taste and slightly warm in nature, and is distributed to the Liver and Kidney Channels.

Action and Indications:

1. Arresting bleeding

In treating metrorrhagia and metrostaxis, the drug is often used in combination with Radix Rubiae, Petiolus Trachycarpi Carbonisatus, Galla Chinensis, Radix Astragali seu Hedysari, Fructus Corni, etc. In treating hemafecia, hemorrhoid, etc., the drug alone can be ground into powder and 6 g of the powder is to be taken as a dose with warm water. In treating bleeding from the lung or stomach, 6 g of the powder of the drug alone or 6 g of the powder of the drug and Rhizoma Bletillae can be taken as a dose with warm water, 3 times a day. In treating bleeding from trauma, the drug powder can be applied to the local area.

2. Controlling seminal emission and leukorrhea

In treating seminal emission and premature ejaculation, the drug can be used in combination with other drugs for tonifying the kidney and controlling seminal emission. In treating abnormal leukorrhea with bloody discharge, the drug can be used in combination with Radix Angelicae Dahuricae and Crinis Carbonisatus.

3. Relieving gastric hyperacidity to alleviate gastralgia

In treating gastric hyperacidity from gastritis and gastric ulcer, 240 g of the drug and 60 g of Bulbus Fritillariae Thunbergii can be ground into powder and 3 g of the powder is to be taken as a dose before meals. In treating gastric perforation from gastric ulcer, the drug can be used in combination with Rhizoma Bletillae.

4. Promoting tissue regeneration and removing dampness

In treating profuse pus over wound surface, eczema, ulceration of the lower limbs, etc., thc drug alone can be ground into powder and applied to the local area, or used in combination with Gypsum Fibrosum, Resina Draconis, Alumen, etc.

Dosage and Administration: Usually, 6–10 g of the drug is used in decoction. Proper amount of the drug can be used in external treatment.

19 Drugs for External Application and Other Purposes

All drugs used on the exterior of the body are called drugs for external application. Although some of the drugs for external application can be taken orally, they are used mainly on the exterior of the body.

Drugs for external application have such different functions as destroying parasites, removing toxin, subduing swelling, relieving pain, promoting tissue regeneration, arresting bleeding, etc. They have, therefore, a wide range of application and can be used respectively to treat various sores, ulceration, pyogenic infections, scabies, tinea, and diseases of the eye, ear, throat, nose, etc. Since diseases occurs in different locations with various manifestations, the form and methods of drug applications are different too, e.g. plaster application, topical application, smearing, fumigation, washing, etc.

Most of the drugs for external application have toxic effect of varying degrees. They should, therefore, be used with care, especially drugs with hypertoxicity, such as Hydrargyrum, Arsenolitum, Mylabris, etc. Overdosage is forbidden and they should not be applied to the head and the five sense organs, in order to avoid reactions caused by strong stimulation on the local area or poisoning due to absorption. When used for oral administration, this kind of drugs are often made into pills or powder, and when used for external application, the drugs are often used in combination, and it is rare for a crude drug to be used alone. In preparing drug agents, certain criteria should be strictly conformed to, so as to ensure safety in drug application.

Red Lead (铅丹 *Qiandan*)
Minium

This drug consists of the lead compound formed by melting black lead with sulphur, nitre, salt and vitriole. The drug is in powder form dark orange or orange in colour. The crude drug is used for medication.

Nomenclature Used in Prescriptions: *Qiandan, Zhangdan, Huangdan*

Properties and Channel Distribution: This drug is pungent in taste and slightly cold in nature with toxicity, and is distributed to the Heart, Spleen and Liver Channels.

Action and Indication:

1. Removing toxin and promoting tissue regeneration

It is used in combination with vegetable oil to form the base of plasters for external application.

2. Promoting expectoration to arrest convulsion

In treating epilepsy due to fright, palpitation, stuffy chest, insomnia, etc., the drug can be used in combination with Os Draconis, Concha, Ostreae, Radix Bupleuri, Radix Scutellariae, etc.

Dosage and Administration: When decocted, 1.5–4.5 g of the drug is used. When taken in pill or powder form, the dosage should not exceed 0.6 g as a dose. Proper amount of the drug is used in external application.

Notes: Overdosage or persistent oral administration are forbidden to avoid cumulative intoxication.

Axsenic Trioxide (砒石 *Pishi*)
Arsenicum

This drug consists of the prepared mineral Arsenolite. The drug may be either red or white in colour, the former being more often on sale in the market. The white powder arsenic trioxide obtained by purifying arsenolite through sublimation is of greater toxicity. The drug is decocted together with mung bean to reduce its toxicity and then ground into powder for medication.

Nomenclature Used in Prescriptions: *Hongpi, Baipi, Pishuang*

Properties and Channel Distribution: This drug is pungent and sour in taste and greatly heat in nature with hypertoxicity, and is distributed to the Lung, Spleen and Stomach Channels.

Action and Indications:

1. Corroding sores and removing slough (external application)

In treating ulcerative gingivitis, the drug can be used in combination with carbonized Fructus Ziziphi Jujubae, Borax, Indigo Naturalis, etc. In treating hemorrhoid, the drug is often used in combination with Alumen, Cinnabaris, etc. In treating scrofula, the drug powder is mixed with Chinese ink and is made into pills as large as the seeds of Chinese parasol tree, which are parched dry. In application, prick the disease area and half of a pill can be applied on the area until the scrofula seems to be corroded and disappear.

2. Eliminating phlegm to relieve asthma

In treating retention of phlegm with frequent attacks of asthma and dyspnea due to invasion of sold, pills made of it and Semen Sojae Preparatum are prescribed.

3. Preventing attacks of malaria

In treating malaria, the drug, Sulfur (decocted with vinegar) and Semen Phaseoli Radiatus (15 g each) can be ground into powder and made into pills (as large as mung beans) with water, and 3–5 pills are to be taken with warm water two hours before the attack.

Dosage and Administration: For external application, the drug powder can be applied to the local area or made into plasters and applied to the local area. For oral administration, the drug is made into pills and 0.002–0.004 g of the drug is used as a dose.

Notes: Persistent oral administration or overdosage are forbidden. The drug should not be taken by pregnant women.

Calomclas (轻粉 *Qingfen*)
Calomelas

This drug consists of the white cystalline powder (mercurous chloride) prepared from mercury, salt and vitriol through the method of sublimation. The crude drug is used.

Nomenclature Used in Prescriptions: *Qingfen*

Properties and Channel Distribution: This drug is pungent in taste and cold in nature with toxicity, and is distributed to the Lung, Large Intestine and Small Intestine Channels.

Action and Indications:

1. Destroying parasites and relieving itching

In treating scabies and tinea with itching of the skin, the drug can be used in combination with other drugs for removing toxin and relieving itching.

2. Relieving edema

In treating tympanites, edema and difficulty in urination and defecation seen in those with strong physiques and excess of *Qi*, the drug can be used in combination with Radix Euphorbiae Kansui, Flos Genkwa, Radix Euphorbiae Pekinensis, etc.

3. Removing toxin to treat external diseases

In treating frostbile, ulceration, syphilis, etc., the drug can be used in combination with other drugs for removing toxin.

Dosage and Administration: For external application, the dry powder or the powder mixed with water can be applied. For oral administration, 0.1–0.2 g of the drugs is used a day, to be taken 3 times. The drug is usually made into pills or powder and should not be decocted.

Notes: This drug has strong toxicity and therefore should be used with care. To avoid poisoning, overdosage or persistent oral administration are forbidden. After oral administration, it is necessary to rinse the mouth to avoid ulceration of the mouth and gum.

Red Mercuric Oxide and Yellow Mercuric Oxide (升药 *Shengyao*) Hydrargyri Oxidum Rubrum and Hydrargyri Oxidum Flavum

This drug consists of the compound prepared from equal amount of mercury, nitre and alum through sublimation. It may be red or yellow in colour, and is ground into powder for use. The drug is more effective if stored over a long time.

Nomenclature Used in Prescriptions: *Shengyao*

Properties and Channel Distribution: This drug is pungent in taste and hot in nature with strong toxicity.

Action and Indications:

Removing toxin and necrotic tissue

In treating ulceration from carbuncle or phlegmon to evacuate pus, remove necrotic tissue and promote regeneration of tissue, the drug is often used in combination with Gypsum Fibrosum Usta (ground into powder)for external application. When the ratio of Gypsum Fibrosum Usta to the drug is 9:1, the mixture is called Nine to One Drug, with relatively weak power of removing toxin. When the ratio of the two is 1:1, the mixture is called Five to Five Drug, with relatively strong power of removing toxin. When the ratio is 1:9, the mixture is called one to nine drug, its power of removing toxin is especially strong. These drugs can be selected according to disease conditions. They can be applied to the local area, or stuck to a paper spill, inserted into the vomica.

Dosage and Administration: The drug should not be taken orally and is only used in external application. Pure drug is usually not used.

Notes: This drug has strong power of removing toxin and necrotic tissues. Therefore it should not be used by those whose necrotic tissues or pus have been already removed, or those with erosion of vulva, chancre, etc. It should not be applied to the hand, foot, back, mouth, eye, nipple, umbilicus, and joints.

Sulphur (硫黄 *Liuhuang*)
Sulphur

This drug consists of the refined product of the natural ore Sulphur. The crude drug is ground into powder or decocted with bean curd (called *Yuzihuang* in Chinese) for medication.

Nomenclature Used in Prescriptions: *Liuhuang, Zhiliuhuang, Yuzihuang*

Properties and Channel Distribution: This drug is sour in taste and warm in nature with toxicity, and is distributed to the gate of life and the Pericardium and Large Intestine Channels.

Action and Indications:

1. Destroying parasites and relieving itching (for external application)

In treating scabies humida, tinea and intractable cellulitis of *Yin* nature, the drug can be used in combination with Calomelas, Realgar, Borneolum Syntheticum, etc.

2. Strengthening *Yang* to relax bowel (for oral adminstration)

In treating coldness and pain of the low back and knee and impotence due to decline of fire of the gate of life, asthma and dyspnea due to failure of the kidney to receive air, etc., the drug can be used in combination with drugs for strengthening *Yang* such as Radix Aconiti Praeparata, Cortex Cinnamomi, etc. In treating constipation of cold type due to cold syndrome of the spleen and stomach of deficiency type, the drug is often used in combination with Rhizoma Pinelliae (made into pills).

Dosage and Administration: The daily dosage is 1.5–6 g. The drug is usually made into pills or powder, Proper amount of the drug is used in external treatment. The crude drug is used for external application and the prepared drug, for oral administration.

Notes: The drug is contraindicated for those with deficiency of *Yin* and hyperactivity of *Yang*, or pregnant women.

Realgar (雄黄 *Xionghuang*)
Realgar

This drug consists of the mineral Realgar (composed of arsenic disulfide). The drug is ground into powder or refined into powder with water for medication.

Nomenclature Used in Prescriptions: *Xionghuang, Cihuang, Xiongjing, Yaohuang*

Properties and Channel Distribution: This drug is bitter and pungent in taste and warm in nature with toxicity, and is distributed to the Liver and Stomach Channels.

Action and Indications:

1. Removing toxin and destroying parasite

In treating carbuncle, sores, furuncle, eczema, scabies, tinea, etc., the drug can be used in combination with Resina Boswelliae Carterii, Resina Commiphorae, Myrrhae, or Cortex Phellodendri, Concha Ostreae, etc. In treating snakebite, equal amount of the drug and Faeces Trogopterorum can be ground into powder, and 6 g of the powder is to be taken at a time with wine. At the same time, the powder is to be applied to the local area.

2. Eliminating dampness and dispelling phlegm

In treating the urgent cases of acute sore throat, inflammation of the throat, and infantile convulsion with accumulation of phlegm, 30 g of the drug, 30 g of Radix Curcumae, 14 grains of Fructus Crotonis (with the shell and oil removed)are ground into powder, which is then cooked with vinegar and flour so as to make the mixture into pills as large as mung beans. Two to five pills (or less for children) is to be taken as a dose with warm water.

Dosage and Administration: The dosage is 0.2–0.4 g, and the drug is taken once or twice a day. The drug is usually made into pills or powder and should not be decocted. Proper amount of the drug can be used in external application.

Notes: Persistent oral administration is not advisable.

Calamine (炉甘石 *Luganshi*)
Calamina

This drug consists of the natural ore Smithsonite (composed mainly of zinc carbonate). The drug is calcined and then ground into fine powder with water, or mixed with decoction of Rhizoma Coptidis for medication.

Nomenclature Used in Prescriptions: *Luganshi, Feiganshi*

Properties and Channel Distribution: This drug is sweet in taste and neutral in nature.

Action and Indications:

1. Removing nebula to improve visual acuity

In treating conjunctival congestion and nebula, the drug is often used in combination with Borax, Borneolum Syntheticum, etc.

2. Removing dampness and promoting tissue regeneration

In treating chronic ulceration with much pus and wounds that does not heal, eczema, etc., the drug is often used in combination with Gypsum Fibrosum Usta, Concha Ostreae Usta, etc.

Dosage and Administration: Proper amount of the drug is used for external application. The drug can be elutriated and used as an eye drops. The drug powder can be applied externally.

Borax (硼砂 *Pengsha*)
Borax

This drug consists of the crystalline substance prepared from the ore Borax. The crude or calcined drug is used for medication.

Nomenclature Used in Prescriptions: *Pengsha*

Properties and Channel Distribution: This drug is sweet and salty in taste and cool in nature, and is distributed to the Lung and Stomach Channels.

Action and Indications:

1. Subduing swelling and removing toxin (for external application)

In treating sore throat and sores of the mouth and tongue, the drug is often used in combination with Borneolum Syntheticum, Natrii Sulfus Exciccatus and Cinnabaris. In treating conjunctival congestion with swelling and pain, the drug can be dipped in water and the liquid is used to wash the local area.

2. Clearing away heat and resolving phlegm

In treating unproductive cough due to accumulation of phlegm–heat, the drug can be used in combination with Cortex Mori Radicis, Fructus Perillae, etc.

Dosage and Administration: Usually, 1.5–3 g of the drug is used in decoction. When the drug is taken in pill or powder form, 0.6–1.5 g can be taken. Proper amount of the drug is used for external application. The crude drug is used to resolve phlegm and the calcined drug is used for external application.

Alum (明矾 *Mingfan*)
Alumen

This drug consists of the refined product of the mineral Alunite. The crude or calcined drug (the latter called *Kufan* in Chinese) is used for medication.

Nomenclature Used in Prescriptions: *Baifan, Mingfan, Kufan*

Properties and Channel Distribution: This drug is sour in taste and cold in nature, and is distributed to the Lung, Liver, Spleen, Stomach, and Large Intestine Channels.

Action and Indications:

1. Removing toxin to treat external diseases

This drug can be used to treat carbuncle, phlegmon, pyogenic infection, sores of the mouth and tongue, otopyorrhea, etc. In treating carbuncle, phlegmon and eczema, equal amount of the drug, Alumen, and Realgar can be ground into powder, mixed with strong tea and applied to the local area. In treating otopyorrhea, the powder of equal amount of the calcined drug and minium can be insufflated into the ear. In treating sores of the mouth and tongue with foul mouth in children, the powder of equal amount of the calcined drug and Cinnabaris can be applied to the local area.

2. Removing dampness to relieve itching

In treating eczema, scabies and tinea, the drug can be used in combination with Sulfur, Borneolum Syntheticum, etc. for external treatment.

3. Arresting diarrhea and bleeding

In treating long–lasting diarrhea, hemafecia, metrorrhagia, metrostaxis, leukorrhea, etc., the drug can be used in combination with Galla Chinensis, outer covering of Fructus Chebulae, etc. In treating hematemesis, equal amount of the drug and Catechu can be ground into powder and 1–1.5 g of the powder is to be taken as a dose with warm water.

4. Dispelling phlegm to induce resuscitation

In treating wind stroke with phlegm syncope, coma, lockjaw and accumulation of phlegm, equal amount of the drug and Spina Gleditsiae can be ground into powder and 1.5 g of the powder is to be taken as a dose with warm water to induce vomiting of phlegm. In treating epilepsy, the drug is often used in combination with Radix Curcumae.

Besides, the drug has the effect of clearing away heat to treat jaundice. It can be used (drug powder) to treat jaundice due to damp–heat.

Dosage and Administration: Proper amount of the drug is used for external application. When taken orally, 1–3 g of the drug is used as a dose. The drug is usually taken in pill or powder form.

Mylabris (斑蝥 *Banmao*)
Mylabris

This drug consists of the dried body of the insect Mylabris phalerata pall. and Mylabris cichorii L. (family Meloidae). The insect is deprived of its head and limbs, and is parched with polished glutinous rise till it turns brown or is parched with bran and decocted with venigar. It is then ground into powder for medication.

Nomenclature Used in Prescriptions: *Banmao*

Properties and Channel Distribution: This drug is pungent in taste and cold in nature with great toxicity.

Action and Indications:

1. Removing toxin and eroding sores

In treating carbuncle and phlegmon without diabrosis, or with diabrosis but without pus, the drug can be ground into paste with garlic and applied to the local area, and the drug paste is to be removed as soon as pus is formed. In treating various kinds of intractable tinea, the drug can be used in combination with Cortex Pseudolaricis, Scolopendra, Scorpio, Cortex Cinnamomi, Herba Asari, etc. In treating scrofula and fistula, the drug can be used in combination with Arsenicum Album, Radix Aconiti Kusnezoffii, Rhizoma Coptidis, etc., or the drug can be parched with polished glutinous rice. In treating bite by rabid dog, 3 mylabrises (with head and limbs removed), 9 g of Rhizoma Coptidis and 9 g of polished glutinous rice are parched and ground into powder and 1.5 g of the powder is to be taken as a dose with millet wine, once a day.

2. Removing blood stasis

In treating amenorrhea, the pills made of it and Semen Persicae and Radix et Rhizoma Rhei are prescribed.

Besides, the drug has been used in recent years to treat various kinds of cancers, with certain effect. For example, it is recorded in the " Dictionary of Traditional Chinese Meteria

Medica" that this drug can be used to treat carcinoma of the liver and stomach. Break the shell of an egg a little and put in 1–3 mylabrises. Bake the egg, remove the mylabrises and eat the egg, one egg each day. This drug can also be used to treat baldness by dippling the drug in wine and then applying the wine to the head, to promote hair growth.

Dosage and Administration: The dosage is 0.03–0.06 g. to be divided into 3 portions and taken. The drug is taken only in pill and powder form and should not be decocted. Proper amount of the drug is used in external treatment.

Notes: When applied to the skin, this drug may cause redness and appearance of blisters. It should, therefore, be taken with care, If poisoning occurs after oral administration, there may appear such symptoms as burning sensation in the throat, nausea, vomiting, abdominal colicky pain, hematuria, toxic nephritis, etc. Dosage for oral administration should be strictly controlled. The drug is contraindicated for pregnant women.

Toad Venom (蟾酥 *Chansu*)
Venenum Bufonis

This drug consists of the white secretion from the retroauricular gland and skin gland of the toad Bufo bufo gargarizans Cantor and B. melanostictus Schneider, etc. (family Bufonidae). The drug is usually made into a cake–form product. The crude drug is ground into powder for medication.

Nomenclature Used in Prescriptions: *Chansu*

Properties and Channel Distribution: This drug is sweet and pungent in taste and warm in nature with toxicity, and is distributed to the Heart and Stomach Channels.

Action and Indicatios:

1. Removing toxin and subduing swelling

In treating all kinds of carbuncle, phlegmon, sores, ulceration and furunculosis with hard swelling and pain, the drug is often used in combination with Calomelas, Borneolum Syntheticum, Moschus, Resina Boswelliae Carterii, Resina Commiphorae Myrrhae, Cinnabaris, etc.

2. Inducing resuscitation and restoring consciousness

In treating sunstroke manifested by coma, vomiting, diarrhea, abdominal colicky pain, distention in the chest and abdomen, etc., the drug is often used in combination with Realgar, Rhizoma Gastrodiae, Rhizoma Atractylodis, Flos Caryophylli, etc.

3. Destroying parasite and relieving pain

In treating toothache due to pathogenic wind or dental caries, a bit of the drug can be ground into powder with pepper and a bit of the powder (about the size of a grain of millet) is wrapped with cotton wool and placed in the painful area once or twice a day, Grit the teeth and spit out the saliva.

Dosage and Administration: The daily dosage for oral administration is 0.01–0.02 g. The drug is made into pills or powder and should not be decocted. This drug has toxicity and therefore should not be taken persistently. Proper amount of the drug is used in external treatment.

Nux–vomica Seed (马钱子 *Maqianzi*)
Semen Strychni

This drug consists of the ripe seed of the arbor Strychnos nux–vomica L. and the liana Strych–nospierriana A. W. Hill (family Loganiaceae). The drug is processed before being used.

Nomenclature Used in Prescriptions: *Maqianzi*

Properties and Channel Distribution: This drug is bitter in taste and cold in nature with strong toxicity, and is distributed to the Liver and Spleen Channels.

Action and Indications:

1. Removing obstruction in the channels and relieving pain

In treating arthralgia due to wind, cold and dampness, spasm, pain or numbness of joints throughout the body, etc., the drug can be used in combination with Herba Ephedrae, Rhizoma Atractylodis, Resina Boswelliae Carterii, Resina Olibani Myrrhae, Lumbricus, etc.

2. Subduing swelling

In treating fracture with stasis of blood, swelling and pain, the drug can be ground into powder with Eupolyphaga seu Steleophaga, Resina Boswelliae Carterii Praeparata, Resina Commiphorae Myrrhae Praeparata, Pyritum, Rhizoma Drynariae, etc. and applied to the local area. In treating inflammation. of the throat, equal amount of the drug, Radix Aristolochiae, Radix Sophorae Tonkinensis, etc. can be ground into powder, insufflated to the local area.

In addition, this drug is now used to treat cancer. Although certain therapeutic effect has been obtained, this is still at the experimental stage.

Dosage and Administration: The daily dosage for oral administration is 0.3–0.6 g. The drug is made into pills or powder and should not be decocted. Proper amount of the drug is used in external treatment.

Notes: This drug has toxicity and therefore it should be processed appropriately. To avoid poisoning, the dosage should be strictly controlled and the drug should not be taken over a long time. Overdosage of the drug may lead to the appearance of such symptoms as tremor of the limbs, paralysis, unconsciousness, or long–lasting contracture of the limbs. The drug is contraindicated in pregnant women.

Cnidium Fruit (蛇床子 *Shechuangzi*)
Fructus Cnidii

This drug consists of the ripe fruit of the annual herbage Cnidium monnieri (L.) Cusson (family Umbelliferae). The crude drug is used for medication.

Nomenclature Used in Prescriptions: *Shechuangzi*

Properties and Channel Distribution: This drug is pungent and bitter in taste and warm in nature, and is distributed to the Kidney Channel.

Action and Indications:

1. Warming the kidney and strengthening *Yang*

In treating impotence and female infertility due to deficiency of the kidney, the drug is often used in combination with drugs for tonifying the kidney and replenishing vital essence such as Semen Cuscutae, Fructus Schisandrae, etc.

2. Destroying parasite and relieving itching

This drug can be used to treat trichomonas vaginalis, eczema of scrotum, rubella, scabies, tinea, cutaneous pruritus, etc. In treating trichomonas vaginalis, steaming method or bathing method can be used by using the decoction of the drug, Radix Sophorae Flavescentis, Pericarpium Zanthoxyli, Radix Stemonae, etc., or 15 g of the drug can be ground into powder with some alum, and the powder is mixed with water, put on gauze and the gauze is inserted into the vagina once a day. In treating pruritus of vulva, 15 g of the drug, 3 g of alum, 6 g of Pericarpium Zanthoxyli and 12 g of Cortex Pseudolaricis can be decocted and the decoction is used to wash the local area. In treating itching due to eczema, the drug can be used in combination with Radix Sophorae Flavescentis, Fructus Kochiae, Rhizoma Atractylodis, etc.

Dosage and Administration: Usually, 3–10 g of the drug is used in decoction. For external application, 15–30 g of the drug is used. The drug is more often used for external application.

Wasp's Nest (露蜂房 *Lufengfang*)
Nidus Vespae

This drug consists of the nest of the insect Polistes mandarinus Saussure (family Vespidae) or other insects of the same genus. The nest is washed with wine or baked and ground into powder for medication.

Nomenclature Used in Prescriptions: *Fengfang, Lufengfang*

Properties and Channel Distribution: This drug is slightly sweet in taste and neutral in nature, and is distributed to the

Liver, Kidney and Stomach Channels.

Action and Indications:

1. Removing toxin to treat external diseases

In treating carbuncle, phlegmon, malignant boil, lumbodosal cellulitis, scrofula, etc., the drug can be used in combination with other drugs for removing toxin. In treating acute mastitis at the onset without suppuration, the drug (torn into pieces) can be baked till it turns brown (not black) and ground into powder, and 1.8–3 g of the powder is to be taken as a dose with 30 g of warm millet wine, to be taken every 4 hours. During drug administration, much water should be drunk. In treating gangrene of finger or toe, the drug can be baked, ground into powder, mixed with vinegar and applied to the local area once a day. In treating scrofula with fistula, the drug powder can be mixed with lard and applied to the local area.

2. Dispelling wind to relieve arthralgia

In treating rheumatic or rheumatoid arthralgia with pain, rigidity or deformity of the joints, the drug can be used in combination with Eupolyphaga seu Steleophaga, Scorpio, Scolopendra, etc. In treating itching from rubella, the drug can be used in combination with Periostracum Cicadae, Herba Spirodelae, Fructus Kochiae, etc.

3. Strengthening kidney–*Yang*

In treating incontinence of urination, equal amount of the drug (baked brown) and Oötheca Mantidis can be ground into fine powder and 3–6 g (or less for children) of the drug is to be taken with millet wine, once or twice a day.

Besides, the drug is often used in combination with Scolopendra, Scorpio, Gekko Swinhoana, etc. to treat carcinoma of the stomach, breast and lung, lymphadenectasis caused by cancerometastasis, etc., with marked therapeutic effect.

Dosage and Administration: For external application, the drug powder or decoction can be applied to or used to wash the local area. For oral administration, 6–12 g of the drug is used in decoction, or 1.5–3 g of the drug powder is taken as a dose.

Dragon's Blood (血竭 *Xuejie*)
Resina Draconis

This drug consists of the red resin of the evergreen trailing plant Daemonorops draco Bl. (family Palmae). The drug is wrapped in cloth, put into hot water to soften it into granules, and then cooled and dried. It is ground into powder for medication.

Nomenclature Used in Prescriptions: *Xuejie, Qilingjie*

Properties and Channel Distribution: This drug is slightly sweet and salty in taste and neutral in nature, and is distributed to the Heart and Liver Channels.

Action and Indications:

1. Removing blood stasis to relieve pain

In treating stasis of blood and swelling due to traumatic injury and fracture, the drug is often used in combination with Resina Boswelliae Carterii, Resina Commiphorae Myrrhae, Catechu, Flos Carthami, etc.

2. Promoting tissue regeneration to treat external diseases

In treating carbuncle, phlegmon and ulceration which do not heal, the drug is often used in combination with elephant's thick skin, Resina Boswelliae Carterii, Resina Commiphorae Myrrhae, Halloysitum Rubrum, Os Draconis, etc. In treating bone tuberculosis, the drug can be used in combination with Colophonium Semen Ricini, Semen Momordicae, Calomelas, etc. In treating epistaxis, gingival hemorrhage, bleeding from incised wound, etc., equal amount of the drug and Pollen Typhae can be ground into powder and the powder can be applied to the local area.

Dosage and Administration: For external application, the drug is ground into powder and applied to the local area. For oral administration. 1−1.5 g of the drug is taken as a dose. The drug is usually made into pills or powder and should not be decocted.

Notes: The drug is contraindicated for those without blood stasis.

Chaulmoogra Seed (大风子 *Dafengzi*)
Semen Hydnocarpi

This drug consists of the ripe seed of the evergreen arbor Hydnocarpus anthelmintica Pier. (family Flacourticeae). The seed (shell removed)is ground into mash or stewed to extract the oil for medication.

Nomenclature Used in Prescriptions: *Dafengzi*

Properties and Channel Distribution: This drug is pungent in taste and hot in nature with toxicity.

Action and Indications:

Removing dampness and destroying parasite

This drug can be used to treat scabies, tinea, leprosy, etc. In treating scabies, the drug is often used in combination with Juglandis Regiae, Hydrargyrum, etc. In treating intractable tinea, the drug can be used in combination with Colophonium, Radix

Sophorae Flavescentis, etc. In treating neurodermatitis, the drug can be used in combination with Semen Momordicae, Fructus Crotonis, Hydrargyrum, etc. In treating leprosy of various types, 30 g of the oil extracted from the drug and 90 g of the powder of Radix Sophorae Flavescentis can be mixed with a bit of wine and made into pills as large as the seeds of Chinese parasol tree and 50 pills are to be taken with warm wine before meals. The decoction of Radix Sophorae Flavescentis is to be used to wash the local area at the same time. In treating leprosy with ulceration and syphilis, 10 g of the drug (calcined) and 45 g of Calomelas can be ground into powder, mixed with sesame oil and applied to the local area.

Dosage and Administration: Proper amount of the drug can be used in external treatment. For oral administration, 0.3–1 g is to be taken as a dose. The drug is not to be decocted.

Dichroa Root (常山 *Changshan*)
Radix Dichroae

This drug consists of the root of the deciduous shrub Dichroa febrifuga Lour. (family Saxifragaceae). The drug is cut into slices and the crude drug, the vinegar–parched drug or the drug steamed with wine may be used for medication.

Nomenclature Used in Prescriptions: *Huangchangshan, Jiguchangshan, Jiuchangshan, Cuchangshan*

Properties and Channel Distribution: This drug is bitter and pungent in taste and slightly cold in nature with slight toxicity, and is distributed to the Lung, Heart and Liver Channels.

Action and Indications:

1. Eliminating phlegm and inducing diuresis

In treating retention of phlegm in the chest, the warm decoction of 9 g of the drug (vinegar–parched) and 4.5 g of Radix Glycyrrhizae (with addition of honey) can be taken to induce vomiting. If it fails, the decoction should be taken again.

2. Destroying parasite and preventing attack of malaria

This drug can be used to treat malaria. If the disease is due to phlegm–dampness, the drug is often used in combination with Semen Arecae, Fructus Tsaoko, etc. in treatment, and if the disease is due to phlegm–heat, the drug can be used in combination with Fructus Tsaoko, Rhizoma Anemarrhenae, Bulbus Fritillariae Thunbergii, Semen Arecae, etc.

Dosage and Administration: Usually, 3–10 g of the drug is used in decoction. The crude drug is rather drastic and the vinegar–parched drug has strong effect of inducing vomiting. The wine–prepared drug is used to treat malaria since this form of the drug is mild in property and does not cause vomiting when small dosage is used.

Luffa (丝瓜络 *Sigualuo*)
Retinervus Luffae Fructus

This drug consists of the reticulate fibre of the ripe fruit of the annual climbing herbage Luffa cylindrica (L.) Roem. or the withered fruit of L. acutangula Roxb. (family Cucurbitaceae). The drug is cut into sections for medication.

Nomenclature Used in Prescriptions: *Sigualuo*

Properties and Channel Distribution: This drug is sweet in taste and neutral in nature, and is distributed to the Lung, Stomach and Liver Channels.

Action and Indications:

Cooling blood, removing toxin, promoting the circulation of blood and removing obstruction from channels

This drug is used to treat chest pain due to stasis of *Qi* and blood, aching pain of muscles and bones, acute mastitis, etc., and can be used in combination with other drugs according to disease conditions.

Dosage and Administration: Usually, 10–15 g of the drug is used in decoction.

Catechu (孩儿茶 *Haiercha*)
Catechu

This drug consists of the extract from the peeled branch and stem of the deciduous arbor Acacia catechu (L.) Willd. (family Leguminosae). It is also called catechu extract and black catechu.

Nomenclature Used in Prescriptions: *Ercha, Haiercha*

Properties and Channel Distribution: This drug is bitter and puckery in taste and slightly cold in nature, and is distributed to the Lung Channel.

Actions and Indications:

Clearing away heat, removing dampness, treating external diseases and arresting bleeding

This drug can be used to treat eczema, aphthae in children, ulcerative gingivitis, bleeding from incised wound, etc. In treating eczema, the drug can be used in combination with Os Draconis, Calomelas, etc. In treating aphthae in children and ulcerative gingivitis, the drug can be used in combination with the natural solid deposit of human urine, Cortex Phellodendri, Indigo Naturalis, etc. In treating chancre, 3 g of the drug, 0.3 g of Calomelas and 0.015 g of Bomeolum Syntheticum can be ground into powder and applied to the local area. In treating bleeding from incised wound, the drug powder can be applied to the local area.

Dosage and. Administration: For external application, the drug powder is used. For oral administration, 0.1–1 g of the drug is taken as a dose in the form of powder, or mixed in the pills, for oral taking directly.

Ark Shell (瓦楞子 *Walengzi*)
Concha Arcae

This drug consists of the shell of the marine mollusc Arca inflata Reeve. or A. granosa L. or A. subcrenata Lischke. The shell is broken into small pieces and the crude or calcined drug is used for medication.

Nomenclature Used in Prescriptions: *Walengzi, Duanwaleng*

Properties and Channel Distribution: This drug is sweet and salty in taste and neutral in nature, and is distributed to the Lung, Stomach, Liver and Spleen Channels.

Action and Indications:

1. Resolving phlegm and softening hard masses

In treating accumulation of stubborn phlegm difficult to be expectorated, the drug can be used in combination with Os Costaziae, Bulbus Fritillariae Thunbergii, Flos Inulae, etc.

2. Removing blood stasis and disintegrating masses

In treating mass in the abdomen of females, the drug can be

used in combination with Rhizoma Sparganii, Rhizoma Zedoariae, Semen Persicae, Carapax Trionycis, etc.

3. Relieving hyperacidity and pain

In treating epigastric pain due to stasis of *Qi* and blood, the drug is often used in combination with Rhizoma Cyperi, Radix Aucklandiae, Faeces Trogopterorum, etc. In treating ulceration and gastralgia with acid regurgitation, 150 g of the drug and 30 g of Radix Glycyrrhizae can be ground into powder, and 9 g of the poeder is to be taken as a dose before meals, 3 times a day.

Dosage and Administration: Usually, 10–15 g of the drug is used in decoction. The crude drug is used to resolve phlegm and disintegrate masses and the calcined drug is used to relieve hyperacidity and pain.

2

中　药　学

序

《英汉实用中医药大全》即将问世，吾为之高兴。

岐黄之道，历经沧桑，永盛不衰。吾中华民族之强盛，由之。世界医学之丰富和发展，亦由之。然而，世界民族之差异，国别之不同，语言之障碍，使中医中药的传播和交流受到了严重束缚。当前，世界各国人民学习、研究、运用中医药的热潮方兴未艾。为使吾中华民族优秀文化遗产之一的岐黄之道走向世界，光大其业，为世界人民造福，徐象才君集省内外精英于一堂，主持编译了《英汉实用中医药大全》。是书之问世将使海内外同道欢呼雀跃。

世界医学发展之日，当是岐黄之道光大之时。

吾欣然序之。

中华人民共和国卫生部副部长
兼国家中医药管理局局长
世界针灸学会联合会主席
中国科学技术协会委员
中华全国中医学会副会长
中国针灸学会会长

胡熙明

1989年12月

序

中华民族有同疾病长期作斗争的光辉历程，故而有自己的传统医学——中国医药学。中国医药学有一套完整的从理论到实践的独特科学体系。几千年来，它不但被完好地保存下来，而且得到了发扬光大。它具有疗效显著、副作用小等优点，是人们防病治病，强身健体的有效工具。

任何一个国家在医学进步中所取得的成就，都是人类共同的财富，是没有国界的。医学成果的交流比任何其他科学成果的交流都应进行得更及时，更准确。我从事中医工作 30 多年来，一直盼望着有朝一日中国医药学能全面走向世界，为全人类解除病痛疾苦做出其应有的贡献。但由于用外语表达中医难度较大，中国医药学对外传播的速度一直不能令人满意。

山东中医学院的徐象才老师发起并主持了大型系列丛书《英汉实用中医药大全》的编译工作。这个工作是一项巨大工程，是一种大型科研活动，是一个大胆的尝试，是一件新事物。对徐象才老师及与其合作的全体编译者夜以继日地长期工作所付出的艰苦劳动，克服重重困难所表现出的坚韧不拔的毅力，以及因此而取得的重大成绩，我甚为敬佩。作为一个中医界的领导者，对他们的工作给予全力支持是我应尽的责任。

我相信《英汉实用中医药大全》无疑会在中国医学史和世界科学技术史上找到它应有的位置。

中华全国中医学会常务理事
山东省卫生厅副厅长

张奇文

1990 年 3 月

出版前言

中国医药学是我中华民族优秀文化遗产之一，建国以来由于党和国家对待中医药采取了正确的政策，使中医药理论宝库不断得到了发掘整理，取得了巨大的成绩。当前，世界各国人民对中国医药学的学习和研究热潮日益高涨，为促进这一热潮更加蓬勃的发展，为使中国医药学能更好地为全人类解除病痛服务，就必须促进中医中药在世界范围内的传播和交流，而要使这一传播和交流进行得更及时、更准确，就必须首先排除语言障碍。因此，编译一套英汉对照的中医药基本知识的书籍，供国内外学习、研究中医药时使用，已成为国内外医药学界和医药学教育界许多人士的迫切需要。

多年来，在卫生部门的号召下，在“中医英语表达研究”方面，已经作出了一些可喜的成绩。本书《英汉实用中医药大全》的编辑出版就是在调查上述研究工作的历史和现状的基础上，继续对中医药英语表达作较系统、较全面的研究，以适应中国医药学对外传播交流的需要。

这部“大全”的版本为英汉对照，共有 21 个分册，一个分册介绍论述中国医药学的一个分科。在编著上注意了中医药汉文稿的编写特色，在内容上注意了科学性、实用性、全面性和简明易读。汉文稿的执笔撰写者主要是有 20 年以上实践经验的教授、副教授、主任医师和副主任医师。各分册汉文稿撰写成后，均经各学科专家逐一审订。各分册英文主译、主审主要是国内既懂中医又懂英语的权威人士，还有许多中医院校的英语教师及医药卫生部门的专业翻译人员。英译稿脱稿后，经过了复审、终审，有些译稿还召开全国 22 所院校和单位人员参加的英译稿统稿定稿研讨会，对英译稿进行细致的研讨和推敲，对如何较全面、较系统、较准确地用英语表达中国医药学进行了探讨，从而推动整个译文达到较高水平，因此，这部“大全”可供中医院校高年级学生作为泛读教材使用。

这部“大全”的编纂得到了国家教育委员会、国家中医药管理局、山东省教育委员会、山东省卫生厅等各部门有关领导的支持。在国家教委高等教育司的指导下，成立了《英汉实用中医药大全》编译领导委员会。还得到了全国许多中医院校和中药生产厂家领导的支持。

希望这部“大全”的出版，对中医院校加强中医英语教学，对国内卫生界培养外向型中医药人才，以及在推动世界各国人民对中医药的学习和研究方面，都将产生良好的影响。

高等教育出版社

1990年3月

前　言

《英汉实用中医药大全》是一部以中医基本理论为基础，以中医临床为重点，较为全面系统、简明扼要、易读实用的中级英汉学术性著作。它的主要读者是：中医药院校高年级学生和中青年教师，中医院的中青年医生和中医药科研单位的科研人员，从事中医对外函授工作的人员和出国讲学或行医的中医人员，西学中人员，来华学习中医的外国留学生和各类进修人员。

由于中国医药学为我中华民族之独有，因此，英译便成了本《大全》编译工作的重点。为确保译文能准确表达中医的确切含义，我们邀集熟悉中医的英语人员、医学专业翻译人员、懂英语的中医药人员乃至医古文人员于一堂，共同翻译、共同对译文进行研讨推敲的集体翻译法，这样，就把众人之长融进了译文质量之中。然而，即使这样，也难确保译文都能尽如人意。汉文稿虽反映了中国医药学的精髓和概貌，但也难能十全十美。我衷心地盼望读者能提出批评和建议，以便《大全》再版时修改。

参加本《大全》编、译、审工作的人员达 200 余名，他们来自全国 28 个单位，其中有山东、北京、上海、天津、南京、浙江、安徽、河南、湖北、广西、贵阳、甘肃、成都、山西、长春等 15 所中医学院，还有中国中医研究院，山东省中医药研究所等中医药科研单位。

山东省教育委员会把本《大全》的编译列入了科研计划并拨发了科研经费，山东省卫生厅和一些中药生产厂家也给了很大支持，济南中药厂的资助为编译工作的开端提供了条件。

本《大全》的编译成功是全体编译审者集体劳动的结晶，是各有关单位主管领导支持的结果。在《大全》各分册即将陆续出版之际，我诚挚地感谢全体编译审者的真诚合作，感谢许多专家、教授、各级领导和生产厂家的热情支持。

愿本《大全》的出版能在培养通晓英语的中医人才和使中医早日全面走向世界方面起到我所期望的作用。

主编　徐象才

于山东中医学院

1990年3月

目　录

说　明

本书是大型系列丛书《英汉实用中医药大全》的第 2 分册。

中药是中医用以防病治病的重要工具之一，中药基础知识是中医临床各科医生所必须学习和掌握的。

本分册分总论和各论两部分。总论主要介绍了中药的炮制、中药的性能、中药的用法等基本理论知识。各论按中药的功效类别共分 19 章，介绍常用药物 363 种，附药 57 种。在每章开头，均以简要文字说明本章所介绍药物的含义、作用、适应证、配伍应用及注意事项。为叙述简要，特将每味药物的来源、炮制等合写成一段，然后再按处方用名、性味归经、功效应用、用量用法及使用注意事项等逐一叙述。在本分册所涉及的中药材中，有些来自濒临灭绝的珍稀动物。由于这些动物已明令禁捕禁杀，这些药材的来源也就因之而断绝。无论在医院里还是在制药厂里，它们均已被具有相同药效的其他药材所替代。本分册仍将其涉及，只是为方便学习探讨。

本分册汉义稿承蒙山东中医学院周凤梧教授审阅。泰安医学院亓秀恒教授、北京中医药大学方廷钰教授审阅了部分英文稿。

编者

总　论

1　中药的炮制

炮制，又称炮炙，是指中药材按照其不同的药性和医疗要求所进行的多种加工方法的总称。也就是药物在应用前或制成各种剂型之前的加工过程。由于中药材大都是生药，其中不少药材必须经过特定的炮制处理，才能更符合治疗需要，确保用药安全，充分发挥药效。

1.1　炮制目的

炮制的目的大致可归纳为以下几点：

1. 消除或减低某些药物的毒性、烈性或副作用。如川乌、草乌炮制后用，可减轻毒性；巴豆经去油用霜，可降低峻烈的泻下作用；常山酒炒可减轻其催吐的副作用等。

2. 增强药物的疗效。有些药物经炮制后，能增强原有效能。如延胡索经醋制后能增强其止痛作用；柴胡醋炙能增强其舒肝解郁之功；款冬花用蜜炙后可增强其润肺止咳功能等。

3. 改变药物的性能。有些药物因生熟而作用不同，经制后可改变原有功效。如地黄生用性寒而凉血，制成熟地黄，则性微温而补血；大黄生用泻下力强，制熟后则泻下力缓等。

4. 便于制剂和贮藏。一般植物类药材，用水浸润后便于切片。矿物类、贝壳类药材，质地坚硬，经煅、淬后则易于研粉。如煅磁石、煅龙骨、醋淬龟板与鳖甲等。药材经过切片或粉碎后，既便于制剂，又易于煎出有效成分。有些药材在贮藏前，要进行烘、炒等干燥处理，使其不易霉变，腐烂，便于长期存放。

5. 矫臭矫味。通过漂洗或经蜜、酒、醋、麸等炒制，以去除咸、腥、臭味，便于服用。如海藻、昆布漂去咸味；紫河车洗去腥味等。

6. 清除杂质和非药用部分，便于服用。如一般植物药的根和根茎当洗去泥沙，捡去杂质，枇杷叶要刷去绒毛，蝉蜕去头足，远志去心等。

1.2 炮制方法

炮制的方法很多，现将常用的 5 类叙述如下：

1. 修制

(1) 纯净处理：采用挑、拣、簸（扬）、筛、刷、刮等方法，去掉灰屑、杂质及非药用部分，以便药物洁净。如剪去合欢花的枝叶，刷去枇杷叶背面的绒毛，刮去厚朴的粗皮等。

(2) 粉碎处理：采用捣、碾、镑、锉等方法，使药物粉碎，以达到制剂和其他炮制方法的要求。如龙骨、牡蛎捣碎便于煎煮；羚羊角刨成薄片或锉成粉末，便于制剂和服用。

(3) 切制处理：采用切或铡的方法，把药物切制成一定的规格，使药物的有效成分易于煎出，且便于进行其他炮制，也有利于干燥、贮藏和配方时进行称量。根据药物性质和医疗的需要，切制有多种规格。如乌药、槟榔宜切薄片；山药、白术宜切厚片；桂枝、黄芪宜切成斜片；木香、苏木宜切成直片；枇杷叶、桑白皮宜切成丝；麻黄、忍冬藤宜切成段；葛根、六神曲宜切成小块等。

2. 水制：水制是用清水或其他液体辅料来处理药材的一类方法。水制的目的主要是清洁药物，减低药物的毒性，和软化药物，便于切制。常用的有洗淘、水漂、浸泡、淋润、水飞等。现介绍 3 种常用的方法。

(1) 润：又称闷或伏。是按照药物质地的软硬，加工时的气温、工具，采用淋润、洗润、泡润、浸润、盖润等多种方法，以使清水或者其它液体辅料渐渐渗透到药内，在不损失或少损失药效的前提下，使药物柔软，便于切制加工。如淋润香薷，酒洗润当归，泡润槟榔，姜汁浸润厚朴，盖润大黄等。

(2) 漂：是将药材置于宽水或长流水中浸渍一段时间，换水宜频，漂洗去药材中的盐分、腥臭味及毒性成分等非药用的杂质。如昆布、海藻、盐苁蓉漂去盐分，紫河车漂去腥味等。

(3) 水飞：是将药物与水同研制取微细粉末的一种方法。操作时，应先将药物打成粗末，然后置于研钵内，加入清水（淹没药面）共研，研至乳钵底部无响声时，再加入多量的清水，搅拌，使药物细浮、粗沉，随即倾出上层混悬液，剩下的粗末继续研磨，如此反复操作，至全部都成混悬液为止。然后将混悬液静置澄清，倾去清水，收取沉淀，晒干备用。此法适于不易溶解于水的矿石和贝壳类药物，目的既能防止研末时粉末飞扬，减少损耗，又能分离出溶解于水的杂质，使药物洁净，尤其能使药材粉研得特别细腻，内服时易于吸收，外用时可以减少刺激。如飞朱砂、飞滑石、飞炉甘石、飞雄黄等。

3. 火制：火制是应用最广泛的一种炮制法，是把药物直接或间接用火（或加入其它辅料）处理药材的一类方法。火制的目的是使坚硬的药材变为松脆，以便于制剂和服用，并可改变药物性能，提高疗效，消除或降低药物的毒性或烈性等。常用的有炒、炙、煅、煨、烫等多种方法。

(1) 炒：是一项多用、常用的炮制方法。炒有加辅料与不加辅料的炒法。不加辅料炒，叫清炒。根据炒的程度不同，又分为炒黄、炒焦、炒炭三种。炒黄、炒焦使药物易于粉碎加工，且缓和药性。种子类药物炒后易于煎出有效成分。炒炭能缓和药性和副作用，或增强收敛止血作用。还有拌固体辅料如土、麸、米炒的，能减少药物的刺激性，增强疗效。如土炒山药，麸炒椿皮，米炒党参等。与砂、滑石粉、海蛤粉等药料同炒的方法习称烫。药物烫炒可使其受热均匀酥脆，使有效成分易于煎出或便于服用。如砂炒穿山甲、蛤粉炒阿胶等。

(2) 炙：亦称制。是用液体辅料拌炒药物，使辅料慢慢渗入药物内部，改变药性，增强疗效或减少副作用的一种炮制方法。常用的液体辅料有蜜、酒、醋、姜汁、盐水、油等。如蜜炙紫菀、冬花可增强润肺止咳之功；酒炙川芎可增强活血作用；醋炙元胡能增强止痛之效；盐炙杜仲可增强补肾作用等。

(3) 煅：是将药物用强火直接或间接烧制的一种方法。可使药物质地松脆，易于碾碎研粉，充分发挥疗效。坚硬的矿物药或贝壳类药物，如海蛤壳、紫石英等多直接用火煅烧到红透时取出晒凉，碾碎即得。间接煅是将药物置于耐火容器中密闭煅烧，至容器底部红透为止，如煅血余炭、陈棕炭等。

(4) 煨：用文火烘烤药材的方法叫煨。是利用湿纸或湿面粉包裹药物，置热火中煨至纸或面焦黑为度，可降低药物的毒性和烈性。如煨肉豆蔻、煨诃子等。

4. 水火共制：水火共制是既用水又用火或同时加入其它辅料的一类综合性的炮制方法。水火共制的目的是改变药性，增强药效，消除或降低药物的毒性和副作用，并能纯净药物，便于切制等。常用的有蒸、煮、燀、淬等。

(1) 蒸：是将药材置于蒸罐或笼中隔水加热利用水热和蒸气蒸制药材的一种方法。如酒蒸大黄可缓和泻下作用。某些药物经反复蒸、晒，才能获得适于医疗需要的作用。如何首乌经反复蒸晒后，不再有泻下之力，而有补肝肾益精血之功。

(2) 煮：是将药物置于清水或液体辅料中加热煮沸的方法。如醋煮芫花可减低毒性；酒煮黄芩能增强清肺热之功等。

(3) 燀：是将药物迅速投入沸水中，经短暂潦过，立即取出的一种方法。常用于需要去皮的种子类和肉质多汁类药物的处理。如燀杏仁、桃仁以去皮；燀马齿苋、天门冬以便于晒干贮存等。

(4) 淬：是将药物煅烧红透后，立即投入冷水或液体辅料中，使之松脆的一种方法。经淬后既易于粉碎，且辅料亦被其吸收，能发挥预期疗效。如醋淬自然铜、鳖甲；黄连煮汁淬炉甘石等。

5. 其它制法：除上述四种类型之外，还有一些较繁杂而特殊的炮制方法，常用的有发芽、发酵、制霜和部分法制法等。其目的是为改变药物原有性能，产生新的疗效，减少毒性或副作用。如稻、麦的发芽；经发酵制取神曲、淡豆豉；巴豆去油取霜；法制半夏等。

2　中药的性能

中药的性能，是指药物的性味和功能，也就是中药的药性理论。其内容主要包括四气、五味，升降浮沉，归经及有毒与无毒等。这些内容都是前人在长期的医疗实践中逐步探索归纳出来的，是从不同方面说明药物作用，以指导临床实践的。所以熟悉中药性能，对临床用药具有重要意义。

中药的药性理论是整个中医理论的组成部分之一。祖国医学认为，每种药物都具有一定的特性，或偏于寒，或偏于热，或升或降，以调整机体阴阳气血的偏胜偏衰，恢复生理平衡，从而达到治疗目的。这就是运用药物治病的基本原理，也是药物性能的基本概念。

2.1　四气和五味

四气、五味，就是药物的性味。每一药物都有性和味两方面。药物的功效与性味又有密切关系。所以，四气和五味是中药性能的主要理论，对指导临床实践具有重要意义。

四气的“气”又称为“性”，所以四气也就是四性，即寒、热、温、凉四种不同的药性。这四种药性，都是我国历代医药学家在长期与疾病作斗争中，经过反复的实践观察，根据药物作用于人体之后，所发生的不同反应和治疗效果而作出的概括性的归纳。例如：能治疗热证的药物，大多属于寒性或凉性；能治疗寒证的药物，大多属于热性或温性。因此，药性的寒、热、温、凉，是与病情的寒热相对而言的。

药性的寒凉与温热，是绝对不同的两类药性。寒与凉，温与热，仅是区别药性程度上的差异，凉次于寒，温次于热。所以在历代本草书籍中常有微寒、大温的记述。所谓微寒，就相当于凉；大温，即相当于热。

寒与凉，温与热，虽然程度上有所不同，但因其属性是一致的，所以在作用上则有它一定的共同点：即寒凉性药具有清热、泻火、解毒等作用，常用于治疗热性病证；温热性药具有散寒、温里、助阳等作用，常用于治疗寒性病证。

除寒热温凉四性之外，还有一种平性药，由于这类药物寒凉或温热之性不甚显著，作用比较平和，不论寒证热证，皆可配用。所以，按药性来说实有五气，但一般则常称四气。

五味，就是辛、甘、酸、苦、咸5种不同的味道。这些味道可由舌感辨别。药物除此五味之外，还有一种淡味，因其药味不甚明显，前人将它附属于甘，故历代本草常甘淡并称，因而也就习称“五味”。但按药味及作用来说，实际上是六味。

前人在长期医疗实践中，发现药物的味和它的功用之间有一定联系，也就是不同味道的药物有不同的治疗作用，从而便总结出来了五味的用药理论。现将辛、甘、酸、苦、咸、淡等味的意义和作用分述如下：

辛：就是辛辣或辛凉的滋味，具有能散能行的作用。一般发汗与行气的药物，大多数有辛味。多用于外感表邪或气血阻滞的病证。

甘：就是甜的滋味，一般具有滋补、和中或缓急作用的药物，大多数为甘味。多用于虚证或调和药性及某些疼痛的疾病。

酸：具有能收能涩的作用。一般酸味的药物大多数能收敛、固涩。多用于虚汗外泄，久泻不止，遗精带下等症。此外，还有不少酸味药物，同时带有涩味，由于涩味作用与酸味相似，故一般均未分列。

苦：具有能泻（能降）、能燥、能坚的作用。一般具有清热、泻火、泻下、燥湿及降逆作用的药物，大多数为苦味。多用于热性病，大便不通，湿盛中满，咳嗽呕逆等症。前人的经验，认为苦能坚阴，如黄柏、知母用于肾阴虚亏而相火亢盛的痿症，即具有泻火存阴（坚阴）的意义。

咸：具有能下能软的作用。一般咸味的药物，能软化坚硬，消散结块或泻下通便。多用于瘰疬、痞块、便秘等症。

淡：就是淡而无味，具有能渗能利的作用。一般能渗利水湿，通利小便的药物大多为淡味。多用于湿邪阻滞，小便不利等症。

随着临床实践的发展，经过概括起来的五味，一旦形成了用药理论，它的含义就超过了直接的舌觉，后来就运用这些道理，把具有收敛作用的药物，统称为酸味；具有软坚作用的药物，统称为咸味等等。所以有的药味就形成本草记载与实际口尝不相符合的情况。例如赤石脂味酸，牡蛎味咸，麻黄味辛等均与口尝不符，这都是参照其疗效而得出来的。

气和味是论述和运用中药的主要依据。每一种药物都具有气和味两个方面，一般气味相同的药物，往往作用相近，如辛温药物，大都有解表散寒作用，这是它的共性。但每一种药物，又各有特性，如紫苏、生姜气味辛温，都能发汗散寒，但紫苏发汗功效较强，并有行气安胎作用，而生姜则发汗功效较弱，另有温胃止呕作用。这是气味相同功效相近而药物作用不同的特点。气味不同的药物，作用则显著不同。如气同味异的黄连、浮萍，都为寒性，但黄连苦寒，可清热燥湿，浮萍辛寒，则发散风热。又如气异味同的黄芪、石斛都为甘味，但黄芪甘温，可温补阳气，石斛甘寒，则养阴清热。此外，还有很多一药兼有数味者，如桂枝辛甘，郁金辛苦等，从药物的发展来看，一般味愈多，说明其作用范围相应的愈大。由于药物气味比较复杂，所以，我们不但要熟悉四气五味的一般规律和药物的共性，还必须掌握每一药物的特性和治疗作用，以便更好地指导临床运用。

2.2 升降浮沉

升、降、浮、沉，是指药物作用于人体上下表里的作用趋向而言。升是上升，降是下降，浮是外行发散之意，沉是内行泻利之意。升与浮，沉与降，其趋向是类似的，升浮药物一般都主上升和向外，有升阳、发表、散寒、涌吐等作用；沉降药物一般都主下行和向内，有潜阳、降逆、清热、渗湿、泻下等作用。药物这种升降浮沉的作用，是与临床病变的部位和病势的趋向相对应的。一般说来，大多是同病位而逆病势，凡病变部位在上在表的，宜升浮而不宜沉降；病变部位在下在里的，宜沉降而不宜升浮；若病势上逆的，宜降而不宜升；若病势下陷的，宜升不宜降。如果倒行逆施，往往导致不良后果。所以药物升降浮沉的理论，对某些药物来说，在治疗上是有一定意义的。

药物升降浮沉的不同作用，一般来说，与药物的气味及质地的轻重有一定的关系。凡味属辛、甘，气属温热的药物，大都具有升浮的作用；凡味苦、酸、咸，性属寒凉的药物，则大都具有沉降的作用。凡质轻的药物，如薄荷、辛夷等花叶类的药材，大都能够升浮，质重的药物，如根茎类、果实种子类、矿物类及介壳类药材，大都能够沉降。但也有不少例外情况，如蔓荆子、苍耳子等皆属果实类药，其性反而升浮；旋复花、番泻叶等皆为花叶类药，其性反而沉降。这说明在一般规律中，有些药物又有其特殊性。

由于升降浮沉的主要依据与药物的气味有关，所以升降浮沉的不同作用，实际上已寓于四气五味的作用之中。因此，就每种药物来说，都有升降浮沉的含义，但在临床实际应用中，除部分药物须注意其升降浮沉的特性外，多数药物的应用还是以性味功效为主。所以药物的升降浮沉，仅是从另一方面说明其作用和另一种归纳形式。

药物的升降浮沉，虽是以气味为基础，但是也每随炮制和配伍而有所转化。如沉降药经酒制或与较多较强的升浮药同用，可随之上升；升浮药经盐制或与较多较强的沉降药同用，也可随之下降。这说明升降浮沉在一定的条件下，可以互相转化而不是一成不变的。因此，在临床用药时，除需掌握一般原则外，还要了解其中的变化，以便运用自如。

2.3 归经

归经，是指药物对于机体某部分的选择性作用——主要对某经（脏腑及其经络）或某几经发生明显的作用，而对其它经则作用较小，或没有作用。也就是指明药物治病的适应范围。

药物在人体所起的作用，皆有一定的适应范围，如同属寒性药，虽然都具有清热作用，但有的偏清肺热，有的偏清肝热；再如同一补药，有的是补肺，有的是补脾。因此，中国医药学便根据脏腑经络学说，结合药物的作用，把所有药物分别归于十二经，以说明某药对某些脏腑经络的治疗作用，这便形成了药物的归经理论。

药物的归经，主要是根据其所作用的脏腑经络来确定的。因为经络能沟通人体内外表里，在病变时，体表的疾病可以影响到内脏；内脏的病变也可以反应到体表。因此，人体各部分发生病变时所出现的证候，便可通过经络获得系统的认识。如肺经病变，每见喘咳等症；肝经病变，每见胁痛、抽搐等症。根据药物的功效，与脏腑、经络密切结合起来，就可以说明某药对某脏腑经络病变起着主要作用。如桔梗、杏仁能治咳喘胸闷，故归肺经；羚羊角、钩藤能熄风止搐，归肝经。这说明归经的理论，具体指出药效的所在，是从疗效观察中总结出来的。

至于一种药物可以归入数经的，是说明对数经都有治疗作用。如石膏归肺胃二经，是说明石膏既能清肺热，也能清胃热；党参归脾肺二经，是说明党参既能补脾气，也能补肺气。

药物的归经，对临床治疗亦有重要意义。例如肝热目赤，在清热药物中，就可选用能清肝热的药物治疗；胃寒腹痛，在祛寒药物中，就可选用温胃止痛药物治疗。从而也就便利了临床的脏腑用药。所以在重点熟悉药物功用的同时，进一步明确和了解某些主要药物的重要归经，仍是必要的。

此外，归经虽然具体指出了药效所在，便利了临床应用，但由于脏腑经络病变，可以互相影响，因此在临床用药时，并不单纯地使用某一经药。如肺病而见脾虚的，除用治肺药外，还可用补脾的药物，因脾能健运，可促进肺病痊愈。总之，既要了解药物的归经，又要掌握脏腑经络之间的相互关系，才能更好地指导临床用药。

综上所述，四气、五味是说明中药性能的主要理论，升降浮沉是指导药物功用的趋向，归经则是药物功能的适应范围。但是四气、五味不是药物作用的唯一根据；升降浮沉和归经理论，有的归经较多，各家记载也不一致；升降浮沉对药物的运用，亦缺乏普遍的指导意义。所有这些理论，都是前人从长期临床实践中总结出来的。我们应当尊重和认真学习，同时还应不断深入研究和整理。

3　中药的用法

中药的用法主要包括药物的配伍、禁忌、用量和服法等几项内容。掌握这些知识和方法，在按照病情、药性和治疗要求使用药物时，对于充分发挥药物疗效和确保用药安全具有十分重要的意义。

3.1　配伍

使用中药治病，能用单味药达到治疗目的的，最好使用单味药。这样既简便、经济，又容易掌握。但往往由于病情复杂，有时数病相兼，或表里同病，或虚实并见，或寒热错杂，单味药不能达到治疗目的，就必须根据药物的性能选用几种药物配伍应用，才能适应复杂多变的病情，收到较好的疗效。所以中药的配伍，就是按照病情需要和用药法度，将两种以上的药物合用，利用药物与药物之间的相互作用，使其互相协同，提高疗效；或使其互相抑制，减低不良作用，更好地发挥药物的效能。配伍的目的就是为了适合病情的需要，照顾全面，充分发挥药物疗效，保证用药安全。

前人把单味药的应用和药与药之间的配伍关系，总结为“七情”。其内容即单行、相须、相使、相畏、相恶、相杀、相反等七个方面。

单行：即主用一种药物单独发挥作用，不配它药辅助。如独参汤。

相须：两种以上功效类似的药物，合用以后，可以明显地增强其原有疗效。如乳香与没药合用，可明显地增强活血止痛的作用。

相使：两种以上功用不同的药物分主辅合用后，能提高主药疗效。如清热泻火的黄芩与攻下泻热的大黄配伍时，大黄能提高黄芩清热泻火的功效。

相畏：即一种药物的毒性反应或副作用，能被另一种药物减低或消除。如生半夏和生南星的毒性能被生姜减轻或消除，所以说生半夏和生南星畏生姜。

相杀：即一种药物能减弱或消除另一种药物的毒性或副作用。如生姜能减轻或消除生半夏和生南星的毒性或副作用，所以说生姜杀生半夏和生南星的毒。由此可见，相畏、相杀实际上是同一配伍关系的两种不同提法，是从药物之间某一方面而言的。

相恶：即两种药物合用，能相互牵制而使原有作用降低甚至丧失药效。如干姜能降低黄芩清热作用。

相反：即两种药物同用后，能产生毒性反应或剧烈的副作用。如"十八反"中的药物。

上述的"七情"，除"单行"外，其它6个方面，主要说明药物与药物配伍之间的关系有着协同、抑制及对抗等作用。其中如"相须"、"相使"，因药物间相互产生协同作用而增进疗效，是常用的配伍方法；"相畏"、"相杀"，因药物之间的相互作用，能减轻或消除原有的毒性或副作用，这是应用具有毒性、烈性药物时的配伍方法；"相恶"与"相反"，前者因互相的拮抗能使其原有功效减弱或消除，后者因相互作用而产生毒性反应或强烈的副作用，二者均属不宜配伍。尤其是"相反"药物，虽然古今医方中某些反药亦有同用之例，但一般多作配伍禁忌，原则上多避免配用。根据前人的经验，现在临床实际常用的配伍方法，主要可概括为相须配伍、相使配伍、相制配伍等3方面。

由上可见，中药的配伍，是使用单味药的进一步发展，也是组合方剂的重要基础，对临床处方用药具有重要意义。

3.2 用药禁忌

药物有防治疾病的一面，也有不利于人体的一面。如寒凉药虽能清热，但又易伤阳；辛热药虽可祛寒，但又能耗阴；攻伐药固可祛邪，但又能伤正；滋补药固能扶正，但又可恋邪等等。因此，我们既要了解它的防治疾病作用，又要了解它可能产生的副作用。特别对药性较猛或有毒的药物，尤须引起重视，或避免使用，或通过炮制、配伍及减轻剂量等方法，以纠正或减少其偏胜之性后再用。这些对人体不利的方面和要注意的问题，就是通常所说的"禁用"（忌用）和"慎用"。属方药禁忌范围的内容较多，大体有如下几个方面：

1. 证候禁忌：由于药物的药性不同，其作用各有所长和一定的适应范围，因此，临床用药也有禁忌。例如麻黄辛温发汗，表散风寒，又能平喘，但必须是外感表实无汗，或肺气不宣的外感咳嗽方能使用，若表虚多汗，或肺虚咳喘就要忌用。所以，除药性极为平和的无须禁忌外，一般药物都有证候禁忌，尤其对偏性较大的药物，更应注意。具体内容详见中药各论每一药物的"使用注意"部分。

2. 配伍禁忌：在传统医药文献中，记载着某些药物不能在同一方中应用，否则就会降低疗效或产生毒性反应，这就是"配伍"一节中所提到的"相恶"和"相反"。历代关于配伍禁忌的认识和发展，在古籍中说法并不一致。影响较大的乃金元时期，所概括的"十八反"和"十九畏"，并编成歌诀，便于习诵。其内容列举于下：

(1) 十八反：甘草反甘遂、大戟、海藻、芫花。乌头反贝母、栝楼、半夏、白蔹、白芨。藜芦反人参、沙参、丹参、玄参、细辛、芍药。

(2) 十九畏：硫黄畏朴硝，水银畏砒霜，狼毒畏密陀僧，巴豆畏牵牛子，丁香畏郁金，川乌、草乌畏犀角，牙硝畏三棱，官桂畏赤石脂，人参畏五灵脂。

“十八反”和“十九畏”中的畏、反诸药，相沿皆为配伍禁忌，但其中部分药物，历代医家亦有同用之例。如甘遂半夏汤，以甘草与甘遂合用；海藻玉壶汤，以甘草和海藻并施；感应丸中巴豆同牵牛相配；十香返魂丹中丁香与郁金互伍等等。现代有些实验研究初步表明，如甘草与甘遂两药合用，毒性的大小主要取决于甘草的用量比例，甘草的用量若与甘遂相等或大于甘遂，则毒性较大；又如半夏和贝母分别与乌头配伍，未见明显毒性增强。而细辛配伍藜芦，则可导致实验动物中毒死亡。对“十八反”和“十九畏”的问题，目前正从文献、临床应用和实验方面不断深入研究，尚无定论，所以要采取慎重态度，对于其中一些药物，若无充分根据和应用经验，应避免盲目配用。

(3) 妊娠用药禁忌：由于有些药物有损害胎元以致堕胎的副作用，所以妇女在怀孕期间，应把这些药物作为妊娠禁忌药，防止引起流产及不良反应。大凡剧毒药、峻泻药、祛瘀药及热性较强和芳香走窜药，皆属妊娠用药禁忌范围。

根据药力峻缓损害胎元的程度不同，一般可分为禁用和慎用2类。凡毒性较强或药性猛烈的药物，如巴豆、斑蝥、牵牛、大戟、甘遂、芫花、商陆、麝香、三棱、莪术、水蛭、虻虫等均属禁用；一般破血、破气或燥热、沉降的药物，如桃仁、红花、大黄、枳实、附子、干姜、肉桂等可斟酌慎用。不论禁用与慎用，如没有特殊必要，应尽量避免使用，以防发生事故。但若遇有孕妇患严重疾病，不使用上述猛烈药物而病不去者，则应慎重考虑，酌情使用。

(4) 服药时的饮食禁忌：饮食禁忌，简称食忌，俗称“忌口”，即服用某些药物或在服药期间，对某些与病情有碍的食物，应注意避免或节制食用。古代文献中记载：常山忌葱；地黄、何首乌忌葱、蒜、萝卜；鳖甲忌苋菜；薄荷忌鳖肉；甘草忌鲢鱼；茯苓忌醋；土茯苓、使君子忌茶；以及蜜反生葱等。此外，有些疾病亦须注意饮食宜忌。如麻疹表证不宜食油腻酸涩之物；疮疖肿毒、皮肤瘙痒不宜食鱼虾、牛羊等腥膻及刺激之品；热证不宜食辛辣膻腻等食物；寒证不宜食瓜果等生冷食物；经常头晕、失眠、性情急躁者，应忌胡椒、辣椒、酒、茶；消化不良者应忌油炸食品等等。

3.3 剂量

由于中药大都是配伍并制成各种剂型来应用的，因此，剂量的涵义就包括每一种药物的用量，方剂中各药物的相对用量，以及制剂的实际服用量等。不过通常所说的用量，大多是指每种药物的用量和全方的剂量而言。

药物剂量的大小与疗效有直接关系，药量过小则起不到治疗作用；药量过大，非但达不到预期疗效，甚至可造成不良后果。所以中药的应用，除应注意配伍外，还要注意方药的剂量。一般说来，中药绝大部分是原生药，药性比较平和，安全剂量的幅度较大，因此用量没有化学药品那样严格。但对某些性质峻烈或剧毒的药物（如乌头、甘遂、马钱子等），用量必须严格掌握，以免发生意外。对于药物剂量大小的掌握，可根据以下 3 方面考虑。

1. 根据药物性能确定剂量：凡有毒、峻烈的药物，用量宜小，并应从小量开始，根据病情需要，再逐渐增加，不要过量。一旦病势减退，应逐渐减量或立即停服。以防中毒或产生副作用。一般药物，质重的如矿物、贝壳类药，用量宜大；质轻的如花、叶类，以及芳香走散的药物，用量宜轻；厚味滋腻的药物，用量可稍重。

2. 根据配伍、剂型确定剂量：一般说来，同样的药物，一味单用剂量较入复方为重；入汤剂用量较作丸剂、散剂为重；在复方中的主药用量较辅助药为重。

3. 根据患者病情、体质、年龄确定剂量：一般重病、急性病及病情顽固的，用量宜重；轻病、慢性病用量宜轻。病人平素体质壮实的用量宜重；年老体弱、妇女和儿童用量宜轻。新病用量宜重，久病用量宜轻。一般6岁以上儿童，可按成人量减半用，5岁以下通常用成人量的$\frac{1}{4}$，乳幼儿应更少。

关于中药的计量单位（重量），以往都沿用16进位的旧制，即10厘为1分，10分为1钱，10钱为1两，16两为1斤。也就是1斤＝16两＝160钱。目前已普遍改用公制，即1公斤＝1 000克。为便于处方和配药时换算起见。按规定采用近似值进行换算。即：1两（16进位制）＝30克　1钱＝3克　1分＝0.3克　1厘＝0.03克。

本书各药所标注的用量，除特别注明者外，都是指干燥后的生药在汤剂中的成人1日内服量而言。若用于小儿，可按上述比例酌情减少。

3.4　用法

中药的用法，有内服和外用之分。这里主要是指常用汤剂的煎煮应当注意的事项与各种药剂的服用方法。

1. 煎药法：为使药物更好地发挥疗效，必须注意药物的煎煮方法。汤剂又叫煎剂，是一种液体制剂，即将药物加水煎煮后，去渣取液而成。这是最常用的一种剂型。具有易于吸收、疗效较速、制备简单等特点，但味苦量大，不便携带服用。

(1) 煎药用具：宜用砂锅、瓦罐或搪瓷器皿。忌用铁器，以防与含有鞣质、有机酸等成分的药材起变化反应，影响质量和疗效。

(2) 煎药用水：用水必须洁净，一般可用清澈的泉水、河水与自来水，井水须选择水质较好的。用水量可视药量大小而定，以漫过药面1寸左右为宜。

(3) 煎药火候：一般宜先武后文，即药液未沸时用武（急）

火，煎沸后用文（慢）火。

(4) 煎煮方法：煎煮前，应先将药物浸泡半小时，以便有效成分的煎出。每剂通常可煎煮两次。头煎水分以高出药物0.5～1寸为宜，加热至沸，不时翻动，煮沸20～30分钟后，倾出药液。二煎时加水以浸没药物为度，煮沸20分钟后，取液去渣。然后再将两次煎取的药液混合在一起分次服用。

煎煮汤剂，不宜用猛火，应先武后文，以使药物有效成分溶出。解表药及其他芳香性药物，用水宜少，煎煮时间宜短（可少煎10分钟），避免香气挥发，药性损失；滋补药，用水宜多，煎煮时间宜长（多煎10分钟），使其有效成分尽量溶出。

由于各种药物的特性不同，在煎汤剂时，还应根据方剂中药物的不同情况而给以不同的处理：

①先煎：有些矿石、贝壳类药物，如生石膏、生牡蛎等，因其质地坚硬，应打碎先煎，即先以武火加热至沸，煎煮15分钟后，再将其它药物倾入同煎，才能充分煎出其有效成分。对某些毒性药物，如天南星、生草乌等，亦应文火先煎或久煎，以降低其毒性。

②后下：有些芳香类药物，如薄荷、砂仁等，因大多含有挥发性成分，煎煮时间宜短，宜后下入锅。即待其它药物煎沸15分钟后，再倾入共煎5～10分钟，以免煎煮过久，有效成分挥发，减低药效。对含蒽甙成分的药物，如大黄、番泻叶等，亦宜后下或短煎，以免影响其泻下作用。

③包煎：有些粘性较强的药物，如车前子等，直接入水煎煮，易使锅底焦糊；有些带毛的药物，如旋复花等，直接入水煎，则药汁中毛不易滤去，服药时刺激咽喉。这些有碍煎煮或不易过滤的药物，应包入纱布袋中，和其它药物入汤同煎。

④另煎：有些贵重药物，如人参、犀角片等，为了保持其有效成分，避免损耗，宜另煎取汁，然后将渣加入其它药中合煎，最后将两次药汁总合服用，以充分发挥药效。

⑤冲服：有些贵重而用量较小或不宜入煎的药物，如琥珀、朱砂、三七、鸡内金等，应研成细粉，随汤剂或用温开水冲服。

此外，还有些胶类、无机盐类药物，如阿胶、芒硝以及饴糖等，因水煎易糊，又难以过滤，宜直接溶于药液或开水中烊化内服。

2. 服药法：服药方法，是根据病情和药性决定的。掌握服法与药物疗效有一定关系。因此，我们必须掌握：

(1) 服药方法：汤剂都宜温服。寒证服热药，可以热服；热证用寒药，可以冷服。但有时寒热错杂，相互格拒，可出现服药反吐的情况，如属真寒假热则又宜热药冷服；如属真热假寒，则又宜寒药热服。对呕吐不止的患者，可少服、频服；对神志昏迷或牙关紧闭的患者，可给予鼻饲。丸、散等固体药剂，除特殊规定外，一般都用温开水吞服。有用酒服者，是取其升提宣通；用淡盐汤送下者，是取其引药入肾。

(2) 服药时间：补益药宜在饭前服；对胃肠有刺激的药物宜在饭后服；杀虫药及泻下药宜在空腹时服；治疟药宜在发作前服；安神药宜在睡前服。当然还须根据病情的缓急而改变服药时间。如急性病应立即服药，不拘时间；慢性病服丸、散、膏、酒者应有定时，如1日3次或每日早晚各1次，以使药物持续发挥治疗作用。此外，根据病情，有的也可煎汤代茶，频频饮服。

无论饭前或饭后服药，都应略有间隔，一般都在饭前后1～2小时左右，否则影响疗效。

一剂中药，通常一天分2～3次服用。病缓者可早晚各服1次，病重病急者可每隔4小时服药1次，使药力持续，利于顿挫病势。在应用发汗、攻下等药时，尚须注意患者体质，若药力较强，一般以得汗、下为度，中病即止，不必尽剂，以免汗、下太过，损伤正气。

各　论

1　解表药

凡通过发汗解肌，能使人体出汗或微出汗以发散表邪，解除表证的药物，称为解表药。

解表药多具有辛味，以入肺、膀胱二经为主。辛能发散，肺外合皮毛，膀胱主一身之表。所以解表药善走肌表，而具有程度不同的发汗解表作用，故适用于邪犯肌表的外感表证。其具体应用，一般有以下几个方面:

1. 感受外邪，具有发热、恶寒、头痛、项强、身痛、无汗、脉浮等表证者。

2. 某些解表药能开宣肺气，而有平喘止咳作用，可用于表邪犯肺，肺气不宣的喘咳。

3. 某些解表药有缓和疼痛作用，除可治有表邪的头痛、身痛外，还可用于风湿痹痛。

4. 某些解表药能促进疹毒透发，故适用于风疹、麻疹等表邪未解，或需要透发者。

5. 解表药通过发汗可以消肿，其中有些药物还兼有行水作用，所以还可用于水肿有表证或腰以上肿者。

解表药虽具有辛散发表的共性，但其药物性质又有温与凉的不同，所以适应的表证也就有所区别。因此，解表药又分为辛温解表药与辛凉解表药两类。辛温解表药适于恶寒重，发热轻的表证；辛凉解表药适用于恶寒轻，发热重的表证。临床应根据症状，选择使用。

解表药虽能通过发汗解除表证，但汗过多亦能耗散阳气，损伤津液，所以凡表虚自汗，阴虚发热，或热病后期，津液亏耗，以及失血等症，均当慎用或禁用。

1.1 辛温解表药

辛温解表药，又称发散风寒药。因其性味多属辛温，发散作用较强。适用于外感风寒，恶寒，发热，无汗，头痛，身痛，舌苔薄白，脉浮紧等风寒表证。有些药物对咳喘、水肿、疮疡兼有风寒表证以及风湿痹痛也可应用。

本类药物大多有较强的发汗作用，体虚者当慎用。

麻　黄

为麻黄科多年生草本状小灌木植物草麻黄 Ephedra sinica Stapf. 中麻黄 E. intermedia phedra Schrenk et C.A.Mey. 或木贼麻黄 Ephedra eguisetina Bunge. 的干燥草质茎。阴干切段，生用或蜜炙用。

处方用名 生麻黄、炙麻黄。

性味归经 辛、微苦，温。入肺、膀胱经。

功效应用

1. 发汗解表：用于外感风寒，发热，头、身疼痛，鼻塞，无汗，脉浮紧等表实证，常与桂枝配用，以增强发汗解表之功。

2. 宣肺平喘：用于风寒外束，肺气不宣所致之喘咳，通常与杏仁配用，以增强平喘作用；若兼内有寒饮，咳喘痰多清稀，可与干姜、细辛、五味子、桂枝等同用，以温肺化饮而平喘止咳；若属热邪壅肺而致喘者，常与石膏配伍，以宣肺清热平喘。

3. 利水消肿：用于水肿实证而兼有表证者，一般常与白术同用。

此外，取麻黄温散寒邪之功，与其它相应药物配伍，亦可治疗风湿痹痛及阴疽等。

用量用法 1.5～9克。煎服。生用发汗力强，多用于发汗解表，利水退肿；炙用发汗力弱，并有润肺作用，多用于止咳平喘。

使用注意 本品发汗力强，用量不宜大。表虚自汗，心悸，失眠，喘咳由于肾不纳气者均应忌用。高血压患者，亦不宜用。

桂 枝

为樟科植物肉桂 Cinnamomum cassia presl 的干燥嫩枝。晒干或阴干，切成薄片或小段用。

处方用名 桂枝、川桂枝、嫩桂枝。

性味归经 辛、甘，温。入心、肺、膀胱经。

功效应用

1. 发汗解肌：用于外感风寒表证，不论有汗无汗皆可应用。如表虚有汗，常与白芍同用，以调和营卫；若表实无汗，常与麻黄相须为用，以增强发汗之力。

2. 温经止痛：用于风寒湿痹，肩臂肢节痠痛。通常配羌活、防风与芍药、附子、白术、知母等同用；若风湿在表，表阳偏虚者，可与附子等配伍；如营卫不足，血痹顽麻者，可与黄芪、芍药等同用。用于胃寒腹痛，喜按喜温，常与芍药、饴糖等配用；用于妇女血寒瘀滞，月经不调或经闭腹痛等症，常与当归、芍药、川芎、桃仁、丹皮等活血通经药配伍。

3. 通阳化气：用于脾阳不运，痰饮内停，背寒胁胀，咳逆头眩等症，常与茯苓、白术等配伍，以温运脾阳，化湿利水；如膀胱气化不行，小便不利，常与茯苓、猪苓、泽泻等同用，以助阳化气利水；如胸痹胸痛，常与瓜蒌、薤白同用；心悸、脉结代，可与甘草、人参、阿胶等配伍，以助阳复脉。

用量用法 3–10克。煎服

紫　苏

为唇形科1年生草本植物紫苏 Perilla Frutescens（L.）Britt.的全草。阴干切段用。如单用叶片，称苏叶。单用茎，称苏梗。生用。

处方用名　紫苏叶、苏叶、老苏梗。

性味归经　辛，温。入肺、脾经。

功效应用

1. 散寒解表：用于感冒风寒，恶寒发热，头痛鼻塞等。常与荆芥、防风、生姜等同用。若兼有肺气不宣之咳嗽，常与杏仁、前胡等同用，以增强宣肺止咳作用；兼气滞胸闷者，每与香附、陈皮等同用。

2. 行气和胃：用于脾胃气滞，胸闷呕吐等症。偏寒者，常与藿香、半夏、生姜等同用；偏热者，常与黄连、竹茹等同用；偏气滞痰结者，又常与半夏、厚朴等同用。还用于气机不利，胎动不安，胸闷气胀，呕吐，恶心等症，常与陈皮、砂仁等同用，以加强止呕、安胎的功效。本品为行气安胎之常用药。

3. 解鱼蟹毒：用治食鱼蟹中毒，呕吐、腹泻、腹痛等症，可配伍藿香、陈皮、生姜等煎服。

用量用法　6～12克，治食鱼蟹中毒，可用30～60克，煎服。本品茎叶分用，苏叶长于发表散寒，苏梗善于理气安胎，故表散风寒，可用苏叶；理气安胎，可用苏梗。

荆　芥

为唇形科1年生草本植物荆芥 Schizonepeta tenuifolia Briq.的干燥地上部分。扎把晒干。茎叶与穗并切段，或单用穗。生用或炒炭用。

处方用名　荆芥、荆芥炭、荆芥穗、炒芥穗、芥穗炭。

性味归经　辛，微温。入肺、肝经。

功效应用

1. 散风解表：用于外感风邪，恶寒发热，无汗头痛等症。其性虽微温，但温而不燥，性质平和，以辛散疏风为主，故既能用于散风寒，又可用以散风热。表证属风寒者，常与防风、白芷、生姜等配伍；属风热者，常与薄荷、银花、连翘等同用；若有目赤咽肿，症属风热所致者，可与薄荷、牛蒡子、柴胡、桔梗、甘草等同用。

2. 宣毒透疹：用于麻疹透发不畅、荨麻疹及疮毒初起，可与防风、蝉蜕、牛蒡子、苦参等随症配用。

3. 散瘀止血：用于吐血、衄血、便血等症，通常用荆芥炭配合其它止血药同用。

此外，用于产后外感邪毒，项强，口噤痉挛，有理血散风止痉作用，可单用炒芥穗6克，研末，用黄酒或童便冲服。

用量用法 3～10克，煎服。发表宜生用，止血宜炒用。

防 风

为伞形科多年生草本植物防风 Ledebouriella divari cata (Turcz) . Hiroe的干燥根。切片，晒干，生用。

处方用名 防风、青防风、口防风。

性味归经 辛、甘，微温。入膀胱、肝、脾经。

功效应用

1. 祛风解表：用于外感表证，头痛身痛。本品为治风通用之品，因其微温而不燥，甘缓而不峻，药力和缓，故有“风药中润剂”之称，表证不论属风寒、风热皆可配用。前者常与荆芥同用；后者常与薄荷、桑叶同用；用于风疹、皮肤瘙痒，常与荆芥、牛蒡子、白蒺藜等同用。

2. 胜湿止痛：用于外感风湿及风寒湿痹，常与羌活、独活、川芎等同用，以增强祛风除湿之功。

3. 祛风止痉：用于破伤风，角弓反张，牙关紧闭，痉挛抽搐等症。常与天南星，天麻、白附子同用。

此外，据方书记载，本品配甘草可解砒石中毒。

用量用法　3～10 克，煎服。

羌　活

为伞形科多年生草本植物羌活 Notopterygium Ting ex H.T. Chang 或宽叶羌活 Notopter ygium forbesii Boiss 的根茎和根。切片晒干用。

处方用名　羌活、川羌活、西羌活。

性味归经　辛、苦，温。入膀胱、肝、肾经。

功效应用

1. 散寒解表：用于外感风寒，恶寒发热，头痛身痛等，常与防风、细辛、川芎等同用。

2. 祛风胜湿：用于风湿痹痛，肩背肢节疼痛或一身尽痛，对上半身肌肉风湿痛，或腰背肌肉有自觉畏冷挛缩者，用之尤宜。本品祛风胜湿，散寒止痛较强。常与独活、防风等同用。

用量用法　3～10 克，煎服。治感冒，用量宜轻；治风湿，用量稍重。一般剂量均不宜过多。

细　辛

为马兜铃科多年生草本植物北细辛 Asarum heterotro poides Fr. var. mandshuricum （Maxim.） Kitag. 或华细辛 Asarum sieboldi Miq. 的干燥全草。阴干切段用。

处方用名　细辛、辽细辛、北细辛。

性味归经　辛，温。入肺、肾经。

功效应用

1. 散寒解表：用于素体阳虚，感冒风寒，恶寒发热，寒重热轻，舌苔水滑，脉沉者，常与麻黄、附子同用，以助阳解表。

2. 祛风止痛：用于头晕头痛，可与羌活、防风、川芎、白芷等配用；用于风冷牙痛，可用本品3克，配川乌1.5克，乳香3克，白芷3克，共研细末，每用少许擦患处，日数次。若属风火牙痛，亦可用本品3克，配石膏30克，水煎服。用于风寒湿痹，关节疼痛，常与羌活、独活、防风、秦艽等同用。

3. 温肺化饮：用于痰饮咳喘，痰多清稀，常与干姜、半夏、麻黄等同用。

4. 宣通鼻窍：用于鼻渊，症见鼻塞头痛，时流清涕，可与白芷、辛夷、薄荷等配伍。

此外，本品外用亦可治疗口舌生疮。以细辛研末，水调敷脐部，另以黄连汁涂患处。

用量用法 入汤剂1～3克。外用适量，可研末吹鼻或外敷。

使用注意 阴虚阳亢头痛，阴虚肺热咳嗽等忌用。用量不宜过大。反藜芦。

白　芷

为伞形科多年生草本植物兴安白芷 Angelica dahurica (Fisch. ex Hoffm.) Benth. et Hook. f. 或杭白芷 Angelica dahurica (Fisch. ex Hoffm.) Benth. et Hook. f. var. formosana (Boiss.) Shan et Yuan 的干燥根。切片晒干用。

处方用名 白芷、杭白芷、香白芷。

性味归经 辛，温。入肺、胃经。

功效应用

1. 散寒解表：用于风寒感冒，头痛偏于额部者，常与荆芥、防风、蔓荆子、羌活等同用。

2. 祛风止痛：用于头风痛、偏头痛、眉棱骨痛、鼻渊头痛、齿痛。治头风头痛，单用或配川芎、菊花、防风、羌活同用；治鼻渊头痛，可配苍耳子、辛夷；治风冷牙痛，可与细辛合用；风火牙痛，可与石膏配伍。

3. 消肿排脓：用治疮疡肿痛，初起能消散，溃后能排脓，为外科所常用；治乳痈肿痛，常与栝楼、贝母、蒲公英等同用；若治其它痈肿，常与银花、连翘等配伍。

4. 化湿止带：用于妇女寒湿带下，色白清稀，常与白术、茯苓、海螵蛸等配伍应用。

用量用法 3～9克。煎服。

藁 本

为伞形科多年生草本植物藁本 Ligusticum sinense Oliv. 或辽藁本 Ligusticum jeholense Nak. et kitaga 的干燥根及根茎。切片晒干，生用。

处方用名 藁本、川藁本。

性味归经 辛，温。入膀胱经。

功效应用

1. 散寒解表：用于感冒风寒，头痛、恶寒无汗，常与羌活、防风、细辛等同用。

2. 祛风胜湿：用于风寒犯脑，巅顶脑后俱痛，连及齿颊，或风湿头痛、头风，尤为巅顶局部性头痛的常用药。本品兼通督脉，善达巅顶而能止痛。常与白芷、川芎、细辛等同用。用于风寒湿邪侵袭所致的痹痛，肢节疼痛等，常与羌活、独活、防风、威灵仙等同用。

用量用法 3～10克。煎服。

使用注意 若头痛属于血虚，非属风寒湿邪者忌用。

苍 耳 子

为菊科一年生草本植物苍耳 Xanthium sibiricum patr. et widd.的干燥成熟带总苞的果实。炒去硬刺用。

处方用名 苍耳子。

性味归经 辛、苦、温。有小毒。入肺经。

功效应用 1. 散风通窍：用于风寒头痛、头风头痛及鼻渊。治风寒及头风头痛，常与防风、白芷、藁本等同用；本品为治鼻渊要药。用治鼻渊头痛，时流浊涕，不闻香臭，常与辛夷、白芷同用。

2. 除湿止痛：用于风湿痹痛，肌肉麻痹，可与羌活、防风、当归、牛膝等同用。

用量用法 3～10克。煎服。

使用注意 本品有小毒，服用过量可引起中毒，出现上腹胀闷，恶心呕吐，有时腹痛腹泻，头痛烦躁等症状。

附药

1. 苍耳草：即苍耳的全草。切段晒干用。苦辛微寒，有毒。功效主治与苍耳子相似，但解毒之力尤强，故善治一切痈疮疔疖，肿毒湿疹及蜂刺、虫咬等症，均可用鲜草洗净捣烂外敷。或用鲜草切细，水煎浓，去渣过滤，文火收膏（万应膏），每服1.5～3克；并可外涂。用量干者5～10克，鲜者10～15克，煎服。外用适量。

2. 苍耳虫：即寄居在苍耳茎中的一种昆虫的幼虫。采取后，浸入麻油中备用。能解毒消肿。治疗疔疮肿毒。每用1～2条，捣烂，放在膏药上，贴患处。

辛 夷

为木兰科落叶灌木植物辛夷 Magnoliq liliflora Desr. 的花蕾。晒干。捣碎生用。

处方用名 辛夷、辛夷苞。

性味归经 辛，温。入肺经。

功效应用

1. 散风寒：用于风寒感冒，头痛鼻塞等症，可与白芷、防风、川芎等同用。

2. 通鼻窍：用于鼻渊头痛，鼻塞流浊涕，不闻香臭。本品为治鼻渊要药。偏于风寒者，常与白芷、细辛等配用；偏于风热者，常与薄荷、黄芩等同用。

现常用治慢性鼻炎、过敏性鼻炎、肥厚性鼻炎、上颌窦炎等鼻腔疾患，除煎服外，尚可制成油剂、乳剂与散剂局部滴用或吹敷，均有良效。

用量用法 3～9克。煎服。外用适量，研末塞鼻。

生　姜

为姜科多年生草本植物姜 Zingiber officinale (Willd.) Rosc.的新鲜根茎。洗净，切片鲜用。捣汁名生姜汁，单独用皮称生姜皮，煨熟名煨姜。

处方用名 生姜、鲜生姜。

性味归经 辛，微温。入肺、脾、胃经。

功效应用

1. 发汗解表：用于风寒感冒，因其发汗之力较弱，故多作辛温发汗剂中之辅助品，以增强发汗作用。一般伤风感冒症轻者，可与红糖煎服或沸水浸泡服。

2. 温胃止呕：用于胃寒呕吐，常与半夏同用。其它某些止呕药，亦每用姜汁炮制，以增强止呕作用。

3. 温肺止咳：用于风寒咳嗽，痰白清稀，常与其它散寒止咳药配伍同用。

4. 解毒：能解半夏、南星毒，故半夏、南星多用姜制；若内服或误食半夏、南星中毒，觉喉舌麻痹者，可捣姜汁冲服或煎汤内服。

用量用法 3～10克。煎服。

附药

1. 生姜汁：辛散之力较强，功能开痰止呕，多用于中风痰迷，口噤昏厥及呕吐不止等症。用量3～10滴，冲服。

2. 生姜皮：辛凉。功能行水。主治皮肤水肿。用量3～6

克。

3. 煨姜：为生姜用纸包润湿入火煨熟而成。辛散之力不及生姜，而温中止呕作用则较生姜为胜，适于脾胃虚寒，腹痛呕吐或大便泄泻等症。用量3～10克。

葱　白

为百合科多年生草本植物青葱 Allium fistulosum L. 近根部的白茎。鲜品生用。

处方用名　葱白、葱白头。

性味归经　辛，温。入肺、胃经。

功效应用

1. 发汗解表：用于感冒风寒初起之轻症，常与豆豉或生姜同用。

2. 散寒通阳：用于阴寒内盛，虚阳上越，四肢厥冷，下利稀便，面赤，脉微，可与干姜、熟附子同用。若寒凝气阻，脘腹疼痛，或小便闭胀者，亦可炒热外熨脐部或小腹部。

用量用法　3～10克，或3～5枚。煎服。外用适量。

使用注意　不宜与蜂蜜同服。

柽　柳

为柽柳科落叶灌木或小乔木植物柽柳 Tamarix chinensis Lour.桧柽柳 Tamarix juniperina Bge. 或多枝柽柳 Tamarix ramossima Ledeb.的细嫩枝叶。切段生用。

处方用名　柽柳、赤柽柳、西河柳、三春柳。

性味归经　辛，平。入肺。胃、心经。

功效应用　解表透疹：用于麻疹初期，透发不出或已出又为风邪外束而内闭者。本品辛散外达，并善解血分之毒，为透发麻疹之专药。常与葛根、牛蒡子、蝉蜕、淡竹叶等同用。

此外，因其又能祛风止痒，故可外用煎汤洗浴，治疗皮肤瘙痒性疾病。

用量用法 3~10克。鲜者加倍。煎服。外用煎汤熏洗，用量不拘，可将药入酒水中煎沸，或先将酒水煮沸后入药，再煎1、2沸，然后用热气熏蒸手足，乘热喷其胸部，或用药汤外洗四肢，促使微汗，使疹易透出。一般头面勿洗，以免头面出疹过多。

使用注意 麻疹已透者不宜用。内服剂量不宜过大，以免患者出现心烦不安。

香　薷

为唇形科多年生草本植物海洲香薷 Elsholtzia splendens Nakai ex F. Maekaw 的全草。切碎生用。

处方用名 香薷、香茹。

性味归经 辛，微温。入肺、脾、膀胱经。

功效应用

1. 发汗解表，和脾化湿：用于夏暑季节，外伤于寒，内伤于湿所致恶寒身热，头重头痛，胸闷，无汗，腹痛吐泻等症。如贪凉饮冷，阳气为阴气所遏，表里同病。常与扁豆、厚朴同用。

2. 利水消肿：头面浮肿，恶寒无汗，小便不利者，用香薷500克，煎汁去渣熬膏，加白术粉250克为丸，每次9克，日2~3次，白水送服。

用量用法 3~10克。煎服。用于解表，煎时宜短；用于消肿，煎时宜长。本品有特殊香气，热饮易呕，可凉服。

使用注意 夏伤暑热，症见高热，大渴，汗多者，为“阳暑”，当忌用。

1.2 辛凉解表药

辛凉解表药，又称发散风热药。本类药物性味多属辛苦寒凉之品，发汗作用比较缓和。适用于外感风热初起，具有一般表症而热象突出的，如恶寒轻，发热重，口渴，无汗或有汗，舌苔薄白而干或薄黄，脉浮数等。有些药还有透疹作用，常用于风疹、麻疹等症。临床多与清热类药物配伍应用。

薄　荷

为唇形科多年生草本植物薄荷 Mentha haplocalyx Briq. 的茎叶。切短段生用，或采鲜者用。

处方用名　薄荷、薄荷梗、薄荷叶、鲜薄荷。

性味归经　辛，凉。入肺、肝经。

功效应用

1. 疏散风热：用于外感风热，发热微寒，头痛无汗，及温病初起而有表证者，常与银花、连翘等同用；热盛者，可与石膏配伍；若夏感暑热，头昏，发热，口渴，小便短赤者，可与滑石、甘草配用。

2. 清头目，利咽喉：用于风热感冒或风火上攻引起的头痛目赤，咽喉肿痛等症，常与荆芥、防风、菊花、牛蒡子、桔梗、甘草等同用。

3. 透疹止痒：用于麻疹初期，透发不畅，或风热外束肌表，麻疹不透、以及风疹，皮肤瘙痒等症，常与连翘、蝉衣、牛蒡子、荆芥、防风等同用。

此外，用治肝郁不舒，胸胁胀痛，亦可少量加入舒肝方中用之。

用量用法　3～10 克，鲜者可用 15～30 克。煎服。因含挥发油，不宜久煎。发散风热多用叶，理气舒肝多用梗。

牛　蒡　子

为菊科 2 年生草本植物牛蒡 Arctium lappa　L. 的成熟果实。微炒，捣碎用。

处方用名　牛蒡子。

性味归经　辛、苦、寒。入肺、胃经。

功效应用

1. 疏散风热：用于感冒风热，喉痒咳嗽，吐痰不爽等症。常与荆芥、桔梗、甘草等同用。

2. 利咽散结：用于咽喉肿痛。属风热者常配疏风解热药同用；属火热者，可与泻火解毒药同用；风火热毒较甚者，二者亦常相互配伍。

3. 宣肺透疹：用于麻疹透发不畅及荨麻疹等。可与荆芥、防风、银花等其他疏风透疹、解毒药同用。

4. 解毒消肿：用于痈肿疮毒兼有风热或便秘症状者。可与清热解毒药配用。

用量用法　5～10克。煎服。

使用注意　本品具有清肠通便作用，便溏者慎用。

桑　叶

为桑科落叶小乔木桑树 Morus alba L. 的叶片。晒干，捣碎生用。

处方用名　桑叶、霜桑叶、冬桑叶。

性味归经　苦、甘，寒。入肺、肝经。

功效应用

1. 疏散风热：用于感冒风热，头痛目赤或风温初起，发热咳嗽等症。常与菊花、连翘、薄荷、杏仁等同用。

2. 清肺止咳：用于燥热伤肺，咳嗽咽干之症。常与杏仁、象贝母、麦冬、石膏等同用。

3. 清肝明目：用于风热目赤涩痛，可配菊花、决明子等同用；用于肝阳上升，头昏目眩，常与菊花、钩藤等配伍；若肝肾不足，目视昏花，亦可用桑叶500克、黑芝麻150克研末蜜丸久服。

用量用法　6～12克。煎服。

菊　花

为菊科多年生草本植物 Chrysanthemum morifolium Ramat. 的头状花序。阴干用。

处方用名　甘菊花、杭菊花、滁菊花、黄菊花、白菊花。

性味归经　甘、微苦、微寒。入肺、肝经。

功效应用

1. 疏散风热：用于外感风热，发热，头痛等，常与桑叶、薄荷、连翘等同用；如风热目赤肿痛，可与防风、白蒺藜等配伍。

2. 平肝明目：用于肝阳上亢，头痛，头晕，目眩等，常与石决明、钩藤、生地、白芍等同用；若肝肾阴虚，血不养目之眼目昏花，可与熟地黄、枸杞子等配伍。

用量用法　9～15 克。煎服。疏散风热，多用杭菊花（黄菊花）；平肝明目，多用滁菊花（白菊花）。

附药　野菊花：为菊科多年生草本植物野菊 Chrysanthemum indicum L. 的干燥头状花序。晒干用或鲜用。性味苦辛微寒。功能清热解毒消肿，根、叶亦有同样疗效。主要用于痈疖肿疡，咽喉肿痛，风火赤眼等。常与清热解毒、明目和利咽喉药物配用，内服外用皆可。用量 10～15 克，大剂可用至 30 克。捣烂外敷或煎汤外洗，用量不拘。

蔓　荆　子

为马鞭草科落叶灌木或小乔木单叶蔓荆 Vitex rotundifolia L. 和 V. trifolia L. 的果实。阴干，炒至焦黑色。

处方用名　蔓荆子。

性味归经　辛、苦、微寒。入膀胱、肝、胃经。

功效应用

1. 疏散风热：用于风热感冒，头痛眩晕，或头风头痛连齿频等症，常与菊花、薄荷、川芎、钩藤、防风、石膏等随症选用。

2. 清利头目：用于风热所致目赤肿痛，头目昏暗，常与菊花、决明子等配伍应用。

用量用法 6～12克。煎服。

葛根

为豆科多年生落叶藤本植物葛 Pucraria lobata (willd.) Ohwi的根。晒干生用。花亦入药，生用。

处方用名 葛根、粉葛根。

性味归经 甘、辛、凉。入胃、脾经。

功效应用

1. 解肌退热：用于外感表证，发热、无汗、头痛、项背发紧等症。如恶寒重者，可与麻黄、桂枝、芍药等同用；发热重者，可与柴胡、黄芩、石膏等配伍。

2. 生津止渴：用于热病表证口渴及消渴证，单用或与清热生津药配用。

3. 透发麻疹：用于麻疹初起或透发不畅，常与升麻、芍药等同用。

4. 升阳止泻：用于脾虚泄泻，常与党参、白术、茯苓等健脾药同用；若热泻、热痢兼有表证者，亦可与黄连、黄芩等配伍。

此外，还用于高血压脑病，对改善头痛，眩晕，项强等症状有效。冠心病心绞痛用之也可获得一定效果。

用量用法 6～15克。煎服。

附药 葛花：为葛的未开放的花蕾。晒干用。性味甘平。能醒胃止渴，解酒毒。可治酒醉呕吐、口渴之症，常与砂仁、豆蔻、泽泻、白术、茯苓、猪苓等同用。用量6～12克。入煎剂。

柴　胡

为伞形科多年生草本植物北柴胡 Bupleurum chinense DC. 和狭叶柴胡 Bupleurum scorzonerifolium Willd. 的根或全草。醋炒用。

处方用名　柴胡、北柴胡、嫩柴胡、春柴胡、醋柴胡。

性味归经　苦、辛，微寒。入肝、胆经。

功效应用

1. 透表泄热：用于感冒发热，常与葛根等同用，以透泄表热；用于寒热往来，常与黄芩配伍，以和解少阳。本品长于疏散少阳半表半里之邪，为治邪在少阳寒热往来的主药。疟疾的寒热往来，亦为常用，每与黄芩、常山、草果等配伍。

2. 升举阳气：用于气虚下陷脱肛、子宫脱垂、胃下垂等，常与人参、黄芪、升麻等补气升阳药同用。

用量用法　3～10 克。用于退热，必要时可用至 15～30 克，且需久煎浓煎。醋炒用能减低散性及增强止痛作用。

使用注意　本品具升发之性，阴虚火旺，肝阳上升之耳鸣、耳聋、头晕、头痛等症，均当忌用。

升　麻

为毛茛科多年生草本植物升麻 Cimicifuga foetida L. 兴安升麻 Cimicifuga dahurica （Turcz.） Maxim.和大三叶升麻 Cimicifuga heracleifolia komar.的根茎。切片晒干。生用或蜜炙用。

处方用名　升麻、绿升麻、炙升麻。

性味归经　辛、甘，微寒。入肺、脾、胃、大肠经。

功效应用

1. 发表透疹：用于麻疹初期，透发不畅，常与葛根同用；如斑疹热毒较甚者，加牛蒡子、紫草等。

2. 清热解毒：用于胃热头痛齿痛、咽痛口疮。治口疮齿痛，可与石膏、黄连等配伍；治咽喉疼痛，可与元参、牛蒡子、桔梗等同用；治头痛，常与石膏、白芷等配用。

3. 升举阳气：用于气虚下陷之脱肛、子宫脱垂等，常与人参、黄芪、柴胡等同用，共奏补气升阳之功。

用量用法 3~9克。煎服。解表宜生用，升提中气宜炙用。

蝉 蜕

为蝉科昆虫黑蚱蝉 Cryptotympana pustulata Fabr.羽化时所蜕之皮壳。晒干，生用。

处方用名 蝉蜕、蝉衣、蝉退。

性味归经 甘，寒。入肺、肝经。

功效应用

1. 疏散风热：用于感冒风热或温病初起有表证者，常与薄荷、甘草、石膏等同用；若风热喉痛，声音嘶哑，可单用或与胖大海同用；用于小儿感冒，发热，烦躁，或夜啼不安等症，可与钩藤、灯心草、薄荷等同用。

2. 透疹止痒：用于麻疹初见或疹出不畅，常与葛根、牛蒡子、薄荷、连翘等同用。

3. 退翳明目：用于风热目赤，翳膜遮睛，常与菊花、谷精草等同用。

4. 祛风解痉：用于破伤风，牙关紧闭，角弓反张，常与天麻、全蝎等熄风止痉药同用；小儿惊风，发热抽搐，常与钩藤、黄芩、羚羊角等同用。

用量用法 3~9克，祛风解痉可用15~30克。煎服。

浮 萍

为浮萍科草本植物紫萍 Spirodela polyrrhiza （L.） Schleid. 或青萍 Lemna minor L. 的带根全草。晒干生用。

处方用名　浮萍草、紫背浮萍。

性味归经　辛，寒。入肺、膀胱经。

功效应用

1. 解表透疹：用于风热表症，身热无汗，可与荆芥、防风、薄荷、连翘等同用；用于麻疹透发不快，常与牛蒡子、薄荷、银花、柽柳、竹叶等同用；用于风热疹块，皮肤瘙痒，常与荆芥、防风、蝉衣、白蒺藜、地肤子、白鲜皮等同用。

2. 利水消肿：用于水肿，小便不利，兼有表证者尤为适宜，常与车前子、冬瓜皮、赤小豆、连翘等同用；单用为末，温开水调服亦效。

用量用法　3～10 克，鲜品可用 15～30 克。煎服。

淡　豆　豉

系用豆科 1 年生草本植物黑大豆加工制成。其制法通常于夏季将黑大豆洗净蒸熟摊席上。用桑叶、鲜青蒿覆盖，使发酵成黄色后取出，去桑叶、青蒿，拌以清水放瓮内，封口置露天晒 3 星期，取出晒干供药用。此法最普遍。

处方用名　淡豆豉、豆豉、香豉。

性味归经　辛、甘、微苦，凉。入肺、胃经。

功效应用

1. 解表：多用于感冒，恶寒发热头痛等症。属风寒者，常与葱白同用；属风热者，常与薄荷、连翘等配伍。

2. 除烦：用于热病后期，余热未尽，胸中烦闷、懊侬不眠，可配栀子煎服。

用量用法　9～15 克。煎服。

附药　大豆黄卷：又名清水豆卷。系用黑大豆湿渍发芽晒干而成。性味甘平，入胃经。功能分利湿热，清解表邪。多用于暑湿、湿温，湿热内蕴，发热汗少，胸闷不舒，风湿热痹，膝胫骨节烦痛等症。用量 15～30 克。煎服。

2 清热药

凡以清解里热为主要作用的药物，称为清热药。

清热药都具有寒凉之性。主要用于热病、瘟疫、热痢、痈肿、疮疡以及目赤肿痛、咽喉肿痛等所呈现的各种里热症。

为了便于掌握各种清热药的特点，现根据各药的专长，分为下列6类。

1. 清热泻火药：多入气分，对气分实热证，有清热泻火的作用。

2. 清热明目药：能清肝火而明目，常用于肝火亢盛，目赤肿痛等证。

3. 清热凉血药：专入血分，能清血分实热，有清热凉血作用。

4. 清热燥湿药：多具苦燥之性，有清热化湿的作用，常用于湿热证。

5. 清热解毒药：清热中兼有解毒之功，常用于一切热毒证。

6. 清退虚热药：能清虚热、退骨蒸，常用于午后潮热，低热不退等症。

以上6类，根据病情需要，可以相互配用。在应用时，应从整个病情来决定主次和先后。如果热而有表证，当先解表，或表里同治；如气分热证而兼有血分热证的，可气血两清；若气分热证而热邪未入营血的，凉血药不宜早用。

清热药性多寒凉，能损伤阳气，故阳气不足，脾胃虚弱者，应慎用。

2.1 清热泻火药

热与火为六淫之一，热为火之渐，火为热之极，两者仅是轻重程度不同。凡能清热的药物，大抵皆能泻火。

清热泻火药，主清气分火热，分别适用于热性病邪在气分，壮热口渴，烦躁或谵语发狂，苔黄或燥，脉洪实有力等里热炽盛的证候。

对于体虚病人使用本类药物时，当考虑照顾正气，勿令克伐太过，必要时可与扶正药配伍同用；并需根据各药作用部位的不同（如清肝热、肺热、胃热），临症时区别使用。

石　　膏

为单斜晶系硫酸盐类矿物石膏 Cypsum 的矿石，主含含水硫酸钙（$CaSO_4 \cdot 2H_2O$）。碾碎生用或煅用。

处方用名　生石膏、煅石膏。

性味归经　辛、甘，大寒。入肺、胃经。

功效应用

1. 清热泻火，除烦止渴：用于温热病，邪在气分，壮热烦躁，口渴欲饮，汗出，脉洪大，甚至神昏谵妄者，常与知母、甘草同用；如热毒壅盛，发斑发疹，色紫黯者，可与犀角、元参等合用；若温热病后期，余热未退，心烦口干，舌红苔少者，亦可与竹叶、麦冬等配用；用于胃热口渴，或胃火上炎引起的头痛、牙痛等症，常与熟地、知母等配伍；治牙痛亦常与细辛配用；用于肺热实喘，呼吸迫促，心烦口渴之症，常与麻黄、杏仁等同用。

2. 生肌敛疮：用于创伤、溃疡、烫火伤等新肉不生，疮口不敛者，火煅研末外用；治溃疡通常配红升丹（9∶1）研末外掺（又称九一丹）；或与龙骨、炉甘石、乳香、没药、血竭等其它吸湿生肌活血药制散外用。

用量用法　15～60克，大剂量可用至120克。煎服，外用适量。清热泻火生用，生肌敛疮煅用。内服宜先煎。

知　母

为百合科多年生草本植物知母 Anemarrhena asphodeloides Bge. 的干燥根茎。生用或盐水炒用。

处方用名　知母、盐知母。

性味归经　苦、甘，寒。入肺、胃、肾经。

功效应用

1. 清热泻火：用于温热病邪在气分，高热烦渴，常辅佐石膏同用；用于肺热咳嗽，或阴虚肺热燥咳痰少，常与贝母同用。

2. 滋阴润燥：用于阴亏火旺，骨蒸潮热、梦遗、盗汗等症，常与黄柏、生地等同用；若咽痛口疮属阴虚火旺者，可配生地、元参同用。

3. 生津止渴：除用于治胃热口渴外，多用于消渴证，常与天花粉、麦冬、葛根等同用。

用量用法　3～12克。多生用；盐水炒制，是取其入肾泻火之义。

栀　子

为茜草科常绿灌木栀子 Gardenia jasminoides Ellis. 的成熟果实。生用、炒用、炒焦或姜汁炒用。亦有将果皮与种子分开使用者。

处方用名　栀子、生栀子、生山栀、炒栀子、姜栀子、栀子炭、黑山栀、栀子仁、栀子皮。

性味归经　苦，寒。入心、肝、肺、胃、三焦经。

功效应用

1. 泻火除烦：用于热病心烦，躁扰不宁，常与淡豆豉同用，以清心除烦。若热毒炽盛，神昏谵语，又常与黄连、黄芩、黄柏等清热泻火解毒药同用；用于肝热目赤肿痛，口苦口干，心中烦热，可与菊花、黄芩、甘草等同用。

2. 清热利湿：用于湿热黄疸，小便短赤。本药有利胆退黄作用，常与茵陈蒿、黄柏等配伍；用于热淋尿血，小便赤涩热痛，常与生地、木通、车前等同用。

3. 凉血止血：用于血热吐血、衄血、血痢下血、血淋涩痛等症，常与清热凉血药同用。

此外，生栀子研末，醋调外敷，可治跌打扭伤，血瘀肿痛；研末与鸡蛋清调涂，用于烫伤、火伤。

用量用法 3～10克。煎服。生用清热泻火，炒用稍减其寒性，炒黑用于止血，姜汁炒用止烦呕。

使用注意 脾胃虚寒，食少便溏者不宜服用。

天 花 粉

为葫芦科多年生宿根草质藤本植物栝楼 Trichosanthes Kirilowii Maxim. 的根。去外皮，切片生用。以质重、粉多、色白者为佳。

处方用名 天花粉、花粉、栝楼根。

性味归经 甘、微苦、微寒。入肺、胃经。

功效应用

1. 清热生津：用于热病伤津，心烦口渴及消渴症，可与沙参、麦冬、知母等配用。本药又能清肺热，润肺燥，可用于肺热咳嗽或燥咳等，常与川贝母、沙参、麦冬、知母等同用。

2. 消肿排脓：用于痈肿疮疡，红肿热痛，可与银花、贝母等同用；亦可研粉外敷。

用量用法 10～15克。煎服。外用适量。

芦 根

为禾本科多年生草本植物芦苇 Phragmites communis Trin.

的干燥或新鲜根茎。切段生用或鲜用。

处方用名 芦根、鲜芦根、活芦根、干芦根。苇根、苇茎。

性味归经 甘，寒。入肺、胃经。

功效应用

1. 清热生津：用于热病伤津，烦热口渴，舌燥津少之症，常与天花粉、麦冬等同用。

2. 清肺泻热：用于肺痈（肺脓疡）咳吐腥臭脓痰，或痰中带血，以及风热感冒咳嗽而有口干舌燥者。前者常与薏苡仁、桃仁、冬瓜仁、鱼腥草等同用；后者常与银花、连翘等同用。

3. 清胃止呕：用于胃热呕哕、反胃、呃逆等症，通常与竹茹、枇杷叶等同用；如配竹茹、姜汁、粳米，水煎服，可治反胃呕哕。

此外，又治麻疹初起，疹透不畅。本品具有宣毒透疹之功。单用或与其他宣毒透疹药同用。

用量用法 15～60克。用鲜者尤佳。煎服。

淡竹叶

为禾木科多年生草本植物淡竹叶 Lophatherum gracile Brongn. 的全草。切段生用。

处方用名 淡竹叶。

性味归经 甘、淡，寒。入心、肺、小肠经。

功效应用

1. 清心除烦：用于热病心烦口渴，可与天花粉、芦根等清热生津药同用；治小儿心热夜啼，常与钩藤、薄荷、蝉蜕、灯心等同用。

2. 利尿通淋：用于小便短赤，淋涩疼痛及口舌生疮等症，常与生地、木通等同用；或与灯心草、车前子等同用。

用量用法 6～12克。煎服。

附药 竹叶、竹叶卷心：为禾本科多年生常绿竹状乔木或灌木植物淡竹 Phyllostachys nigra（Lodd.）Munro var·henonis (Mitf.) ex Rendle 的新鲜或干的叶片；初出的卷状嫩叶，称“竹叶卷心”。一般以鲜用为好。功效基本与淡竹叶相似，但清心除烦之功较淡竹叶为强，而利尿之力较淡竹叶为弱。竹叶卷心主要用于清心热，故清宫汤中用之，以治温病神昏谵语等症。用量用法同淡竹叶。

2.2 清热明目药

清热明目药有清肝火、退目翳的功效。适用于肝火亢盛，目赤肿痛，目生翳膜等症；其中有些药物尚可用于肝阳上扰的证候。

夏 枯 草

为唇形科多年生草本植物夏枯草 Prunella Vulgaris L.的干燥带花的果穗。晒干生用。

处方用名 夏枯草。

性味归经 苦、辛，寒。入肝、胆经。

功效应用

1. 清肝明目：用于肝火目赤肿痛，可与菊花、蒲公英等同用；若肝郁目珠疼痛，至夜尤甚，可配香附 30 克，甘草 6 克，共研末，早晚各服 6 克；如偏肝虚目珠疼痛者，可与当归、白芍等同用；用于肝阳上亢或肝火上升，头痛目眩，性情急躁，烦热失眠，为临床之常用药，可单用或与草决明、野菊花、石决明、黄芩等清热平肝潜阳药同用。

2. 清火散结：用于痰火郁结所致之瘰疬、瘿瘤，及乳肿、痄腮等，可单用熬膏常服，或与玄参、浙贝母、昆布等随症配用。

现常用于治疗高血压、甲状腺肿大、淋巴结结核、乳腺增生症等。此外，还可用于肺结核、淋巴肉瘤及纵膈肿瘤等。

用量用法 10～12克。煎服。

决 明 子

为豆科一年生草本植物草决明 Cassia tora L. 的成熟种子。微炒打碎用。

处方用名 决明子、草决明。

性味归经 甘、苦，微寒。入肝、肾经。

功效应用

1. 清肝明目：用于肝热或肝经风热所致的目赤肿痛，羞明多泪等。属肝热，可配夏枯草、栀子；属风热，可配桑叶、菊花。亦可用于肝肾不足之青盲内障，视物昏花，目暗不明，常与生地、枸杞、玄参、山药等同用。

2. 润肠通便：用于肠燥便秘，可单用或与火麻仁、郁李仁等同用。

此外，亦常用于肝阳上亢所致的高血压头痛，有一定效果。

用量用法 6～10克。煎服。单味亦可用开水泡服。

使用注意 大便泄泻者忌用。

青 葙 子

为苋科1年生草本植物青葙 Celosia argentea L. 和鸡冠花 Celosia cristata L. 的成熟种子。微炒用。本品与鸡冠花子相似，俗名野鸡冠花子。

处方用名 青葙子。

性味归经 苦，微寒。入肝经。

功效应用 清肝明目，退翳：用于肝火上炎之目赤肿痛，目生翳膜，视物昏暗等，常与决明子、夏枯草等同用。

此外，现临床还用于高血压头晕目眩，属于肝阳上亢型者，每与决明子、夏枯草、钩藤等同用。

用量用法 6～10克。煎服。

使用注意 本药清热之力较强，且有扩散瞳孔作用，对虚性目疾和青光眼的患者忌用。

密 蒙 花

为马钱科落叶灌木植物密蒙花 Baddleja officinalis Maxim. 的干燥花蕾及其花序。酒浸晒干后，蜜拌蒸用。

处方用名 密蒙花。

性味归经 甘，微寒。入肝经。

功效应用 清热养肝，明目退翳：用于肝热目疾，赤肿多眵，可与石决明、菊花等同用；用于肝虚目昏干涩或生翳障，可与枸杞、菟丝子等配伍。本品对目疾，虚证，实证，皆可应用。尤以肝肾阴虚而有热者，最为适宜。

用量用法 6～10 克。煎服。

谷 精 草

为谷精草科 1 年生草本植物谷精草 Eriocaulon buergerianum koern. 的干燥带花茎的头状花序。切段生用。

处方用名 谷精草、谷精珠。

性味归经 辛、甘、平。入肝、胃经。

功效应用 疏散风热，退翳明目：用于风热目疾，肿痛羞明，或目生星翳，常与菊花、决明子、木贼、夏枯草等同用；治痘（麻疹）后目翳，亦可配猪肝、蛤粉同用。

用量用法 6～12 克，煎服。

木 贼 草

为木贼科多年生常绿草本植物木贼 Eguisetum hiemale L. 的全草。切段、晒干，生用。

处方用名 木贼、木贼草。

性味归经 甘、苦，平。入肺、肝经。

功效应用　疏散风热，明目退翳：用于风热目赤，翳膜遮睛，常与谷精草、蝉蜕等同用；若眼花多泪，亦可与苍术、防风、夏枯草等配用。

用量用法　3～10克。煎服。

使用注意　久翳及血虚者不宜用，多服令人目肿。

2.3 清热凉血药

清热凉血药，常用于血热妄行的吐血、衄血、血热发斑发疹及温热病邪入营血，热甚心烦、舌绛神昏等症。

热邪入营分、血分，往往伤阴耗液。本节药物中除生地兼有养阴滋液作用外，在热病伤阴之时，还可与滋阴药如元参、麦冬之类配伍，应用此类药物还有标本兼顾之效。

清热凉血药，一般适用于热在血分的病症，如果气血两燔，可配清热泻火药同用。血热证而火毒炽盛，可配清热解毒药。

犀　角*

为犀科动物印度犀 Rhinoceros unicornis L.、爪哇犀 Rhinoceros sondaicus Desmarest 或苏门犀 Rhinoceros sumatrensis (Fischer) 等的角。除上述品种外，尚有下列2种：①广角：为非洲产黑犀 Rhinoceros bicornis L.或白犀 R.simus Burchell 的角；②小犀角，亦称“蘑菇头”，为犀角顶上的小角。捕捉后，截取其角。均系进口药材。药用锯成小条，名犀角条，刨成薄片，名犀角片，或锉为细末，名犀角粉，或磨汁服。

处方用名　犀角片（花）、犀角粉、广角片、广角粉。

性味归经　苦、咸、寒。入心、肝、胃经。

功效应用

1. 清心安神：用于急性热病，热入心营之神昏谵语，常与

*参见本分册之说明。

生地、元参、连翘等同用；若热陷心肝、痉厥抽搐者，又常与牛黄或羚羊角等熄风开窍药同用。

2. 凉血止血：用于血热妄行之吐血、衄血等症，常与生地、丹皮、芍药等同用。

3. 解毒化斑：用于温热病，热毒炽盛，发斑发疹，其色紫暗者，每与石膏同用。

用量用法 1.5～6克。煎服。宜制散剂为佳；亦可另煎汤兑服。散剂冲服每次1～3克。广角价廉力弱，用量宜加倍。今多以水牛角代用。

使用注意 非热入营血者，不宜轻用；孕妇亦当慎用。且不宜与川乌、草乌同用。

附药 水牛角：为牛科动物水牛 Bubalus bubalis·L. 的双角。有类似犀角的性能。可用于急性热病壮热，斑疹，神昏谵语，惊厥等。用量宜大，有谓应为犀角的8～10倍，内服量30～150克，锉碎先煎。锉末服，每次1.5～6克，本品在《本草纲目》已有记载："治时气寒热头痛。煎汁，治热毒风及壮热"。近据临床报道，用牛角代替犀角治疗温热病及小儿热症，效亦良好。其药理作用与犀角相似。

生 地 黄

为玄参科多年生草本植物地黄 Rehmannia glutinosa (Gaertn.) Libosch. 和怀庆地黄 Rehmannia glutinosa Libosch F. hueichingensis（chao et Schih）Hsiao. 的根茎。切片，晒干用或鲜用，亦可炒炭用。

处方用名 生地黄、干生地、生地、生地炭、鲜地黄。

性味归经 甘、苦，寒。入心、肝、肾经。

功效应用

1. 清热滋阴：用于温热病，热入营血，身热口干，舌红或绛等症，常与元参、犀角等同用；如热盛伤阴，津亏便秘者，可重用生地与元参、麦冬等配伍；用于热病后期，低热不退，或慢性病阴虚发热，常与青蒿、鳖甲、地骨皮、知母等同用。

2. 凉血止血：用于血热妄行，吐血、衄血、尿血、便血、崩漏下血等症，常与侧柏叶、茜草根等其他凉血止血药同用；用于血热毒盛，斑疹紫黑，可与犀角、丹皮等凉血解毒药同用。

3. 生津止渴：用于热病伤津，舌红口干或口渴唇燥，常与麦冬、玉竹、沙参等益胃生津药同用；用于消渴症，口渴多饮，可与天冬、枸杞、山药、山萸肉等滋补肝肾药同用。

此外，若荨麻疹、皮癣等症而有血热现象者，可与白蒺藜、白鲜皮、防风等配用。

用量用法　10～30克。煎服。清热生津宜生用，止血可炒炭用。

使用注意　凡脾虚有湿，腹满便溏者忌用。

牡　丹　皮

为毛茛科多年生落叶小灌木牡丹 Paeonia suffruticosa Andr. 的根皮。切片，晒干。生用、酒炒或炒炭用。

处方用名　牡丹皮、粉丹皮、酒丹皮、丹皮炭。

性味归经　苦、辛，微寒。入心、肝、肾经。

功效应用

1. 清热凉血：用于热病发斑发疹，血热吐血、衄血等症，通常与生地同用，重者可与犀角配伍；用于热病后期，热伏阴分，夜热早凉，常与青蒿、鳖甲或地黄、山萸肉同用；若妇女虚热或经前发热，可与山栀、当归、地黄、芍药、川芎等随症配伍。

2. 活血消瘀：用于血瘀经闭、痛经，或瘀血积聚，腹中包块等症，常与桂枝、茯苓、芍药、桃仁等同用；用于跌打损伤(尤以胸腹挫伤)，瘀阻作痛，常配入赤芍、乳香、没药等理血方中同用；用于肠痈腹痛，大便秘结，常与大黄、桃仁、冬瓜子等同用。对其他痈疡肿毒，亦可配伍用之。

此外，现临床还用于治高血压及动脉硬化，可与野菊花、石决明、银花藤等同用。

用量用法 5～10克。煎服。清热凉血宜生用；活血消瘀可酒炒用；用于止血，宜炒炭用。

使用注意 月经过多，孕妇不宜用。

赤 芍 药

为毛茛科多年生草本植物芍药（野生种）Paeonia lactiflora pall. 草芍药 Paeonia obovata Maxim. 川赤芍 paeonia veitchii lynch 等的根。切片晒干生用。

处方用名 赤芍药、赤芍。

性味归经 苦，微寒。入肝经。

功效应用

1. 凉血活血：用于血热瘀滞，经闭、痛经等，常与当归、丹参、桃仁、红花等同用；用于血热痈肿，焮热疼痛，常与当归、川芎、银花、连翘等同用；用于血热吐衄，斑疹色赤，常与生地、丹皮等同用。

2. 祛瘀止痛：用于血瘀症积，或产后瘀滞腹痛，通常与当归、川芎等配伍；瘀积重者，可配桃仁、红花；产后瘀痛，亦可酌配炮姜等温化药同用；用于跌打损伤，血瘀肿痛，常与乳香、没药、当归、桃仁等同用。

3. 清肝明目：用于肝热目赤肿痛，常与菊花、薄荷等配伍。

用量用法 6～12克。煎服。

使用注意 不宜与藜芦同用。

紫 草

为紫草科多年生草本植物紫草 Lithospermum erythro rhizon

Sieb. et. Zucc. 新疆紫草 Arnebia euchroma（Royle）Johnst.或滇紫草 Onosma paniculatum Bur. et Franch.的根。晒干，切段生用。

处方用名 紫草、紫草根。

性味归经 甘，寒。入心、肝经。

功效应用

1. 凉血活血，解毒透疹：用于血热毒盛，斑疹不透，或斑疹紫黑，色不红活，可与赤芍、蝉蜕等同用；用于疮疖、湿疹、皮炎、阴痒及水火烫伤等症，可用紫草研末入植物油（3∶6）浸泡数天，滤取油液，涂敷患处；如治一切痈疽疮疡肿毒，可与当归、白芷、血竭、轻粉等制膏用。

2. 利尿滑肠：用于血热毒盛之小便淋痛或大便秘结，多与清热解毒药同用；亦可单用为末，温开水送服。

用量用法 3～10克。煎服。外用适量。

2.4 清热燥湿药

清热燥湿药性味多为苦寒，苦能燥湿，寒能清热，常用于湿热内蕴或湿邪化热之症，如烦热，口苦，胸痞，黄疸、泄痢，以及痈肿疮毒，小便黄赤等症。

本节中黄芩、黄连、黄柏、龙胆草等，亦为常用的泻火解毒药，宜互相参症。

清热燥湿药虽可用治火热之症，但苦燥之性，易于伤阴败胃，故一般不适用于津液亏耗及脾胃虚弱的患者，如须使用，亦应分别配养津和益胃药同用。

黄　芩

为唇形科多年生草本植物黄芩 Scutellaria baicalensis Georgi 的干燥根。切片晒干，生用，酒炒或炒炭用。

处方用名 黄芩、酒黄芩、枯芩、条芩、子芩、黄芩炭。

性味归经 苦，寒。入肺、大小肠、脾、胆经。

功效应用

1. 清热燥湿：用于湿热下痢，里急后重，常与芍药、甘草等同用；若腹泻，可与葛根、黄连等配伍；用于湿热黄疸，多作辅助药，可与茵陈、山栀等配用；用于膀胱湿热、小便涩痛，常与生地、木通等同用。

2. 泻火解毒：用于急性热病，高热烦躁，苔黄，脉数等，常与黄连、栀子等同用；用于肺热咳嗽，咳吐黄痰，常与桑白皮、知母、麦冬等同用；用于痈疮肿毒，烫火灼伤，可与其它泄火解毒药同用。内服外用均可。

3. 清热安胎：用于怀胎蕴热，胎动不安，常与白术、当归等同用。

此外，还常用于热盛迫血妄行的吐血、衄血、便血、血崩等症。对动脉硬化、高血压，属于肝阳亢盛，有头痛、口苦、面红、心烦等症者，可与夏枯草、菊花、石决明等同用。

用量用法 3～12克。煎服。清热多用生黄芩、安胎多用炒制品；清上焦热可用酒芩；止血则多炒炭用。

使用注意 脾胃虚寒，少食，便溏者忌用。

黄　连

为毛茛科多年生草本植物黄连 Coptis chinensis Franch. 三角叶黄连 Coptis deltoidea C. Y. Cheng et Hsiao. 或云连 Coptis teetoides C. Y. Cheng 的根茎。晒干。生用、炒用、或酒炒、姜汁炒、吴茱萸水炒用。用时捣碎。

处方用名 黄连、川黄连、川雅连、炒黄连、姜连、酒连、萸连。

性味归经 苦，寒。入心、胃、肝、胆、大肠经。

功效应用

1. 清热燥湿：用于肠胃湿热，泄泻下痢，里急后重，有清肠止痢之功；常与木香、黄芩、白头翁等同用；若赤痢而兼有身热表症，可与葛根、黄芩配用；用于肠胃湿热，脘腹痞满，呕吐恶心，可与黄芩、半夏、生姜等同用；若由胸有积热，肠中有寒，寒热不调，以致腹痛欲呕者，亦可与干姜、桂枝、半夏等配伍。

2. 泻火解毒：用于急性热病，火热炽盛，高热烦躁，神昏谵语，或心火内炎，胸膈热闷，心烦失眠，或口舌生疮等症，常与黄芩、山栀等同用；若因火热内盛，迫血妄行而致吐血、衄血并有便秘尿赤者，可与大黄、黄芩及其他凉血止血药同用；若治心烦失眠，常与朱砂，枣仁或阿胶等配伍；用于肝火上升，目赤肿痛，羞明多泪等症，有清肝明目作用，可与黄芩、山栀、菊花、薄荷等同用；亦可单用切碎，用人乳浸汁点眼，每日 2～3 次；用于胃热呕吐苦水、酸水，能清胃止呕，常与吴茱萸或苏叶同用；用于疔毒痈肿，口舌生疮，湿疮瘙痒等症，随症配伍，内服外用均可。

用量用法　1.5～4.5 克。煎服。研末服，每次 0.6～1.5 克，每日 2～3 次。外用适量。清心与大肠火宜生用，清肝胆火宜吴茱萸水炒，治上焦火宜酒炒，治胃火呕恶宜姜汁炒。炒制诸法，既能增强疗效，又可缓解苦寒性，可随症而施。但不宜多用。

使用注意　脾胃虚寒，无湿热实火者忌用。

黄　柏

为芸香料落叶乔木黄檗（关黄柏）Phellodendron amurense Rupr. 和黄皮树（川黄柏）P. chinense Schneid. 除去栓皮的树皮。切片生用或盐炒用。

处方用名　黄柏、盐黄柏。

性味归经　苦，寒。入肾、膀胱、大肠经。

功效应用

1. 清热燥湿：用于湿热泻痢，身热后重，常与白头翁、秦皮等同用；用于湿热黄疸，身黄发热，常与山栀及其他清热燥湿药同用；用于湿热带下，秽浊黄稠，常与芡实、白果等同用；用于湿热下注，腿足湿肿热痛及热淋，小便赤涩热痛等症。前者常与苍术、牛膝同用；后者可与山栀、车前子等配伍。

2. 泻火解毒，用于湿疹、热毒疮疡等，内服外敷均可。湿疹，可与荆芥、苦参同用；治疮疡肿毒，内服多与黄连、栀子等同用；外用以本品研细末调猪胆汁外涂。

3. 退虚热：用于阴亏火旺，潮热骨蒸、遗精、盗汗等症，常与知母同用。

用量用法　3～10克。煎服。外用适量。内服多盐水炒用，外科多生用。

使用注意　脾胃虚寒者忌用。

龙　胆　草

为龙胆科多年生草本植物龙胆 Gentiana scabra Bge.或三花龙胆 Gentiana triflora Pall. 的根及根茎。切段生用。

处方用名　龙胆草、胆草。

性味归经　苦，寒。入肝、胆经。

功效应用

1. 清热燥湿：本品为清利肝胆及下焦湿热的常用药。用于湿热黄疸，可与茵陈、郁金、黄柏等配用；用于湿热下注，囊肿阴痒，常与车前子、滑石等利湿清热药同用。

2. 泻肝降火：用于肝胆实火，头痛头胀，目赤肿痛，耳聋耳肿，胁痛口苦等症，常与黄芩、山栀等同用；用于肝热生风，高热不退，急惊抽搐，可与石决明、芦荟、钩藤等清热凉肝药同用。

用量用法　3～6克。煎服。

使用注意　脾胃虚寒者忌服；不宜过量使用。

苦　参

为豆科多年生落叶亚灌木植物苦参 Sophora flarescens Ait. 的干燥根。晒干，切片生用。

处方用名　苦参。

性味归经　苦，寒。入心、肝、大肠、膀胱经。

功效应用

1. 清热燥湿：用于湿热痢疾，可与黄芩、马齿苋同用，或与葛根、山楂配伍；若便血、痔血，亦可与地榆、槐角配用。

2. 杀虫止痒：用于疥癣、湿疹、皮肤瘙痒等症，常与白鲜皮、蛇床子等同用；如治脂溢性皮炎、脓泡疮等，可用苦参 60 克、当归 45 克，蜜丸久服；如治阴道滴虫，阴痒带下，可与白头翁、蛇床子等同用；治麻风，可与大风子、苍耳子等同用。

此外，尚可用于黄疸。并兼有利尿作用，可用治湿热蕴结，小便不利之症。

用量用法　3～10 克。煎服。外用适量。

白　鲜　皮

为芸香科多年生宿根草本植物白鲜 Dictamnus dasycarpus Turcz. 的根皮。晒干。切片生用。

处方用名　白鲜皮。

性味归经　苦，寒。入脾、胃、膀胱经。

功效应用　清热燥湿，祛风止痒：用于湿热疮毒，风疹疥癣，皮肤瘙痒等症，常与苦参、蝉蜕、地肤子、防风等同用；用于妇女阴痒带下，可与苦参、蛇床子、川椒等煎汤，外洗。

此外，亦治湿热黄疸及湿热痹痛等症。

用量用法　6～12 克。煎服。外用适量。

秦 皮

为木樨科落叶乔木苦枥白蜡树 Fraxinus rhynchophylla Hance. 小叶白蜡树 Fraxinus bungeana DC.或秦岭白蜡树 Fraxinus paxiana Lingelsh.的树皮。晒干。切段生用。

处方用名 秦皮，北秦皮。

性味归经 苦、涩，寒。入肝、胆、大肠经。

功效应用

1. 清热燥湿：用于湿热下痢属急性者，常与白头翁、黄连、黄柏或苦参、木香等配伍；属慢性者，可与生地榆、椿根皮等同用。

2. 清肝明目：用于肝胆有热，目赤肿痛，或生翳膜。单用煎水洗眼，可治目赤生翳，与竹叶、黄连煎服，可治眼暴肿痛；亦可配黄连各 6 克、滑石 12 克，为末泡汤乘热熏洗。

用量用法 6～10 克。煎服。外用适量。

2.5 清热解毒药

毒的含义很广，这里所称的毒，主要系指因火热壅盛以致发生红、肿、热、痛等痈疡肿毒，各种化脓性感染而言。亦通称热毒或火毒。本类药物具有清火热、消肿毒的特点，即具有不同程度的消炎、抗感染（抗菌、抗病毒）等作用，故称清热解毒药。

热毒在人体不同的脏腑、经络、部位所呈的证候各有不同，本类药物在清热解毒方面亦具有不同特长，故可分别适用于疮痈、疖肿、斑疹、丹毒、急性热病以及喉痹、痢疾等症。因此，临床应用时，应根据热毒表现的不同证候，分别选用适宜的药物，或与其它有关药物相互配用。如热毒在血分者，清热解毒药应配伍凉血药用；火热炽烈者应配伍泻火药用；挟湿者应配伍燥湿或利湿药用，疮痈属虚者应配伍补养药同用。此外，疮痈喉痹诸症，还当与外用药配合使用。

由于本类药物，均为寒凉之品，若疮疡、喉痹、痢疾、发斑等症属于阴症、寒症者，则不宜使用。

金 银 花

为忍冬科多年生半常绿缠绕灌木忍冬 Lonicera japonica Thunb.的花蕾。晾晒或阴干。生用。

处方用名 金银花、银花、双花、二宝花、忍冬花。

性味归经 甘，寒。入肺、心、胃经。

功效应用

1. 清热解毒：用于各种热性病初起，耳热或微感恶风及发斑发疹等症。本品兼有宣风散热作用，可与连翘、豆豉、薄荷等同用；若热毒较重，并发喉痛、腮肿，亦可与黄芩、大黄、黄柏、板蓝根等同用；用于热毒疮痈，咽喉肿痛等症，通常与连翘配用；若肿痛较重，为促使消散或加速溃破，亦可与穿山甲、皂角刺等配伍；如治疔毒，常配紫花地丁、蒲公英、野菊花之类；治喉痛，可配山豆根、薄荷等品，又可治肠痈，常配薏苡仁、黄芩、当归等。

2. 凉血止痢：用于热毒泄痢，便脓血，或便血之症，可与黄芩、芍药等配用；单用浓煎服亦可。

用量用法 10～15 克，热盛毒重者，可用 30～60 克，煎服。

附药 忍冬藤：为忍冬科植物忍冬的干燥茎枝。又叫银花藤。切段晒干用。功效同花，兼清经络风热，常用于痈肿疮毒，咽喉肿痛。关节红肿热痛或风热痹痛等经络不利之症。用量 15～30 克，煎服。

连 翘

为木犀科落叶灌木植物连翘 Forsythia suspensa（Thunb.）Vahl 的干燥果实。晒干用。

处方用名 连翘、青连翘、连翘壳、连翘心。

性味归经 苦，微寒。入心、小肠经。

功效应用

1. 清热解毒：用于各种热性病初起，身热或微恶风及发斑发疹等症。本品有轻清透热作用，常与银花、薄荷等清热透表药同用；若热在胸膈，烦热不安者，可配黄芩；如热入心包，烦热神昏者，可配犀角，或银花、大青叶、黄芩等；用于热毒所致各种疮疡肿毒，乳痈等，常与银花、紫花地丁、薄公英、野菊花等配伍。本品为疮家要药。用于清热解毒，常与银花相须为用。

2. 清火散结：用于瘰疬结核，常与元参、夏枯草等同用。

此外，亦治过敏性紫癜，可用本品配赤芍 10 克，麻黄、甘草各 6 克。水煎服。

用量用法 6～15 克。煎服。

附药 连翘心：为连翘的种子。性味苦，微寒。能清心热。主要用于温热病热入心包，神昏谵语，常与玄参心、连心麦冬、莲子心等同用。用量 3～6 克。煎服。

大 青 叶

为十字花科 2 年生草本植物菘蓝 Isatis indigotica Fort. 的干燥叶。晒干用或鲜用。

此外，全国各地作大青叶用的植物还有：马鞭草科 1 年生草本植物路边青 Clerodendron cyrtophyllum Turcz.蓼科植物蓼蓝 Polygonum tinctorium Ait.的叶。

处方用名 大青叶。

性味归经 苦，寒。入心、肝、胃经。

功效应用

1. 清热解毒：用于瘟疫热病，高热头痛及热毒所致咽喉肿痛，口疮、肿毒，丹毒等。可单用或与石膏、黄芩、元参及银花、山栀等配用。

2. 凉血化斑：用于热毒发斑，血热吐衄等，可与犀角、山栀等同用。

现代多用于上呼吸道感染，流行性感冒等引起的发热、咽部充血、扁桃体肿大，流行性乙型脑炎，流行性腮腺炎，病毒性肺炎，病毒性肝炎等，有良效。本品亦为解毒要药。

用量用法 9～15克。煎服。

附药 板蓝根：为菘蓝的根。切片用。性味苦，寒。有类似大青叶的功用，而尤以解毒散结见长。主要用治大头瘟，头面红肿，或咽喉肿痛，烂喉丹痧等症，常与大青叶、生石膏、黄芩、黄连以及银花、连翘、生地、元参等随症配用。现代临床多用于流行性乙型脑炎、流行性腮腺炎、流行性感冒、病毒性肝炎等。用量9～15克。煎服。

紫花地丁

为堇菜科多年生草本植物紫花地丁 Viola yedoensis Makino 的全草。切段。晒干用或鲜用。

除此，全国各地作紫花地丁用的植物还有：豆科多年生草本植物米口袋 Gueldensta edtia multiflora Bge. 小米口袋 G.pauciflora（Rall.）Fisch.的全草。堇菜科1年生草本植物犁头草 Viola japonica Langsd 的全草。

处方用名 紫花地丁、地丁。

性味归经 苦、辛，寒。入心、肝经。

功效应用 清热解毒：用于疔疮痈肿。本品以治痈肿疔毒为特长，为治疗痈疮疖通用之药。常与蒲公英、银花、连翘等同用；或用鲜者捣汁服或捣烂外敷患处皆可；治毒蛇咬伤，亦可取鲜者捣烂外敷；若治内痈，可随症配伍。

用量用法 10～30克，大量用30～60克。煎服。外用适量。

蒲 公 英

为菊科多年生草本植物蒲公英 Taraxacum mongolicum Hand-Mazz.、碱地蒲公英 Taraxacum sinicum Kitag.或同属数种植物的全草。切碎，生用或鲜用。

处方用名 蒲公英、公英。

性味归经 苦、甘，寒。入肝、胃经。

功效应用

1. 清热解毒：用于乳痈肿痛，疔毒，痈肿，肺痈，肠痈等。本品与地丁均为外科痈肿疔毒常用药，二者相须为用。尤为治乳痈要药。如乳痈早期，红肿坚硬，可与银花、连翘、炒山甲、天花粉等配伍，亦可取鲜品捣烂外敷；肠痈热毒壅盛，可与银花、大黄、桃仁等同用；治疔毒，常与紫花地丁、野菊花、金银花等配用；治其它痈肿疮疖，亦常加入清热解毒方中用之。

2. 清肝明目：用于肝火上炎，目赤肿痛，可与黄芩、菊花、夏枯草等配用；亦可单味或与菊花煎汤熏洗。

此外，本品尚有利尿作用，可治尿路感染，湿热黄疸。对上呼吸道感染、急性扁桃体炎及慢性胃炎等，亦为临床所常用。

用量用法 15～30克。大剂量可用至60克。煎服。但过多应用，有时可致缓泻。

败 酱 草

为败酱科多年生草本植物黄花败酱 Patrinia scabiosaefolia Fisch. ex Link.或白花败酱 P.villosa Juss.的带根全草。阴干，切段用。

此外，我国北方地区习惯以菊科多年生草本植物苣荬菜 Sonchus brachyotus DC. 的带根全草作败酱用。南方地区习惯以十字花科植物菥蓂Thlaspi arvens L. 的带果全草作败酱用。

处方用名 败酱、败酱草。

性味归经 辛、苦，微寒。入胃、大肠、肝经。

功效应用 清热解毒，行瘀排脓：用于肠痈。古方与薏苡仁、附子同用，治肠痈有脓；现代常与薏苡仁、冬瓜子、桃仁以及银花、连翘等清热解毒药同用；用于肺痈，可与鱼腥草、芦根、桔梗等配用；用于热毒疮疖，可单用内服，并以鲜品捣烂敷患处，或与金银花、连翘、紫花地丁等配用。本品善消内痈，为治肠痈要药。不论有脓无脓，均可应用。用于血热瘀滞，心腹疼痛，单用煎服或配当归、川芎、乳香等同用。

此外，亦可用治急性肠炎、急性菌痢、急性黄疸型肝炎及肝脓疡等。

用量用法 10～30 克。煎服。

红 藤

为木通科落叶木质藤本植物大血藤 Sargentodoxa cuneata Rehd. et wils. 的藤茎。趁鲜切片，晒干用。

处方用名 红藤、省藤、大血藤。

性味归经 苦，平。入胃、大肠经。

功效应用

1. 清热解毒，消痈散结：用于肠痈腹痛，常与银花、连翘、大黄、丹皮等同用；用于乳痈肿痛，可与蒲公英、花粉、银花、贝母等同用。本品历来为治痈肿之要药，现临床专用治肠痈。

2. 活血通经，祛风除湿：用于血瘀经闭，可与当归、益母草、香附等水煎配红砂糖调服；用于风湿筋骨酸痛，四肢麻木拘挛，可与五加皮、威灵仙等同用。

用量用法 10～15 克。

鱼 腥 草

为三白草科多年生草本植物蕺菜 Houttuynia cordata

Thunb. 的干燥地上部分。阴干用或鲜用。

处方用名 鱼腥草。

性味归经 辛，微寒。入肺经。

功效应用

1. 清热解毒，消痈排脓：用于肺痈，痰热壅盛，咳吐脓血及肺热咳嗽，痰黄而稠等。前者，常与桔梗、芦根、冬瓜子等同用；后者，常与黄芩、贝母、桑白皮等同用；用于痈疮肿痛，可单用内服或取鲜品捣烂外敷。治痔疮肿痛，可煎外洗。本品虽内痈外痈均治，但为治肺痈之要药。

2. 利尿通淋：用于湿热淋症，小便涩痛，常与木通、滑石、车前子等同用。

现代多用治肺脓疡，肺炎，急、慢性气管炎，尿路感染等。

用量用法 15～30 克，鲜者加倍，煎服。不宜久煎。外用适量。

射　　干

为鸢尾科多年生草本植物射干 Belamcanda chinensis (L.) DC. 的根茎。晒干。切片生用。

处方用名 射干、射干片。

性味归经 苦，寒。入肺经。

功效应用

1. 解毒利咽：用于咽喉肿痛。本品为治咽痛喉痹之要药。属于痰热者最宜，常与忍冬藤、马勃、桔梗、甘草等同用。

2. 消痰散结：用于肺热多痰，咳嗽上气。如风热咳嗽，痰涎壅盛，可与前胡、杏仁、贝母同用；如风寒咳嗽痰多，或因风寒寒饮而致咳逆喘息，呼吸不畅，喉中有哮鸣音者，可与麻黄、细辛、生姜、五味子等同用。

用量用法 3～10 克。煎服。

马 勃

为马勃科植物脱皮马勃 Iasiosphaera fenzlii Reich. 大马勃 Calvatia gigantea（Batsch ex Pers.）LIoyd 或紫色马勃 Calvatia lilacina（Mont. et Berk.）Lloyd 的子实体。晒干用。

处方用名 马勃、轻马勃、马勃绒。

性味归经 辛，平。入肺经。

功效应用

1. 清肺利咽，解毒消肿：用于肺火上炎，咽喉肿痛，咳嗽失音，可与元参、桔梗、板蓝根、甘草等同用。

2. 收敛止血：用于外伤出血，单用其粉敷压伤口；此法亦治冻疮。若吐血、衄血，亦可与其他清热止血药同用。

用量用法 2～6 克。宜包煎内服。外用适量。

锦 灯 笼

为茄科多年生草本植物 physalis alkekengi L. var. franchetii (Mast.) Makino 的宿萼或带果实的宿萼。晒干用或鲜用。

处方用名 锦灯笼、金灯笼、挂金灯。

性味归经 苦，寒。入肺、心、膀胱经。

功效应用

1. 清热解毒，利咽消肿：用于咽喉肿痛，常与射干，牛蒡子、桔梗、元参等同用。本品为治咽喉肿痛常用之药。

2. 降气化痰：用于风热咳嗽，气逆痰多，可与杏仁、桔梗、前胡等同用。

3. 利尿通淋：用于热淋尿痛，小便赤涩，常与车前子、木通、淡竹叶等同用。

用量用法 6～12 克。煎服。

山　豆　根

为豆科蔓生性矮小灌木植物越南槐 Sophora tonkinensis Gapnep. 的根及根茎。切片，晒干用。

处方用名　山豆根。

性味归经　苦，寒。入肺、胃经。

功效应用　清热解毒，利咽消肿：用于肺胃火毒上攻所致咽喉或牙龈肿痛，可与元参、桔梗或射干、牛蒡子等配用，内服或含漱均可。本品为治热毒咽喉肿痛的要药。

此外，现代尚用治口腔炎、宫颈炎及皮肤溃疡，内服或研粉外用。

用量用法　3～10 克。煎服。外用适量。

青　果

为橄榄科常绿乔木橄榄 Canarium album（Lour.）Raeusch. 的成熟果实。鲜用或阴干生用。

处方用名　青果、干青果、橄榄。

性味归经　甘、涩、酸，平。入肺经。

功效应用

1. 清肺利咽：用于咽喉肿痛、肺热咳嗽等症，常与银花、胖大海、杏仁、桔梗、甘草等配用；若时行风火咽喉肿痛，可用鲜青果、鲜莱菔，水煎服。

2. 解毒：用治河豚鱼鳖及酒中毒，可单用鲜青果榨汁频服或煎浓汤饮。

附药　金果榄：为防已科多年生常绿小藤本植物金果榄 Tinospora capillipes Gagn 的块根。形似橄榄，故名。性味苦寒。功能解毒、利咽。适用于咽喉肿痛，肺热咳嗽，疮痈肿毒。用量 3～10 克。煎服。

漏　芦

为菊科多年生草本植物祁州漏芦 Rhaponticum uniflorum (L.) DC.和禹州漏芦 Echinops latifolius Tausch.的根。晒干。切片生用。

处方用名　漏芦。

性味归经　苦，寒。入胃经。

功效应用　清热解毒，消痈下乳：用于痈疮肿痛，乳汁不下等症。如时疫丹毒。面喉红肿，可与升麻、大青叶、大黄等同用；治乳痈初起，可与栝楼、蒲公英、银花、白芷等同用；治妇女乳汁不下，可与王不留行、穿山甲等同用。

用量用法　6～10 克。煎服。

贯　众

为鳞毛蕨科多年生草本植物粗茎鳞毛蕨 Dryoptevis crassirhizoma Nakai 或蹄盖蕨科多年生草本植物蛾眉蕨 Lunathyrium acrostichoides（Sw.）Ching、球子蕨科植物荚果蕨 Matteuccia struthiopteris（L.）Todaro.紫萁科植物紫萁 Osmunda japonica Thuub.和乌毛蕨科多年生草本植物乌毛蕨 Blechnum orientale L.、苏铁蕨 Brainia insignis（Hook.）J.Sm.狗脊蕨 Woodwardia japonica（L.f.）Sw.等的根茎及叶柄残基。晒干，切片，生用或炒炭用。

处方用名　贯众、贯仲、贯众炭。

性味归经　苦，微寒。有小毒。入肝、肾、肺、胃经。

功效应用

1. 清热解毒：用于湿热疮毒，痄腮肿痛等症，可单用研末，油调涂；用于防治疾病，在瘟疫流行时，民间用本品与菖蒲、苍术、雄黄等浸入水缸中，为生活用水，以防传染；防治麻疹，可用贯仲 10 克，丝瓜络 15 克，煎汤代茶。

2. 凉血止血：用于妇女崩漏，产后出血，可炒炭单用，煎服或为末服；或与旱莲草、阿膠等其他止血药同用；亦可用治血痢，便血等。

3. 杀虫消积：用于蛔虫、蛲虫、绦虫、钩虫等虫积腹痛，肛门瘙痒，多配入其他杀虫方中同用。

此外，现代常用预防流感，单用贯众10克，水煎服，每天1剂，1次服完，或研粉每服1.5～3克，日3次；亦可与银花、甘草煎汤服。预防流脑，可配甘草、野菊花煎服，连服3～7天。

用量用法 3～10克，煎服。解毒宜生用，止血宜炒炭用。

土 茯 苓

为百合科多年生攀援灌木土茯苓（光叶菝葜）Smilax glabra Roxb.的根茎。鲜用，或鲜时切片，晒干生用。

处方用名 土茯苓。

性味归经 甘、淡，平。入肝、胃经。

功效应用 利湿解毒：用于梅毒或梅毒服用汞剂而致肢体拘挛者，本品清血解毒，历来为治梅毒要药，且能利关节，并可解轻粉、银朱中毒，故对梅毒筋骨拘挛者，尤为适用有效。可单用大剂量煎服，或与金银花、白鲜皮、威灵仙、甘草等配用；若因服轻粉导致肢体拘急者，重用本品配大皂荚、牵牛各3克应用；用于痈肿疮疖，或反复发作的慢性疮疡，可与银花、连翘、蒲公英等配用；用于慢性湿疹，可配生地、赤芍、地肤子等同用。

此外，亦常用于银屑病，单用30克，水煎当茶常饮；并治风湿关节疼痛。

用量用法 15～60克。煎服。

使用注意 服药期间忌饮茶，饮茶能致脱发，用时当注意。

蚤　休

为百合科多年生草本植物七叶一枝花 Paris polyphylla Smith 或金线重楼 Paris Chinensis Franch.的根茎。晒干。切片生用。

处方用名　蚤休、重楼、七叶一枝花。

性味归经　微苦，凉，有小毒。入肝经。

功效应用　清热解毒，消肿止痛：用于一切疔疮肿毒，咽喉肿痛，毒蛇咬伤等症。治一切疮毒，可单味醋磨汁涂患处；亦可与银花、川连、蝉蜕、僵蚕等同用；如治毒蛇咬伤，单味研末，每次 3 克，每日 2～3 次服；另醋磨汁涂伤口周围肿疡处。

此外，尚可用于小儿高热惊风痉挛，单味研末，每次 1 克，凉开水送服；或与其它清热解毒，熄风止痉药同用。

现代有配大青叶、板蓝根等清热解毒药，防治流行性乙型脑炎、腮腺炎等病，有一定疗效。

用量用法　5～10 克。煎服。外用适量。

马　齿　苋

为马齿苋科 1 年生肉质草本植物马齿苋 Portulaca oleracea L. 的全草。晒干。切段生用或鲜用。

处方用名　马齿苋。

性味归经　酸，寒。入心、大肠经。

功效应用　清热解毒，治痢疗疮：用于热痢血痢，可单用煎服，或鲜者捣汁，入蜜和服；亦可用作预防痢疾；用于痈肿疔疮，可单用煎汤服，并以鲜品捣敷患处。

此外，尚用于月经过多、崩漏和产后出血，单用煎服，或与益母草、地榆、茜草等止血药配伍；用于百日咳，单用 60 克，水煎分 3 次服。

用量用法　15～30 克，鲜品 30～60 克，煎服。外用适量。

白 头 翁

为毛茛科多年生草本植物白头翁 Pulsatilla Chinensis (Bge.) Regel 的根。晒干。切片生用。

处方用名 白头翁。

性味归经 苦，寒。入胃、大肠经。

功效应用 清热解毒，凉血止痢：用于热毒血痢，赤痢腹痛。如热痢下重，常与黄连、秦皮等同用；若下痢血虚，或产后血虚下痢，可配阿胶、甘草同用。

现代临床用本品治细菌性痢疾和阿米巴痢疾均有良效。此外，治阴道滴虫，与苦参、蛇床子煎汤熏洗，亦有一定效果。

用量用法 6～12 克。煎服。外用适量。

穿 心 莲

为爵床科 1 年生草本植物穿心莲 Androgaphis paniculata (Bum.f.) Nees 的全草或叶。切段。晒干生用。

处方用名 穿心莲、一见喜、榄核莲。

性味归经 苦，寒。入肺、胃、大肠、膀胱经。

功效应用

1. 清热解毒：用于肺热咳喘，肺痈，咽喉肿痛，可与金银花、黄芩等配伍；用于疮疗肿毒，可与金银花、野菊花、七叶一枝花、白花蛇舌草等同用。

2. 清热燥湿：用于湿热泻痢、热淋、湿疹等。用于湿热泻痢，可单用或与黄连、黄芩、马齿苋等同用；热淋，小便短赤涩痛，可与车前子、海金沙、石苇等利尿通淋药同用；治湿疹，可研粉用甘油调涂。

穿心莲为近年临床应用的新品种，具有较强的清热解毒、抗感染的作用，可广泛用于呼吸道、消化道、泌尿系及皮肤化脓性多种感染性疾病。

用量用法 干品 3～10 克。煎服。粉剂 1.5～3 克，每日 3 次；因味极苦，如用粉剂，宜装入胶囊吞下，或糖水送服。现多用片剂，每次 6～8 片，每日 3 次。

使用注意 本品苦寒，不宜多服久服，以免损伤胃气。

白花蛇舌草

为茜草科 1 年生草本植物白花蛇舌草 Oldenlandia diffusa (Willd.) Roxb 的全草。晒干，切段用。

处方用名 白花蛇舌草。

性味归经 甘、淡，凉。入胃、肺、大肠、膀胱经。

功效应用

1. 清热解毒，散瘀消痈：用于肠痈，肺痈，疔疮，痈疖，毒蛇咬伤等。内服外用均可。治肠痈，可与金银花、红藤等同用；治肺痈，可与鱼腥草、桔梗、芦根等同用；治疔疮痈疖，常与金银花、连翘、野菊花等同用；毒蛇咬伤，可捣敷患处，或配伍紫花地丁、半边莲等内服。

2. 利尿通淋：用于热淋小便淋涩热痛，可与金银花、车前草、黄柏、石苇等配用。

此外，尚可用治急性肾炎浮肿，尿有蛋白，可用本品配车前草各 15 克，白茅根 30 克，山栀子 9 克，苏叶 6 克，煎服，对小儿肾炎退肿较好。试用治疗胃癌、食道癌、直肠癌多种癌症，但其疗效有待进一步观察。

白　蔹

为葡萄科多年生攀援性藤本植物白蔹 Ampelopsis japonica (Thunb.) Mak.的根。斜切成片，晒干，生用。

处方用名 白蔹、白蔹根。

性味归经 苦、辛，微寒。入心、肝、胃经。

功效应用 清热解毒，消肿生肌：用于痈肿疮毒。治痈肿未脓，可配赤芍、连翘，亦可研末外敷；治痈疮已脓，可配白芷、花粉；溃疡脓净，疮口不敛，可与当归、乳香等养血活血生肌药同用。用于烫伤、火伤，可单用为末，水调涂，或配赤小豆为末，以鸡蛋白调敷；亦可单用煎服。

此外，尚可用治疝气腹痛，单用本品 30 克，水煎加红糖调服。

用量用法 3～10 克，大剂量可用至 30 克。煎服。外用适量。

使用注意 反乌头。

半 边 莲

为桔梗科多年生蔓生草本植物半边莲 Lobelia chinensis Thunb.的全草。晒干或阴干。生用或鲜用。

处方用名 半边莲。

性味归经 甘、淡，微寒。入肺、肝、肾经。

功效应用

1. 清热解毒：用于毒蛇、蜈蚣咬伤或蜂、蝎螫伤。治蛇伤可用鲜品 120 克，捣烂，加甜酒或温开水擂汁内服，服后盖被取微汗，日服 1 次，重症日服 2 次，外用鲜全草捣烂，加食盐少许，敷伤口周围及肿处，或用鲜草煎服，渣外敷；治蜂、蝎螫伤，可用鲜品捣烂外敷。

2. 利水消肿：用于水肿腹胀，小便不利，可与其他利尿药同用。

现代多用治晚期血吸虫病腹水、肝硬化腹水等，用鲜品捣烂取汁，加烧酒少许滴耳，可治急性脓耳；近年亦常试用于癌症。

用量用法 15～30 克，鲜品 30～60 克，煎服。

2.6 清退虚热药

清退虚热药，性多寒凉，具有凉血退虚热的功效，适用于骨蒸潮热，低热不退等症。

应用本类药物时，通常要配伍养阴药，标本兼顾。

青 蒿

为菊科1年或2年生草本植物青蒿 Artemisia apiacea Hance 或黄花蒿 Aretemisia annua L.的茎叶。阴干。切碎生用。

处方用名 青蒿、嫩青蒿、南青蒿。

性味归经 苦、微辛，寒。入肝、胆经。

功效应用

1. 清热退蒸：用于热病后期，热伏阴分，夜热早凉，热退无汗之症，常与鳖甲、生地、知母等同用；用于阴虚潮热，骨蒸盗汗，常与鳖甲、地骨皮等同用；或加入滋阴药中以助解热。

2. 清热解暑：用于暑温外感，发热汗出，可与连翘、滑石、甘草等同用；若小儿夏季发热，也可与地骨皮、白薇、知母等配伍。

3. 清胆截疟：用于疟疾寒热往来，可单用较大量的鲜品，加水捣汁服。因其又能清解暑热，故历来对疟疾兼感暑邪者尤为常用。若疟疾发热心烦，胸闷苔腻等兼暑湿之邪者，则又常与黄芩、淡竹茹、赤茯苓等配伍同用。

4. 凉血止血：用于鼻衄、紫斑。治鼻衄可用鲜品捣汁加凉开水冲服；治紫斑可与升麻、鳖甲、当归、生地等同用。

用量用法 6～15克。大量可用18～30克。煎服，或鲜用绞汁。

使用注意 不宜久煎。

白　薇

为萝藦科多年生草本植物直立白薇 Cynanchum atratum Bge.或蔓生白薇 Cynanchum versicolor Bge.的根及根茎。晒干。切段生用。

处方用名　白薇、香白薇。

性味归经　苦、咸，寒。入胃、肝经。

功效应用

1. 凉血退蒸：用于阴虚血热，午后身热，或低热不退，或骨蒸潮热，及一切原因不明的虚性发热等症，常与生地、青蒿、地骨皮等同用；纯阴虚者，可与滋阴药配伍。若配当归、人参、甘草，可治产后血虚发热、昏厥。

2. 利尿通淋：用于热淋、血淋，小便赤涩热痛，常与木通、滑石、石苇等同用。

此外，本品尚可治乳痈疮疖、毒蛇咬伤疼痛，可用白薇全草适量，捣烂外敷患处。亦可与其他清热解毒药配伍同用。

用量用法　6～12克。煎服。

银 柴 胡

为石竹科多年生草本植物银柴胡 Stellaria dichotoma L. var. lanceolata Bge.的根。晒干。切片生用。

处方用名　银柴胡、银胡。

性味归经　甘，微寒。入肝、胃经。

功效应用

1. 凉血退蒸：用于阴虚血热，劳热骨蒸，本品善于退虚热，为治虚热之良药。常与青蒿、鳖甲、地骨皮等配伍；若久疟不止，体虚低烧，或热病后期，余热未尽者，亦可随症配用。

2. 清疳热：用于小儿疳积，消瘦发热，烦渴躁急，可与胡黄连、鸡内金、党参、白术等配用。

用量用法 3～10克。煎服。

使用注意 外感风寒，血虚无热者忌用。

地 骨 皮

为茄科落叶蔓生灌木枸杞 Lycium chinense Mill.的根皮。晒干。切段生用。

处方用名 地骨皮。

性味归经 甘，寒。入肺、肾经。

功效应用

1. 凉血退蒸：用于阴虚血热，劳热骨蒸，盗汗及小儿疳积发热等症，本品善清虚热。常与鳖甲、知母等同用。

2. 清泻肺火：用于肺热咳喘或咳血之症，常与桑白皮、甘草等同用。

此外，本品可用治糖尿病，烦热消渴、多尿之症。

用量用法 6～12克。煎服。

胡 黄 连

为玄参科多年生草本植物胡黄连 Picrorrhiza scrophulariiaeflora Punnell 的根茎。晒干，切片，生用。

处方用名 胡黄连。

性味归经 苦，寒。入心、肝、胃、大肠经。

功效应用

1. 清热退蒸：用于阴虚发热，劳热骨蒸，常与银柴胡、地骨皮等配用。

2. 清热消疳：用于小儿疳积，时有腹胀，午后潮热，可与党参、白术、使君子、山楂等同用；或与芜荑、干蛤蟆等配用；若有疳眼，视物不清，可配鸡肝蒸服。

3. 清热燥湿：用于湿热下痢，有类似黄连功效。亦可用治痔疮肿痛，内服外敷皆可。

用量用法 3～10 克。煎服。

3 泻下药

凡能引起腹泻或滑利大肠，促使大便排出的药物，统称泻下药。

泻下药适用于里实之证，其主要作用大致可分为3点：

1. 清除肠内宿食燥屎以及其他有害物质，使从大便排出。

2. 清热泻火，使体内热毒通过泻下而得到缓解。

3. 逐水消肿，使水有出路，则水肿、停饮得以消除。

此外，泻下药在临床上还用于以下几个方面：

1. 对于上部充血、出血等病症兼见便秘者，用泻下药可使病情缓解，这是"上病下取"的方法。

2. 如痢疾初起，里急后重，泻而不畅者，虽无便秘现象，也可酌用泻下药，可促使病情减轻，这是"通因通用"的方法。

3. 近些年来，中、西医结合治疗急腹症，在内服药方面，根据中医的"不通则痛"，"通则不痛"以及"六腑以通为用"等原理，对某些急腹症属于实热结滞的证候，应用通里泻下、清热泻火的方法，获得良好效果，从而免除手术治疗减轻病人痛苦。

根据泻下药作用的不同，分为攻下药、峻下逐水药、润下药3类。攻下药与峻下逐水药力量较猛，而后者尤为峻烈，奏效迅速，但易伤正气。故凡久病正虚、年老体弱，妇女胎前产后、月经期，皆应慎用。润下药力量缓和，其润滑作用，能解除排便困难，但不致引起大泻，故对年老体弱患者，以及妇女胎前产后等由于血虚或津液不足所致的肠燥便秘，皆可应用。

使用泻下药，还应注意以下几点：

1. 泻下作用的强度与剂量有关。如病情较重需要急下者，可选用攻下药，应用大剂量，并煎汤剂内服，以取速效；病情较缓，只需缓下者，药量不宜过重，或制成丸剂内服。缓下药用大剂量时，其效等于峻下药，峻下药用小剂量时，也可相当于缓下药的作用，所以剂量的掌握十分重要。

2. 本类药物经不同的方法处理后，其疗效差异较大，因此，对炮制和煎煮方法应予注意。

3.1 攻下药

本类药物，性味大多苦寒，具有较强的泻下作用，适用于宿食停滞，大便不通所致的各种里实证候，以其性偏寒凉，具有清热泻火作用，故尤以实热壅滞，燥粪坚积者为适宜。如治寒积便秘，须配温里药；如便秘症腹部胀满而气滞者，可与理气药同用；如属体虚不胜攻下的，可配补益药，攻补兼施，使泻不伤正；如里实而兼表邪者，当先解表，然后攻里。必要时可与解表药同用，表里双解，以免表邪陷里。

大　黄

为蓼科多年生草本植物掌叶大黄 Rheum palmatum L.唐古特大黄 R. tanguticum Maxim. ex Reg.，或药用大黄 R. officinale Baill.的根和根茎。切片或小块入药。生用，黄酒合蜜蒸熟用，酒炒或炒炭用。

处方用名　生大黄、熟大黄、酒大黄、大黄炭。

性味归经　苦、寒。入胃、大肠、脾、肝、心包经。

功效应用

1. 攻下积滞：用于胃肠积滞，大便秘结。本品苦寒沉降，力猛善走，泻下之力较强，为治积滞便秘之要药。以其苦寒泻火，故热结便秘用之尤宜。若热结便秘，腹痛胀满，高热不退，烦躁神昏谵语，常与芒硝、枳实、厚朴同用；里实热结而兼有气血虚者，常与人参、当归等补气养血药配伍；热结阴伤者，可与生地、玄参、麦冬等养阴生津药配伍；脾阳不足，冷积便秘者，可与党参、附子、干姜等补气温阳药配用；若肠胃湿热下痢，或大便溏而不爽的，常与芍药、黄芩、黄连、木香等同用，此为“通因通用”之法。

2. 泻火解毒：用于火热亢盛所致血热妄行之吐血、衄血，以及火邪上炎引起的咽喉肿痛、牙龈肿痛、目赤。常与黄芩、黄连同用；亦可与枯矾同研细末涂口腔，以治口疮；用于痈疡肿毒，可单味为末醋调涂；亦可与其他清热解毒药配用；用于烫火烧伤，常与地榆等量，为末，香油调涂患处；治肠痈，可配芒硝、丹皮、桃仁等同用。

3. 逐瘀通经：用于血瘀经闭，产后瘀滞腹痛者，可与桃仁、䗪虫同用；若治跌打损伤，血瘀胀痛，可与当归等量为末服。

此外，本品尚能清泄湿热，故亦用于湿热黄疸和淋症。前者，常配茵陈、栀子；后者，常配木通、车前子、栀子等。

用量用法　3～15克。煎服。外用适量。泻下攻积用大量，活血化瘀用小量。生用力猛，熟用力缓；欲攻下者，宜生用；入汤剂应后下，或沸水浸泡服。酒制善清上部火热，炒炭则化瘀止血。

使用注意　孕妇或妇女经、产、哺乳期宜慎用或忌用。

芒　硝

为含硫酸钠的天然矿物，经精制加工而成的结晶体。秋冬之间，扫取含硫酸钠的天然矿物，用热水溶解，过滤，放冷析出结晶，此结晶称为朴硝或皮硝，再取萝卜洗净切片，置锅内加水与朴硝共煮，取上层液，放冷，析出结晶，即为芒硝（结晶形如马牙者，又称为牙硝）。芒硝经风化成粉者，名风化硝。

处方用名　芒硝、风化硝。

性味归经　咸、苦，寒。入胃、大肠经。

功效应用

1. 软坚泻下：用于胃肠实热积滞，大便燥结不通，常与大黄、甘草同用。

2. 清热泻火：用于咽喉肿烂，口疮，可与冰片、硼砂配用；用于乳痈，可以本品外敷，消散肿块，尚可用于回乳。

此外，用于皮肤湿疹、荨麻疹，可用芒硝、白矾各30克，沸水溶化乘热烫洗。

用量用法　3～10克。入汤剂溶化服。外用适量。

附药　元明粉：又称玄明粉。系芒硝经风化后，同甘草再煎炼，凝浮上面之硝块，风化后为元明粉。性味甘、咸、微苦，性寒。有如芒硝类似的功效，但作用较缓和。主要用于口腔溃烂，咽喉肿痛，目赤红肿，疮疡等症。常与冰片、硼砂等同用，研末吹患处，或化水点眼，敷疮、洗疮等。用量3～10克。外用适量。孕妇禁用。

番　泻　叶

为豆科草本状小灌木狭叶番泻树 Cassia angustifolia vahl 或尖叶番泻树 Cassia acutifolia Delile 的小叶片。原药生用。

处方用名　番泻叶、泻叶、泻叶茶。

性味归经　甘、苦，寒。入大肠经。

功效应用

1. 泻热通便：用于热结食积，肠燥便秘，可与枳实、厚朴同用；亦可单味沸水泡汤服或研末蜜丸服。

2. 行水消胀：用于腹水臌胀（较甘遂稳妥），可与二丑、大腹皮同用；亦可单味沸水泡汤服。

用量用法　缓下1～2克；峻下3～6克。入煎剂宜后入，一般泡服即可，研末蜜丸服，奏效较缓。

使用注意　孕妇、月经期及哺乳期及下部出血者均忌用。剂量过大，可引起恶心、呕吐、腹痛等副作用。

芦　荟

为百合科多年生常绿植物库拉索芦荟 Aloe vera L.好望角芦荟 Aloe ferox Mill.或斑纹芦荟 Aloe vera L. var. chinensis (Haw.) Berger 叶片基部的液汁所制成的黑色或暗绿色透明或半透明的干膏硬块。原药研末用。

处方用名　芦荟。

性味归经　苦，寒。入肝、胃、大肠经。

功效应用

1. 泻热通便：用于肝胆实热而兼大便秘结者，常与龙胆草、山栀、黄芩等同用；若治肠道实热津亏心烦之便秘，可用芦荟 22 克，朱砂 15 克，共研末，调和为丸，每次 3 克，温水送服。

2. 杀虫疗疳：用于小儿蛔虫病，疳积，可与胡黄连、芜荑、木香等同用。

现代，临床用于治疗白血病，多与青黛、当归等清热补血药用，取得了一定的效果。

用量用法　1～2 克。入丸散剂，不入煎剂。

使用注意　脾胃虚寒，孕妇忌用。

3.2　峻下逐水药

本类药物性较猛峻，能引起强烈腹泻，而使大量水分从大小便排出，达到消除肿胀的目的。

本类药物适用于水肿、胸腹积水及痰饮结聚等病情比较严重，出现喘满呕逆等壅实之症。现代用于晚期血吸虫病腹水，在改善症状方面效果良好。

本类药物非但药性峻烈，且多具有毒性，不宜过服。对于炮制、配伍、剂量、运用方法以及禁忌等，都必须严格掌握使用，以保证用药安全。

严重水肿患者用逐水药时，应酌情与补益药同用，宜一攻九补之法，攻补兼施，或先攻后补，注意顾护正气。

甘　遂

为大戟科多年生肉质草本植物甘遂 Euphorbia kansui Liou 的根。醋炒或麸炒用。

处方用名　炒甘遂、制甘遂、甘遂。

性味归经　苦，寒。有小毒。入肺、脾、肾经。

功效应用

1. 泻水逐饮：用于胸腹水饮内停所致的痰饮积聚，胸胁引痛，咳逆喘满，心下痞硬，腹水胀满等症，常与大戟、芫花、白芥子、二丑、木香等同用。

2. 消肿散结：用于湿热肿毒，研末水调涂。

现代治疗重型肠梗阻、肠腔积液较多者，常与大黄、厚朴、桃仁等同用。

用量用法　0.6～1.5克。炮制后用，多入丸散剂。外用生品适量。

使用注意　体虚者、孕妇均忌用。反甘草。

大　戟

为大戟科多年生草本植物京大戟 Euphorbia pekinensis Rupr.及茜草科多年生草本植物红芽大戟 Knoxia valerianoides Thorel 的根。醋炒醋煮，或入豆腐同煮后用。

处方用名　大戟、红芽大戟。

性味归经　苦，寒。有毒。入肺、脾、肾经。

功效应用

1. 泻水逐饮：用于胸腹水饮内停所致的痰饮喘咳，胸胁引痛及腹水胀满等症，常与甘遂、芫花同用。

2. 消肿散结：用于疮肿、瘰疬等症，单用熬膏外敷。

用量用法 0.6～1.5克。多入丸散剂。

使用注意 虚弱者及孕妇忌用。反甘草。

芫　花

为瑞香科落叶灌木芫花 Daphne genkwa sieb. et zucc.的花蕾。醋炒或醋煮用。

处方用名 醋芫花、陈芫花、芫花。

性味归经 辛、苦，寒，有毒。入肺、脾、肾经。

功效应用

1. 泻水逐饮：用于痰饮喘咳，胸胁引痛以及腹水胀满等症，常与甘遂、大戟同用。

2. 杀虫疗疮：用于顽癣、头疮、白秃等，单用或与雄黄共研细末，猪脂调敷患处；用于冻疮，与甘草煎汤外洗。

用量用法 0.6～1.5克，多入丸散剂。外用适量。

使用注意 孕妇忌用，反甘草。

牵　牛　子

为旋花科1年生攀援草木植物牵牛 Pharbitis nil（L.）Choisy 或毛牵牛 Pharbitis purpurea（L.）Voigt 等的种子。生用或炒用，打碎入药，或研细取头末用。

处方用名 牵牛子、黑丑、白丑、黑白丑、二丑。

性味归经 苦，寒，有毒。入肺、肾、大肠经。

功效应用

1. 泻下逐水：用于水肿胀满，二便不利，可与红糖、生姜、大枣同用；用于湿热壅滞之大便秘结，单用为末，姜汤送服；亦可用于痰饮喘咳，多与葶苈子、杏仁、厚朴同用。

2. 杀虫消积：用于蛔虫腹痛，牵牛子、槟榔、大黄各等分，研末，早晚空腹服2～3克，开水调下；用于蛲虫，牵牛子、雷丸各9克，生大黄3克，研末，分3次于临睡时用温开水送服。

用量用法 3～9克，煎服。丸散减半。研细去皮用。

使用注意 孕妇忌用，畏巴豆。

商　陆

为商陆科多年生草本植物 Phytolacca acinosa Roxb.的根。晒干。生用或醋煮用。

处方用名 商陆、商陆根。

性味归经 苦，寒，有毒。入肺、脾、肾经。

功效应用

1. 逐水消肿：用于遍身水肿，胸腹胀满，二便不利，可与茯苓皮、椒目、槟榔、赤小豆等同用；亦可与瘦猪肉炖服。

2. 解毒消肿：用于疮痈肿毒，以鲜品加食盐捣外敷。

用量用法 2～4.5克，煎服。外用适量。内服宜醋煮，外治可生用。

使用注意 脾虚水肿及孕妇忌用。

巴　豆

为大戟科常绿乔木巴豆树 Croton tiglium L.的成熟种子。生研碎压去油取霜用，或炒焦黑用。

处方用名 巴豆霜、焦巴豆。

性味归经 辛，热，有大毒。入胃、大肠经。

功效应用

1. 泻下冷积：用于寒积便秘，腹满胀痛，甚至气急暴厥者，可与干姜、大黄各等分，蜜丸如梧桐子大，每次0.6～0.9克，开水送服。用于小儿痰食积滞，疳积等，常与胆南星、神曲等同用。

2. 逐水消胀：用于腹水臌胀，焦巴豆90枚，炒杏仁60枚，共捣泥为丸，每次0.3～0.6克，开水送服，以下为度。现代用治晚期血吸虫病肝硬化腹水，可用巴豆霜9克，绛矾30克，神曲糊为丸，小豆大，每次1～1.5克，日1次，开水送服。

3. 豁痰利咽：用于喉痹、痰壅咽喉，呼吸急促，喉闭肿塞，窒息欲死，本品能祛痰涎以利呼吸，可用巴豆霜少量灌服，或用巴豆与白矾同炒，待矾枯，去巴豆，研矾为细末，水调灌服或将末吹入喉中，促使吐出痰涎，开通闭塞。

4. 解毒疗疮：用于疮疡疔毒脓成未溃者，以焦巴豆、乳香适量，捣为膏，敷贴患处；或用焦巴豆、雄黄、大黄各等份，为末糊丸，小豆大，每次2～4丸，日2次，开水送服。

现代用治白喉、喉炎引起的喉梗阻，可用巴豆霜吹喉，引起呕吐，排出痰涎，或伴有腹泻，使梗阻症状得以解除。

用量用法　每次0.1～0.2克。只入丸散剂。外用适量。炒焦则泻力较缓，用霜则泻力较峻。

使用注意　服用巴豆时，不宜进食热粥、饮热开水等，以免泻下加剧。本品得热则助泻，如服后欲泻不泻者，可进热粥以助药力；若泻下不止，速进冷粥或冷水以解药力。中其毒而腹痛大泻不止者，急用黄连或绿豆煎汤以解之。体虚及孕妇均当忌服。

3.3 润下药

本类药物多为富含脂肪的植物种子或种仁，具有润滑肠壁和粪便，促进泻下的作用。适宜于老年津枯的便秘，或产后血虚，或病后津液未复，以及亡血病人，大肠燥结，以致排便困难者。

若热盛伤津而便秘者，可配养阴药用；兼血虚者宜与补血药同用；兼气滞者可与理气药同用。

火　麻　仁

为桑科1年生草本植物大麻 Cannabis sativa L.的种仁。取净仁微炒打碎用。

处方用名 火麻仁、大麻仁、麻子仁。

性味归经 甘，平。入脾、胃、大肠经。

功效应用 润肠通便，滋阴补虚：用于老人或体虚者之肠胃燥热，大便秘结，常与大黄、枳实等同用；若治老人或妇女产后血虚之便秘，可与肉苁蓉、当归等同用。

此外，尚可用于习惯性便秘和痔疮便秘。

用量用法 10～15克。煎服。

使用注意 剂量不宜过大，一次内服60～120克以上，可致中毒，出现吐泻，四肢麻木，甚至昏睡。

郁 李 仁

为蔷薇科落叶灌木植物欧李 Prunus humilis Bge.或郁李 P. japonica Thunb.的种子。去壳取仁，微炒捣碎用。

处方用名 郁李仁。

性味归经 辛、苦，平。入大肠、小肠、脾经。

功效应用

1. 润肠通便：用于津枯肠燥便秘，常与杏仁、柏子仁等同用。

2. 行水消胀：用于实满胀急之腹水症，可与二丑、甘遂等同用；若治脚气浮肿，二便不利，可用郁李仁10克，生薏仁30克，水煎服。

用量用法 6～12克。煎服。

使用注意 孕妇慎用。

4 祛风湿药

凡能祛除肌肉、经络以及筋骨之间的风湿之邪，以解除痹痛的药物，称为祛风湿药。

当人体遭受风寒湿邪侵袭之后，经络阻滞，气血流行不畅，便能形成痹证。痹证的主要症状是：肢体关节等处疼痛，酸楚麻木，重着，筋脉拘挛等。但由于风寒湿邪各有偏胜，所表现的症状也就各异，如风气偏胜，多见拘挛掣痛，游走不定，称为行痹；寒气偏胜，疼痛较剧，称为痛痹；湿气偏胜，多见麻痹肿痛，重着不移，称为着痹。此外，尚有热痹，是痹证兼有热象，属风寒湿邪化热所致。

本类药物分别具有祛风、散寒、除湿及通络、行痹、止痛的作用。其中，部分药物还有补肝肾、壮筋骨的功效，在临证时须根据痹证的症状，选择应用。

由于痹痛一证较为复杂，在使用本类药物时，还应根据各种不同症状，作适当配伍，才能增强疗效。如风寒湿邪在表者，当配解表药同用，使邪易从外解；如风寒湿邪入于筋骨经络，便当配合活血通络药同用，使邪不易稽留；如病证偏风者，可配祛风止痛药同用；病证偏寒者，应配辛温祛寒药同用；病证偏湿者，应与利湿药同用；病证偏热者，宜配苦寒清热药同用；如病久气血亏虚，又当配合补气养血药同用，以扶正达邪。这些配伍原则，必须重视。

一般祛风湿药，大都辛散、温燥、能伤阴耗血，故阴亏血虚者，宜慎用。

独　活

为伞形科多年生草本植物重齿毛当归 Angelica pubescens Maxim.f. biserrata shan et Yuan.毛当归 Angelica pubescens Maxim.的根。晒干，横切片生用。

处方用名　独活、川独活。

性味归经　辛、苦，微温。入肾、肝经。

功效应用

1. 祛风胜湿止痛：用于风湿痹痛，腰膝两足偏重者，常与桑寄生、秦艽、牛膝等同用。本品善治在下在里之风，对下半身的肌肉关节疼痛用之最宜。

2. 散寒解表：用于风寒感冒，头痛，全身肢节酸痛，可与羌活、防风、白芷、川芎、甘草、生姜等同用。

用量用法　3～10 克。煎服。

秦　艽

为龙胆科多年生草本植物大叶秦艽 Gentiana macrophylla pall.和麻花秦艽 G.straminea Maxim.粗茎秦艽 G.crassicaulis Duthie ex Burk.或小秦艽 G.dahurica Fisch.等的根。切片生用。

处方用名　秦艽、西秦艽、左秦艽。

性味归经　苦、辛，平。入胃、大肠、肝、胆经。

功效应用

1. 祛风止痛：用于风湿痹痛，关节拘挛，筋骨不利，及感受风邪所致的肢体酸痛等症，常与独活、防风、川芎、防己、海桐皮等同用。

2. 清热退蒸：用于骨蒸潮热，常与青蒿、地骨皮、鳖甲等同用。

此外，尚具清湿热，利二便之功，可用于湿热黄疸；又为治肠风便血之要药。

用量用法 6～10克。煎服。

威灵仙

为毛茛科多年生攀援性灌木威灵仙（软灵仙）Clematis chinensis Osbeck.棉团铁线莲 Clematis hexapetala pall.或东北铁线莲 Clematis manshurica Rupr.的根及根茎。晒干，切片，生用。

处方用名 威灵仙、铁灵仙。

性味归经 辛、咸、温。入膀胱经。

功效应用

1. 祛风除湿，通络止痛：用于风湿痹痛，风邪偏胜，拘挛掣痛，可与其他祛风活血药同用；若治寒湿脚气入腹，胀闷气急，用威灵仙为末，每次6克，黄酒送服。

2. 行气化滞：用于妇女气血凝滞之腹痛，可与当归、肉桂等同用。

此外，还可用于诸骨鲠喉，可单用本品或与米醋、砂糖同煎去渣，待温，徐徐咽下。

用量用法 6～10克。煎服。

片姜黄

为姜科多年生宿根草本植物郁金 Curcuma aromatica salisb.的根茎。又称片子姜黄、毛姜黄。趁鲜时切片，晒干用。

处方用名 片姜黄。

性味归经 辛、苦，温。入肝、脾经。

功效应用 温经散寒，除风燥湿，行气止痛：用于风湿痹证，关节不利，肩臂酸痛。本品辛散横行，长于行肢臂而能通利筋脉。常与羌活、当归、赤芍等同用；用于气滞血瘀之胸胁脘腹诸痛及血瘀经闭、腹中包块，常与当归、白芍、川芎、莪术、红花等配用。

用量用法 3～10克。煎服。

木 瓜

为蔷薇科落叶灌木贴梗海棠 Chaenomeles lagenaria (Loisel.) Koidz.的果实。水浸入笼蒸软即切片用。

处方用名 木瓜、宣木瓜、陈木瓜。

性味归经 酸，温。入肝、脾经。

功效应用

1. 舒筋活络：用于湿痹脚气，足胫肿大，腰膝酸痛，关节肿胀，筋挛足痿等症。若属寒湿脚气，常与苏叶、吴茱萸、生姜等同用；若属湿热脚气，可与黄柏、萆薢、石斛等同用；若治腰膝酸痛，常与续断、杜仲等同用。

2. 化湿和胃：用于夏月伤暑，饮食不调，霍乱吐泻，甚或转筋腿痛等症，常与藿香、厚朴、半夏等或与吴茱萸、紫苏等同用。本品善于温通肌腠之湿滞，走筋而舒挛急，所以为治湿痹、脚气和一切转筋腿痛之要药。

此外，还能消食止渴，亦属和中祛湿，酸以生津的效用。

用量用法 6～10克。煎服。

防 己

为防己科多年生缠绕藤本植物粉防己 Stephania tetrandra S. Moore、木防己 Cocculus trilobus （Thuub.）DC.及马兜铃科多年生攀援藤本植物广防己 Aristolochia fangchi Wu 的根。刮去外皮，切片晒干生用。

处方用名 防己、汉防己、木防己。

性味归经 苦、辛，寒。入膀胱、脾、肺经。

功效应用

1. 祛风止痛（木防己较佳）：用于风湿关节疼痛。治风寒湿关节疼痛，可与白术、桂心、川乌、生姜等同用；若治湿热阻滞经络，关节疼痛，或脚气肿痛，可与牛膝、黄柏、木瓜、薏苡仁等同用。

2. 利水退肿（汉防己较佳）：用于下焦湿热，水肿、腹水、小便不利等症。治遍身水肿，脉浮身重，汗出恶风者，可与黄芪、白术、甘草同用；若治皮水四肢浮肿，小便不利者，可与茯苓、黄芪、桂枝、甘草同用；若用于痰饮，肠间有水气，腹胀满而口舌干燥，可与椒目、葶苈、大黄各等分，研末蜜丸，每次6克，日服3次。

用量用法　3～10克。煎服。

使用注意　本品苦寒较甚，不宜大量使用，以免损伤胃气。体弱阴虚及胃纳不佳者忌用。

桑　枝

为桑科落叶小乔木桑树 Morus alba L.的嫩枝。切片生用。

处方用名　桑枝、嫩桑枝。

性味归经　苦，平。入肝经。

功效应用　祛风通络：用于风湿手臂指麻，常与威灵仙、防己、当归等同用；若用于风湿热痹，又常与络石藤、忍冬藤、地龙等同用。

用量用法　15～30克。煎服。

桑寄生

为桑寄生科常用小灌木寄生植物槲寄生 Viscum coloratum (kom.) Nakai.桑寄生 Loranthus Parasiticus（L.）Merr.的干燥带叶茎枝。切片或切段生用。

处方用名　桑寄生。

性味归经　苦、甘，平。入肝、肾经。

功效应用

1. 祛风湿，强筋骨：用于风湿腰膝酸痛。本品长于补肝肾，强筋骨。故对痹痛日久，损及肝肾，筋骨不利，腰膝酸痛，用之最宜。常与独活、牛膝、杜仲、当归等同用。

2. 补肝肾，养血安胎：用于肝肾虚损，冲任不固之胎漏，胎动不安，常与当归、阿胶、续断等同用。本品祛邪之力有余，补养之功不足，故不能专恃为滋补药。

此外，本品尚有降血压作用。

用量用法　15～30克。煎服。

五　加　皮

为五加科落叶小灌木细柱五加 Acanthopanax gracilistylus W.W. Smith 的根皮，习称“南五加皮”。切段生用。

处方用名　五加皮。

性味归经　辛、苦，温。入肝、肾经。

功效应用

1. 祛风除湿：用于风湿关节痛，湿邪偏胜，腰脚酸重肿痛或兼筋骨拘挛者，常与木瓜、松节、牛膝等同用；或单用五加皮60克，白干酒500毫升，浸7天，去渣，日3次，适量饮服。

2. 强壮筋骨：用于筋骨软弱，小儿脚痿行迟，并可用于外伤骨折等症，可与其他舒筋活络药同用。

此外，本品尚有利水消肿之效，可治水肿。

用量用法　6～10克。煎服。外用适量。宜入酒剂。

虎　骨*

为脊椎动物猫科虎 Panthera tigris L.的全身骨骼。香油炸酥，或砂炙成黄色，乘热醋淬用。

处方用名　炙虎骨、虎胫骨。

性味归经　辛，温。入肝、肾经。

---

*参见本分册前之说明。

功效应用 搜风定痛，强筋健骨：用于风寒湿痹，筋骨酸痛，常与木瓜、当归、牛膝、秦艽等同用；若治肝肾不足，筋骨痿软，行步无力等症，常与熟地、知母、黄柏等同用。

用量用法 3～10克。煎服。多入丸散或浸酒服用。

附药 豹骨：为脊椎动物猫科豹 Panthera pardus L.的骨骼，铁砂炙后供药用。一般认为性味、功效、用量均同虎骨，惟药力稍弱。

白 花 蛇

为蝮蛇科动物尖吻蝮（五步蛇）Agkistrodon acutus (Guenther) 的干燥全体。酒浸3日，去皮骨用。

处方用名 白花蛇、蕲蛇肉。

性味归经 甘、咸、温、有毒。入肝经。

功效应用 祛风通络，定痉止痛：用于中风伤湿，肌肉麻痹，骨节疼痛等症，可与羌活、秦艽、五加皮等同用；用于麻风厉毒，手足麻木，可与乌梢蛇、雄黄等同用；用于破伤风，可与蜈蚣等同用。

用量用法 3～6克。多用于丸、散、酒、膏剂，一般不入汤剂。

附药 乌梢蛇：为游蛇科动物乌梢蛇 Zaocys dhumnades (Cantor) 除去内脏的干燥全体。性味甘平，无毒。功效同白花蛇而力较缓。用量3～12克。

海 桐 皮

为豆科常绿乔木植物刺桐 Erythrina variegata L. var. orientalis (L.) Merr.的干燥树皮。晒干，切片生用。

处方用名 海桐皮。

性味归经 苦、辛，平。入肝、肾经。

功效应用

1. 祛风湿，通经络：用于风湿痹痛，腰膝疼痛，手足拘挛等症，常与独活、川芎、牛膝、当归等活血通络药同用。

2. 本品尚用治疥癣、湿疹，因其能杀虫止痒。多外用煎汤洗，或研末调敷。

用量用法 6～10克。煎服。外用适量。

豨 莶 草

为菊科1年生草本植物腺茎豨莶 Siegesbeckia orientalis L. var. Pubescens Mak.或毛梗豨莶 S.glabrescens Mak.的全草。晒干切段，生用或黄酒蒸用。

处方用名 豨莶草。

性味归经 辛、苦，寒。入肝、肾经。

功效应用

1. 祛风湿，利筋骨（制用）：用于筋骨疼痛，四肢麻痹，腰膝酸软，本品一味为末，酒蒸制后，蜜丸，每丸9克重，每次1丸，日2～3次服；若风痹走注疼痛，或半身瘫痪，可与苍耳子、五加皮、海风藤、当归等同用。

2. 化湿热，除风痒（生用）：用于皮肤风疹，湿疮瘙痒，可与白鲜皮、苍耳子等同用。

此外，本品有降压作用，现代应用治疗高血压。

用量用法 10～15克。煎服。

臭 梧 桐

为马鞭草科落叶灌木或小乔木臭梧桐树 Clerodendron trichotomum Thumb. 的嫩枝及叶。原药生用。

处方用名 臭梧桐、八角梧桐。

性味归经 辛、苦，平。入肝经。

功效应用 祛风湿：用于风湿四肢筋络不利及中风之半身不遂，可与豨莶草为丸服；用于周身风痒，可煎汤洗浴。

此外，本品有降压之功，可用于肝阳上升之高血压头晕头痛，可单味为末常服，或配复方用。用时宜采未开花以前之生药，疗效较高，用时不宜高热煎煮，以免降低降压之功效。

用量用法 10～15克。煎服。散剂每次服3克。外用适量。

伸 筋 草

为石松科多年生常绿蔓茎匍匐植物石松 Lycopodium clavatum L.的全草。晒干，切段生用。

处方用名 伸筋草。

性味归经 辛、苦，温。入肝、肾经。

功效应用 祛风通络：用于风湿痹痛，四肢关节酸痛，伸屈不利，皮肤不仁等症，可随症配伍。

用量用法 10～15克。煎服。

海 风 藤

为胡椒科常绿攀援藤本植物细叶青蒌藤 Piper kadsura (choisy) Ohwi 的藤茎。切片生用。

处方用名 海风藤。

性味归经 辛、苦，微温。入肝经。

功效应用 祛风湿，通经络：用于风寒湿痹，关节疼痛，筋脉拘挛等症，常与羌活、独活、当归、桂枝等同用。

用量用法 10～15克。煎服。

络 石 藤

为夹竹桃科常绿攀援灌木藤本植物络石 Trachelospermum jasminoides (Lindl.) Lem.的带叶藤茎。切段生用。

处方用名 络石藤。

性味归经 苦，微寒。入心、肝经。

功效应用

1. 祛风通络：用于风湿筋骨酸痛，常与千年健、独活、威灵仙、防己、防风、秦艽等同用。

2. 凉血消肿：用于痈疽肿痛，可与皂刺、乳香等同用；用于咽喉肿闭，可与桔梗、射干、木通等同用；或以本品30克煎汤，细细呷之。

用量用法 15～30克。煎服。

钻 地 风

为虎耳草科落叶木质藤本植物钻地风 Schizophragma integrifolium（Franch.）Oliv.的根皮。晒干。切段生用。

处方用名 钻地风、追地风、地风。

性味归经 淡，凉。入肝、肾经。

功效应用 祛风除湿，舒筋活血：用于风湿筋骨疼痛，足膝痿软麻木等症，常与千年健同用；若治四肢关节酸痛，可用钻地风750克，千年健、五加皮、丹参各250克，川牛膝180克，生麻黄15克。切细，入黄酒12斤，红糖、红枣各500克，装入小坛内密封，再隔水缓火炖4小时。每天早晚空腹饮100毫升左右。头汁服完后，可再加黄酒10斤，如上法烧炖，服用。

用量用法 6～12克。煎服。

千 年 健

为天南星科多年生草本植物千年健 Homalomena occulta（Lour.）Schott的肉质根茎。切片生用。

处方用名 千年健、千年见、年健。

性味归经 苦、辛，温。入肝、肾经。

功效应用 祛风湿，强筋骨：风寒湿痹，筋骨疼痛，拘挛麻木等症，常与钻地风相须为用。

此外，本品还可用治风寒性坐骨神经痛，常配桂枝、芍药、炙川乌、伸筋草、地风、牛膝、当归、甘草、姜、枣等，疗效较好。颇宜于老人。

用量用法 6～12克。煎服。制酒剂良。

松　节

为松科常绿大乔木油松 Pinus tabulaeformis Carr.的枝干的结节。切片生用。

处方用名 松节、油松节。

性味归经 苦，温。入肝、肾经。

功效应用 祛风燥湿：用于筋骨关节风湿痹痛，单用一味浸酒服。或与羌活、独活、防风、海风藤、桑枝、当归、川芎等同用。

用量用法 10～15克。煎服。制酒剂良。

蚕　沙

为昆虫纲鳞翅目蚕娥科家蚕 Bombyx mori L.的干燥粪便。原药晒干生用。

处方用名 蚕沙、晚蚕沙。

性味归经 甘、辛，温。入肝、脾、胃经。

功效应用

1. 祛风除湿：用于久病风寒湿痹，关节疼痛，可与蕲蛇、地风、土鳖、全蝎等同用；或用蚕沙装两袋，蒸热轮熨患处。

2. 和胃化浊：用于内伤饮食，吐泻腹痛转筋等症，可与薏苡仁、半夏、木瓜等同用。

用量用法 6～10克。布包入煎。外用适量。

徐 长 卿

为萝藦科多年生草本植物徐长卿 Cynanchum Paniculatum (Bge.) Kitag.的根及根茎。阴干。切段生用。

处方用名 徐长卿。

性味归经 辛，温。入肺、胃、肝、肾经。

功效应用 祛风止痛、止痒：用于风湿关节腰腿疼痛，可与防己同用；用于跌仆血肿，单用内服外洗均可；用于胃痛、腹痛，单用或与延胡索等分研末，每次1.5～3克，水冲服；亦可配香附煎服；用于龋齿牙痛，可单用10克，煎汤漱口。用于荨麻疹，周身瘙痒，顽癣，单用水煎外洗内服均可；亦可加入少量白矾洗浴。

此外，本品还可用于慢性哮喘，可单用水煎服；用于登山呕吐、晕车、晕船。可为末，每服1.5克，水冲下。因其还能解蛇毒，又治毒蛇咬伤。可与半边莲同用内服或外敷。

用量用法 10～15克。煎服。

寻 骨 风

为马兜铃科多年生攀援草本植物绵毛马兜铃 Aristolochia mollissima Hance 的全草及根茎。切段，晒干生用。

处方用名 寻骨风。

性味归经 辛、苦，平。入肝经。

功效应用 祛风湿，通络止痛：用于风湿关节疼痛，筋骨不利，跌打损伤肿痛。可单用煎服，浸酒或制成浸膏、片剂服用；亦可配伍其他风湿药同用。

用量用法 15～30克。煎服。外用适量。

此外，本品亦可用于胃痛、疝气、睾丸肿痛。

5 芳香化湿药

凡是气味芳香，而以化湿运脾为主要作用的药物，称为芳香化湿药。

芳香化湿药，其气芳香，性偏温燥，具有疏畅气机，宣化湿浊，醒脾开胃。适用于湿浊阻中，脾为湿困，运化失职所致的脘腹痞满，食少体倦，呕吐泛酸，口甘多涎，大便溏薄，舌苔白腻等症。至于湿温、暑湿等证，亦可选用。

在使用本类药物时，当根据湿的不同性质和成因或兼症，进行配伍。属寒湿者，配温里药；属湿热者，配清热燥湿药；因脾虚生湿者，配补脾药；痰湿阻滞者，配燥湿化痰药；湿阻气滞者，配行气药。

本类药物，辛温香燥，易伤阴耗气，故对阴虚津少，舌绛及气虚者应慎用。又因其芳香，含挥发油，入煎剂时宜后下，不宜久煎，以免降低药效。

苍　术

为菊科多年生草本植物茅苍术（茅术、南苍术）Atractylodes lancea（Thunb）或北苍术 A.chinensis（DC.）Koidz.的根茎。烘干。水浸切片，再用米泔水焖透，炒至微黄用。

处方用名　制苍术、苍术、茅苍术。

性味归经　辛、苦，温。入脾、胃经。

功效应用

1. 燥湿健脾：用于湿阻中焦，脾为湿困，脘腹胀满或泄泻，舌苔浊腻者，常与厚朴、陈皮同用。对于痰饮、水肿等脾湿偏盛之症，亦可随症选用。

2. 祛风湿：用于风湿或寒湿所致的关节肢体疼痛。若属风寒湿痹，可与羌活、防风、桂枝、秦艽等同用；若属热痹，可与黄柏、牛膝同用。

3. 散寒解表：用于外感风寒，头痛无汗者，可与藁本、白芷等同用。

此外，本品尚能除障明目，用于目疾内外翳障、青盲、夜盲等症，可单用，或与猪肝或黑芝麻同用。

用量用法 6～10克。煎服。

使用注意 凡阴虚内热，气虚多汗者忌服。

厚　朴

为木兰科落叶乔木厚朴 Magnolia officinalis Rehd. et Wils. 或凹叶厚朴（又名庐山厚朴）Magnolia biloba（Rehd. et Wils）cheng 的干皮、根皮及枝皮。晒干，切片生用或与生姜同煮切条用或姜汁炒用。

处方用名 厚朴、川朴、制川朴、姜厚朴。

性味归经 苦、辛，温。入脾、胃、肺、大肠经。

功效应用

1. 行气燥湿：用于湿困脾胃，或食积气滞，脘腹胀闷，或腹痛、泄泻等症。若治脾胃寒湿，胸腹气滞胀满，可与生姜、半夏等同用；若治肠胃湿热，气滞胀满便秘者，可与枳实、大黄同用。

2. 温中止痛：用于脘腹寒滞疼痛，胀满少食等，可与干姜、草豆蔻、木香等同用。

3. 降逆平喘：用于湿痰壅肺，咳嗽气喘，可与杏仁、麻黄、半夏等同用。

用量用法 3～10克。煎服。

附药 厚朴花：系厚朴的花蕾，性味同厚朴，功能健胃止痛，利气宽中。适用于肝胃气滞，胸闷腹胀等症。用量同厚朴。

藿　香

为唇形科多年生草本植物广藿香 Pogostemon cablin (Blanco) Benth.或藿香 Agastache rugosus (Fisch. et Mey) O. Ktze. 的全草。晒干。切段入药，或鲜用，亦有单用其梗或叶者。

处方用名　广藿香、藿香叶、藿香梗、鲜藿香。

性味归经　辛，微温。入脾、胃、肺经。

功效应用

1. 化湿止呕：用于寒湿内阻，脘痞呕吐，可与半夏、陈皮等同用；用于湿温病，体倦胸闷，可与半夏、厚朴、杏仁等同用；若偏气虚者，可配党参、白术；偏热者，可配黄连；若孕妇胎气不安，呕吐酸水，可与砂仁、香附配用。

2. 发表解暑：用于暑月内伤生冷，外感风寒，出现寒热头痛，胸闷，腹胀，呕恶，便泻等症，常与紫苏、半夏、厚朴、大腹皮、茯苓等同用；用于夏季伤暑，头昏胸闷，恶心，口中粘腻，不欲饮食等症，可与佩兰、薄荷泡水饮服。均用鲜者更佳。

3. 行气止痛：用于脾胃气滞，脘腹胀痛，可与厚朴、砂仁、陈皮、木香、枳实等同用。

此外，还可治鼻渊，可与猪胆配用。

用量用法　6～12 克，鲜者 15～30 克，煎服。藿香叶偏于发表，藿香梗偏于和中，鲜藿香清暑化湿辟秽之力尤强。均不宜久煎。

佩　兰

为菊科多年生草本植物兰草 Eupatorium fortunei Turcz. 的地上部分。晒干。切段入药，亦可鲜用。

处方用名　佩兰、南佩兰、香佩兰、鲜佩兰。

性味归经 辛，平。入脾、胃、肺经。

功效应用 化湿解暑，醒脾和中：用于湿浊内蕴。郁于中焦，胸痞腹胀，口甘，口臭，苔腻等症；常与藿香、半夏、厚朴、陈皮等同用；用于夏伤暑湿，发热头痛，胸闷不饥，可与藿香、厚朴、荷叶等同用。

用量用法 6～12 克，鲜者可用 15～30 克。煎服。不宜久煎。

砂 仁

为姜科多年生草本植物阳春砂 Amomum villosum Lour. 海南砂 A. longiligulave T. L. Wu 或缩砂 A. xanthioides Wall. 的成熟果实。用时打碎，随用随打。

处方用名 砂仁、春砂仁、缩砂仁、阳春砂。

性味归经 辛、温。入脾、胃、肾经。

功效应用

1. 化湿行气：用于湿浊阻中和脾胃气滞，腹痛胀满，常与木香、枳实同用；用于脾虚气滞者，配党参、白术等同用。

2. 温胃止呕：用于脾胃虚寒，胸痞呕吐，可与木香、半夏、陈皮等同用；若治妊娠呕吐，可单用砂仁末 1.5～3 克，日 3 次，生姜汤送服。

3. 温脾止泻：用于脾虚寒湿积滞之泻痢症，可与干姜、肉豆蔻、诃子肉等同用。

此外，本品尚有安胎之效，用于气滞之胎动不安，常与白术、桑寄生、续断等配用。

用量用法 3～6 克。煎服。以研末作丸散剂或随汤剂冲服为宜，如入煎剂当后下。

附药 砂仁壳：为砂仁之果壳。气淡味清，但温性略减，功效薄弱，一般用于胸痞胃呆，仅取其宽中开胃而已。用量同。

白 豆 蔻

为姜科多年生草本植物白豆蔻 Amomum cardamomum L. 的种子。打碎生用，随用随打。

处方用名　白豆蔻、白蔻仁、紫蔻、空白蔻。

性味归经　辛，温。入肺、脾、胃经。

功效应用

1. 化湿行气：用于湿阻中焦与脾胃气滞，胸脘痞满，可与厚朴、陈皮、砂仁等同用；若湿温初起，胸闷不饥，苔浊腻者，常与薏苡仁、杏仁、厚朴等同用。

2. 温胃止呕：用于脾胃虚寒，恶心呕吐，呃逆噫气等症。如治反胃呕吐，可与藿香、陈皮等同用；亦可与姜汁配丸用。

此外，本品尚能解酒毒，酒醉不醒者可用之。

用量用法　3～6克。煎服。宜研末作丸散剂或随汤剂冲服，如入煎剂宜后下。

附药　豆蔻壳：为白豆蔻的果壳。气味淡薄，温燥之性大减，具有宽中利气，和胃化浊之效。用量同白豆蔻。

草 豆 蔻

为姜科多年生草本植物草豆蔻 Alpinia Katsumadai Hayata 的干燥近成熟的种子。晒干生用，用时打碎。

处方用名　草豆蔻。

性味归经　辛，温。入脾、胃经。

功效应用　燥湿，暖胃止呕，行气：用于寒湿阻滞中焦，脘腹胀满疼痛，呕吐，常与高良姜、生姜、半夏、吴茱萸等温胃散寒药同用；用于脾胃虚寒。饮食不思，大便溏薄，苔厚腻等，常与川厚朴、砂仁、陈皮、苍术等同用。

用量用法　3～6克。煎服。入煎剂后下。

草　果

为姜科多年生草本植物草果 Amomum tsao-ko Crevost et Lem.的果实。取仁捣碎用。

处方用名　草果仁、煨草果。

性味归经　辛，温。入脾、胃经。

功效应用

1. 燥湿温中：寒湿内积，胸腹胀痛，可与良姜、丁香、厚朴等同用；用于湿浊郁伏，脘腹胀痛，或呕吐者，可与苍术、厚朴等同用；用于湿滞痰饮，头痛背痛，饮食欲呕者，可与半夏、陈皮、南星等同用。

2. 截疟：用治疟疾。本品既燥湿、散寒，又能截疟，而以寒湿偏盛者为宜。对于脾寒疟疾，寒多热少，或但寒不热，或腹泻不食等症，可与附子、生姜、大枣同用；正疟，寒热往来，1日或间日1发，头痛、面赤口渴者，可与柴胡、黄芩、常山等同用。

用量用法　3～6克。

使用注意　脾胃虚弱而无寒湿及素体阴虚者忌用。

6 利水渗湿药

凡以通利水道，渗除水湿为主要功能的药物，称为利水渗湿药。服用这类药物之后，能使小便畅通，尿量增多，所以又称利尿药。这类药物大都味淡，又称淡渗利湿药。

本类药物，大致分为3类。一是属于利水消肿的，有渗利水湿，通利小便的作用，主要适用于水湿壅盛，小便不利，水肿之症；一是属于利尿通淋的，适用于小便涩痛或浑浊之淋症；一是属于利湿退黄的，适用于湿热黄疸及结石之症。其中部分药物还可兼治痰饮、疮疹、关节疼痛、泄泻等症。总之，皆以通利导下为用。

本类药物，能伤阴耗液，故凡阴虚津亏，尿源不足之小便不利或短涩者，水肿症之属虚性者，以及滑精、遗精无湿热者，皆不宜单独使用。

6.1 利水消肿药

茯　苓

为多孔菌科真菌茯苓 Poria cocos（schw.）Wolf 的干燥菌核。切片或切方块，生用。菌核的外皮称茯苓皮；皮内侧呈淡红色者，为赤茯苓；内部抱有松根者称茯神；白色部分称白茯苓，即茯苓。因以云南产者著名，故又称云苓。

处方用名　茯苓、白茯苓、云苓。

性味归经　甘、淡，平。入心、脾、肺、肾经。

功效应用

1. 利水渗湿：用于水湿仃滞之小便不利，水肿胀满等症，常与白术、猪苓、泽泻、大腹皮等同用。

2. 健脾补中：用于脾虚不能运化水湿，痰饮内停，或大便泄泻等症，常与党参、白术、山药等同用。

3. 宁心安神：用于心脾不足之心悸，失眠，常与党参、龙眼肉、酸枣仁等同用；若用于痰浊内阻，或心肾不交之惊悸失眠，又常与菖蒲、远志等同用。

用量用法 10～30克。煎服。

附药 茯苓皮：本品性味同茯苓，但长于利水消肿，专行皮肤水湿，治皮肤水肿。用量同茯苓。

猪　苓

为多孔菌科真菌猪苓 Polyporus umbellatus (Pers.) Fries 的菌核。阴干，润透切片，生用。

处方用名 猪苓、粉猪苓。

性味归经 甘、淡，平。入肾、膀胱经。

功效应用 利水渗湿：用于小便不利，淋痛，水肿，腹泻，白带等症。多与茯苓、泽泻等同用。本品专主渗泄，其利水渗湿之功比茯苓强。因其性偏凉，故以水湿为病之偏热者，用之最宜。

本品一味单用亦可，如妊娠足肿，取猪苓散剂，温开水调服。

用量用法 10～15克。煎服。

泽　泻

为泽泻科多年生沼泽植物泽泻 Alisma orientalis (Sam) Juzep.的块茎。切片晒干，生用或麸炒、盐炒用。

处方用名 泽泻、盐泽泻。

性味归经 甘、淡，寒。入肾、膀胱经。

功效应用 利水渗湿泄热：用于小便不利，水肿，泄泻，停饮等症。治小便不利，水肿，常与猪苓、茯苓同用；若治水饮、眩晕，可用泽泻24克，白术30克，水煎服；而治泄泻，又常与白术、猪苓、车前子等同用。

用量用法 10～15克。煎服。一般多盐水炒用。

薏苡仁

为禾本科1年生或多年生草本植物薏苡仁 Coix lacryma-jobi L. var. ma-yuen（Roman）Stapf.的成熟种仁。生用或炒用。

处方用名 薏苡仁、生薏仁、炒薏仁。

性味归经 甘、淡，微寒。入脾、肺、肾经。

功效应用

1. 利水渗湿：用于小便不利，水肿，脚气等，可配防已、苍术、郁李仁等同用。

2. 祛湿除痹：用于湿热痹症，常与苍术、忍冬藤、黄柏等同用。

3. 排脓消痈：用于肺痈、肠痈。前者常与桃仁、丹皮、苇茎等同用；后者常与桃仁、丹皮、红藤、银花等同用。

4. 健脾止泻：用于脾虚有湿的泄泻症，常与白术、茯苓、山药等同用；如治妇女湿盛白带，可与山药、芡实等配用

用量用法 15～30克。煎服。利湿热可生用，止泻可炒用。亦可作羹或与粳米煮粥、饭食用，为食疗佳品。

车前子

为车前科多年生草本植物车前 Plantago asiatica L.或平车前 P.depressa Willa.的成熟种子。晒干，生用或盐水炒用。

处方用名 车前子、炒车前。

性味归经 甘，微寒。入肝、肾、肺、小肠经。

功效应用

1. 利水通淋：用于水肿，小便不利，或赤涩热痛等症，常

与瞿麦、木通、扁蓄、滑石等同用。

2. 渗湿止泻：用于暑热吐泻，小便不利，常与香薷、茯苓、猪苓等同用。

3. 清肝明目：用于肝热目赤肿痛，可与菊花、密蒙花、黄芩、龙胆草等同用。

4. 清肺化痰：用于咳嗽痰多，可与桔梗、杏仁、紫菀等同用。

用量用法 9～15克。煎服。

冬瓜皮

为葫芦科1年生草本植物冬瓜 Benincasa hispida (Thunb.) Cogn.的外层果皮。生用。

处方用名 冬瓜皮。

性味归经 甘，微寒。入肺、小肠经。

功效应用 清热利水消肿：用于皮肤水肿，胀满，小便不利，常与茯苓、车前子等同用。

用量用法 15～30克。煎服。

附药 冬瓜子：为冬瓜的种子，生用或炒用，捣碎入药。性味与皮相同，功能清肺化痰，利湿排脓，并有缓泻作用，适用于肺热咳嗽、肺痈、肠痈、淋浊、带下等症。用量15～30克。

赤小豆

为豆科1年生半攀援草本植物赤小豆 Phaseolus cal caratus Roxb.或赤豆（饭赤豆）P.angularis Wight 的成熟种子。晒干。生用。

处方用名 赤小豆、红小豆。

性味归经 甘、酸，平。入心、小肠经。

功效应用

1. 利水消肿：用于水肿，小便不利，脚气等症，常与鲤鱼同煮服；用于一般虚肿，可与落花生、红枣等煎汤，长期服用。

2. 解毒排脓：用于痈肿初起，红肿热痛，研末，水调，或以醋调外敷患处；亦可内服。

此外，本品尚用于湿热黄疸。现代用本品治疗肾炎水肿、肝硬化腹水及营养不良性水肿。

用量用法 15～30克。煎服。外用适量。

6.2 利尿通淋药

萹 蓄

为蓼科1年生草本植物萹蓄 Polygonum aviculare L. 的全草。切碎生用。

处方用名 萹蓄、萹蓄草。

性味归经 苦，微寒。入膀胱经。

功效应用

1. 利尿通淋：用于小便短赤，淋漓不畅，尿道热痛，常与瞿麦、滑石、木通等同用。若与大、小蓟、白茅根等同用，亦可治血淋。

2. 杀虫止痒：用于皮肤湿疹，阴道滴虫，阴部瘙痒，可煎汤外洗。

用量用法 10～30克。煎服。

瞿 麦

为石竹科多年生草本植物瞿麦 Dianthus superbus L. 和石竹 Dianthus chinensis L. 的带花全草。切碎生用。

处方用名 瞿麦、瞿麦穗。

性味归经 苦、寒。入心、小肠经。

功效应用

1. 利尿通淋：用于热淋，小便淋沥热痛，或尿血者，常与萹蓄、栀子、滑石等同用。

2. 活血通经：用于血瘀经闭，可与丹参、赤芍、益母草、红花等同用。

用量用法 10～30克。煎服

使用注意 孕妇忌服。

木 通

为木通科落叶木质藤本植物白木通 Akebia trifoliata (Thunb.) Koidz.var. australis (Diels) Rehd. 的木质茎和马兜铃科藤本植物木通马兜铃（关木通）Hocguartia manshuriensis (Komar.) Nakai 或毛茛科常绿攀援灌木小木通（川木通）Clematis armandii Franch 及同属的绣球藤 C. montana Buch.-Ham.的藤茎。切片生用。

处方用名 木通、细木通。

性味归经 苦，寒。入心、肺、小肠、膀胱经。

功效应用

1. 降火利尿：用于小便赤涩热痛，口舌生疮，心烦等症；常与生地、竹叶、甘草梢同用；用于湿脚气，小便不利，可与猪苓、苏叶、槟榔等同用。

2. 宣通血脉：用于乳汁不通，可与通草、漏芦、王不留行、猪蹄等同用；用于血瘀经闭，可与丹参、牛膝、桃仁、生蒲黄等同用；用于湿热痹痛，关节不利，可与忍冬藤、海桐皮、桑枝等同用。

用量用法 3～6克。煎服。

使用注意 据临床报道，有服大剂量（60克）而致急性肾功能衰竭者，故用量不宜过大。孕妇慎用。

通 草

为五加科灌木通脱木 Tetrapanax papyriferus (Hook.) K.

Koch.的茎髓。晒干，切片生用。

处方用名 通草、白通草、方通草。

性味归经 甘、淡、寒。入肺、胃经。

功效应用

1. 清热利水：用于湿热之小便不利，常与竹叶、滑石等同用。

2. 通乳：用于妇女产后乳汁不多，常与猪蹄、穿山甲、川芎、甘草配伍。

用量用法 6～10克。煎服。

使用注意 孕妇慎用。

灯 心 草

为灯心草科多年生草本植物灯心草 Juncus effusus L. var. decipiens Buchen.的茎髓。切段生用。

处方用名 灯心草、灯心、灯草。

性味归经 甘、淡，微寒。入心、肺、小肠经。

功效应用

1. 清热利水：用于热症之小便淋涩，可与栀子、滑石、甘草梢等同用。由于本品药力单薄，只宜于病情轻浅者，或辅助其它清热利尿药同用。

2. 清心除烦：用于小儿心热烦躁，夜啼，可与淡竹叶同用，开水泡代茶喝。

用量用法 3～6克。煎服。

地 肤 子

为藜科1年生草本植物地肤 Kochia scoparia（L.）Schrad.的种子。生用。

处方用名 地肤子。

性味归经 辛、苦，寒。入肾、膀胱经。

功效应用

1. 清湿热，利小便：用于湿热小便不利，常与瞿麦、猪苓、滑石、甘草等同用。

2. 祛风止痒：用于皮肤瘙痒、湿疹、荨麻疹、疥癣等症，常与白鲜皮、蝉蜕、薄荷、荆芥等同用；如妇女阴道炎、外阴炎、可与蛇床子、苦参、白矾、川椒等煎汤熏洗患处。

用量用法　10～12克。煎服。外用适量。

冬　葵　子

为锦葵科1年生或多年生草本植物冬葵 *Malva verticillata* L. 的种子。打碎生用。

处方用名　冬葵子。

性味归经　甘，寒。入小肠、大肠经。

功效应用

1. 利尿通淋：用于小便不利，淋漓涩痛，可与茯苓、车前子、木通等配合；用于石淋，可与滑石、地龙等同用；若用于妊娠水肿，身重，小便不利，可与茯苓同用。

2. 通乳：用于产后乳少，乳房胀痛，用冬葵子12克，王不留行12克，漏芦15克，猪蹄2个，水煎，吃蹄喝汤。

此外，本品尚能滑肠，可治大便秘结。

用量用法　10～15克。煎服。

石　　苇

为水龙骨科多年生常绿草本植物石苇 *Pyrrosia lingua* (Thunb.) Farw.或芦山石苇 *Pyrrosia sheareri* (Bak.) Ching 或有柄石苇 *P. petiolosa* (christ) Ching.的叶片。切碎，生用。

处方用名　石苇。

性味归经　甘、苦，微寒。入肺、膀胱经。

功效应用

1. 利尿通淋：用于热淋，或血淋及石淋尿血等症，常与车前子、滑石、木通、瞿麦等同用。

2. 清热止血：用于血热崩漏，吐血，可单味30克。水煎服。

此外，单用水煎配冰糖和服，可用于肺热咳喘，如支气管炎或支气管哮喘有一定疗效。

用量用法 6～10克。煎服。

海 金 沙

为海金沙科多年生攀援蕨类植物海金沙 Lygodium japonicum (Thunb.) Sw.的成熟孢子。生用。

处方用名 海金沙。

性味归经 甘、咸，寒。入膀胱、小肠经。

功效应用 利尿通淋：用于膏淋、石淋、砂淋、热淋等症。本品功专通利水道，而为治淋病尿道作痛之要药。可与滑石、甘草、金钱草等同用。

此外，现代临床尚用于肾炎水肿。

用量用法 6～12克。煎服。布包入煎。

萆 薢

为薯蓣科多年生缠绕草质藤本植物萆薢 Dioscorea hypoglauca palib.和绵萆薢 Dioscorea officinalis Tsi, mss.的根茎。切片，晒干生用。

处方用名 萆薢、粉萆薢。

性味归经 苦，平。入肾、胃经。

功效应用

1. 利湿祛浊：用于膏淋的小便混浊，色白如米泔，淋涩频数及女子带下属于湿胜者。本品有分清去浊之功，常与茯苓、石菖蒲、乌药等同用。

2. 除痹止痛：用于风湿痹症，腰脊关节肌肉疼痛者，可与牛膝、白术、附子等同用。

用量用法 6～10 克。煎服。

滑　石

为单斜晶系滑石的矿石。主含含水硅酸镁。打碎研末用，或研细水飞用。

处方用名 滑石、飞滑石。

性味归经 甘、淡，寒。入膀胱、胃经。

功效应用

1. 利尿通淋：用于热淋，石淋，可与木通、海金沙，金钱草等同用。

2. 清热解暑：用于感受暑热，心烦口渴，小便赤涩，或有水泻等症，常与甘草配用。

3. 祛湿敛疮：用于湿疹、湿疮，常与枯矾、黄柏等研粉外用。本品亦为制作痱子粉的主药。

本品用治泌尿系结石，因其性寒而滑，滑能利窍，便于结石排出。

用量用法 10～15 克。治泌尿结石，可重用至 24～30 克。煎服。外用适量。

6.3 利湿退黄药

茵 陈 蒿

为菊科多年生草本植物茵陈蒿 Artemisia capillaris Thunb.或滨蒿 Artemisia scoparia waldst. et kit.的幼苗。晒干生用。

处方用名 茵陈蒿、茵陈、绵茵陈。

性味归经 苦，微寒。入脾、胃、肝、胆经。

功效应用 清热除湿，利疸退黄：用于湿热黄疸。本品善清热除湿退黄，为治黄疸专药，属于湿热薰蒸而发黄者，身目黄色鲜明，发热，小便短赤，可与栀子、大黄同用；若属寒湿阴黄，色黄晦暗，纳少脘闷，神疲畏寒，可与附子、干姜等同用。

此外，本品亦可用于湿疮瘙痒，流黄水，常与苦参等用同。

现代用于急、慢性黄疸型传染性肝炎、肝硬变、胆石症及胆囊炎等。以其有利胆作用。配乌梅可治胆道蛔虫。

用量用法 15～30克。煎服。

金 钱 草

为报春花科多年生草本植物过路黄（四川大金钱草）Lysimachia christinae Hance 的全草。鲜用或阴干后切碎用。

处方用名 金钱草。

性味归经 甘、淡，平。入肝、胆、肾、膀胱经。

功效应用

1. 利湿退黄：用于湿热黄疸。可与茵陈、栀子等同用。

2. 通淋排石：用于热淋、砂淋、石淋。本品为治泌尿系结石要药。治膀胱、输尿管结石，单用金钱草60克，煎汤代茶，每天常饮，或与海金沙，滑石、鸡内金等配用；治肾结石，可与石苇、鱼脑石、杜仲、胡桃肉等配用。本品功能利胆排石，故亦常用于肝胆管结石，每与茵陈、郁金、栀子等配用。用治结石，本品须长期坚持服用，一般需1个月以上。

3. 解毒消肿：用于疔疮肿毒，可用鲜者捣汁1小杯（约50毫升），分2次饮服；若烫伤烧伤，亦可用鲜者捣汁擦患处。

用量用法 30～60克。单用最大量120～150克。鲜用150～300克。煎服。外用适量。

7　温里药

凡能温散里寒，补火回阳的药物，称为温里药，又称祛寒药。

温里药性味辛热，能温中祛寒，温肾回阳。适用于里寒之证。所谓里寒，包括两个方面：一为寒邪内侵，阳气受困，而见呕逆吐利，胸腹冷痛，食欲不振等脏寒证，必须温中散寒，以消阴翳；一为元阳衰微，阴寒内生，而见汗出畏寒，口鼻气冷，下利清谷，四肢厥逆，脉微欲绝等亡阳虚脱证，必须温肾回阳，益火之源。

使用本类药物，可根据不同情况，作适当配伍。如外寒内侵兼有表证者，配解表药；寒凝气滞者，配行气药；寒湿内蕴者，配健脾化湿药；脾肾阳虚者，配温补脾肾药；亡阳气脱者，配伍大补元气药。

温里药性均温热燥烈，能伤阴助火，故凡阳盛阴虚，或内真热而外假寒之证均禁用。又本类药物的用量，亦当根据季节气候的寒暖酌情增减为宜。

附　子

为毛茛科多年生草本植物乌头 Aconitum carmichaeli Debx. 的子根的加工品。切片用或生用。

处方用名　熟附子、炮附子、川附子、淡附片、生附子。

性味归经　辛，大热，有毒。入心、肾、脾经。

功效应用

1. 回阳救逆：用于阳气衰微，四肢厥冷，脉微欲绝，冷汗淋漓，或大吐、大下所致的上述亡阳虚脱证，常与干姜、甘草同用；若治寒邪入里，四肢厥冷，腹痛吐泻等症，可与干姜、肉桂、人参等同用；若治阳衰而表不固，冷汗不止者，可与炙黄芪同用；若治血脱亡阳者，可与人参同用。

2. 助阳行水：用于肾阳衰微，身面浮肿，腰以下肿甚，腰痛酸重，尿少之症，常与白术、茯苓等同用；若治脾阳不足，肢体浮肿，腹胀便溏等症，常与干姜、白术、草果等同用。

3. 祛寒止痛：用于风寒湿痹，骨节疼痛，常与桂枝、白术等同用；用于阴寒内盛，脘腹冷痛，常与干姜、党参、白术等同用。

用量用法　3～12克。煎服。生用作用峻烈，宜于回阳救逆；熟用毒性减弱，宜于助阳散寒。不论生用或熟用，必须久煎（1小时以上），以减其毒性。

使用注意　本品性燥烈，故非阴盛阳虚之证不宜服用，阴虚内热及孕妇忌用。反半夏、栝楼、白蔹、白及、贝母、畏犀角。

附药　川乌头、草乌头：为毛茛科多年生草本植物乌头的块根。乌头分川乌、草乌两种。川乌属卡氏乌头 Aconitum carmichaeli Debx.，系栽培；草乌属北乌头 A. kusnezoffii Reichb.，系野生。其炮制方法与附子相同。乌头性味功效与附子相近，可以散在表之风邪，逐在里之寒湿，但补阳之功不及附子，而祛风通痹之力则较附子为胜。所以古有"附子逐寒，乌头去风"之说。用治风寒湿痹，酸痛麻木，脘腹冷痛之症，功效卓著。但其性毒烈（草乌更甚），故宜慎用。用量3～9克。用法、使用注意同附子。

干　姜

为姜科多年生草本植物姜 Zingiber officinale Rosc.的根茎。切片用。切方块炮焦用，称为炮姜。

处方用名　干姜、淡干姜、干姜片。

性味归经　辛，热。入心、肺、脾、胃经。

功效应用

1. 温中回阳：用于脾胃阳虚，下利清谷，四肢厥冷，脉微欲绝并见面赤烦躁者，可与附子、葱白同用；若脾胃虚寒泄泻，清稀无臭，肠鸣腹痛，可与高良姜等分，水丸，每次 3～6 克。温开水送服；亦可与党参、白术、甘草同用。

2. 温肺化痰：用于寒饮喘咳，常与麻黄、半夏、细辛、五味子等同用。

用量用法 3～10 克。煎服。

使用注意 热证、阴虚者及孕妇均忌服。

附药 炮姜：又名黑姜、炮姜炭。性味苦温，散烈之性已减弱。功能温经止血，主治虚寒性的吐血、便血、血崩等症。阴虚血热妄行的出血症忌服。用量 1.5～6 克。

肉　桂

为樟科常绿乔木桂树 Cinnamomum cassia Presl 的树皮。切片用或研末用。

处方用名 肉桂、紫油桂、桂心。

性味归经 辛、甘，大热。入肝、肾、心、脾、胃经。

功效应用

1. 补火助阳：用于肾阳衰微，下元虚冷，畏寒肢冷，腰脚软弱，阳萎，小便不利等症，常与附子、熟地、山药、山萸肉等同用；用于脾肾阳虚所致的腹痛泄泻，可与干姜、附子、肉豆蔻、茯苓等同用。

2. 散寒止痛：用于虚寒性胃痛，腹痛，疝痛等症，可单用研末服；亦可与其他温中散寒药同用；若用于妇女虚寒痛经，可与当归、干姜、熟地等同用。

此外，本品亦可在治气血衰少的方中少量用之，有鼓舞气血生长的功效，如治气血两虚的人参养荣汤、十全大补汤；治寒性疮疡久不愈合或内陷不起的托里散、阳和汤，及下焦湿热，小便不通的通关丸等方中均用适量肉桂。

用量用法 1.5～5 克。煎服。多研末冲服，作煎剂当后入。

使用注意 阴虚火旺，里有实热，血热妄行者及孕妇均当忌用。

高良姜

为姜科多年生草本植物高良姜 Alpinia officinarum Hance 的根茎。切片生用。

处方用名 高良姜、良姜、良姜片。

性味归经 辛，热。入脾、胃经。

功效应用

1. 散寒止痛：用于时发时止的胃脘寒痛，常与香附等分为丸，每次 6 克，开水送服；若脘腹感寒绞痛如刺，两胁胀满，常与厚朴、桂心等同用；亦可与五灵脂配用；若寒疝腹痛，可与小茴香同用。

2. 温中止呕：用于胃寒气逆，呕吐清水，四肢冰冷等症，可用高良姜 6 克，大枣 6 枚，水煎服。

用量用法 3～6 克。煎服。

吴茱萸

为芸香科常绿灌木或小乔木吴茱萸 Evodia rutaecarpa (Juss.) Benth.接近成熟的果实。盐水炒用，或甘草水炒用。

处方用名 吴茱萸、吴萸、淡吴萸。

性味归经 辛、苦，热。入肝、肾、脾、胃经。

功效应用

1. 散寒止痛：用于头额冷痛，经常发作，日久不愈，兼吐涎沫者，常与党参、生姜等同用；用于寒疝作痛，可用吴茱萸 5 克，小茴香 6 克，金铃子 9 克，木香 3 克，水煎服；用于寒湿脚气上逆，腹痛，闷乱不识人，可与木瓜、槟榔、生姜同用。

2. 下气止呕：用于胃中虚寒，食后欲吐；腹痛，或干呕吐涎沫，亦可用之，每与党参、生姜配用；若饭后吞酸，胸腹冷痛，可与炮姜等分为末服。若肝火犯胃之胁痛，吞酸、呕吐等症，常与黄连为丸用。

此外，本品研末醋调外敷足心，可以引火下行，治口舌生疮。

用量用法 1～5 克。煎服；外用适量。一般甘草水炒用，治疝气可用盐吴茱萸。

使用注意 阴虚火旺者忌用。

小茴香

为伞形科多年生草本植物茴香 Foeniculum vulgare Mill.的成熟果实。盐水炒用。

处方用名 小茴香。

性味归经 辛、甘，温。入肝、肾、脾、胃经。

功效应用

1. 祛寒止痛：用于阴寒腹痛，疝痛，可与肉桂、沉香、乌药等同用；若疝气睾丸肿大，痛不可忍，可与荔枝核，川楝子等同用；若阴囊水肿，睾丸胀痛，可用小茴香 30 克，车前子 30 克，食盐 6 克，共为细末，每次 6 克，温黄酒下，日 2 次服。

2. 理气和胃：用于胃寒腹痛，呕逆少食。可用小茴香 30 克，生姜 60 克炒黄为末，酒糊为丸，每次 6 克，日 2 次服。

用量用法 6～10 克。煎服。

使用注意 阴虚火旺者忌用。

丁香

为桃金娘科常绿乔木丁香树 Syzygium aromaticum（L.）Merr. et Perry 的花及果实。生用。

处方用名 公丁香、母丁香。

性味归经 辛，温。入肺、胃、脾、肾经。

功效应用

1. 温中降逆：本品为治虚寒呃逆之要药。用于胃寒呕吐呃逆，以及小儿吐乳等症，可用丁香1.5克，柿蒂5枚，党参9克，生姜9克，水煎服；若脾胃虚寒，吐泻食少，可与丁香、砂仁、白术等同用。

2. 下气止痛：用于奔豚气逆，胸腹疼痛，可与五味子、莪术同用；若少腹寒疝疼痛，可与附子、川楝子、小茴香等同用。

3. 温肾助阳：用于阴冷、阳萎等症，可与雄蚕蛾、茴香、附子、肉桂等温肾助阳药同用。

此外，丁香研细末，可敷妇女乳头破裂，或用香油调涂。

用量用法 1～3克。煎服。

使用注意 热证忌用。畏郁金。

花　　椒

为芸香科落叶灌木或小乔木花椒 Zanthoxylum bungeanum Maxim.或同属植物香椒子（青花椒）Zanthoxylum schinifolium Sieb. et Zucc.的果壳。产于四川者，特称川椒。微炒去仁取壳用。

处方用名 川椒、蜀椒、花椒。

性味归经 辛，温。有小毒。入脾、胃、肾经。

功效应用

1. 温中止痛：用于脾胃虚寒，脘腹冷痛，呕吐不能食，可与干姜、党参等同用；用于久寒腹痛下痢而有冷沫者，可用川椒6克，附子9克，干姜6克，水煎服；用于胃脘寒痛引背，可用川椒5克，附子、半夏各9克，研末为丸，每次6克，日2次，温水送服。

2. 杀虫止痒：用于因蛔虫引起的腹痛，呕吐或吐蛔等症。

挟寒者，可用川椒6克，乌梅、生姜、榧子各9克，水煎服；挟热者，可用川椒6克，乌梅9克，黄连3克，黄柏9克，枳实6克，水煎服；用于皮肤湿疹瘙痒，常与苦参、地肤子、白矾各适量，煎水熏洗，以增强杀虫止痒之功。

用量用法 2～6克。煎服。外用适量。

附药 椒目：为花椒的种子，性寒，味苦，辛，有小毒。入脾、膀胱经。具有行水，平喘之功。用于水肿胀满，痰饮喘咳之实证。

荜 茇

为胡椒科多年生草质藤本植物荜茇 Piper longum L.未成熟的果穗。晒干，生用。

处方用名 荜茇、荜拨。

性味归经 辛，热。入胃、大肠经。

功效应用 温中止痛：用于胃寒引起之脘腹疼痛，吐泻等症，可与肉桂、高良姜等分为丸用。

此外，本品又能治寒邪外凝，火郁于内的头痛、牙痛，可用荜茇6克，细辛3克，升麻6克，生大黄9克，水煎服。亦可单味为末涂患处，再以苍耳汤漱口，可治牙痛。

用量用法 1.5～6克。煎服。外用适量。

使用注意 实热郁火，阴虚火旺者均忌用。

荜 澄 茄

为胡椒科常绿攀援藤本植物荜澄茄 Piper cubeba L. 或樟科落叶小乔木或灌木山鸡椒 Litsea cubeba（Lour.）Pers.的果实。均打碎生用。

处方用名 荜澄茄。

性味归经 辛，温。入脾、胃、肾、膀胱经。

功效应用 温中散寒，行气止痛：用于胃寒疼痛，呕吐哕逆，食欲不振等症。可与吴茱萸、半夏等同用；用于寒疝腹痛，可与吴茱萸、香附等同用；用于下焦虚寒，小便不利，可与椒目、桂枝等同用；若下焦虚寒，膀胱冷气，小便频数，可与乌药、芡实等同用。

用量用法 1.5～6克。煎服。

胡　椒

为胡椒科常绿木质藤本植物胡椒 Piper nigrum L.的果实。商品有2种：当果实由绿变红时，采下未成熟的果实，晒干或烘干，名黑胡椒；采下红色完全成熟的果实，渍后去果皮，晒干，名白胡椒，作用较黑者为佳。多研末生用。

处方用名 胡椒、白胡椒。

性味归经 辛，热。入胃、大肠经。

功效应用 温中散寒，行气止痛：用于胃脘疼痛，可与丁香、木香、五灵脂等同用；若胃寒吐泻，可与干姜、丁香、半夏、陈皮等同用；也可单研粉放膏药中，外贴脐部，治受寒腹痛泄泻。

胡椒又是调味品，少量使用，能增进食欲。

用量用法 1.5～3克，煎服；散剂每次0.3～0.6克，吞服。外用适量。

8 理气药

凡能调理气分，疏畅气机的药物，统称为理气药。

理气药大多辛香苦温，善于行散或泄降，具有理气健脾，行气止痛，顺气降逆，疏肝解郁或破气散结等功效，适用于气机不畅所致的气滞、气逆等症。

气分的病变，大多与肝、脾（胃）、肺三脏有关。因肺主气，肝疏气，脾（胃）调气，若饮食不节，寒温失调，情志抑郁，忧思过度等，则常可导致肝气失疏，脾（胃）气失调，肺气壅滞而出现各种气滞病症。其它如痰湿、宿食、瘀血等，也皆能影响气机的运行。气滞的程度与部位不同，所表现的症状也各异。一般地说，气滞轻的为满，稍重的为胀，再重的为痛。脾胃气滞，则脘腹胀满，嗳气泛酸、恶心呕吐，便秘或腹泻；肝气郁滞，则胁肋胀痛，胸闷不舒，男子疝气疼痛，女子乳房胀痛及月经不调等；肺气壅滞，则胸闷不畅，咳嗽气喘等。

使用本类药物时，还需针对病情作适当配伍，如脾胃气滞，而兼有湿热困脾者，宜并用清热利湿药；兼有寒湿困脾者，当配温中燥湿药；有饮食停滞者，加消食导滞药；兼脾胃虚弱者，又当配健脾药。肝郁气滞之临床表现及兼夹证候较多，可根据具体病情配伍养肝、柔肝、止痛、健脾及活血调经等药。肺气壅实兼有痰饮者，须配祛痰化饮之品。

理气药大都辛温香散，虽可治气滞疾病，但易耗气伤阴，故对阴虚，气虚患者当慎用。

香　附

为莎草科多年生草本植物莎草 Cyperus rotundus L.的干燥

根茎。生用或醋炒用。

处方用名 生香附、制香附、香附子、香附米。

性味归经 辛、微苦、微甘，平。入肝、三焦经。

功效应用

1. 疏肝理气：用于肝郁气滞，胸胁痞闷，脘腹疼痛等症，常与其它理气药配用。

2. 调经止痛：用于月经不调，痛经，本品为妇科常用要药；属肝气郁结者，用之尤宜。常与当归、川芎、乌药或艾叶等同用。

用量用法 6～12克。煎服。理气解郁可生用，调经止痛可制用。

木　　香

为菊科宿根草本植物云木香 Saussurea lappa Clarke、川木香 Vladimiria souliei（Franch.）Ling 等的根。原药打碎生用或煨用。

处方用名 木香、云木香、广木香、煨木香。

性味归经 辛、苦，温。入脾、胃，大肠、三焦经。

功效应用

1. 行气止痛：用于胃肠气滞，脘腹胀痛，泻痢后重等症，治脘腹胀痛，呕逆等症，常与砂仁、藿香、丁香等同用；若治食积气滞，脘腹胀满，大便秘结，或泻痢后重等症，常与黄连、槟榔、大黄等同用。

2. 健胃消食：用于消化不良，食欲不振，呕吐，慢性腹泻等症，常与砂仁、白术、茯苓、半夏、陈皮等同用。

现代用于胆囊炎，胆石症，胰腺炎，阑尾炎，肠梗阻等多种急腹症。胆囊炎，胆石症，胰腺炎，可与柴胡、黄芩、大黄等同用；阑尾炎，可与金银花、大黄、牡丹皮配用；肠梗阻，可与甘遂、桃仁、牛膝等配用。

用量用法 3～6 克。煎服。理气多生用，止泻多煨用，入汤剂不宜久煎。

附药 青木香：又名土木香。为马兜铃科多年生缠绕草本植物马兜铃 Aristolochia contorta Bge.的根。切片生用。味辛苦，性寒，有小毒。有催吐，解毒，消肿之功。可治食物中毒，热毒肿痛及毒蛇咬伤等症，可以内服，亦可外用。多服有涌吐之弊。用量 3～6 克，煎服。外用适量，研末敷患处。

乌　　药

为樟科常绿灌木或小乔木乌药 Lindera strychnifolia（Sieb. et Zuce.）Villar 的根。晒干，切片生用。

处方用名 乌药、台乌药。

性味归经 辛，温。入脾、肺、肾、膀胱经。

功效应用

1. 行气止痛：用于胸腹闷胀疼痛，及疝气、痛经等症。治中寒气滞，腹部冷痛，可与沉香、生姜、党参等同用；若治胸膈痞闷，食欲不振，可与沉香、槟榔等同用；若治寒凝气滞所致的小肠疝气，可与小茴香、川楝子、木香等同用；若治气滞腹胀，经期腹痛，可与木香、当归等同用。

2. 温肾散寒：用于虚寒性小便频数，可与益智仁、山药各等分，研末，黄酒为丸，每次 10 克，每日 2～3 次，淡盐水送服。

用量用法 6～10 克。煎服。

橘　　皮

为芸香科常绿小乔木橘树 Citrus reticulata Blanco 的成熟果实之果皮。切丝生用。

处方用名 橘皮、陈皮、广皮、广陈皮、新会皮。

性味归经 辛、苦，温。入脾、肺经。

功效应用

1. 燥湿化痰：用于痰湿滞塞，咳嗽痰多，胸闷不畅，常与半夏、茯苓、甘草同用。

2. 理气健脾：用于脾胃气滞，消化不良，腹胀脘闷，食欲不振，恶心呕吐等症，常与厚朴、白术、生姜等药同用。

用量用法 3～10克。煎服。

使用注意 本品性偏温燥，津亏实热之证，不宜使用。

附药

1. 橘红：橘皮去内层橘白者名橘红。性较燥烈，功效与橘皮相似，以祛痰化湿为胜，主治肺寒咳嗽，喉痒痰多。用量3～6克。煎服。

2. 橘络：橘瓤上之筋膜。性味甘苦而寒，功能通络化痰，主治咳嗽胸胁作痛，痰热积滞经络，取其宣通络道。用量3～5克。煎服。

3. 橘核：系橘的种子。性味苦平，入肝经。功能理气散结止痛，专治小肠疝气及睾丸肿痛。用量6～12克。煎服。

4. 橘叶：为橘树之叶。味苦性平，入肝经，功能疏肝解郁，行气散结。适用于肝气郁结，胸胁疼痛，乳腺肿痛等症。用量6～12克。煎服。

青　皮

为芸香科常绿小乔木橘树 Citrus reticulata Blanco 的未成熟的果实或青色果皮。剖开，除去瓤肉，晒干。生用或醋炒用。

处方用名 青皮、小青皮、均青皮。

性味归经 苦、辛，温。入肝、胆、胃经。

功效应用

1. 疏肝破气：用于肝气不舒，胸胁胀痛，常与柴胡、郁金、香附等同用；若肝脾肿大者，再加鳖甲、党参等药；属痰饮胁痛者，可与白芥子同用；治乳痈肿痛者，可与蒲公英、栝楼、橘叶等同用；亦可单用青皮研末，每次1.5克，日服2次，以治因气郁所致的乳核、乳肿、胸痞、嗳呃、胁痛、腹痛等症。用于寒疝腹痛，可与乌药、小茴香 木香等同用。

2. 散积化滞：用于食积佇滞，脘腹胀痛。常与山楂、麦芽、草蔻等同用。

用量用法 3～6克。煎服。用于疏肝，醋炒为好。

使用注意 本品性峻烈，能伤气，气虚者当慎用。

枳　实

为芸香科常绿小乔木枸橘 Poncirus trifoliata (L.) Raf.、酸橙 Citrus aurantium L.或香橼 Citrus wilsonii Tanaka 的幼果。夏至前后采取幼果，名枳实，秋季采摘成熟果实，名枳壳。切片晒干，麸炒用。

处方用名 小枳实、炒枳实。

性味归经 苦，微寒。入脾、胃、大肠经。

功效应用

1. 破气消积：用于肠胃湿热积滞，腹痛便秘或泻痢后重等症，可与大黄、黄连、白术等同用；若治妇女产后气血凝滞，腹痛，烦闷不安，可用枳实、白芍各10克，研末，每次6克，日2次服。

2. 化痰除痞：用于胸胁痰饮，痞满不适，常与半夏、茯苓、陈皮等同用；用于心下痞满，食欲不振，或胸腹胀满，大便不畅者，可与黄连、干姜、厚朴等同用；若用于脾虚胸痞腹胀，消化不良，常与白术同用。

此外，现临床常用本品治胃下垂，子宫脱垂，脱肛等症。可与黄芪、升麻等同用。

用量用法 3～6克。煎服。

使用注意 脾胃虚弱者慎用。

附药 枳壳：即酸橙等成熟后的果实，去瓤，压扁，切片，晒干，麸炒用。性味、功效与枳实同，惟力量较弱。以理气宽中、消除胀满为主。

川楝子

为楝科落叶乔木川楝树 Melia toosendan Sieb. et Zucc.的果实。捣开去核，生用或盐炒用。

处方用名 川楝子、金铃子。

性味归经 苦，寒。入肝、胃、小肠、膀胱经。

功效应用

1. 行气止痛：本品苦寒性降，兼能疏泄肝热，以症见热象者较宜。用于肝气郁滞，肝胆火盛所致的胸腹胀痛及疝痛等症。前者常与玄胡索同用，可增强止痛之功；后者疝痛，症见寒象者，可配木香、小茴香、吴茱萸等，以散寒理气止痛。

2. 驱虫：用于虫积腹痛，多与其它杀虫药，如使君子、槟榔等同用。

此外，本品外用可治头癣，以川楝子适量，焙黄研末，用熟猪油或麻油调成油膏，涂于患处。涂药之前，先用食盐泡温开水，将患处洗净。

用量用法 5～10克。煎服。一般生用，治疝气可用盐炒。

使用注意 脾胃虚寒者不宜用。

薤白

为百合科多年生草本植物小根蒜 Allium macrostemon Bge 或薤 A. chinense G. Don. 的地下鳞茎。蒸熟用。

处方用名 薤白、薤白头。

性味归经 辛、苦，温。入肺、胃、大肠经。

功效应用

1. 通阳散结：用于寒痰凝滞，胸阳不宣，胸脘痞闷，咳喘痰多，胸背刺痛等症，本品辛散苦降，温通滑利，能宣通胸中之阳，以散阴寒之结，为治胸痹之要药。常与瓜蒌及其它理气活血药同用。

2. 下气导滞：用于肠胃气滞，泻痢后重，可与柴胡、白芍、枳实等同用。

现代亦常用于冠心病心绞痛，每与丹参、红花、栝楼等同用，能活血，宽胸，定痛。

用量用法　5～10克。煎服。

使用注意　气虚无滞者，及胃弱纳呆，不耐蒜味者不宜用。

甘　松

为败酱科多年生矮小草本植物甘松香 Nardostachys chinensis Batal.的根及根茎。切段生用。

处方用名　甘松、甘松香。

性味归经　甘，温。入脾、胃经。

功效应用　行气止痛，开胃醒脾：用于脾胃受寒，气郁不舒，脘腹满痛，食欲不振等症，常与藿香、麦芽、砂仁等同用。

用量用法　3～10克。煎服。

佛　手

为芸香科常绿亚乔木佛手 Citrus medica L. var. sarcodactylis（Noot.）Swingle的果实。切片晒干生用。

处方用名　佛手片、陈佛手、鲜佛手、佛手柑。

性味归经　辛、苦、酸，温。入肝、脾、胃、肺经。

功效应用

1. 疏肝理气止痛：用于肝胃气郁，脘腹胀痛等症，常与木香、青皮等理气药同用。

2. 健胃止呕：用于消化不良，食欲不振，嗳气，呕吐等症，本品为治呕良药。可与砂仁、白蔻、半夏等同用。

此外，尚有止咳化痰作用，可治咳嗽痰多之症。

用量用法　6～10 克。煎服。

沉　香

为瑞香科常绿乔木沉香 Aguilaria agallocha Roxb.或白木香 A.sinensis（Lour.）Gilg.含有棕黑色树脂的木心，经干燥后加工而成。研末用。

处方用名　沉香、盔沉香。

性味归经　辛、苦，温。入脾、胃、肾经。

功效应用

1. 行气止痛：用于气滞胸胁痞满疼痛，及妇女月经不调，少腹疼痛，可与香附、砂仁等同用；治痰饮内停而致气滞胸痞疼痛者，可与木香、半夏、茯苓等同用。

2. 降逆平喘：用于胸膈痞闷，上气喘急，可与乌药、木香、槟榔同用；本品性温，既降逆气，又纳肾气，故可用治下元虚冷，肾不纳气之虚喘，与附子、生姜同用，共奏温肾纳气之功。

3. 温中止呕：用于胃寒呕吐、呃逆，可与白蔻、丁香、柿蒂等同用。

用量用法　1～3 克。研末冲服，不宜入煎。

使用注意　本品辛温助热，阴虚火热者慎用。

檀　香

为檀香科常绿小乔木檀香 Santalum album L.的木质心材。水洗后镑成片，或劈碎入药。

处方用名　檀香、白檀香。

性味归经　辛，温。入脾、胃、肺经。

功效应用

1. 行气止痛：用于气滞寒凝所致的脘腹冷痛及神经性胃痛，可与沉香、木香、丁香、乌药等同用；若治气滞血瘀之胃脘疼痛、心绞痛等症，可与丹参同用。

2. 温胃止呕：用于胃寒疼痛，呕吐清水，可与菖蒲、丁香、木香等同用。

此外，近年常用其治疗冠心病属于气滞血瘀者，每与荜茇、延胡索、细辛等同用。

用量用法 1～3克。煎服。

柿 蒂

为柿树科落叶乔木柿树 Diospyros kaki, L. f.的宿存花萼。晒干生用。

处方用名 柿蒂。

性味归经 苦、涩，微温。入胃经。

功效应用 降气止呃：用于胃寒呃逆，可与丁香、生姜同用；若属胃热呃逆，可与竹茹、赭石等同用。

用量用法 6～10克。煎服。

荔 枝 核

为无患子科常绿乔木植物荔枝树 Litchi chinensis Sonn.的成熟种子。生用或盐水炒用。用时捣碎。

处方用名 荔枝核。

性味归经 甘，温。入肝、肾经。

功效应用 行气止痛：用于肠疝、睾丸肿痛，及妇女少腹气血刺痛等症。治疝气，常与橘核、小茴香、川楝子等同用；若治妇女气血刺痛，可用荔枝核、香附各等分，研末，每次6克，淡盐汤或温水送服。

用量用法 6～10克。煎服。

使用注意 无寒湿气滞者不宜用。

玫 瑰 花

为蔷薇科落叶小灌木玫瑰 Rosa rugosa Thunb.的花蕾。晒干入药。

处方用名 玫瑰花。

性味归经 甘、微苦，温。入肝、脾经。

功效应用 行气活血，疏肝止痛：用于肝胃不和，脘胁胀痛，可与香附、川楝子等同用。

此外，尚用于妇女月经不调，及损伤瘀痛等症。现临床治心绞痛方中，亦常配用。不外取其理气活血之功。

用量用法 3～10 克。煎服。

9 消食药

凡以消食化积为主要功效的药物，称为消食药。又称消导药。

本类药物主要具有消食导滞，促进消化的作用。其中有的药物尚能健运脾胃。适用于饮食积滞，消化不良，脘腹胀满，不思饮食，嗳酸、恶心、呕吐，大便失常等症。

应用本类药物时，须根据不同的病情，适当配伍其他药物，如食滞而兼气滞者，配行气药；如食积已化热者，配苦寒轻下药；如食积而脾胃虚弱，不能运化，兼有气虚症状者，应与补气健脾药同用。

山　楂

为蔷薇科落叶灌木山楂 Crataegus pinnatifida Bge. var. major N. E. Br.的成熟果实。去核生用，炒焦或炒炭用。

处方用名　生山楂、炒山楂、焦山楂、山楂炭。

性味归经　酸、甘，微温。入脾、胃、肝经。

功效应用

1. 消食化积：用于食积停滞，油腻肉积，胸腹胀满，小儿伤乳等症，常与麦芽、神曲、莱菔子等同用。

2. 活血散瘀：用于血瘀经痛及产后瘀滞腹痛，恶露不尽等症，常与当归、川芎、元胡、益母草等同用；若治产后宫缩痛，可用山楂炭 30 克，水煎加红糖、童便服。

此外，本品尚有活血松肌透疹作用，若麻疹初出，透发不快，症见气血郁滞或消化不良者，与青皮同用甚效。近年，常用其治高血压，与决明子、白糖泡水代茶，天天饮服。本品亦常用于冠心病、高脂血症及细菌性痢疾的治疗。

用量用法 10～15克。煎服。消食多炒用，止痢、化瘀多炒炭用，降压，透疹多生用。

附药 山楂核：功能软坚散结，下气消胀。用于肠疝胀痛、睾丸疝肿，常与橘核、荔枝核同用；若治呃逆，可用山楂核30克，白蔻仁9克，共研细末，每次3克，日服2次。

神　曲

为全麦粉和其他药物（青蒿、苍耳、辣蓼、杏仁、赤小豆芽）混合后经发酵而成的加工品。原药生用、麸炒用或炒焦用。

处方用名 生神曲、六神曲、炒神曲、焦神曲。

性味归经 甘、辛，温。入脾、胃经。

功效应用 消食和胃：用于饮食积滞，消化不良，或伤食腹泻，腹胀等症，常与山楂、麦芽、莱菔子、鸡内金等同用。

此外，丸剂中有金石药品，难于消化吸收者，常用生六曲打糊为丸，以助消化，如磁朱丸、万氏牛黄清心丸等。

用量用法 6～12克，煎服。和胃消食多炒用，止泻痢多炒焦用，配丸制糊则生用。

附药 建曲：又名范志曲。系以六曲加其他药物而制成，并不发酵。其功效与六曲同中有异，能治感冒风寒，食滞胸闷。用量6～12克。

麦　芽

为禾本科1年生草本植物大麦 Hordeum vulgare L.的成熟果实经发芽而成。生用或炒至微焦用。

处方用名 生麦芽、炒麦芽。

性味归经 甘，平。入脾、胃、肝经。

功效应用

1. 健胃消食：用于饮食积滞，消化不良，脘腹胀闷等症，常与山楂、神曲等同用。小儿乳积不化之吐乳，可单用麦芽煎服。

2. 舒肝回乳：用于肝气不舒，脘胁胀闷，嗳气等症，常与川楝子、青皮等同用；若乳汁郁积，乳房胀痛或需断乳者，可单用生麦芽60～120克。水煎服。

用量用法 10～15克。大剂可用至30～120克。煎服。舒肝、回乳宜生用，消食宜炒用。

使用注意 妇女授乳期不宜用。

谷 芽

为禾本科1年生草本植物稻 Oryza sativa L.的成熟果实，发芽晒干而成。生用或炒至微焦用。

处方用名 生谷芽、炒谷芽、香稻芽、炒稻芽。

性味归经 甘，平。入脾、胃经。

功效应用 健脾开胃，消食和中：用于食欲减退，消化不良之因于脾胃虚弱者，常与党参、白术、砂仁等同用。

用量用法 10～15克。煎服。生用养胃，炒用消食。

莱 菔 子

为十字花科1年生或2年生直立草本植物莱菔 Raphanus sativus L.的成熟种子（萝卜种子）。微炒捣碎用。

处方用名 莱菔子。

性味归经 辛、甘，平。入肺、脾经。

功效应用

1. 导滞消食：用于食积不化，脘腹胀闷，嗳气食臭，或腹痛泄泻等症，常与山楂、麦芽、神曲等同用，以助消化之力。有湿者可配茯苓，有热者可配连翘。

2. 降气化痰：用于咳嗽痰喘，常与苏子、白芥子同用。

用量用法 3～10克。煎服。

使用注意 本品能损耗正气，气虚无食积和痰滞者慎用。

鸡 内 金

为雉科动物家鸡 Gallus gallus domesticus Brisson 的砂囊角质内膜（鸡肫内的黄皮）。生用或砂炮鼓起后，研末用。

处方用名 鸡内金、炙内金。

性味归经 甘、涩，平。入脾、胃、膀胱经。

功效应用

1. 健胃消食：用于饮食停滞，消化不良及小儿疳积等症，单用，或与六曲、麦芽、山楂同用。

2. 固摄缩尿：用于遗尿、小便频数，可与桑螵蛸、黄芪、龙骨、牡蛎等随症配用。

3. 消结石：用于胆、肾及膀胱结石等症。治胆结石常与金钱草、郁金等配伍；治肾及膀胱结石常与胡桃、海金砂等同用。

用量用法 1.5～3 克。宜散剂冲服，或入丸剂服。入煎剂，其有效成分不易溶解。

10 驱虫药

凡以驱除或杀灭人体寄生虫为主要作用的药物，称为驱虫药。

驱虫药主要用于蛔虫、蛲虫、绦虫、钩虫和姜片虫等肠寄生虫病。虫病的一般临床表现为腹痛时作，腹胀，善饥多食，或不思饮食，或嗜食异物，肛门、耳、鼻瘙痒。久则出现面色发黄，形体消瘦等。当用驱虫药从根本上治疗。

使用本类药物，必须根据患者的兼症，体质等分别选用和适当配伍。如便闭者当配泻下药，有积滞者配消导药，脾胃虚弱者配健脾药，体质虚弱者，可先补后泻，或攻补兼施。

本类药物，具有毒性者，使用时应注意用量。

使 君 子

为使君子科藤本状灌木使君子 Quisqualis indica L.的种子。去壳取仁，生用，炒香用，或连壳打碎用。

处方用名 使君子、使君肉。

性味归经 甘，温。入脾、胃经。

功效应用 杀虫消积：用于蛔虫、蛲虫等症。本品味甘美，气香可口，故尤宜于小儿。症轻者，单用炒香嚼服即有效；如蛔虫多，症较重者，常与槟榔、苦楝皮、乌梅等同用。若治小儿疳积，常与槟榔、胡黄连、木香等同用。

用量用法 6～12 克。煎服。宜入丸散剂。炒香嚼服，成人每次 10～20 粒；小儿每岁每天 1 粒半，总量不得超过 20 粒。

使用注意 大量服食，可引起呃逆，头晕，呕吐，恶心等反应；与茶同用，亦可引起呃逆。

苦 楝 皮

为楝科落叶乔木苦楝树 Melia azedarach L.和川楝树 M. toosendan S. et Z.的根皮或树皮。生用或鲜用。

处方用名 苦楝根皮、苦楝皮。

性味归经 苦，寒，有小毒。入肝、脾、胃经。

功效应用 杀虫消积：用于蛔虫、蛲虫、钩虫等虫积腹痛。本品杀虫之功较强，疗效颇佳。可单用，亦可与槟榔等其他杀虫药配伍同用。

用量用法 6～10 克，鲜者 15～30 克，煎服。外用适量。

使用注意 性寒有毒，不宜持续服用，体虚者慎用，肝炎患者忌用。

槟 榔

为棕榈科常绿乔木槟榔树 Areca catechu L.的成熟种子。晒干，捣碎或用冷浸法浸透切片生用。

处方用名 花槟榔、槟榔片。

性味归经 苦、辛，温。入胃、大肠经。

功效应用

1. 杀虫消积：用于绦虫、蛔虫、蛲虫、姜片虫等多种肠道寄生虫病。其中对绦虫驱虫疗效较佳。可与其他驱虫药同用。

2. 下气通便：用于食积气滞，腹胀，腹痛，便秘，或泻痢后重等症，常与大黄、木香等同用。

3. 利水消肿：用于脚气肿痛，常与紫苏、吴茱萸、生姜等同用。

此外，尚可用于疟疾。

用量用法 6～10 克。单味大量可用 30～120 克。煎服。

使用注意 脾虚便溏者不宜服用。

附药 大腹皮：为槟榔的果皮。味辛，性微温。入脾、胃、大、小肠经。功能下气宽中，利水消肿。用于湿阻气滞，脘腹胀闷，大便不爽，水肿胀满，脚气浮肿，小便不利等。近年临床多用于肝硬变腹水、肾病水肿等。用量6～12克。煎服。

南瓜子

为葫芦科1年生缠绕草本植物南瓜 Cucurbita moschata Duch.的种子。研粉生用，以新鲜者良。

处方用名 南瓜子。

性味归经 甘，温。入胃、大肠经。

功效应用 杀虫：用于绦虫病。常用本品60～120克，连壳生用，洗净，研细，冷开水调服，于2小时后用槟榔60～120克煎汤服下，再过30分钟用开水冲服芒硝15克，促使泻下，以利于虫体排出体外。

此外，本品对血吸虫、蛔虫、蛲虫亦有治疗效果。

用量用法 60～120克。嚼烂吞服。

鹤虱

为菊科多年生草本植物天名精 Carpesium abrotanoides L.或伞形科2年生草本植物野胡萝卜 Daucus carota L.的成熟果实。晒干，生用或炒用。

处方用名 鹤虱。

性味归经 苦、辛，平，有小毒。入大肠经。

功效应用 杀虫消积：用于蛔虫、蛲虫、绦虫、钩虫等虫积腹痛，肛门瘙痒。常与其它杀虫药同用。

用量用法 3～10克。煎服。入丸散宜炒用，入煎剂可生用。

榧子

为红豆杉科常绿乔木榧树 Torreya grandis Fort.的成熟种

子。去壳生用或炒用。

处方用名 榧子、榧子仁、榧子肉。

性味归经 甘，平。入肺、胃、大肠经。

功效应用 驱虫润燥：用于蛔虫、丝虫、绦虫、钩虫、姜片虫等虫积腹痛诸症，常与槟榔、芜荑等杀虫药同用。

此外，本品能润肠通便，可用于痔疮便难。

用量用法 30～50克。炒熟去壳，取种仁嚼服，或入丸散剂。亦可连壳生用，打碎入煎。治钩虫每天30～40个，空腹1次嚼服，连服至大便虫卵消失为止。

芜　荑

为榆科落叶小乔木或灌木植物大果榆 Ulmus macr ocarpa Hance 果实的加工品。生用。

处方用名 臭芜荑、白芜荑。

性味归经 辛、苦、温。入脾、胃经。

功效应用 杀虫消积：用于蛔虫、绦虫等虫积腹痛及小儿疳积泄泻等症。本品功专杀虫，可单用，或与其它杀虫药同用。若用于小儿疳积，腹痛有虫，形瘦面黄而经常泄泻者，可与白术、山药、鸡内金、木香等同用。

用量用法 3～10克．煎服．

雷　丸

为多孔菌科植物雷丸 Polyporus mylittae Cook. et Mass.的菌核。切片生用，或干燥后研粉末用。

处方用名 雷丸。

性味归经 苦，寒，有小毒。入胃、大肠经。

功效应用 杀虫消积：用于绦虫、钩虫、蛔虫等症。实验证明，本品有杀虫之功，用于驱绦虫，能使虫体分解，单用即效，常与槟榔、牵牛、木香等同用；若用于小儿疳积，可与使君子、胡黄连等同用；若治脑囊虫病，可与半夏、茯苓等同用。

用量用法 研末吞服，每次3～6克。驱杀绦虫，每次服粉剂12～18克，日3次，用冷开水调，饭后服。连服3天。

使用注意 宜作丸散剂，不入煎剂。

鹤草芽

为蔷薇科多年生草本植物龙芽草 Agrimonia pilosa Ledeb.的冬芽。晒干研末用。

处方用名 鹤草芽。

性味归经 苦、涩，凉。入肝、小肠、大肠经。

功效应用 杀虫：用于绦虫病。本品驱杀绦虫，疗效颇佳，为驱杀绦虫的要药。单用研粉，于早晨空腹1次顿服，多在服后5～6小时内即可排出虫体。

用量用法 研末服，成人每次30～50克，用温开水送服。小儿按每公斤体重用0.7～0.8克计算。

鸦胆子

为苦木科常绿灌木或小乔木植物鸦胆子 Brucea javanica (L.) Merr.的成熟果实。晒干，去壳取仁用。

处方用名 鸦胆子、鸦胆油。

性味归经 苦，寒。入大肠，肝经。

功效应用

1. 杀虫止痢：用于热毒血痢，下脓血，里急后重等。本品为治热毒血痢与休息痢的要药。可单用本品，用龙眼肉包裹服，每次15粒，每日3次，连服10～14日。现临床用治急、慢性阿米巴痢。

2. 杀虫截疟：用于间日疟、3日疟及恶性疟，鸦胆子仁，用龙眼肉包，每次10～15粒，日3次，连服5～7天。

3. 腐蚀赘疣：用于鸡眼、寻常疣，可用本品捣烂涂敷患处，或以鸦胆子油涂擦，日 2 次。皆能使赘疣脱落。

用量用法 治痢内服，成人每次 10～30 粒；治疟疾内服，每次 10～15 粒，小儿每岁 1 粒，但不得超过成人量。去壳取仁(不宜敲碎)，外用龙眼肉包裹，饭后吞服，以减少胃肠刺激症状。外用适量。

使用注意 本品有小毒，对胃肠道及肝、肾均有损害，不宜多用久服，胃肠出血及肝、肾病患者，应慎用或忌用。

11 止血药

凡以制止人体内外各种出血为主要作用的药物，称为止血药。

本类药物主要适用于各种出血的病症，如咯血，衄血，吐血，便血，尿血，崩漏，紫癜，以及创伤出血等。及时并有效地制止出血，可减少血液的耗损。同时对于防止大失血或气随血脱，都具有重要的意义。

止血药有凉血止血，收敛止血，化瘀止血，温经止血等不同作用。出血只是某些疾病的一个现象，引起出血的原因很多，而止血药为治标的药物。因此，治疗出血性疾病时，不可盲目的止血，当根据出血的原因选择配伍，以治其本。如出血属血热妄行的，当与清热凉血药同用；属于阴虚阳亢，血随气逆的，当与养阴潜阳降气药配伍；属于气虚不能摄血的，当与补气药同用。这样标本兼顾，方能药到病除。

此外，使用止血药必须注意有无瘀血，如有瘀血未尽，单纯止血，则有留瘀之弊。故在出血病初期宜选用化瘀作用的止血药或与行血药同用。大失血而有虚脱现象者，当先补气，即“血脱益气”之法。

蒲　黄

为香蒲科多年水生草本植物狭叶香蒲 Typha angustifolia L. 或香蒲属其他植物的花粉。生用或炒炭用。

处方用名　生蒲黄、炒蒲黄、蒲黄炭。

性味归经　甘，平。入肝，心包经。

功效应用

1. 止血（炒用）：用于咳血、吐血、衄血、尿血、便血及崩漏下血等症，单用内服或随症配伍。若外伤出血，可单用外敷。

2. 行血消瘀（生用）：用于血瘀，胃痛，腹痛，痛经，产后瘀滞腹痛等症，常与五灵脂同用；用于木舌、重舌、舌肿，以生蒲黄敷之，数分钟后，漱去。

此外，本品有利尿之功生用常治血淋涩痛。可配冬葵子、生地黄等。现代尚用于冠心病心绞痛。

用量用法 3～10 克。包煎。外用适量。

使用注意 生蒲黄有收缩子宫作用，故孕妇忌用，但对产后子宫收缩不良的出血，可以使用。

仙鹤草

为蔷薇科多年生草本植物龙芽草 Agrimonia pilosa Ledeb. var. japonica（Miq.）Nakai 的全草。切段生用。

处方用名 仙鹤草。

性味归经 苦、涩，平。入心、脾、胃、大肠经。

功效应用

1. 收敛止血：用于咯血、吐血、衄血、便血、尿血以及妇女崩漏等各种出血症。本品可广泛用于治疗身体各部分出血，不论虚实寒热，皆可应用。单用或与其他药配伍应用。如属于血热妄行，可配凉血止血药，如生地、丹皮、侧柏叶、赤芍、藕节等；如用于虚寒性出血，可配党参、黄芪、熟地、当归、炮姜、艾叶、灶心土等。

2. 收敛止泻：用于腹泻、痢疾，以慢性泻痢为宜。可用本品 30 克、木槿花 10 克同用，亦可视症情与它药配伍同用。

3. 杀虫：用于滴虫性阴道炎引起之阴部瘙痒。可用仙鹤草 120 克，水煎浓汁，冲洗阴道，再用带线棉球浸汁放入，约 3 小时后取出，每日 1 次，连用 1 周。有杀灭滴虫作用。

此外，本品尚可用于劳力过度所致的脱力劳伤，见有神疲乏力而纳食正常者，每天30克与等量红枣水煎服，有调补气血之功，有助于体力恢复。用于疖疮痈肿、痔疮等，可用茎叶熬膏调蜜外涂，并可同时内服。

用量用法 10～15克，大剂量可用30～60克。外用适量。

白　及

为兰科多年生草本植物白及 Bletilla striata（Thunb.）Reichb. f.的地下块茎。切片生用。

处方用名 白及。

性味归经 苦、甘、涩，微寒。入肺、肝、胃经。

功效应用

1. 收敛止血：用于肺胃出血，可单用研末冲服，如治肺出血，亦可与海蛤粉、枇杷叶等同用；治肺结核空洞咯血，又可与松香、知母、百合等同用；治胃出血，或胃及十二指肠溃疡穿孔等症，可与乌贼骨等同用。用于外伤出血，疮口不敛，可单用或与煅石膏等研末外用；治烫伤或手足皲裂，可用麻油调涂。

2. 消肿生肌：用于痈肿溃疡，常与银花、穿山甲、皂刺等同用。

用量用法 3～10克。煎服。散剂吞服1～3克。外用适量。

使用注意 反乌头。

藕　节

为睡莲科多年水生草本植物莲 Nelumbo nucifera Gaertn.的地下茎之节。生用或炒炭用。

处方用名 生藕节、藕节炭。

性味归经 甘、涩，平。入肝、肺、膀胱、胃经。

功效应用 收敛止血，凉血化瘀：用于咳血、吐血、衄血、尿血、血痢、血崩等症，对血热有瘀滞者尤为适宜。鲜者捣汁服有效，常与生地、侧柏等其它止血药配伍应用。

用量用法 10～15克，鲜者可用30～60克煎服。凉血化瘀宜生用，收涩止血宜炒炭用。

棕　榈

为棕榈科常绿乔木棕榈树 Trachycarpus Wagnerianus Becc. 的叶鞘纤维。一名棕榈皮。切成小片，煅炭用。

处方用名 棕榈、棕榈炭、陈棕榈。

性味归经 苦、涩、平。入肺、肝、大肠经。

功效应用 收涩止血：用于吐血、衄血、便血、崩漏下血、赤白下痢等症而无瘀滞者，临床以治妇科崩漏居多。单用有效，或复方配用。

用量用法 3～10克。煎服。

灶　心　土

为久经草或木柴熏烧的灶心土。剁成小块入药。

处方用名 灶心土、伏龙肝。

性味归经 辛，微温，入脾、胃经。

功效应用

1. 收敛止血：用于虚寒性吐血、便血等症见血色黯淡、面色萎黄、四肢不温、舌淡脉细者。本品温中收涩以止血，可配白术、生地、附子等同用。

2. 温中止呕：用于虚寒性呕吐，妊娠恶阻等症，可与陈皮、生姜等同用。

此外，还可用于脾虚泄泻，有温脾止泻之效。

用量用法 15～30克。煎服。布包，先煎。或用60～120克煎汤代水。

三　七

为五加科多年生草本植物人参三七 Panax pseudoginseng Wall. Var. notoginseng（Burkill）Hoo　& Tseng 的根。磨粉入药。

处方用名　三七粉。

性味归经　甘、微苦，温。入肝、胃经。

功效应用

1. 止血化瘀：用于吐血、衄血、血痢、便血、血崩以及产后出血过多等症。本品为止血要药，具有止血不留瘀的特长，不论内服外用均有殊效，对出血兼有瘀滞者尤为适宜。可单用研末，米汤或温开水送服，每次 1.5～3 克，或与花蕊石等药配用；用于创伤出血，研末敷于伤口。

2. 消肿定痛：用于跌打损伤，瘀滞疼痛，痈肿疮疡等症，可单用适量，研末，米醋调涂。

此外，近年用治冠心病心绞痛，有一定疗效。

用量用法　1.5～3 克。宜作丸散剂，入汤剂宜研粉冲服。外用适量。

使用注意　本品性温，凡出血而见阴虚口干者，常配滋阴凉血药同用。

茜　草　根

为茜草科多年蔓生草本植物茜草 Rubia cordifolia L.的根。晒干切段入药，生用或炒炭用。

处方用名　茜草根、茜草炭。

性味归经　苦，寒。入肝经。

功效应用

1. 止血化瘀：用于热征吐血、衄血、便血，及崩漏下血等症，可与生地、侧柏叶、阿胶等随症选用；如治血痢，可与黄芩、黄连等配伍；若治虚寒性崩漏，亦可与乌贼骨、牡蛎、黄芪等收敛补虚药同用；如治过敏性紫癜，可与紫草、丹参等同用。

2. 凉血行血：用于血热瘀滞，痛经，经闭等症，可与丹参等同用；若用于跌打损伤，常与红花、赤芍等同用。

用量用法 6～10克。煎服。

花 蕊 石

为矿石类含蛇纹石大理岩 Ophicalcite 的石块。经火煅，研细，水飞用。

处方用名 花蕊石。

性味归经 酸、涩，平。入肝经。

功效应用 止血化瘀：用于吐血、衄血，及产后血晕，胎衣不下等症，本品凡内出血而兼有瘀滞者皆可应用。可单用花蕊石，每次6克，合童便，另加酒或醋调服，亦可与三七、血余炭等同用；用于外伤出血，可用花蕊石，研细末，擦伤处。

用量用法 3～10克。煎服，以入丸散为宜。如入汤剂宜先煎。外用适量。

血 余 炭

为人发洗净后，经加工焖煅之炭。碾成小块或研极细末用。

处方用名 血余炭、发炭。

性味归经 苦，平。入肝、肾经。

功效应用 止血散瘀：用于吐血、衄血、尿血、血淋、血痢、便血、崩漏等症，常与其它止血药同用，如治创伤出血或溃疡不敛，可研末或熬膏外敷。

此外，尚有利尿之效。

用量用法 3～10克。煎服。外用适量。

小　蓟

为菊科多年生草本植物刺儿菜 Cephalanoplos Segetum (Bge.) Kitam.的全草。切段，生用或炒用。

处方用名　小蓟、小蓟炭。

性味归经　甘，凉。入心、小肠、膀胱经。

功效应用　凉血止血，破血化瘀：用于血分有热的吐血、衄血、尿血、血淋、便血、妇女崩漏等症。本品兼可利尿，故擅治血淋。常与生地、山栀、藕节、滑石、蒲黄等同用；若治吐血，常与大蓟、侧柏叶、茅根、山栀、茜草根等同用。

用量用法　10～15克。鲜品可用30～60克。煎服。

附药　大蓟：为菊科多年生宿根草本植物大蓟 Cirsium japonicum DC.的根、茎及叶。性味功能用量均同小蓟，唯能消痈肿，兼治痈疮肿毒。无论内服外敷皆可。但以用鲜品为佳。

侧　柏　叶

为柏科常绿乔木侧柏 Biota orientalis （L.） Endl.的带叶枝梢。生用或炒炭用。

处方用名　生侧柏、侧柏炭。

性味归经　苦、涩，微寒。入肺、肝、大肠经。

功效应用

1. 凉血止血：用于血分有热之咳血、吐血、衄血、尿血、便血及血崩下血等症。本品为收敛凉血止血药。可单用或与生地、荷叶等凉血止血药同用；若属虚寒出血，可与艾叶、炮干姜同用。

2. 生发乌发：用于青、中年血热血虚，病后脱发或发色早白，常与何首乌、女贞子、生地等同用。

此外，本品尚能止咳祛痰，用于咳喘痰多之症。其燥湿之功，又可治湿热带下。外用可治脂溢性皮炎，用鲜品60克，加

60%酒精（或白酒）适量，浸泡7天，取药液涂擦。

用量用法　6～10克。煎服。

白　茅　根

为禾本科多年生草本植物白茅 Imperata Cylindrica（L.）Beauv. var. major（Nees）C. E. Hubb.的根茎。切段，生用或鲜用。

处方用名　白茅根、茅根、鲜茅根。

性味归经　甘，寒。入心、肺、胃、膀胱经。

功效应用

1. 凉血止血：用于血热失血，如吐血、衄血、尿血等症，可单用或与生地、黑山栀、藕节等同用。

2. 清热利尿：用于热淋涩痛及水肿，小便不利等症，可单用或与车前子等同用：若与赤小豆煎汤，可用于治黄疸。

3. 清热生津：用于热性病，胃热口渴，呕哕，或肺热咳嗽，咳吐黄痰，本品味甘性寒，能清心、肺、胃之热，故热症而有阴津不足者，用之最宜。可与芦根、石膏等配用；若麻疹初起，疹发不畅，并有高热口渴或有咳嗽者，亦可单用或与芦根及其它透疹药同用。

用量用法　10～30克，鲜用30～60克。煎服。以鲜品为佳。

地　　榆

为蔷薇科多年生草本植物地榆 Sanguisorba officinalis L.的根茎和根。晒干切片，生用或炒炭用。

处方用名　生地榆、地榆炭。

性味归经　苦、酸、涩，微寒。入肝、胃、大肠经。

功效应用

1. 凉血止血：用于吐血，衄血，尿血、崩漏等症，常与茜草根、藕节等同用；若治便血，痔血，血痢等症，常与槐角、生地、芥穗、防风等同用；若治胃及十二指肠溃疡，呕血及便血，可与白及等同用。

2. 消肿止痛：用于烫火烧伤。本品能收敛泻火，为治烫伤之要药。取生地榆研末，麻油调敷，可使渗出液减少，疼痛减轻，愈合加速；亦可用生地榆、生大黄各 30 克，冰片 1.5 克，共研末香油调涂。用于痈肿疮疡，可与银花，蒲公英等同用。

用量用法 10～30 克。煎服。外用适量。治烧伤肿毒可生用，止血可炒炭。

槐 角

为豆科植物落叶乔木槐树 Sophora japonica L.的果实。生用或炒炭用。

处方用名 槐角、槐实、槐角炭。

性味归经 苦、寒。入肝、大肠经。

功效应用

1. 凉血止血：用于便血、痔疮出血、血痢等症。本品善治下部出血，以治肠出血为主。常与地榆、黄芩同用；若用于湿热下注，黄带，漏血，可与生侧柏、生地榆、鱼腥草、银花、甘草等同用。

2. 清肝明目：用于肝热，头昏目赤，常与黄连同用。

用量用法 6～12 克。煎服。清热凉血明目可生用，止血可炒炭。

附药 槐米、槐花：槐之花蕾称槐米，花盛开时采者称槐花。二者味苦性微寒，功能凉血止血，作用较槐角为强，适用于大便下血、痔血，亦治吐衄等症。本品生用能降压，又常用于高血压。用量与槐角同。

苎 麻 根

为荨麻科多年生草本植物苎麻 Boehmeria nivea（L.）Gaud.的根。切片或段生用。

处方用名 苎麻根。

性味归经 甘，寒。入肝、心经。

功效应用

1. 止血安胎：用于妊娠胎动不安或胎漏下血等症。本品为安胎专药，为临床所常用。可与地黄、当归、阿胶等同用。

2. 清热解毒：用于痈疽初起，痔疮肿疼，脱肛不收等症，可用鲜苎麻根皮适量，洗净捣烂外敷，每日换 2 次；捣烂外敷亦可治毒蛇、毒虫咬伤。

3. 利尿：用于淋病尿血，可与滑石、瞿麦、萹蓄等同用。

用量用法 6～12 克。煎服。外用适量。

艾 叶

为菊科多年生草本植物艾 Artemisia argyi Lévl. et Vant.的叶片。生用或炒炭用。

处方用名 生艾叶、艾叶炭、艾绒。

性味归经 辛、苦，温。入肝、脾、肾经。

功效应用

1. 温经止血：用于虚寒性崩漏下血，胎动不安及月经不调等症。常与阿胶、地黄等药配伍；若治血热妄行之吐血、衄血，亦可用生艾叶与生侧柏、生地黄、生荷叶等同用。

2. 散寒除湿：用于妇女宫冷带下，月经不调，腹痛，不孕等症，常与香附、吴茱萸、肉桂等同用。

此外，本品配白鲜皮、地肤子，煎汤外洗，可治湿疹皮肤瘙痒。又可炒热熨少腹，治临产寒甚，胎衣不下。艾叶捣为绒着体表穴位烧灸，能使热气内注筋骨，以治寒痹关节疼痛，故又为温灸的主要药料。

用量用法 3～10 克。煎服。外用适量。散寒湿，理气血宜生用；暖宫止血宜炒炭用。

12 活血化瘀药

凡以通利血脉、促进血行、消散瘀血为主要作用的药物，称为活血化瘀药或称活血祛瘀药。其中活血逐瘀强烈者，又称破血药。

活血化瘀药多偏辛温，辛能散瘀化滞，温可通行血脉，促进血行，故能消瘀肿，解疼痛。适用于气血瘀滞所致之疼痛，跌仆损伤，腹中包块，痈疽肿痛，月经闭止，痛经等症。

形成瘀血证的原因很多，应辨证审因，选择适当的药物，并作适宜的配伍。由于气血关系密切，气行则血行，气滞则血瘀，血凝气亦滞，故活血化瘀药常与理气药配伍应用。

活血化瘀药有促进血行的作用，故月经过多，血虚无瘀滞者，不宜用。此外，通经药物有促进子宫收缩作用，故孕妇尤当禁用，以免引起流产。

川　芎

为伞形科多年生草本植物川芎 Ligusticum chuanxiong Hort. 的根茎。切片生用。

处方用名　川芎、抚芎。

性味归经　辛，温。入肝、胆、心包经。

功效应用

1. 活血行气：用于冠心病心绞痛，可与红花、丹参等活血化瘀药同用；用于气血瘀滞，妇女月经不调，经闭，痛经，难产，胞衣不下等症，常与当归、白芍、地黄等同用；用于损伤瘀肿，气郁胸胁作痛，痈肿疮疡等症，可与桃仁、红花、乳香、没药等同用。

2. 祛风止痛：用于头痛。本品祛风止痛作用颇佳，能上行头巅，为治头痛之良药。对感冒头痛。属风寒者，可与荆芥、白芷、防风等同用；属风热者，可与菊花、薄荷等同用；属风湿者，可与羌活、藁本、防风等同用。治血瘀或血虚头痛，可与活血药或补血药同用。用于风湿痹痛，可与羌活、独活、防风等同用。

用量用法 3～6克。煎服。

使用注意 本品辛温升散，凡阴虚火旺，舌红口干，肝阳头痛，妇女月经过多及出血性疾病，均不宜使用。

丹　参

为唇形科多年生草本植物丹参 Salvia miltiorrhiza Bge.的根。切片生用。

处方用名 丹参、紫丹参、血丹参。

性味归经 苦，微寒。入心、肝经。

功效应用

1. 活血祛瘀：用于血热瘀滞，月经不调，痛经，经闭，腹中包块以及产后恶露不尽等症。可单用，研末，黄酒送服，每次6克，日3次。或与其它活血、养血药同用；用于冠心病心绞痛，可与川芎、红花等同用；用于肝郁胁痛，可与大青叶、蒲公英、鳖甲、牡蛎、赤芍、青皮等随症配用；用于血瘀气滞的胃痛，可与檀香等同用。

2. 除烦安神：用于热病伤营，心烦不寐之症，常与生地、元参、竹叶等药同用；若神经衰弱，症见长期失眠、头痛、头晕、精神不振等，可用丹参50克（研粗末）泡入95%酒精500ml中，再加开水500ml，浸泡1～2天，搅匀过滤，每晚睡前服10ml。严重者，可早晚各服1次。

3. 消肿止痛：用于痈疮肿痛，常与银花、连翘、乳香、没药等活血解毒药同用；用于热痹关节肌肉肿痛，可单味30～60

克，水煎服。

现代常用于慢性肝炎、早期肝硬变有肝脾肿大者。还用于治疗血栓闭塞性脉管炎较轻者和宫外孕等。

用量用法 10～15 克，治脉管炎，热痹等可大量用 30～60 克。煎服。如有出血倾向者不宜用大量。

桃 仁

为蔷薇科落叶小乔木桃 Prunus persica (L.) Batsch.的成熟种仁。取种仁晒干，水煮去皮，捣碎用。

处方用名 桃仁、桃仁泥。

性味归经 苦、甘，平。入心、肝、大肠经。

功效应用

1. 破瘀行血：用于血瘀经闭，痛经，腹中包块等症，常与红花、川芎、当归、熟地、白芍等同用；用于跌打损伤，瘀血肿痛等症，常与红花、山甲珠、酒大黄等活血消肿药同用；用于肺痈，肠痈等症。治肺痈，常与苇茎、冬瓜子、薏苡仁等同用；治肠痈，常与大黄、丹皮等同用。

2. 润肠通便：用于肠燥便秘，常与杏仁、火麻仁等同用。

此外，尚可治上气喘咳，与杏仁同用。现代临床常用于肺脓疡、急性阑尾炎等。

用量用法 6～10 克。煎服。

使用注意 血枯经闭及孕妇均忌用。

红 花

为菊科 1 年生草本植物红花 Carthamus tinctorius L. 的筒状花冠。生用。

处方用名 红花、南红花、草红花。

性味归经 辛、温。入心、肝经。

功效应用

1. 活血通经：用于血瘀经闭，痛经，腹中包块等症，常与桃仁、当归、川芎等同用。

2. 祛瘀止痛：用于冠心病心绞痛，可与川芎、丹参等同用；用于瘀血胁痛，痈肿及吐血而有瘀滞者，可与桃仁、乳香、没药等同用；用于跌打损伤，挫伤，扭伤的皮下瘀血，青紫肿痛，可配酒精（红花酒）外擦；用于血栓闭塞性脉管炎，患肢足部呈暗红或青紫色，属于气滞血瘀型者，常与当归、桃仁、赤芍、乳香、没药等同用。

用量用法　3～10克，稍大量用10～15克。煎服。

使用注意　孕妇忌用，月经过多，有出血倾向者亦不宜用。

附药　藏红花：又称西红花或番红花。为鸢尾科多年生草本植物番红花 Crocus sativus L.的干燥花柱头。性味甘寒。入心、肝经。功能活血祛瘀，效用与红花相同，而药力较胜。惟兼有清血解毒之功，故尚可用于温病热入营分，发斑发疹大热之症。用量1～3克。煎服。

益 母 草

为唇形科1年或2年生草本植物益母草 Leonurus heterophyllus Sweet 的全草。生用或熬膏用。

处方用名　益母草、坤草。

性味归经　辛、微苦，微寒。入肝、心、肾经。

功效应用

1. 活血行瘀：用于血脉瘀滞，月经不调，痛经，产后血滞腹痛，恶露不尽及崩漏下血等症，单用本品砂糖熬膏服；或与当归、赤芍等同用。

2. 利尿退肿：用于水肿，小便不利，可单用或与白茅根、云苓、桑皮等同用。

3. 清热解毒：可配用于肿毒疮疡，皮肤痒疹等。

现代尚用于急慢性肾炎水肿，高血压和冠心病。

用量用法 12～30克。煎服。治肾炎入煎剂，干品可用60～120克，鲜品120～240克。

附药 茺蔚子：即益母草的种子。生用。味甘，微寒。功能活血化瘀，凉肝明目。多用于肝热目赤肿痛，血灌瞳子，或生云翳等症，常与青葙子、决明子等同用。用量3～10克。如肝血不足，瞳子散大者忌用。

泽 兰

为唇形科多年生草本植物地瓜儿苗 Lycopus lucidus Turcz. 或毛叶地瓜儿苗 Lycopus lucidus Turcz. var. hirtus Regel 的茎叶。亦有单用叶者。生用。

处方用名 泽兰、泽兰叶。

性味归经 苦、辛、微温。入肝、脾、肾经。

功效应用

1. 活血祛瘀：用于血瘀经闭，痛经，月经不调，腹中包块，产后血滞腹痛等症，可与当归、芍药、甘草等同用；用于损伤瘀肿，可用鲜者捣烂外敷。

2. 行水消肿：用于妇女产后小便淋漓腹痛，身面浮肿，肝硬化腹水等症，可与利水消肿药同用。

用量用法 6～12克。煎服。

三 棱

为黑三棱科多年生草本植物黑三棱（荆三棱）Sparganium stoloniferum Buch-Ham.的块茎。醋炒或麸炒用。

处方用名 三棱、荆三棱、醋三棱。

性味归经 苦，平。入肝、脾经。

功效应用

1. 破血行气：用于血瘀经闭，腹中包块，产后瘀滞腹痛等症，常与莪术、川芎等同用；用于肝脾肿大，常与莪术、青皮、麦芽等同用。

2. 消积止痛：用于食积腹痛，常与莪术、青皮、麦芽等同用。

用量用法 3～10克。煎服。醋炒能增强止痛消瘀之效。

使用注意 月经过多与孕妇均忌用。

莪　术

为姜科多年生草本植物莪术（温郁金）Curcuma wenchowensis Y.H. chen et C. Ling.的根茎。蒸熟切片，醋炒用。

处方用名 莪术、蓬莪术、醋莪术。

性味归经 苦、辛，温。入肝、脾经。

功效应用

1. 行气破血：用于血瘀经闭，腹中包块等症，常与三棱、川芎等同用；用于肝脾肿大，常与三棱、红花、赤芍、香附等同用；用于跌打肿痛，可用鲜根茎捣烂加酒炒热外敷。

2. 消积止痛：用于饮食积滞，胸腹痞胀作痛，呕吐酸水等症，常与三棱、青皮、谷芽等同用。

此外，现临床尚用治癌肿。用莪术注射治疗子宫颈癌，每日在病灶局部注入药液10～30毫升，疗程3个月左右，亦可配合口服水煎剂，用醋莪术、醋三棱各10克，水3碗煎成1碗，早饭前及晚饭后各服半碗。也可用莪术挥发油软膏外用局部敷治。上述治疗方法对外阴癌和皮肤癌也有一定疗效。

用量用法 3～10克。煎服。

使用注意 月经过多及孕妇忌用。

郁　金

为姜科多年生宿根草本植物郁金（毛姜黄）Curcuma aromatica salisb.和莪术 C. zedoaria（Berg）Rosc.或姜黄 C.

longa L.或广西莪术 C. kwangsiensis S. Lee et C. F. Liang.的块根。煮透晒干，切片用。

处方用名 郁金、玉金、广郁金、黄郁金、川郁金、黑郁金。

性味归经 辛、苦，寒。入心、肺、肝、胆经。

功效应用

1. 行气祛瘀：用于气血郁滞，胸胁脘腹胀闷作痛，痛经等症，可与柴胡、香附、当归、白芍等同用。

2. 清心解郁：用于湿温病，痰浊蒙蔽清窍，神志不清，常与菖蒲、山栀、滑石等同用；用于痰热蒙蔽清窍之癫痫、狂症，常与白矾同用，或与香附、蜈蚣等同用。

3. 凉血止血：用于血热瘀滞之吐血，衄血，尿血及妇女倒经等症，可与生地、丹皮、山栀等凉血止血药同用。

此外，本品又可用于胆石症，黄疸。因其尚有利胆作用，常与金钱草、茵陈、山栀等药配用。慢性肝炎、肝硬变所致的肝区痛、肾结核尿血，"乙脑"、"流脑"症见神昏，精神分裂症的躁狂状态等也为临床所常用。

用量用法 3～10 克。煎服。

使用注意 畏丁香。

色 姜 黄

为姜科多年生宿根草本植物姜黄 Curcuma longa L.的根茎。又称姜黄、硬姜黄、子姜黄。擦去外皮，切薄片或捣碎用。

处方用名 色姜黄、姜黄。

性味归经 辛、苦，寒。入肝、胆、脾、胃经。

功效应用

1. 凉血止血：用于血热月经先期，可与黄芩、延胡索、熟地等同用。

2. 破瘀消肿，行气止痛：用于跌打损伤，瘀血肿痛，可与桃仁、苏木、乳香等同用；用于气滞血瘀之胸胁脘腹诸痛，常与当归、白芍、川芎、莪术等同用；用于风热壅闭，咽喉肿痛，常与僵蚕、蝉蜕、大黄等同用；用于疮疡肿毒，又常与花粉、黄柏、大黄等制散外用。

用量用法 3～10 克。煎服。外用适量。

延 胡 索

为罂粟科多年生草本植物延胡索 Corydalis yanhusuo W. T. Wang 的小圆球形块茎。醋炒捣碎用，或研粉用。

处方用名 延胡索、玄胡、元胡、醋元胡。

性味归经 辛、苦，温。入肝、脾、心经。

功效应用 活血散瘀，利气止痛：用于气血瘀滞，脘腹胁痛，常与川楝子同用；用于瘀血痛经，腹中包块，产后血滞腹痛等症，常与当归、白芍、三棱、莪术等同用；用于疝气疼痛，常与川楝子、小茴香等同用；用于气血凝滞，遍体作痛，跌打肿痛等症，可与当归、桂枝等同用。

近年，常以本品配活血行气药，治冠心病心绞痛，亦用于心律失常等。

用量用法 3～10 克。煎服。宜研末吞服，每次 1.5～3 克，温水或随汤剂送服。醋炒则功效更强。

五 灵 脂

为哺乳脊椎动物鼯鼠科滑翔兽类橙足鼯鼠（寒号鸟）Trogopterus xanthipes Milne—Edwards 的粪便。晒干，醋炒或炒炭用。

处方用名 五灵脂、醋灵脂、灵脂炭。

性味归经 甘，温。入肝经。

功效应用

1. 通利血脉，散瘀止痛：用于气血瘀滞之心腹胁肋诸痛及瘕痛，经闭，痛经，产后瘀阻，儿枕痛等症。本品止痛之功甚强，与乳没相仿，凡一切血瘀气滞作痛之症，都有良效。可单用为末酒服，又常与蒲黄同用。

2. 祛瘀止血：用于妇女崩漏，可与生地、熟地、阿胶、丹参等同用。

此外，现临床用治冠心病心绞痛及胃与十二指肠溃疡病出血疼痛等症。

用量用法　3～10克。煎服。活血宜醋炒用，止血宜炒炭用。

使用注意　孕妇慎用。

乳　香

为橄榄科矮小灌木卡氏乳香树 Boswellia carterii Birdw.皮部采得的胶状树脂。入药多炒用。

处方用名　制乳香、明乳香。

性味归经　辛、苦，温。入心、肝、脾经。

功效应用

1. 活血止痛：用于跌打损伤，瘀血肿痛或筋脉拘挛，常与没药、血竭、红花等同用；用于心血瘀阻之心绞痛及血滞胃痛、腹痛、痛经，产后腹痛等症。本品止痛力强，凡内、妇、外、伤诸科见有瘀滞疼痛之症者，用之其效颇佳。尤为外、伤二科常用要药。常与没药等活血祛瘀药同用。

2. 消肿生肌：用于痈疽肿痛或溃久不敛，可内服，常与没药、雄黄、麝香等同用；亦可外用，与没药共研细末，掺疮面后，以膏贴之。

3. 伸筋活络：用于痹症之筋脉拘挛，常与羌活、当归等祛风胜湿药同用。

用量用法　3～10克。煎服。外用适量。

使用注意　本品味苦，入煎剂汤液混浊，故用量不宜过多。

胃弱者服后易呕吐，尤应慎用。无瘀滞者及孕妇不宜用。

附药 没药：为橄榄科乔木植物没药树 Commiphora myrrha Engl.或其他同属植物的茎干皮部渗出的油胶树脂。加工方法同乳香。性味苦平。归经功效同乳香。前人实践经验，认为乳香功擅活血伸筋，没药偏于散血化瘀。用治痹症的方剂中，选用乳香而不用没药。气血凝滞疼痛之症，二者相伍应用，取效尤捷。

本品消肿生肌之功，外用，每与乳香配伍。

用量 3～10 克。煎服。外用适量。使用注意同乳香。

苏 木

为豆科落叶灌木或小乔木苏木 Caesalpinla sappan L.的心材。刨成薄片，或砍成小块。

处方用名 苏木、苏方木。

性味归经 甘、咸、辛，平。入心、肝、脾经。

功效应用 活血祛瘀，消肿止痛：用于跌打损伤，瘀肿疼痛，常与乳香、没药、血竭、红花等同用；用于妇女血滞经闭腹痛，产后瘀阻等症，常与赤芍、归尾、桃仁、红花、川芎等同用。

用量用法 3～10 克。煎服。外用适量。

使用注意 孕妇忌用。

降 真 香

为豆科植物乔木降香檀 Dalbergia odorifera T. Chen 的根部心材。用时镑片或刨片。

处方用名 降香、降真香、紫降香。

性味归经 辛，温。入心、肝经。

功效应用 行瘀止血定痛：用于跌打损伤，瘀肿作痛，或体内、外出血等症，可单用研末外敷，或与乳香、没药、三七等活血理气药同用；用于冠心病心绞痛，常与川芎、红花、赤芍等同用。

此外，本品与藿香、木香等配伍，可用于秽浊内阻，呕吐腹痛。

用量用法 3～6 克，治冠心病心绞痛可用至 12 克。煎服。

使用注意 凡阴虚火盛，血热妄行而无瘀滞者不宜用。

牛 膝

为苋科多年生草本植物怀牛膝 Achyranthes bidentata Blume 和川牛膝（甜牛膝）C. officinalis Kuan 的根。切小段生用。

处方用名 牛膝、怀牛膝、川牛膝。

性味归经 苦、酸，平。入肝、肾经。

功效应用

1. 活血通经：用于妇女血滞经闭、痛经、月经后期、腹中肿块及难产等症，常与当归、桃仁、赤芍、丹皮等同用；若与冬葵子配用可治胞衣不下。

2. 舒筋利痹：用于腰膝关节酸痛，下肢风湿痹痛。症偏湿热者，常与苍术、黄柏同用；症偏于寒者，常与独活、木瓜等同用；属肾虚者，常与杜仲、川断等同用。

3. 引血下行：用于阴虚火亢之齿龈肿痛、吐血、咯血、衄血等症，常与熟地、麦冬、石膏、知母等滋阴泻火药同用；用于高血压、属于肝阳上亢者，及脑血管痉挛之头痛，可与代赭石、龙骨、牡蛎、玄参等同用。

4. 利尿通淋：用于热淋茎痛，尿血，常与瞿麦、滑石、通草等同用。

用量用法 6～12 克。大剂可用至 30 克。煎服。本品有川、怀之分。活血通经，舒筋利痹，消肿止痛，宜用川牛膝；补益肝肾，强壮筋骨，宜用怀牛膝。

穿山甲

为脊椎动物鲮鲤科食蚁兽鲮鲤 Manis pentadactyla L.的鳞甲。用时以沙烫至松泡呈黄色时，筛去沙子。称炮甲珠。

处方用名 穿山甲、炙山甲、炮甲片、山甲珠。

性味归经 咸，微寒。入肝、胃经。

功效应用

1. 消肿排脓：用于痈肿初起，或脓成不溃等症。本品性善走窜，可透达经络直达病所，治痈肿未成可消，已成可溃，尤以脓成将溃之际最为适宜。常与皂角刺、银花、乳香、没药等同用。

2. 通经下乳：由于乳汁不通，可单用为末，每次6克，日2次，黄酒送服，或与王不留行、瞿麦等同用；用于瘀血经闭，可与当归、赤芍、红花、大黄等破血通经药同用。

此外，还常用治风湿痹痛，肢体拘挛，常与当归、川芎、羌活、防风等同用。

用量用法 3～10克。煎服。亦可研末吞服，每次1～1.5克，研末吞服效果较好。

使用注意 孕妇忌用。

皂角刺

为豆科落叶乔木皂荚树 Gleditsia sinensis Lam.茎枝上的棘刺。切片生用。

处方用名 皂角刺、皂刺、皂针。

性味归经 辛、温。入肝、胃经。

功效应用

1. 消肿排脓：用于痈疽疮肿，乳痈，瘰疬痰核等症，常与山甲、银花、生甘草等同用。

2. 治风杀虫：用于麻风，皮癣等症。若治麻风，可与大枫子油、大黄等同用；治皮癣，以本品与醋浓煎，外涂。

用量用法 3～10克。煎服。外用适量。

鸡 血 藤

为豆科植物攀援灌木密花豆（三叶鸡血藤）Spatholobus suberectus Dunn 和香花崖豆藤（山鸡血藤）Millettia dielsiana Harms 等的藤茎。切片生用，或熬制鸡血藤胶用。

处方用名 鸡血藤。

性味归经 苦、微甘，温。入肝、肾经。

功效应用 行血补血，舒筋活络：用于风湿痹痛，腰膝酸痛，筋骨麻木，多与桑椹子、白术、当归、川牛膝、防已、海风藤等补气养血、祛风湿药同用；用于血虚月经不调，经闭腹痛等症，常与当归、川芎、白芍、地黄等同用。

用量用法 10～15克，大量可用至60克。煎服。亦可浸酒服。鸡血藤胶用6～10克。服汤药时，可溶化调匀后温服，或用温开水溶化后服。

王 不 留 行

为石竹科1年生或2年生草本植物麦蓝菜 Vaccaria segetalis (Neck.) Garcke 的成熟种了。生用。

处方用名 王不留行、王不留。

性味归经 甘、苦，平。入肝、肾经。

功效应用

1. 通乳消肿：用于乳汁不通，常与穿山甲、瞿麦等同用；2. 用于乳痈初起，尚未化脓者，可与公英、白芷同用。

2. 活血通经：用于瘀血经闭不通，可与当归、川芎、桃仁、红花等同用。

此外，尚可治睾丸炎。如流行性腮腺炎合并睾丸炎时可与川楝子、板蓝根、黄芩、生地、丹皮等同用。

用量用法 6～10克。煎服。

使用注意 孕妇慎用。

自 然 铜

为天然矿石类等轴晶系铁矿 Pyrite 的硫化铁矿石。以火煅透，醋淬，复煅复淬，反复2、3次，置地下退火毒，研末水飞。

处方用名 自然铜、煅自然铜。

性味归经 辛，平。入肝经。

功效应用 散瘀止痛，接骨续筋：用于跌打损伤，筋断骨折，瘀肿疼痛。本品行血散瘀，能接骨续筋，以疗折伤，为伤科接骨之要药。可与乳香、没药、当归、羌活等同用；用于闪腰岔气，腰痛，可用煅自然铜、土鳖虫各30克，共研末，每次2克，温水送服，日2次。

用量用法 1～3克。入丸散剂，不宜入煎。

水 蛭

为环节动物水蛭科宽体金钱蛭（蚂蟥）Whitmania pigra (Whitman)、茶色蛭（柳叶蚂蟥）Whitmania acranulata (Whitman) 和水蛭 Hirudo nipponica Whitman 等的干燥全体。切段，滑石烫炙用。

处方用名 水蛭。

性味归经 咸、苦，平，有小毒。入肝经。

功效应用 破血逐瘀：用于血滞经闭，腹中肿块，蓄血等症，常与虻虫、桃仁、大黄等同用；用于跌打损伤，瘀肿作痛，心腹胀痛，大便不通，常与大黄、牵牛共研细末，温酒调服。

此外，本品与活血祛瘀药同用，可治血小板增多症，短期煎服，有一定疗效。

用量用法 3～6克。煎服。入丸散剂每次1～1.5克。

使用注意 孕妇忌服。

虻 虫

为昆虫类虻科复带虻 Tabanus bivittatus Mats.的雌虫体。生用或炒用。

处方用名 虻虫。

性味归经 苦，微寒，有小毒。入肝经。

功效应用 破血逐瘀：用于血滞经闭，腹中肿块蓄血，常与水蛭、桃仁、大黄同用；用于跌打损伤，瘀肿作痛等症，可与丹皮为末酒服。

用量用法 1.5～3 克。煎服。焙干，制散剂，每次服 0.3～0.6 克。

使用注意 孕妇忌服。

䗪 虫

为鳖蠊科昆虫土鳖虫 Eupolyphaga sinensis Walker 雌成虫的干燥全体。

处方用名 䗪虫、地鳖虫、土元。

性味归经 咸，寒，有小毒。入肝经。

功效应用

1. 破血逐瘀：用于血滞经闭，月经不调及产后瘀阻，常与大黄、桃仁等破血逐瘀药同用；用于宫外孕之急性腹痛，腹部包块不消者，可与炮山甲、桃仁泥、海藻、全当归、元胡、没药、生牡蛎等同用；用于慢性肝炎之肝肿大或早期肝硬变，肝区闷痛者，可与党参、紫河车、姜黄、广郁金、参三七、鸡内金等共研细末，饭前服；用于木舌强肿，土鳖虫 5 个，食盐 15 克，煎汤热含，吐涎，瘥则止；用于肿舌塞口，用活地鳖和鲜薄荷捣汁，纱布吸收，贴舌下肿处。

2. 续筋接骨：用于跌打筋骨折伤，可用䗪虫 20 个，自然铜

(醋淬)、龙骨、乳香，没药各 6 克，麝香 0.3 克。共研细末，每服 1.5 克，日 3 次，黄酒送下。

用量用法 5～10 克。煎服。入丸散剂，每次 1～2 克。

使用注意 孕妇忌服。

13 止咳平喘化痰药

凡以止咳平喘为主要作用的药物，叫止咳平喘药，以化痰祛痰为主要作用的药物，叫化痰药。由于止咳平喘药大多能用来化痰，而化痰药又多兼有止咳作用，故统称为止咳平喘化痰药。

咳嗽与痰，在病机上有密切的关系。一般咳嗽每多挟痰，而痰多亦每致咳嗽，因而治疗上应用止咳平喘药时，常与化痰药配伍。化痰药也常与止咳平喘药配伍应用。止咳平喘药主要用于咳嗽，哮喘及久咳劳嗽等病症。化痰药主要用于痰多咳嗽，或痰饮气喘，咳痰困难，以及由痰所引起的癫痫惊厥，瘰疬流注等病症。

凡内伤外感的病症，均能引起痰多与咳嗽，因而治疗时除应针对病情，选用适宜的止咳平喘化痰药外，还应根据各种致病原因，综合观察其表里、虚实、寒热而作必要的配伍，方能增强疗效。如外感咳嗽，当配解表药；虚劳咳嗽，需配补养药；热痰燥痰宜清宜润；寒痰湿痰可温可燥。倘外感而用收敛，虚劳过于耗散，热痰燥痰再用温燥，寒痰湿痰而予清润等，则均可引起不良后果。

咳嗽而有咳血的，不宜用强烈的化痰药，否则有促进出血之可能。

根据止咳化痰药的主要性能，又把它分为止咳平喘药，清化热痰药，温化寒痰药3类。

13.1 止咳平喘药

本类药物止咳或平喘是其主要功效，分别具有宣肺祛痰、润肺止咳、下气平喘等作用，适用于肺气不利的咳嗽喘息等症。

咳喘的症状多端，有干咳者，有咳吐稀痰或稠痰者，有外感咳逆者，有虚劳咳喘者，寒热虚实各异，必须辨证施治，选用适宜的配伍，不可单用止咳平喘药。

麻疹初期，或外感病而有发斑疹趋势的，虽有咳嗽症状，但不宜应用温性而带有收涩作用的止咳药，以免影响斑疹透发，变成逆证。

杏　仁

为蔷薇科落叶小乔木杏树 Prunus armeniaca L.的成熟种子的核仁。晒干生用或炒用，捣碎入药。

处方用名　苦杏仁、杏仁泥。

性味归经　苦、辛，温，有小毒。入肺、大肠经。

功效应用

1. 止咳平喘：用于风寒感冒，咳嗽气喘，可与苏叶、半夏、茯苓等同用；用于风热咳嗽，常与桑叶、菊花、桔梗等同用；用于肺燥咳嗽，常与沙参、川贝母、桑叶等同用；用于久嗽，咳逆气喘，可与桑皮、紫菀、五味子等同用。

2. 润肠通便：用于老人或产后大便燥结，常与火麻仁、桃仁等同用。

用量用法　6～10 克。煎服。

附药　甜杏仁：又名巴旦杏仁，为同属植物巴旦杏 Prunus amygdalus Batsch 的种仁。性味甘平，无毒。功能滋润养肺，下气止嗽。专治虚劳久咳，胸闷不畅，大便秘结等症。用量同苦杏仁。

百　部

为百部科多年生草本植物蔓生百部 Stemona japonica (BL.) Miq.直立百部 Stemona sessilifolia (Miq.) Franch. et Sav.或对叶百部 Stemona tuberosa Lour.等的地下块根。切段入

药，生用或蜜炙用。

处方用名 百部、炙百部。

性味归经 甘、苦，微温。入肺经。

功效应用

1. 润肺止咳：用于外感咳嗽或感冒后遗之咳嗽。本品温而不燥，可治新久咳嗽，尤以久咳为良。常与紫菀、桔梗、荆芥等同用；若用于肺虚久咳，可与沙参、黄芪、百合等同用；若治肺痨（肺结核空洞）咳嗽痰血，可与白及、贝母、三七等同用。近有百部糖浆制剂，可治小儿顿咳。

2. 灭虱杀虫：单用本品酒浸液外擦，可治头虱、体虱、阴虱、衣虱（对虱卵无效；喷烟可灭臭虫）。内服可用于蛲虫病，亦可单用本品水煎液灌肛用。

用量用法 6～10克。煎服。外用适量。

紫　菀

为菊科多年生草本植物紫菀 Aster tataricus L. f.的根茎及根。生用或蜜炙用。

处方用名 紫菀、炙紫菀。

性味归经 辛、苦，微温。入肺经。

功效应用 润肺下气，化痰止咳：本品质润而不燥，为化痰止嗽要药，不论肺寒肺热皆可应用。用于肺结核阴虚劳热，痰中带血，可与知母、川贝、阿胶等同用；若用于久嗽，可与款冬花、百部等同用；若用于肺气衰弱，寒咳喘息而无热者，可与党参、黄芪、干姜同用；若用于外感风寒，痰多咳嗽，可与荆芥、白前、陈皮等同用。

用量用法 6～10克。煎服。外感咳嗽宜生用，久咳虚嗽宜炙用。

款 冬 花

为菊科多年生草本植物款冬 Tussilago farfara L.的花蕾。生用或蜜炙用。

处方用名 款冬花、炙款冬。

性味归经 辛、甘，温。入肺经。

功效应用 润肺止咳，消痰下气：本品为润肺化痰止嗽之良药。凡咳嗽，不论外感内伤，寒热虚实，皆可用之。用于痰嗽哮喘，遇冷即发，可与麻黄、杏仁、紫苏子等同用；若用于咳嗽带血，可与百合研末蜜丸用；若用于暴咳，可与杏仁、贝母、五味子等同用。

用量用法 6～10 克。煎服。外感咳嗽宜生用，久咳虚嗽宜炙用。

桑 白 皮

为桑科植物落叶乔木桑树 Morus alba L.除去栓皮的根皮。切条生用或炙用。

处方用名 生桑皮、炙桑皮。

性味归经 甘，寒。入肺经。

功效应用

1. 泻肺平喘：用于肺热咳嗽喘促。本品功专泻肺火以平喘。可与地骨皮、粳米、甘草等同用。

2. 行水消肿：用于浮肿，小便不利之水肿实症，常与大腹皮、茯苓皮、生姜皮等同用。

此外，本品尚可用治高血压病，因其具有一定的降压作用。

用量用法 6～12 克。煎服。行水宜生用，平喘止嗽宜炙用。

使用注意 肺寒咳嗽及风寒咳嗽均不宜用。

枇 杷 叶

为蔷薇科常绿小乔木枇杷树 Eriobotrya japonica（Thunb.）Lindl.的叶片。刷去毛，洗净切条，生用或蜜炙用。

处方用名 生杷叶、炙杷叶。

性味归经 苦，平。入肺、胃经。

功效应用

1. 化痰止咳：用于肺热咳喘，口苦咽燥等症。本品苦平偏凉而性善降，能清肃肺气以化痰止咳。可与沙参、桑皮、栀子等同用；若治顿咳（百日咳），可与百部、大蒜头等同用。

2. 降逆止呕：用于胃气上逆，恶心呕哕，可与半夏、茯苓等同用；若用于胃热呕吐，可与竹茹、橘皮、生姜同用。

用量用法 6～12克。煎服。止咳宜炙用，止呕宜生用。

马 兜 铃

为马兜铃科多年生蔓草缠绕或葡匐状细弱草本植物马兜铃 Aristolochia debilis Sieb. et Zucc.或北马兜铃 Aristolochia contorta Bge.的果实。生用或蜜炙用。

处方用名 马兜铃、炙兜铃。

性味归经 苦、微辛，寒。入肺、大肠经。

功效应用 清肺降气，止咳平喘：用于肺虚火盛，咳嗽气喘，可与阿胶、杏仁、糯米等同用；若用于麻疹末期，余热未清，干咳声喑，可与浙贝、牛蒡子、麦冬等同用。

此外，还用于痔疮下血，肛门周围肿胀疼痛，可煎汤熏洗。本品有缓慢而持久的降压作用，用于高血压病肝阳上亢，头晕面赤者较为适宜。可与夏枯草、钩藤、黄芩等同用。

用量用法 3～10克。煎服。外用适量。止咳炙用，外洗生用。

使用注意 虚寒喘咳及感冒咳嗽均忌用。本品尚有涌吐之弊，孕妇恶阻期及胃气虚弱者，虽有肺热痰咳之症，即用少量，每易引起呕哕，因而不宜服用。

葶苈子

为十字花科1年生或2年生草本植物独行菜（北葶苈子）Lepidium apetalum Willd.或播娘蒿（南葶苈子）Descurainia sophia（L.）Webb.的成熟种子。生用或微炒打碎用。

处方用名 葶苈子、苦葶苈、甜葶苈。

性味归经 辛、苦，寒。入肺、膀胱、大肠经。

功效应用

1. 泻肺平喘：用于痰饮壅滞，胸满胀喘不得卧，一身面目浮肿，可与大枣水煎服；近年用于渗出性胸膜炎及胸腔积液有效。

2. 下气行水：本品能泻肺气之闭塞，以利尿消肿。用于水饮停留肠间引起的腹满，口舌干燥之症，可与防己、椒目等配丸用；用于胸胁积水，大便燥结，小便短少，可与杏仁、大黄等蜜丸用。

用量用法 3～10克。煎服。

使用注意 肺虚喘咳，脾虚肿满者忌用。

紫苏子

为唇形科1年生草本植物紫苏 Perilla frutescens（L.）Britt. var. crispa（Thunb.）Hand-Mazz.的种子。微炒捣碎用。

处方用名 苏子、紫苏子、炒苏子。

性味归经 辛、温。入肺、大肠经。

功效应用 下气消痰，止咳平喘：用于痰涎壅盛，胸闷气逆，咳嗽喘息，常与前胡、厚朴、半夏、陈皮等同用；亦常与白芥子、莱菔子同用。

此外，尚有润肠之功，用于肠燥便秘，常与麻子仁、杏仁、枳壳等润肠降气之品同用。

用量用法 6～10 克。煎服。

使用注意 脾虚便滑者忌服。

白 果

为银杏科落叶乔木银杏树 Ginkgo biloba L.的成熟种子。捣碎生用或煨熟用。

处方用名 白果仁、白果肉、炒白果。

性味归经 甘、苦、涩，平，有小毒。入肺经。

功效应用

1. 敛肺定喘：用于痰热内蕴，痰多气急，咳嗽哮喘，常与麻黄、杏仁、黄芩等同用。

2. 止带除浊：用于妇女湿热带下，色黄稠腻者，常与黄柏、山药等同用；用于慢性淋浊而尿无涩痛者，炒白果仁、炒山药等分为细末，每次 10 克，日服 3 次。

此外，尚有缩尿作用，若小便频数，可煨熟嚼食。

用量用法 6～10 克，或 5～10 枚。煎服。入煎剂可生用，制散剂或嚼食宜煨熟用。

使用注意 生食有毒，过食亦可中毒，不可过量。感冒咳嗽应忌用。

洋 金 花

为茄科 1 年生草本植物白蔓陀罗 Datura metel L.或毛蔓陀罗 Datura innoxia Mill.的花。晒干生用。

处方用名 洋金花。

性味归经 辛，温。有大毒。入肺经。

功效应用

1. 止哮喘：用于哮喘咳嗽无痰或痰少等，可作散剂单用，或制成卷烟（掺入等量烟叶）燃吸。

2. 止痛：用于胃痛、腹痛，可单用 0.3 克，水煎服；用于风寒湿痹，关节疼痛，可单用 10 克，煎汤外洗。

3. 解痉：用于癫痫及慢惊风之痉挛抽搐，可与天麻、全蝎等同用。

现代有关中药麻醉的研究，亦多以本品为主，与川乌、草乌、防己等制成注射剂用。

用量用法 内服 0.3 克，煎服。吸烟 0.6～1 克。外洗适量。

使用注意 外感及热痰咳嗽，青光眼，高血压患者忌用。本品有剧毒。应控制剂量，以免中毒。

13.2 清化热痰药

本类药物多属寒性，具有清化热痰作用，适用于咳嗽，痰液浓稠、黄臭、咯痰不利，及癫痫惊厥，瘰疬流注等症，常与清热药配伍同用。

除礞石的作用较强烈外，一般作用多属缓和。凡属寒痰及脾胃虚弱者，不宜使用。

桔　梗

为桔梗科多年生草本植物 Platycodon grandiflorum (Jacg.) A. DC.的根。切片生用。

处方用名 桔梗、苦桔梗、白桔梗。

性味归经 苦、辛，平。入肺经。

功效应用

1. 宣肺祛痰：本品既升且降，善于开提肺气，宣胸快膈，并有较好的祛痰作用。治咳嗽痰多，不论肺寒、肺热，皆可配用。用于肺热咳嗽，痰稠难咯，可与桑叶、杏仁、杷叶、薄荷、甘草等同用；若用于风寒咳嗽，痰稀色白，鼻塞流涕等症，可与苏叶、杏仁、半夏、陈皮、白前、甘草等同用；用于肺气不宣，咽喉肿痛，可与甘草同用，亦可加锦灯笼、忍冬藤等同用。

2. 排脓消痈：用于肺痈，可与鱼腥草、生薏仁、冬瓜仁等同用。

用量用法 6~10克。煎服。

前 胡

为伞形科多年生草本植物白花前胡 Peucedanum praeruptorum Dunn.或紫花前胡 Peucedanum decursivum (Mig.) Maxim.的根。生用。

处方用名 前胡、嫩前胡。

性味归经 苦、辛，微寒。入肺经。

功效应用 降气消痰：用于肺热咳嗽，痰黄稠粘，胸部满闷不舒等症，可与杏仁、桑皮等同用；若用于肺气壅实，咳逆短气，或呕吐不食，可与半夏、陈皮、苏子等同用。

用量用法 6~10克。煎服。

川 贝 母

为百合科多年生草本植物乌花贝母 Fritillaria cirl-hosa D. Don. var. ecirrhosa Franch.和卷叶贝母 F. cirrhosa D. Don.或棱砂贝母 F. delavayi Franch.或罗氏贝母 F. roylei Hook.或甘肃贝母 F. przewalskii Maxim.的地下扁圆锥球形鳞茎。捣碎入药。

处方用名 川贝母、川贝。

性味归经 苦、甘，微寒。入心、肺经。

功效应用

1. 润肺化痰：用于阴虚肺热，咳嗽痰少，贝母、知母各等分，蜜丸用；若用于肺燥咳嗽，吐痰稠粘，常与紫菀、款冬等同用。

2. 泄热散结：用于瘰疬痰核，常与玄参、牡蛎同用；用于乳痈初起肿痛，常与蒲公英、连翘、天花粉等同用。

用量用法　3～10克。煎服。

使用注意　不宜与乌头同用。

附药　浙贝母：又名象贝、大贝。为百合科多年生草本植物浙贝母 F. thunbergii Mig.的地下鳞茎。切厚片入药。味苦性寒，功能宣肺化痰止咳，清热散结。因其开泄力胜，大多用于外感风邪、痰热郁肺所引起的咳嗽，以及疮痈肿毒，瘰疬痰核等症。用量6～12克，煎服。不宜与乌头同用。

栝　楼

为葫芦科多年生宿根草质藤本攀援性植物栝楼 Trichosanthes kirilowii Maxim.的果实。整个栝楼入药者，名全栝楼；如分开入药，果壳称栝楼壳或栝楼皮；种子又名栝楼仁，炒打碎用；压去油者，名楼仁霜。

处方用名　全栝楼、瓜蒌、瓜蒌皮、瓜蒌仁、蒌仁霜。

性味归经　甘，寒。入肺、胃、大肠经。

功效应用

1. 清热化痰：用于肺气壅遏，痰热咳嗽之症，常以瓜蒌皮与贝母、杏仁、桔梗等宣肺化痰药同用；若用于停饮积痰，胸闷气急，可与半夏、枳实等同用；如小儿喘急，可单用全瓜蒌15克，水煎服。

2. 宽胸散结：用于胸痹胸痛，常与薤白等同用；若用于痰热互结之胸膈满闷，或作痛，可与半夏、黄连水煎服。

3. 消肿疗痈：用于肺痈，咳吐脓血，常与银花、鱼腥草、芦根等同用；用于乳痈初起，红肿热痛者，常与蒲公英、银花、连翘等同用。

4. 润肠通便：用于肠燥便秘，以全瓜蒌30克，甘草6克，水煎，加白蜜调服。若用于食滞便秘，可以瓜蒌仁、六曲、山楂、半夏各等份蜜丸用。

现代常用于冠心病心绞痛、乳腺癌。

用量用法 全栝楼12～30克，瓜蒌皮6～12克，瓜蒌仁3～10克，蒌仁霜3～10克，煎服。治胸痹，痈肿，便燥，多用全栝楼；清热化痰，下气宽胸，多用瓜蒌皮；润肺涤痰，滑肠通便，则用瓜蒌仁；蒌仁霜功用与仁相同，而滑肠之力，大为减缓。

使用注意 反乌头。

竹 茹

为乔木科多年生常绿竹状乔木或灌木淡竹 Phyllostachys nigra（Lodd.）Munro var henonis（Mitf.）Stapfex Rendle 的茎杆除去外皮后刮下的二层细条状竹皮。生用或姜汁微炒用。

处方用名 淡竹茹、姜竹茹。

性味归经 甘，微寒。入肺、胃、胆经。

功效应用

1. 清热化痰：用于胆虚痰热郁结，烦闷不宁，不得眠等症，常与枳实、半夏、茯苓等同用；若用于中风痰迷心窍，舌强不能言，常与胆星、菖蒲、茯苓、半夏等同用；治热痰咳嗽，常与黄芩、瓜蒌配用。

2. 清热止呕：用于湿热呕吐，可与黄连、半夏等同用；若用于胃虚热所致的呕吐或呃逆，可与橘皮、党参、甘草、生姜、大枣同用。

用量用法 6～12克。煎服。一般祛痰多生用，止呕多姜汁炒用。

附药 竹沥：又名竹油、竹沥水、竹沥膏。系由鲜淡竹经火炙沥出之液汁。甘寒滑润，能清心、肺、胃三经之火而涤痰除烦，定惊透络。凡中风不语、癫痫、惊厥等痰壅闭症，或痰热壅肺而致之咳嗽喘急，或痰留经络，致使肢体麻木、拘急等症，均可配生姜汁用之或随方冲服。然性寒伤胃滑肠，故有寒湿及便溏者忌服。用量30～60克。

天竺黄

为乔木科多年生常绿植物大节竹 Indosasa crassiflora Mcclure 等因被寄生的竹黄蜂咬洞后，而于竹节间贮积的伤流液，经干燥凝结而成的块状物。晾干打碎用。

处方用名 天竺黄、竺黄。

性味归经 甘，寒。入心、胃、肝经。

功效应用

1. 清热豁痰：用于小儿痰热壅盛，气急咳喘，可与黄连、僵蚕、朱砂等同用。

2. 凉心定惊：用于小儿惊风，身热昏睡，痰壅抽搐，常与胆星、朱砂等同用；若用于小儿惊风夜啼，可与蝉衣、僵蚕、郁金等同用。

用量用法 3～10 克。煎服。研粉吞服，每次 0.6～1 克。

海浮石

本品药材分海浮石和海石花两类。海浮石为火山喷发出的岩浆所形成的石块；海石花为胞孔科动物脊突苔虫 Costazia aculeata canuet Bassler 或瘤苔虫 Costazia costazii Audouin 等的骨骼。晒干打碎用。

处方用名 海浮石、浮海石。

性味归经 咸、寒。入肺经。

功效应用

1. 清肺化痰：用于痰热喘咳，顽痰胶结，可与胆星、贝母等同用；若用于肺结核咳血、吐黄痰，海浮石 60 克，白及 180 克，三七 60 克，共为末，每次 3 克，日服 2～3 次。

2. 软坚散结：用于瘰疬结核，单用力弱，常入于复方中应用。

3. 消石通淋：用于砂淋、石淋、血淋尿痛等症，海浮石研细末，每次3克，日服3次，甘草煎汤送下。

用量用法 6～10克，煎服。宜入丸、散剂。

海蛤壳

为帘蛤科动物青蛤 Cyclina sinensis (Gmelin) 或文蛤 Meretrix meretrix L.的贝壳。碾碎生用或煅用。

处方用名 海蛤壳、海蛤粉、煅蛤壳。

性味归经 咸，寒。入肺、肾经。

功效应用

1. 清肺化痰：用于痰火咳嗽，或痰结胸满等症，可与青黛、天冬、黄芩等同用；若治热痰积结胸痛，以蛤粉、瓜蒌仁等分为丸用。

2. 软坚散结：用于瘿瘤、瘰疬，可与昆布、海藻等同用。

3. 利水消肿：用于湿热水气浮肿，小便不利，可与木通、滑石、猪苓等同用；用于臌胀腹水，小便不利，可与防己、葶苈、郁李仁等同用。

此外，还能制酸止痛，同于胃痛泛酸。油调外用可治烫火伤、湿疹等。

用量用法 10～15克。煎服。蛤粉宜包煎。多入丸、散剂。一般内服宜生用，制酸、外敷宜煅用。

海藻

为海产马尾藻科多年生植物羊栖菜 Sargassum fusiforme (Harv.) Setch.或海蒿子 Sargassum pallidum (Turn.) C. Ag.的全草。漂洗后切段入药。

处方用名 海藻、淡海藻。

性味归经 苦、咸，寒。入肝、胃、肾经。

功效应用 消痰散结：用于瘰疬结核瘿瘤结肿，常与昆布、海蛤、僵蚕等同用；用于睾丸肿痛，可单味煎服。

此外，本品尚治脚气浮肿及水肿。因其有利水退肿之功。

用量用法 15～30克。煎服。

使用注意 不宜与甘草同用。

昆 布

为海产翅藻科植物鹅掌菜（昆布）Ecklonia kurome Okam. 裙带菜 Undaria pinnatifida（Harv.）Suring 或昆布科植物海带 Laminaria japonica Aresch.的叶状体。漂洗后，切丝或小块入药。

处方用名 昆布、淡昆布。

性味归经 咸，寒。入肝、胃、肾经。

功效应用 消痰散结：用于瘿瘤瘰疬，常与海藻等同用。本品作用与海藻相同而较强，二者并用可增强疗效，均为治瘿瘤瘰疬之主药。用于肝脾肿大，常与三棱、莪术、鳖甲等同用。

此外，亦常用于水肿胀满、脚气。因其能利水退肿。又治睾疝。近年用治地方性甲状腺肿大及腺瘤、淋巴结核、肝硬变。

礞 石

为变质岩类岩石绿泥石片岩（青礞石）Chlorite-schist 或云母片岩（金礞石）Mica-schist 的石块或碎粒。与火硝拌匀，煅至硝尽，色变金黄，再水飞其硝毒，晾干用。

处方用名 礞石、金礞石。

性味归经 甘、咸，平。入肺、肝经。

功效应用 下气坠痰，平肝镇惊：用于顽痰内结，喘逆不得平卧，大便秘结，或痰积癫痫、狂躁烦闷等症，常与沉香、大黄等同用；若治小儿痰热急惊，用本品一味研末，每次1.5～3克，薄荷煎汤加白蜜冲服。

用量用法 6～10克。煎服。多入丸散剂，每次1.5～3克。

13.3 温化寒痰药

本类药物，药性偏于温燥，具有温化寒痰或燥湿化痰之功。适用于痰涎稀薄清冷，易于咯出的寒痰、湿痰及由此而引起的咳嗽哮喘、肢节酸痛、阴疽流注等症。为增强疗效，应与温散寒湿药同用。如属阴虚燥咳，或有咯血、吐血病史者，应慎用。

半　夏

为天南星科多年生草本植物半夏 Pinellia ternata（Thunb.）Breit.的块根。生用或制用。因泡制方法不同，又有清半夏：以生半夏加白矾共煎，切片晒干；法半夏：以生半夏与甘草、石灰共制而成；姜半夏：以生半夏加生姜、白矾共煮，切片晒干。

处方用名　清半夏、姜半夏、法半夏、生半夏。

性味归经　辛，温，有小毒。入脾、胃经。

功效应用

1. 燥湿化痰：用于湿痰咳嗽，痰多清稀，或痰逆头眩，常与陈皮、茯苓等同用；若用于风痰吐逆，头痛头眩，胸膈烦满，饮食不下，可与生南星等同用。

2. 降逆止呕：用于胃寒或痰饮呕吐，半夏 15 克，生姜 10 克，水煎服；若用于胃虚呕吐，半夏 12 克，党参 15 克，白蜜 30 克（兑入），水煎服；若用于痰热胸痞呕吐，常与黄连、干姜同用。

3. 消痞散结：本品有辛散消痞，化痰散结之功。用于痰热互结的胸脘痞闷，可与黄连、栝楼仁同用；气郁痰结，咽中如有物阻的梅核气，可与厚朴、苏叶、茯苓等同用；用于瘿瘤痰核，可与昆布、海藻、浙贝母等软坚散结药同用；用治痈疽肿毒，以生半夏研末，用鸡蛋白调敷患处。

用量用法　3～10 克。煎服。习惯上以清半夏长于化湿痰；姜半夏善于止呕；法半夏用于燥湿和胃；生半夏多外用于痈疽肿毒。

使用注意 反乌头。因其性温燥，对阴亏燥咳，血证、热痰等证，当慎用或忌用。

天 南 星

为天南星科多年生草本植物的天南星 Arisaema consanguineum schott. 东北天南星 Arisatma amurense Maxim. 或异叶天南星 Arisaema heterophyllum Bl.的地下扁圆型球状块茎。洗净晒干即为生南星；用白矾水浸泡，再与生姜共煮，切片晒干则为制南星。生用或制用。

处方用名 生南星、制南星。

性味归经 苦、辛，温，有毒。入肺、肝、脾经。

功效应用

1. 燥湿化痰：用于顽痰湿痰所致的咳嗽，胸膈胀满等症，常与半夏、茯苓、枳实等同用；亦可与白术、半夏配丸用；若用于肺热痰多黄稠而粘，可与半夏、黄芩同用；若用于寒痰咳嗽，痰涎清稀，可与半夏、肉桂为丸，生姜汤下。

2. 祛风解痉：用于痰涎壅盛，手足顽麻，半身不遂，口眼㖞斜之属于风痰留滞经络之症，可与半夏、白附子、川乌等同用；用于破伤风之肢搐，口噤，项强等症，可与防风等分为末，内服或外用。

3. 解毒医疮：用于疮疖痈肿，瘰疬结核，生南星以醋研浓汁，涂患处；用于蛇咬伤，鲜南星捣烂敷患处；或用干南星与雄黄为末，白酒敷患处。

此外，近代用本品治子宫颈癌，经药理研究证实其有抗肿瘤作用。

用量用法 3～10克。煎服。外用生品适量。生者外用。

使用注意 孕妇慎用。

附药 胆南星：取生南星研末，与牛胆汁加工制成小块状或圆柱状，即为胆南星，简称胆星。味更苦，而性转凉。功能熄风化痰定惊。适用于热痰蒙蔽清窍而致的神昏痉厥，惊痫抽搐等症。用量 3~6 克，煎服。

白附子

为天南星科多年生草本植物独角莲 Typhonium giganteum Engl.的块茎（禹白附）。生用或制用。

处方用名 白附子、制白附子。

性味归经 辛、甘，大温，有毒。入肝、脾经。

功效应用

1. 祛痰止痛：用于风痰眩晕，痰厥头痛，可与南星、半夏煎服。

2. 祛风止痉：用于中风口眼歪斜，常与全蝎、僵蚕同用；用于风痰壅盛，抽搐呕吐，可与南星、全蝎、僵蚕等同用；用于破伤风之口噤痉挛，可与南星、防风、天麻等同用。

3. 解毒散结：用于毒蛇咬伤，可单用本品外敷，也可与其他解蛇毒药合用，外敷或内服；治瘰疬痰核，可用鲜品捣敷。

用量用法 3~5 克。煎服。外用适量。

使用注意 孕妇忌服。生者一般不作内服。

白芥子

为十字花科植物白芥 Brassica alba（L.）Boiss.或芥 B. juncea（L.）Czern. et Coss.的成熟种子。前者习称白芥子，后者习称黄芥子。生用或炒用。

处方用名 白芥子、炒芥子。

性味归经 辛，温。入肺、胃经。

功效应用

1. 豁痰利气：用于寒痰壅肺，痰多清稀，咳嗽气喘，胸胁胀满等症，常与紫苏子、莱菔子同用；用于痰饮气逆，咳喘胸痛，胸胁积水等症，常与甘遂、大戟同用；用于气滞痰凝之肢体关节疼痛，白芥子、没药、桂心、木香各10克，木鳖子3克，共为细末，每次3克，日2次，温酒送服。

2. 散结消肿：用于瘰疬痰核、阴阻漫肿等症，可与葱白各等量，捣成泥状，敷患处，每日1次。单味为末，醋调涂，可治肿毒初起之症。

此外，近年用其治疗渗出性胸膜炎，有消除胸腔积液的作用。

用量用法 3～10克。煎服。外用适量。

使用注意 外敷有发泡作用，皮肤过敏者忌用。

白　前

为萝藦科多年生草本植物柳叶白前 Cynanchum stauntoni (Decne.) Schltr. ex Levl.或芫花叶白前 Cynanchum glaucescens (Decne.) Hand-Mazz.的根茎及根。切段生用或蜜炙用。

处方用名 白前、炙白前。

性味归经 苦、辛，微温。入肺经。

功效应用 宣肺降气，祛痰止咳：本品善于降气，气降则痰涎自消，咳嗽自止，为肺家咳嗽要药。用于肺气壅实，咳嗽痰多，胸满气急喘息等症，可与麻黄、款冬花、杏仁、甘草等同用；若用于肺热咳喘，痰黄稠不易咳出等症，可与桑皮、生地、地骨皮等同用；用于外感风寒咳嗽、常与荆芥、桔梗、陈皮等同用。

用量用法 6～10克。煎服。久咳或稠痰难咯者可蜜炙用。

旋　复　花

为菊科多年生草本植物旋复花 Inula britannica L. Nar. chinensis (Rupr.) Reg.或大花旋复花 Inula britannica L.的头状花序。生用或蜜炙用。

处方用名 旋复花。

性味归经 苦、辛、咸，微温。入肺、胃、大肠经。

功效应用

1. 开结消痰：用于痰饮蓄结的胸膈痞闷，气逆喘促等症，可与桔梗、桑白皮、槟榔等同用；若用于感冒伤寒，咳嗽痰喘，常与荆芥、细辛、前胡等同用。

2. 降气止噫：用于胸痞噫气之由于脾胃气虚，或痰湿上逆者，常与代赭石、半夏等同用。

用量用法 6～12克。布包入煎。

14　安神药

凡以安神定志为主要功效的药物，称为安神药。

安神药按其性能可分为 2 类：属于质重的金石药及介类药，取其重则能镇，重可去怯的，为重镇安神药；属于植物药而取其养心滋肝的，为养心安神药。

重镇安神药，多用于阳气躁动，心神不安属于实证者，有镇定安神之功。然这类药物虽能镇定浮阳，但不能消除导致浮阳的其它因素，故在应用时作适当配伍。养心安神药，多用于心肝血虚神志不宁的虚证，多与滋阴养血药配伍应用。

重镇安神药虽然大多较适宜实证，养心安神药大多适宜虚证，但若虚实相兼，亦常相互配用，提高疗效。

14.1　重镇安神药

重镇安神药，是为质重镇坠之品，具有镇静安神作用，适用于阳气躁动，心悸，失眠，惊痫，狂妄，烦躁易怒等症。如因邪热炽盛，须合清热降火药同用；若肝阳上越，应与平肝潜阳药配伍。

朱　　砂

为天然硫化汞矿石辰砂 Cinnabar 的矿石。研细水飞入药。

处方用名　朱砂、飞朱砂、丹砂、辰砂。

性味归经　甘，寒。入心经。

功效应用

1. 镇心安神：用于心血不足，心火偏胜而引起的心神不安，烦躁不眠，常与黄连、生地或琥珀等同用；用于癫痫，可与南星、琥珀、白矾等同用。

2. 解毒医疮：用于疮疡肿毒，及口鼻生疮，咽喉肿痛等症。前者，可配雄黄等研末外敷。后者，常配冰片、硼砂等研末吹患处。

此外，研末作丸剂外衣，有防腐作用。

用量用法 0.3～1克。只入丸散剂，不宜入煎，入汤剂当研末冲服。外用适量。入药只宜生用。

使用注意 忌用火煅，见火则析出水银，尤易中毒。内服不宜过量，也不可持续服用，防止汞中毒。对肝肾功能异常者，当慎用之，以免病情加重。

龙 骨

为古代多种大型哺乳动物的骨骼化石。如东方剑齿象、三趾马、犀类、鹿类、牛类等的骨骼化石。用时打碎，生用或煅用。

处方用名 生龙骨、煅龙骨。

性味归经 甘、涩，平。入心、肝经。

功效应用

1. 镇心安神：用于神志失常，心悸健忘，失眠多梦等症，常与龟板、菖蒲、远志各等分，研末水丸，每次3克，日服3次。

2. 平肝潜阳：用于肝阴亏损，虚阳浮越所致头晕目眩，烦躁惊狂等症，常与牡蛎、白芍、白薇、菊花、钩藤、玄参等同用。

3. 收涩固脱：用于遗精带下、自汗、盗汗、月经过多等症，常与牡蛎、山药、海螵蛸、茯苓等同用。

4. 生肌敛疮：用于疮疡溃腐，久不愈合，及脐疮流水，金疮出血等症，龙骨、枯矾各等分，研细末，掺敷患处。

用量用法 10～30克。入汤剂宜先煎。外用适量。镇心、平肝宜生用，收敛固脱宜煅用。

琥　　珀

琥珀 Amber 为古代枫树、松树的树脂埋藏地层中经多年而成的化石，研末入药。

处方用名　琥珀、血珀、老琥珀。

性味归经　甘，平。入心、肝、膀胱经。

功效应用

1. 镇惊安神：用于惊悸，怔忡，健忘，多梦，失眠，癫痫等症，可与朱砂、南星、茯苓、远志、菖蒲等同用。

2. 利尿通淋：用于小便癃闭，以及血淋、热淋、砂淋等症，常与其它利尿化瘀药同用。

3. 活血化瘀：用于妇女血瘀气滞，经闭不通，可与当归、莪术等同用。

此外，也可用于疮疡肿毒，能活血消肿。外用可作生肌收敛药。近代配伍三七研末服，治冠心病。又用于阴囊及阴唇血肿或子宫郁血，单味为散服有效。

用量用法　1.5～3 克。不入煎剂。研末冲服，或入丸散剂。

磁　　石

为天然的等轴晶系磁铁石 Magnetite 的矿石。击碎生用，或醋淬研细用。

处方用名　磁石、灵磁石、活磁石、煅磁石。

性味归经　辛、咸、微寒。入肝、肾经。

功效应用

1. 潜阳安神：用于阴虚阳亢引起的头晕头痛，心悸失眠，烦躁不宁及癫痫等，常与朱砂同用。

2. 聪耳明目：用于肝肾不足引起的耳鸣、耳聋、目视不明等症，可与熟地、山茱萸、五味子等同用。

3. 纳气平喘：用于老年气喘之由于肾气虚弱者，可与熟地、山茱萸、山药等同用。

用量用法 10～30克。煎服。入汤剂宜生用打碎先煎。如入丸散内服，必须煅透，否则服后腹痛。

使用注意 因妨碍消化，入丸散剂，不可多服久服。

14.2 养心安神药

本类药物，具有养心柔肝，滋阴养血之功，适用于心肝血虚，心神失养以及七情所伤的心悸怔忡，不眠多梦，喜笑失常，神志不宁等症。在复方中每与补血滋阴药配伍，以提高疗效。

酸 枣 仁

为鼠李科落叶小灌木或小乔木酸枣 Ziziphus jujuba Mill.的种子。取核仁，生用或炒用。

处方用名 酸枣仁、炒枣仁。

性味归经 甘、酸，平。入心、肝、胆、脾经。

功效应用

1. 养心安神：用于血虚不能滋养心肝引起之烦热不眠，惊悸怔忡，常与知母、茯苓、川芎、甘草同用；若用于神经衰弱、健忘、多梦易醒、饮食减少，疲倦乏力之由于心脾气虚者，可与党参、茯苓、远志、菖蒲同用。

2. 益阴敛汗：用于阴虚多汗，可与人参、茯苓为末，米汤送服；或与生地黄、白芍、麦冬、五味子、龙眼肉等同用。

用量用法 10～15克。煎服。亦可研末，于临睡前吞服，每次1.5～3克。

柏 子 仁

为柏科常绿乔木侧柏 Biota orientalis（L.）Endl.的种仁。碾去种皮，原药生用，或去油取霜用。

处方用名 柏子仁、侧柏仁、柏子霜。

性味归经 甘，平。入心、脾经。

功效应用

1. 养心安神：用于心血不足，神志不宁，失眠多梦，惊悸怔忡，记忆衰退等症，常与熟地、当归、茯苓、菖蒲等同用。兼盗汗者，亦可与人参、五味子、牡蛎同用。

2. 益脾润肠：用于阴虚患者、老人及产后的肠燥便秘，常与松子仁、郁李仁等同用。

用量用法 6～10克。煎服。大便稀者用柏子霜。

远　志

为远志科多年生草本植物远志 Polygala tenuifolia Willd.或宽叶远志 P. sibirica L.的根皮。生用或炙用。

处方用名 远志、远志肉、炒远志。

性味归经 苦、辛，温。入心、肾、肺经。

功效应用

1. 养心安神：用于惊悸恐惧，心神不安，健忘等症，常与党参、茯苓、菖蒲、枣仁等同用。

2. 祛痰开窍：用于痰阻心窍引起的精神错乱，神志恍惚，惊痫等症，常与郁金、菖蒲、白矾等同用，以增强祛痰开窍之力；用于痰多咳嗽，或稠粘不爽等症，可与陈皮、甘草同用。

此外，还可用于湿痰壅滞所致的痈疽肿毒，乳房肿痛，单用研末，酒送服或外用调敷。

用量用法 3～6克。煎服。外用适量。

使用注意 本品性温燥，痰热及溃汤病、胃炎者慎用。

合　欢　皮

为豆科落叶乔木合欢树 Albizzia julibrissin Durazz.的树皮。切片生用。

处方用名 合欢皮。

性味归经 甘，平。入心、脾经。

功效应用

1. 安神解郁：用于虚烦不安，忧郁忿怒，健忘失眠等症，可单用，亦可与白芍、柏子仁、龙齿、琥珀等同用。

2. 活血消肿：用于肺痈，咳吐痰浊，可单用煎服，亦可配白蔹同服；用于跌打损伤，瘀血肿痛，可与当归、赤芍、川芎、桃仁等同用。

3. 生肌续骨：用于筋骨折伤，可与白芥子为末，黄酒调服，并可用药末外敷患处。

用量用法 10～15克。煎服。

附药 合欢花：为合欢树的花。功用与皮相同，长于理气解郁，和中开胃。用量6～12克。

15. 平肝熄风药

凡具有平熄肝风或潜阳镇静作用的药物，称为平肝熄风药。

本类药物，分别具有清肝，潜阳，镇痉等作用，适用于高热引起的神志昏迷，痉厥抽搐，甚至角弓反张；或因肝阳偏亢、肝风上旋而致的头目眩晕，脑中热痛，颜面色红，甚至猝然昏倒，口眼㖞斜，半身不遂等肝风内动者。其中虫类药还可用于顽固性的风湿关节痛、肌肉麻木等症。

应用平肝熄风药时，当根据病变原因予以不同的配伍：如因高热引起者，配以清热泻火药，因风痰引起者，配以化痰药；因肾不养肝引起者，配以滋肾养阴药；因血虚引起者，配以补血养肝药等。须知风证变化很快，风火相煽，每火升气升痰亦升，则易出现痰涎上涌，神志昏迷等现象，此时，宜先豁痰开窍以救急，待神志清醒后，再进行辨证论治。另外，惊痫痉厥的患者，多有惊悸、失眠等症，故熄风药又常配伍安神药同用。

本类药物性能各异，应区别应用。凡脾虚慢惊，则非寒凉药所宜；而阴虚血亏者，温燥之品，又宜慎用。

羚 羊 角

为洞角科动物赛加羚羊 Saiga tatarica L.的角。锯角镑片或锉末入药，或磨汁服。

处方用名 羚羊片、羚羊粉。

性味归经 咸，寒。入肝、心、肺经。

功效应用

1. 凉肝熄风：用于温病热盛，引动肝风，肢体痉挛抽搐，甚至角弓反张，可与钩藤、菊花、贝母或全蝎、蜈蚣等同用。

2. 清肝明目：用于肝火炽盛所致的头痛、目赤，可与龙胆草、栀子、黄芩等同用。

此外，尚有散血解毒之功，用于热毒发斑，红肿痒痛，及麻疹热毒内陷，不能透发，均可磨汁内服。

用量用法　3～6克。入煎剂宜另煎汁冲服，亦可磨汁或锉末服，每次0.6～1.5克。

石决明

为鲍科动物九孔鲍 Haliotis diversicolor Reeve 或盘大鲍 Haliotis gigantea discus Reeve 等的贝壳。生用或煅用。

处方用名　石决明、生石决、煅石决。

性味归经　咸，寒。入肝、肺经。

功效应用

1. 平肝潜阳：用于头目眩晕，烦扰不寐及阴虚肝阳上升者，常与生牡蛎、生白芍、生地、女贞子、菊花、牛膝等同用。

2. 退翳明目：用于目生翳障，青盲雀目，及肝热目赤肿痛，可与菊花、谷精草、蛇蜕等同用；若单用石决明研细面，每次10克，入羊肝内，以线缚扎，砂罐煮熟，食肝饮汁，每日服之，可治青盲。

用量用法　10～30克。煎服。入汤剂宜先煎，久煎。

使用注意　脾胃虚寒，消化不良，及胃酸缺乏者慎用。

牡蛎

为特蛎科动物长牡蛎 Ostrea gigas Thunb.和大连湾牡蛎 O. talienwhanensis Crosse 或近江牡蛎 O. rivularis Gould，等的贝壳。打碎，生用或煅用。

处方用名　生牡蛎、煅牡蛎。

性味归经　咸、涩，微寒。入肝、肾经。

功效应用

1. 平肝潜阳：用于阴虚阳亢之头痛，头晕，耳鸣，肢麻等症，常与龙骨、代赭石、龟板、白芍等同用。

2. 镇静安神：用于心悸不安，胆怯惊恐，烦躁不寐等症之属于肝阴不足者，常与龙骨、枣仁、远志、夜交藤等安神药同用。

3. 收敛固涩：用于结核病潮热，盗汗，自汗，单用牡蛎30克，水煎服；用于遗精滑精，常与莲须、芡实等同用；用于崩漏带下，可与阿胶、赤石脂、续断等同用。

4. 软坚散结：用于痰火郁结所致的瘰疬，痰核等，常与玄参、浙贝母等同用。

此外，近代亦以本品作制酸剂，治胃痛反酸有效。

用量用法 15～30克。入汤剂。宜先煎。潜阳、软坚宜生用；收敛、制酸宜煅用。

珍　珠

为珍珠贝科动物马氏珍珠贝 Pteria martensii（Dunker）和蚌科动物三角帆蚌 Hyriopsis cumingii（Lea）、褶纹冠蚌 Cristaria plicata Leach.或背角无齿蚌 Anodonta woodiana Lea.等贝类动物珍珠囊中所形成的无核珍珠。临用时，以绢包入豆腐内同煮4小时，然后取出研粉水飞入药。

处方用名 珍珠粉，真珠粉、濂珠粉。

性味归经 甘、咸，寒。入心、肝经。

功效应用

1. 镇心定惊：用于惊悸，癫痫，急热惊风等症，可与朱砂、琥珀、胆星、天竺黄等同用。

2. 清肝除翳：用于目赤翳障涩痛之由于肝虚有热者，可与炉甘石、冰片等配合点眼。

3. 生肌敛疮：用于溃疡不合，疮口不敛，可与冰片、象皮、血竭等同用；若治咽喉腐烂及牙疳蚀烂，可用珍珠9克，牛黄 3 克，共研细粉，吹患处。

用量用法 0.3～1 克，只作丸散，不入煎剂。外用适量。

附药 珍珠母：为珍珠贝的贝壳，性味相同，功能平肝潜阳，清肝明目。主治头痛，眩晕，耳鸣，目翳，惊痫等症。用量 15～30 克。煎服。须先煎，久煎。

代赭石

为三方晶系赤铁矿 Hematite 的矿石。砸碎生用，或火煅醋淬后粉碎晒干用。

处方用名 生赭石、煅赭石。

性味归经 苦、甘，寒。入肝、心经。

功效应用

1. 平肝泻热：用于肝阳上亢所导致的头痛眩晕，可与石决明、夏枯草、牛膝等同用。

2. 镇逆降气：用于气逆引起的呕吐，噫气，痞胀，吐粘涎等症，常与旋复花、半夏等同用；若治胆火上冲之呕吐呃逆，可与青黛、龙胆草、吴茱萸等同用。

3. 凉血止血：用于血热妄行的吐血、衄血，可与白芍、竹茹、牛蒡子等同用；用于妇女崩漏下血，煅赭石为末，每次 10 克，日服 3 次。亦可将本品煅研外敷，治外伤出血。

用量用法 10～30 克。煎服。平肝镇逆凉血宜生用，敛血止血宜煅用。

天麻

为兰科多年生寄生草本植物天麻 Gastrodia elata Bl.的地下块茎。擦去粗皮，热水渍透切片，晒干生用。

处方用名 天麻、明天麻、天麻片。

性味归经 甘，平。入肝经。

功效应用

1. 熄风止痉：用于破伤风之抽掣痉挛，常与南星、防风等同用；用于痰湿内蕴引起的头目眩晕，常与半夏、白术等同用；若治偏正头风头痛，眼目昏花，可用天麻、川芎各等分，水丸，每次 3 克，日服 3 次。

2. 通络止痛：用于风寒湿所致关节疼痛，麻木不仁，可与牛膝、全蝎等同用；若治肝肾亏虚，肢体萎弱无力，麻木不遂，可与杜仲、牛膝、生地、当归等同用。

用量用法 3～6 克。煎服。

钩　藤

为茜草科常绿木质藤本植物钩藤 Uncaria rhynchophylla (Miq.) Jacks.的带钩茎枝。晒干生用。

处方用名 钩藤、双钩藤、嫩钩藤。

性味归经 甘，微寒。入肝、心包经。

功效应用

1. 熄风止痉：用于肝热生风，惊痫抽搐，及破伤风等症，常与天麻、菊花、蝉蜕、羚羊角等同用。

2. 平肝清热：用于肝热头痛，风热头痛，头目眩晕等症，常与桑叶、菊花、薄荷等同用。

此外，本品尚有良好的降血压作用，对高血压病而属肝热阳亢者，疗效较佳。

用量用法 10～15 克。煎服。

使用注意 本品经水煮沸 20 分钟以上，降压作用减弱，故不宜久煎。

白　蒺　藜

为蒺藜科 1 年生或多年生平卧地面草本植物刺蒺藜 Tribulus terrestris L.的果实。晒干，盐水炒黄去刺用。

处方用名 白蒺藜、刺蒺藜。

性味归经　苦、辛，平。入肝、肺经。

功效应用

1. 祛风疏肝：用于头目眩晕，头风头痛，可与桑叶、菊花、蔓荆子、钩藤等疏散风热药同用；若用于肝肾虚热生风，目赤多泪，可与菊花、决明子、青葙子等同用；用于风疹瘙痒，每与蝉衣、荆芥等同用；用于胸胁不舒，乳汁不通之属于肝气郁结者，可与青皮、郁金、橘叶等舒肝药同用。

2. 行气活血：用于少腹胀痛，可与乌药、白芍、金铃子、香附等同用。

用量用法　6～10克。煎服。

僵　蚕

为蚕蛾科昆虫家蚕 Bombyx mori L.的幼虫在未吐丝前，因感染白僵菌而发病致死的僵化虫体。生用或麸皮炒黄用。

处方用名　僵蚕、姜蚕、白僵蚕、炙姜蚕、制天虫。

性味归经　咸、辛，平。入肝、肺经。

功效应用

1. 化痰止痉：用于小儿急惊，痰喘痉挛，可与全蝎、胆星、天麻等同用；若治发热头痛咳嗽而兼发热惊痫抽搐者，可与蝉蜕、钩藤、菊花等同用。

2. 祛风泄热：用于风热头痛，迎风流泪及风热喉痛等症，可与桑叶、荆芥、薄荷、木贼等同用；用于皮肤瘙痒，可单味研末服，但一般仍宜入复方应用。

3. 消肿散结：用于瘰疬痰核，可单味研末服；用于乳痈初起，以本品研末，醋调为稀糊，敷肿块上。

用量用法　3～10克。煎服。一般多炙用，散风热宜生用。

全　蝎

为钳蝎科节足动物问荆蝎 Buthus martensi Karsch 的全体。

全用或单用尾部（后腹部）。

处方用名 全蝎、蝎尾、全虫。

性味归经 甘、辛，平，有毒。入肝经。

功效应用

1. 熄风止痉：本品有良好的熄风止痉作用。用于湿温病，破伤风，癫痫，小儿急惊风等引起之痉挛抽搐，角弓反张而属于实证者，可与僵蚕、蜈蚣各等分为末，每服1～1.5克，每日1～2次；用于中风口眼㖞斜，常与僵蚕、白附子同用。

2. 活络止痛：用于风湿骨节挛痛，以全蝎3克，麝香0.06克，共研细末，每服1.5克，温酒调服；亦可单用全蝎研末，每服1.5克，酒调下。若治慢性关节炎，可与制川乌、乳香、山甲珠等同用。

3. 解毒散结：用于疮疡肿毒，瘰疬结核，痄腮等症，可与山栀、白芷等同用；若单用全蝎2条，油炸食，可治小儿痄腮。

用量用法 全蝎1.5～5克，蝎尾3～8条。煎服。宜入散剂，用量可酌减。

使用注意 本品有毒。用量不宜过大。血虚生风者慎用。

蜈　蚣

为蜈蚣科节足动物少棘蜈蚣 Scolopendra subspinipes mutilans L. Koch.的全体。晒干或烘干，剪碎或研末用。

处方用名 蜈蚣、金头蜈蚣。

性味归经 辛，温，有毒。入肝经。

功效应用

1. 熄风止痉：用于肝风引起的肢体抽搐，口噤，甚至角弓反张，及小儿惊厥，癫痫，破伤风，颜面神经麻痹等症，常与僵蚕、全蝎等熄风药同用。

2. 解毒散结：用于疮疡肿毒，瘰疬结核等症，可与其它解毒药同用。

3. 活络止痛：用于顽固性头部抽掣疼痛，风湿痹痛等症。本品有良好的活络止痛作用。每与全蝎相伍，或与僵蚕、天麻、川芎等同用，治头痛，痹痛甚效。

用量用法 2～5克，或1～3条，煎服。研末吞服，每次0.6～1克。外用适量。

使用注意 血虚发痉，孕妇忌用。

地　龙

为巨蚓科环节动物参环毛蚓 Pheretima asiatica Michaelsen 和缟蚯蚓 Allolobophora caliginosa trapezoides（Duges）的干燥全体。生用或焙用，亦可鲜用。

处方用名 地龙、干地龙、地龙肉、鲜地龙。

性味归经 咸，寒。入肝、肾、肺经。

功效应用

1. 清热止痉：用于高热烦躁，惊风抽搐，可与钩藤、全蝎、石膏等同用；或用地龙10克，朱砂3克，为末，分2次服；若治乙脑高热持续不退，昏厥较甚者，用鲜地龙六条（洗净），皂矾18克，共捣烂，敷于患者囟门（头发剃净）。5小时后如发热仍未下降者，可洗去续敷1次。

2. 通络疗痹：用于风湿热痹关节红肿热痛，常与络石藤、忍冬藤、海桐皮等同用；若治风寒湿痹，可与乌头、附子、桂枝等同用；若治湿痰瘀血窒塞经络之肢节疼痛，或半身不遂，可与乌头、南星、或桃仁、红花、当归等同用。

3. 清肺平喘：用于火热灼肺的咳喘及小儿百日咳等症，用鲜地龙100条，水煎熬，去渣，加白糖收膏，每次1小茶匙，开水冲服；或用干地龙末，每次3克，日服2次。

4. 利尿通淋：用于热结尿闭，及砂石淋痛，单味研末服，或与其它利尿药配伍同用。

用量用法 6～10克。煎服。鲜品10～20克。入丸、散剂，每次 1～3 克。外用适量。

罗 布 麻

为夹竹桃多年生草本植物罗布麻 Apocynum venetum L.的叶。晒干切段用。

处方用名 罗布麻。

性味归经 微苦，凉。入肝经。

功效应用

1. 平肝安神：本品经实验证明有降血压之功。用于肝阳上亢或肝热型的高血压，症见头痛眩晕及烦躁失眠等。单用以开水泡汁代茶饮，或与夏枯草、钩藤、野菊花等同用。

2. 清热利水：用于小便不利，水肿等有热象者，可与车前子、泽泻等利尿药同用。

用量用法 6～15 克。煎服或开水泡服。

16　开窍药

凡以通关开窍，醒神为主要作用的药物，称为开窍药。

本类药物多气味芳香，善于走窜，具有通关开窍、启闭醒神之功。主要用于中风，中气，中痰以及惊痫等病的卒然昏厥，或热病引起的神志昏迷等内闭实证。有的药可通鼻窍。

神志昏迷，不仅见于闭证，也可见于脱证。闭证以口噤握拳、气色有神，脉搏有力为辨证依据；脱证则恰恰相反，可见口开手撒，气色无神，脉搏无力等。闭是邪实内闭，宜本类芳香开窍之品以通其闭。脱是气虚外脱，当大补元气，回阳救脱，禁用芳香开窍，以免耗伤元气，促使病情恶化。另外，闭证有寒闭，热闭之分。寒闭，面青身凉，苔白脉迟；热闭，面赤身热，苔黄脉数。寒闭开窍宜配祛寒药；热闭开窍宜配清热药。

开窍药只可暂用，不可久服，久服泄人元气。本类药物仅个别药可入煎剂外，其它只入丸散剂。

牛　黄

为牛科动物黄牛 Bos taurus domesticus Gmelin 或水牛 Bubalus bubalis L.的胆囊、胆管或肝管中的结石。用时研为细末入药。

处方用名　牛黄、西黄。

性味归经　苦、凉。入心、肝经。

功效应用

1. 豁痰开窍：用于热病神昏谵语，烦躁不安，以及小儿急惊，中风窍闭，痰热壅盛者，常与朱砂、山栀、黄连等同用。

2. 熄风定惊：用于热甚所致的惊厥，抽搐等症，常与朱砂、麝香、蝎尾等同用。

3. 清热解毒：本品又为防腐解毒要药。用于乳岩、瘰疬、痰核，肺痈，肠痈等症，可与麝香、乳香、没药同用；用于火热上炎所致的咽喉肿痛，白喉，口舌疮疡等症，常与麝香、冰片、朱砂等同用；用于一切痈疡肿毒，及小儿胎毒疮疖，常与银花、甘草、草河车同用。

用量用法 0.15～0.3 克。入丸、散剂，不入煎剂。外用适量。

麝　香

为鹿科动物雄麝 Moschus moschiferus L.的脐下腺囊中的分泌物干燥品。研细入药。

处方用名 麝香、射香、寸香、元寸、当门子。

性味归经 辛，温。通行十二经。

功效应用

1. 开窍醒神：用于热病神昏，痉厥，及中风痰厥、气厥，卒然昏倒之内闭证，常与犀角、冰片、牛黄、朱砂等同用。

2. 活血消肿：用于跌打损伤，瘀血阻滞，遍身疼痛，常与血竭、乳香、儿茶等同用；用于咽喉肿痛，常与牛黄、雄黄、冰片等同用；用于痈疽肿毒，常与解毒药配伍。

3. 通经达络：用于癥瘕，经闭，可与三棱、莪术、肉桂同用。

4. 催产下胎：用于胎死腹中，胞衣不下，麝香 0.15 克，肉桂 1.5 克，研末分 2 次冲服。

用量用法 0.1～0.15 克，入丸、散剂，不宜入煎。外用适量。

使用注意 孕妇忌用。

冰　片

为龙脑香科常绿乔木龙脑香树 Dryobalanops aromatica Gaertn. f.树脂的加工结晶品。或以松节油为主要原料经化学方法加工而成，俗名机片。另一种，还有用菊科植物艾纳香 Blumea balsamifera DC.加工制成的艾片。用时研细末入药。

处方用名　冰片、梅片。

性味归经　辛、苦，微寒。入心、肝经。

功效应用

1. 开窍醒神：用于一切暴病或重伤神昏息微者，可与朱砂、雄黄、芒硝等同用；用于暑热秽浊、霍乱痧气所致的头目昏晕，吐泻昏迷不省者，常与牛黄、雄黄、芒硝等同用。

2. 散热止痛，防腐消肿：用于咽喉肿痛，口腔溃疡，常与硼砂等同用；用于疖毒肿痛，常与银朱（朱砂）、轻粉、蓖麻仁等同用；用于火眼肿痛，常与炉甘石、黄连等同用。

此外，现代又用于冠心病心绞痛，与苏合香相伍，有一定疗效。

用量用法　0.15～0.3 克，入丸散剂，不入煎剂。外用适量。

使用注意　孕妇慎服。

苏　合　香

为金缕梅科落叶乔木苏合香树 Liguidambar orientalis Mill. 的树脂，系黄色胶质如饴糖的浓稠液体。原药入丸剂。

处方用名　苏合香。

性味归经　辛，温。入心、脾经。

功效应用　开窍醒神，豁痰逐秽：用于中风，中气，卒然昏倒，牙关紧闭，不省人事，及痰壅气闭，突然昏迷，或胸腹满痛，时疫，瘴疟等症，可与安息香、麝香、冰片、丁香、檀香等同用。

近年来，以本品与檀香、冰片、乳香等配伍，用于冠心病心绞痛，可较快的缓解疼痛。以本品与冰片制成苏冰滴丸，亦有同样效果。

用量用法 0.3～1克。宜作丸剂，不入煎剂。

菖　蒲

为天南星科多年生草本植物石菖蒲 Acorus gramineus Soland.和毛茛科多年生草本植物阿尔泰银莲花 Anemone altaica Fisch.的根茎。晒干成段入药。

处方用名 石菖蒲、九节菖蒲。

性味归经 辛，苦，温。入心、脾、胃经。

功效应用

1. 开窍除痰：用于浊痰蒙闭心窍，神昏谵语，可与郁金、半夏、竹茹、竹沥、姜汁等同用。

2. 醒神健脑：用于惊恐不得卧，癫痫，健忘等症，常与远志、龙齿、朱砂、茯苓等同用。

3. 化湿开胃：用于痰多食少，可与郁金、半夏、佩兰等同用；用于痢疾噤口不食，可与黄连、石莲子、茯苓等同用。

此外，对于耳聋耳鸣，配方内服外用均可，亦可单用。

用量用法 3～6克。煎服。

17 补虚药

凡能补益人体气血阴阳不足，以治疗各种虚弱证候的一类药物，统称为补虚药或补益药，亦称补养药。

虚证有气虚、阳虚、血虚、阴虚之分，而补虚药根据其性能与应用范围也大致可分为补气、助阳、养血、滋阴四类。由于人体的气血阴阳有着相互依存的关系，阳虚多兼有气虚，而气虚易导致阳虚，气虚和阳虚是表示人体生理功能的不足；阴虚者每兼血虚，而血虚者亦常导致阴虚，血虚和阴虚是表示体内津液的损耗。因此，补气和助阳，养血和滋阴往往相须为用。至于气血两亏，阴阳俱虚的证候，则须统筹兼顾，用气血并补或阴阳兼补的方法。

补虚药对实邪未尽的不宜应用，以免“闭门留寇”。如病邪未清而正气已虚的，可于祛邪药物中，酌加补虚药协助，增强抵抗力，扶正以祛邪。

17.1 补气药

补气药具有强壮作用，能增强人体的生理功能和体力，主要适用于气虚之证，而尤以脾肺气虚为主。脾为后天之本，生化之源，脾气虚则倦怠，饮食不振，胸腹胀满，大便泄泻；肺主一身之气，肺气不足，则气短，少气，言微，自汗。凡呈现以上证候，皆可用补气药。

临床应用补气药，应根据不同的气虚证加以选择。若兼有阴虚或阳虚者，可与补阴药或补阳药配用。由于气血关系密切，气旺可以生血，故补气药亦常用于血虚之证。

补气药味多甘，一般比较腻滞，多服易致胸膈胀满，影响食欲，必要时可加入少许理气药如木香、枳壳等同用。

人　参

为五加科多年生草本植物人参 Panax ginseng C. A. Mey.的根。野生者称野山参，人工培植者称园参（或养参）。本品由于产地和加工方法不同。而有不同规格和名称。切片或研粉用。

处方用名　人参、吉林参、辽东参、红参、大力参、白参、别直参、人参须。

性味归经　甘、微苦，微温。入脾、肺、心经。

功效应用

1. 补气救脱：用于大病久病或大出血后，气短神疲，脉微欲绝，虚极欲脱之证，本品能大补元气，而有挽救虚脱之功。可单用本品一味，浓煎取汁服，即独参汤；若气脱兼见肢冷，自汗而有亡阳之象者，可配附子同用。

2. 补益脾肺：本品为治虚劳内伤之要药。用于脾胃气虚，精神疲乏，四肢无力，短气食少，或上腹痞满，泄泻，及各种原因所致气虚体弱之证，通常与白术、甘草等同用；若气血两虚，可配熟地、当归等，若脾虚有湿，便溏泄泻，可与山药、扁豆、莲子肉等健脾利湿药配伍；如中气下陷，久泄脱肛，亦可与黄芪、升麻、柴胡等补气升阳举陷药同用；用于肺肾虚喘，常与胡桃肉、五味子、蛤蚧等同用。

3. 生津止渴：用于热病热伤气津，短气口渴或亡津失水，心力衰竭，脉虚微细之症，常与麦冬、五味子配伍，近年有制成生脉注射液，用于抢救感染中毒性休克，亦有一定作用；用于消渴症，口渴多尿，常与熟地黄、天花粉等同用。

4. 宁神益智：用于心脾两虚，惊悸健忘，疲劳乏力等症，常与黄芪、白术、龙眼肉、酸枣仁等同用；若心肾不交，惊悸失眠，精神恍惚者，可与茯苓、远志、枣仁、龙骨、牡蛎等配伍；如有自汗又常与五味子、白芍、浮小麦等合用。

此外，亦可用治血虚、阳痿之证，可与补血药或温补肾阳药配用。其它对体虚外感或里实体虚不耐攻泻驱邪之患者，亦可少配本品于解表或攻下药中，以加强抗病能力，扶正驱邪。

用量用法 3～10克，大量15～30克。宜文火另煎兑服。研末吞服，每次1～2克，日服2～3次。一般用作补剂，用量宜轻；用于救急，用量宜重。又吉林参药效较缓，用量可稍大；朝鲜参药效较大，用量可稍轻。平素体虚，须服人参调补者，可5～7日服1次。

使用注意 实证、热证而正气不虚者忌服。反藜芦，恶皂荚，均忌同用。服人参不宜喝茶与吃萝卜，以免影响药力。

党 参

为桔梗科多年生草本植物党参 Codonopsis pilosula (Franch.) Nannf.的根。野生者习称野台参，栽培者称潞党参。切片生用。

处方用名 党参、台参、潞党参、野台参、防党。

性味归经 甘，平。入脾、肺经。

功效应用

1. 补中益气：本品善于补脾养胃，健运中气，为临床所常用。治脾胃虚弱，食少便溏，或肺虚咳嗽，气短倦怠，以及各种原因所致气虚体弱之证，多与白术、茯苓、炙甘草同用。本品补气之功类似人参，在一般补气与健脾方中，每以本品代用。唯补气之力较弱，气脱危证不能胜任，仍以人参为宜。

2. 养血生津：用于血虚头晕，或面黄浮肿，可配熟地、当归、白芍、鸡血藤等同用；用于热伤气津，短气口渴，常与麦冬、五味子等同用。

此外，亦可用治肾炎浮肿，可减轻尿蛋白的排出。

用量用法 10～15克。大量可用至30克。煎服。

使用注意 中满邪实者不宜用。

太 子 参

为石竹科多年生草本假繁缕属植物孩儿参 Pseudostellaria heterophylla（Mig）Pax ex Pax et Hoffm 的块根。生用。

处方用名 孩儿参、太子参、童子参。

性味归经 甘、微苦，平，入脾、肺经。

功效应用 健脾补肺，益气生津：用于气虚体弱，疲倦乏力，食欲减退，津少口干，阴虚肺燥，咳嗽痰少，及儿童病后瘦弱无力，体虚自汗等症。为增强疗效，常与其它补气、生津药配用，若用于脾气虚弱，胃阴不足，可与党参、玉竹、山药合用；气阴不足，自汗口渴，可与五味子、黄芪合用；小儿自汗，可与浮小麦配用；阴虚肺燥，咳嗽痰少，可与沙参、麦冬同用。

本品益气生津，补益脾肺之功与人参近似，但药力较弱，是补气药中的一味清补之品。

用量用法 10～30 克。煎服。

黄 芪

为豆科多年生草本植物黄芪 Astragalus membranaceus（Fisch.）Bunge.和内蒙黄芪 A.mongholicus Bunge.的根。切片生用或蜜炙用。

处方用名 生黄芪、炙黄芪。

性味归经 甘，温。入脾、肺经。

功效应用

1. 补气升阳：用于气虚衰弱，体倦乏力，懒言食少等症，常与人参同用，以增强补气之力；若兼阳虚者，可配附子；兼血虚者，可配当归；若血虚发热，或大失血后虚极欲脱之证，需补气生血者，可重用本品与当归同用；用于气虚血滞，四肢麻木及中风后遗症之半身不遂，神清脉弱等症。治血痹，常与桂枝、白芍等同用。若肩臂肢节痹痛者，可加配防风、片姜黄；治半身不遂，可重用本品与桃仁、红花、川芎、地龙等同用。用于中气下陷，内脏下垂，子宫脱垂，久泻脱肛等症，常与人参、升麻、柴胡等同用。

2. 固表止汗：用于体弱表虚，肌表不固之自汗盗汗等症，常与白术、防风同用；亦可与牡蛎、浮小麦、麻黄根等同用。

3. 托毒生肌：用于痈肿疮疡，因气血不足，内陷不起，常与当归、川芎、山甲、皂刺等配伍；若小儿体虚，痘疹内陷，亦可与透疹药同用；用于疮疡溃久，脓稀不愈，常与党参、肉桂同用；如糖尿病并发痈肿、疮疖，可用生黄芪180克、生甘草30克，研末，每次冲服9克，日服2～3次，或水煎服。

4. 利尿消肿：用于心肾阳虚，面目四肢浮肿，小便不利，心悸气短等症，常与白术、防己等同用；若慢性肾炎，尿有蛋白，身面浮肿，可重用本品15～30克煎服。

此外，亦治消渴症，可与山药、生地、天花粉、五味子等配用。

用量用法 10～15克。大剂量可用30～60克，煎服。黄芪蜜炙，补气力强，故专用于补气，宜炙用；用于止汗，利水，托疮生肌，宜生用。

使用注意 本品功偏温补，易于助火，内有实热，肝阳上亢，气火上冲或湿热气滞，或痈疽初起或溃后热毒尚盛，或表实邪盛，须当忌用。

白　术

为菊科多年生草本植物白术 Atractylodes macrocephala Koidz.的根茎。生用、炒用，炒焦用或土炒用。

处方用名 生白术、炒白术、焦白术、土白术。

性味归经 甘、苦，温。入脾、胃经。

功效应用

1. 补脾益气：用于脾胃气虚，运化失常所致的饮食减少，脘腹虚胀，倦怠乏力，大便溏泻等症。本品为健脾补气之要药。常与人参、茯苓、炙甘草同用，如虚寒较甚，可配党参、干姜。

2. 燥湿利水；用于脾不健运，水湿停蓄，症见肢体浮肿，面色苍黄，食欲不振，大便稀溏，神疲肢冷，舌苔薄白，脉沉者，常与渗湿利水药配伍，轻者配茯苓、泽泻、桂枝等，以增强利尿作用；如脾肾虚寒显著者，则需配附子、干姜、或生姜；如水湿内停，结为痰饮，致胸胁支满，头眩者，可与茯苓、桂枝、甘草同用。

3. 固表止汗：用于表虚自汗，尤其是治小儿病后食欲不振，体弱自汗，白术常不可少，可与山药、浮小麦、麻黄根等配用；如阳虚自汗，平日易于伤风感冒者，可与黄芪、防风配伍。

此外，配黄芩可治胎热之胎动不安。还常用于风湿关节疼痛，主要取其祛风湿，镇痛之功。

用量用法 3～10克。煎服。健脾和胃宜用炒白术或焦白术；健脾止泻宜用土白术；利水消肿，固表止汗，风湿痹痛宜用生白术。

使用注意 本品性燥伤阴，阴虚内热，津液不足，烦渴者，皆不宜用。

山　药

为薯蓣科多年蔓生草本植物薯蓣 Dioscorea opposita Thunb. 的块根。切片晒干，生用或炒用。

处方用名 怀山药、生山药、炒山药。

性味归经 甘，平。入脾、肺、肾经。

功效应用

1. 补脾止泻：用于脾胃虚弱，食少体倦，或脾虚泄泻，大便稀溏等症，常与党参、白术、茯苓等同用；如治小儿脾胃虚弱，消化不良，形体消瘦，大便不实等症，可与藿香、半夏、谷芽、建粬等同用。

2. 养肺益阴：用于肺虚喘咳，虚劳咳嗽等症，常与党参、川贝等同用，亦可单用煮汁，代茶常饮。

3. 益肾固精：用于肾虚遗精，或带下尿频等症，可与莲子肉、芡实、白术等同用；如肾阴虚损，又常与熟地、山萸肉等配伍。

4. 养阴生津：用于消渴或阴虚津亏，烦热口渴之症。治轻型消渴，可每日单用本品150克，煎水代茶，长期服用，或与黄芪、葛根、天花粉、知母等配伍；如治津亏口渴，可与麦冬、玉竹等同用。

用量用法 10～30克，大剂量可用60～120克。煎服。如炒研细粉，每次6～10克，吞服。用于养阴宜生用，用于健脾止泻或入丸散剂可炒黄用。

使用注意 脾虚湿盛，胸腹满闷者，不宜应用。

扁　豆

为豆科1年生蔓生草本植物扁豆 Dolichos lablab L.以开白花植株的种子入药。生用或炒用，用时捣碎。

处方用名 白扁豆、生扁豆、炒扁豆。

性味归经 甘、微温。入脾、胃经。

功效应用

1. 健脾止泻：用于脾虚泄泻，妇女带下，常与白术、山药等健脾药同用；亦可单用炒扁豆为末，每服6克，治赤白带下。

2. 消暑化湿：用于夏月暑湿内伤所致的吐泻腹痛，可用炒扁豆、藿香各等分，共为末，每次6克，白水送服；若防治暑病，可与藿香、厚朴、甘草同用。

用量用法 10～15克。煎服。治暑湿，解毒宜生用，健脾和胃宜炒用。

附药

1. 扁豆衣：即白扁豆的干燥种皮，又称扁豆壳。功效与扁豆相同，但药力较差。多用于暑湿吐泻之症。用量 6～10 克。

2. 扁豆花：为扁豆盛开之花，功能解暑化湿，多用于夏令感冒吐泻，暑温发热，痢疾以及妇女崩漏，带下等症。干扁豆花单味可治泻痢脓血。用量同扁豆衣。

甘　草

为豆科多年生草本植物甘草 Glycyrrhiza uralensis Fisch.的根和根茎。切片晒干，生用或蜜炙用。

处方用名　甘草、生甘草、粉甘草、炙甘草、甘草梢。

性味归经　甘，平。入脾、胃、心、肺经。

功效应用

1. 补中益气：用于脾胃气虚诸证，常以炙甘草辅助党参、白术等同用；若用于虚弱劳损，元气不足，体倦乏力，又常辅助党参、黄芪等同用；用于气虚血少，心悸自汗，脉结代等症，常用炙甘草与生地、麦冬、党参、桂枝等配伍。

2. 祛痰止咳：用于咳嗽气喘。治风寒犯肺之咳喘，可配麻黄、杏仁；风热咳嗽，可配桔梗、牛蒡子、前胡、桑叶等；风寒咳嗽，可配麻黄、苏叶、杏仁等；热痰咳嗽，则配瓜蒌、贝母、黄芩、桑皮；寒痰咳嗽，可配干姜、细辛、五味子。

3. 缓急止痛：用于胃痛、腹痛及筋肉挛急疼痛等症。治胃脘剧烈疼痛，服其他药不止者，可用甘草 120 克，白术 30 克，水煎频服；治胃及十二指肠溃疡，可单味熬膏服，或与煅瓦楞子研末服；治脘腹及小腿腓肠肌痛，常与白芍配伍。

4. 清热解毒：用于疮疡肿毒、咽喉肿痛及农药、食物中毒。治肿毒常与银花、连翘等同用；治咽痛，常与桔梗或忍冬藤等配伍；如治农药、食物中毒，常配绿豆煮汤服或与防风水煎服。

5. 调和药性：都于复方中用之，以减低或缓解药物的偏性或毒性。

此外，本品尚兼有利尿作用，传统上用甘草梢作治疗热淋尿痛的辅佐药。

用量用法 3～6克，作主药可用10～30克。煎服。本品生用则通，炙用则补，凡入清泻药中宜生用，入补益药中宜炙用。

使用注意 久服或服量过大，易引起水肿。湿盛胸满腹胀及呕吐不宜用。反大戟、芫花、甘遂。

大　枣

为鼠李科落叶灌木或小乔木枣树 Ziziphus jujuba Mill. var. inermis (Bge.) Rehd.的成熟果实。晒干生用。

处方用名 大枣、红枣。

性味归经 甘，微温。入脾、胃、心、肝经。

功效应用

1. 补脾和营：用于脾胃虚弱，食少倦怠，或脾虚泄泻，营卫不和等症。补脾胃，常与党参、白术同用；调营卫每与生姜配伍。

2. 养心安神：用于虚烦失眠，常与酸枣仁、远志等同用；治脏躁，常与甘草、浮小麦等配伍。

3. 缓和药性：用于药力过猛或辛苦药物较多的方中，取其缓和峻烈之性，以免过烈伤及脾胃，且有矫味作用。

此外，近些年来尚用于血小板减少症及过敏性紫癜等，可单用大剂量持续服用有一定疗效。

用量用法 3～12枚，大量可用30～60克。煎服。入煎剂可劈开。用于缓和矫味或制丸剂时，随方配用。

使用注意 本品能助湿，凡湿阻腹胀满闷，龋齿疼痛等，均不宜服用。

饴　糖

为糯米粉、粳米粉或面粉煮熟，加入麦芽搅合均匀，微火煎熬而成。入药以软饴为主。

处方用名 饴糖。

性味归经 甘，微温。入脾、胃、肺经。

功效应用

1. 补脾缓痛：用于中气虚乏，劳倦伤脾，或虚寒腹痛，喜温喜按等症，通常与桂枝、芍药等配伍；若气虚甚者，可配人参、黄芪；血虚者，可配当归；寒重者，可配干姜、花椒。

2. 润肺止咳：用于肺虚咳嗽，干咳无痰，常与蜂蜜、百部等药同用。

用量用法 30～60克。入汤剂宜溶化服。不入煎。

使用注意 本品味甘易滞，多服易致胀满，故湿热腹满呕吐及痰热咳嗽者忌用。

蜂　蜜

为蜜蜂科昆虫中华蜜蜂 Apis cerana Fabricius 等所酿的蜜糖。原品过滤后生用或经加热炼去水分用。

处方用名 蜂蜜、生蜜、白蜜、黄蜜、炼蜜。

性味归经 甘，平。入肺、脾、大肠经。

功效应用

1. 补中缓急：用于脾胃虚弱，倦怠食少，脘腹作痛。若治胃及十二指肠溃疡，可用蜂蜜60克（冲兑），芍药、甘草各10克，陈皮6克，水煎服。本品因能补养、矫味及调和药性，故滋补药多用蜜丸或收膏，某些补养药用蜜炙后服用，可增强补虚之功。

2. 润肠通便：用于肠燥便秘难解，蜂蜜2汤匙，开水冲服，每天空腹1次，或加香油1汤匙亦可；或制成栓状，纳入肛门内。

3. 润肺止咳：用于肺虚久咳及肺燥干咳。若治干咳无痰，咽喉干燥，可用蜂蜜1茶匙，开水冲服，每日2次。许多止咳化痰药用于润肺止咳，常蜜炙。

此外，本品可用以涂敷疮肿，烫伤，有解毒之功。内服又可解乌头、附子等药物的毒性。

用量用法 15～30 克。入汤剂冲服。不入煎。外用适量。润肠通便解毒宜生用，止咳止痛宜炼用。

使用注意 本品究属滑润之品，湿热积滞，胸痞不舒及脾虚便溏者均不宜用。

17.2 助阳药

助阳药主要用于阳虚病证。阳虚包括心阳虚，脾阳虚，肾阳虚等。由于肾阳为元阳，故阳虚通常多指肾阳虚而言，助阳也都从补肾着手，所以助阳药主要就是温补肾阳。

肾阳虚常表现为全身功能衰退及阳萎、遗泄等症状。助阳药一般具有温肾助阳，补精髓，强筋骨等作用，故主要适用于神倦畏寒，四肢不温，腰膝酸软，阳萎滑精，尿频遗尿等肾阳不足等症。此外，肾火衰微，不能温运脾胃，可以引起泄泻；肾气不足，摄纳无权，每易引起喘促。故助阳药中某些药物，亦可治疗虚性泄泻和气喘。

助阳药性多温燥，阴虚火盛者忌用，以免引起助火劫阴之弊。

鹿　茸

为脊椎动物鹿科梅花鹿 Cervus nippon Temminck 或马鹿 Cervus elaphus L.的雄鹿头上未骨化而带毛茸的幼角。前者习称“花鹿茸”，后者习称“马鹿茸”。切片或研粉生用。

处方用名 鹿茸、鹿茸片、鹿茸粉。

性味归经 甘、咸，温。入肝、肾经。

功效应用 补肾阳，益精血，强筋骨：用于肾阳不足，畏寒乏力，阳萎滑精，遗尿尿频，女子不孕等症。单用或与熟地、山茱萸、巴戟天、补骨脂、淫羊藿等同用；用于虚寒崩漏，可与阿胶、乌贼骨等同用；用于精亏血虚，腰脊酸疼，骨软无力，精神疲倦，眩晕耳鸣等症，常与补肾养血药同用；用于小儿肝肾不足，发育不良，筋骨痿软，行迟齿迟，囟门不合等症，可与熟地、山茱萸、山药等同用。

此外，亦治阴疽久溃，因气血亏虚，脓稀不敛之症。现代亦有用治心脏衰弱，心悸腰酸以及神经衰弱而有肾虚见症者。

用量用法 0.5～1克。研末吞服。或入丸散剂。

使用注意 本品服用宜从小量开始，渐增，不宜骤用大量，以免阳升风动，头晕目赤。凡阴虚阳亢，血分有热者忌用。

附药

1. 鹿角：为梅花鹿和各种雄鹿已成长骨化的角。处方名称鹿角片、鹿角屑。味咸性温，入肾经。炒黄熟用。能补肾壮阳，强健筋骨，可作鹿茸之代用品，惟效力薄弱。生用能活血消肿，多用治疮疡肿毒等症，内服或醋磨涂敷均可，但皆以气弱虚寒之症为宜。用量6～10克，煎服。

2. 鹿角胶：为鹿角煎熬成胶。味甘、咸，性温。入肝肾经。功能温补肝肾，益精养血，惟效能不及鹿茸，但有止血作用。适用于精血不足，虚损劳伤，吐衄崩漏，女子子宫虚寒及阴疽内陷等症。用量6～10克，用开水、黄酒或入药液中化服。

3. 鹿角霜：为熬胶剩余的骨渣。味咸性温，功同鹿角，惟力较逊，可治肾阳不足，血虚精寒，崩中漏下以及脾胃虚寒，呕吐食少等症；外用有收敛止血之功。用量6～10克。煎服。

巴 戟 天

为茜草科多年生缠绕或攀援藤本植物巴戟天 Morinda officinalis How 的根。切段，再以盐水炒用。

处方用名 巴戟、巴戟天、巴戟肉。

性味归经 辛、甘，微温。入肾经。

功效应用

1. 补肾壮阳：用于男子肾阳虚衰，阳萎不举，女子宫冷不孕，经寒不调，下焦虚寒，少腹冷痛以及小便失禁或小便频数等症。通常与补肾固涩药同用。

2. 强筋骨，逐寒湿：用于腰膝风湿疼痛或肌肉萎缩无力，常与杜仲、牛膝、川断、山茱萸等同用。

用量用法 6～10 克。煎服。

使用注意 阴虚火旺，口干舌燥，小便不利者均忌服。

肉 苁 蓉

为列当科 1 年生寄生草本植物苁蓉 Cistanche salsa (G. A. Mey.) G. Beck.的肉质茎。晒干切片入药。

处方用名 淡苁蓉、甜苁蓉。

性味归经 甘、咸，温。入肾、大肠经。

功效应用

1. 补肾壮阳：用于肾虚阳萎，腰膝冷痛及妇女不孕等症，常与补骨脂、菟丝子、蛇床子、巴戟天、沙苑子、山萸肉等同用。

2. 润肠通便：用于老人、体虚，肠燥便秘，常与火麻仁、沉香等同用；若血虚津亏，可配生地、当归。

用量用法 10～18 克，大剂量可用至 30 克。煎服。

使用注意 肾火旺盛，脾虚便溏及实热便秘者忌用。

仙 茅

为石蒜科多年生草本植物仙茅 Curculigo orchioides Gaertn 的根茎。晒干生用。

处方用名 仙茅。

性味归经 辛，热。有小毒。入肾经。

功效应用

1. 温肾壮阳：用于肾阳不足，阳萎精寒，遗精早泄，常与熟地、淫羊藿、枸杞子等同用。

2. 祛寒湿，强筋骨：用于肾虚腰膝酸软，寒湿痹痛，常与通痹止痛药同用。

此外，近年亦常用治妇女更年期高血压病，常与淫羊藿同用。

用量用法 3～10 克。煎服。

使用注意 不宜作补药长期服用。若阴虚火盛，或阳亢之体均忌服。

淫羊藿

为小檗科多年生草本植物淫羊藿 Epimedium grandiflorum Morr.和心叶淫羊藿 Epimedium brevicornum Maxim 或箭叶淫羊藿 E. sagittatum（S. et Z.）Maxim.的茎叶。阴干或晒干，切丝羊脂炙用。

处方用名 淫羊藿、仙灵脾。

性味归经 辛、甘，温。入肝、肾经。

功效应用

1. 补肾壮阳：用于肾阳虚衰，阳萎不举，腰膝无力，小便不禁及妇女不孕等症，可单用本品 30 克，浸米酒 1 斤，每次 5 毫升，日服 3 次，或与其他补肾药同用。

2. 祛风除湿：用于风寒湿痹，下肢瘫痪，筋骨拘挛，手足麻木等症，可与桑寄生、秦艽等通痹止痛药同用。

此外，本品又治妇女更年期高血压而有阴阳两虚见症者，可与仙茅、巴戟天、黄柏、知母等补阳滋阴药同用。

用量用法 6～10 克。煎服。

使用注意 本品性较燥烈，能伤阴助火，故阴虚火盛，阳强易举者忌用。

杜　仲

为杜仲科落叶乔木杜仲 Eucommia ulmoides Oliv.的树皮。晒干，切块，盐水炒断丝用。

处方用名　杜仲、杜仲炭。

性味归经　甘，温。入肝、肾经。

功效应用

1. 补肝肾，强筋骨：用于肝肾不足，腰膝酸痛，筋骨无力及阳萎，尿频等症，通常与续断、牛膝、熟地、山茱萸等补肝肾药配伍；若寒湿腰痛，可配桂枝、独活、秦艽等；妇女经期腰痛，可与当归、川芎、白芍等同用。

2. 固经安胎：用于妇女崩漏及孕妇体虚，胎漏胎动等症，常用杜仲炭、续断与其他补益固经药同用。

此外，又治高血压病而有肾虚见症者，因其有降压之功，可与桑寄生、牛膝及夏枯草等配伍。

用量用法　10～15 克。大量可用至 30～60 克。煎服。

使用注意　阴虚火旺者不宜用。

续　断

为山萝卜科多年生草本植物川续断 Dipsacus asper Wall.或续断 Dipsacus japonicus Miq.的根。晒干，切片生用。

处方用名　续断、川断、川断肉。

性味归经　苦、甘、辛，微温。入肝、肾经。

功效应用

1. 补肝益肾，活络止痛：用于肝肾不足，血脉不利之腰腿酸痛，足膝无力，或风寒湿痹，筋骨拘挛等症。常与杜仲、牛膝、木瓜等同用。

2. 续筋骨，疗折伤：用于跌打损伤，挫伤，扭伤及闭合性骨折，常与乳香、没药、自然铜、土鳖虫、骨碎补等同用。

3. 固经止痛：用于妇女崩漏带下及胎动胎漏等症，常与当归、熟地、阿胶、艾叶等同用。

用量用法 10～15克。煎服。

狗 脊

为蚌壳蕨科大形蕨类多年生草本植物金毛狗脊 Cibotium barometz (L.) J. Sm.的根茎。除去根及毛茸，砂烫切片用。

处方用名 狗脊、金毛狗脊。

性味归经 苦、甘，温。入肝、肾经。

功效应用

1. 补肝肾，壮腰脊：用于肝肾不足，腰痛脊强，俯仰不利，膝痛脚弱，筋骨无力以及小便失禁，妇女带下等症，常与杜仲、桑寄生、菟丝子、牛膝、熟地、山茱萸、鹿角胶等配用。

2. 祛风湿，利关节：用于风湿痹痛，肢体麻木，腰膝酸软，足弱无力等症，常与补养气血，通痹活络药同用。

用量用法 3～10克。煎服。

骨 碎 补

为水龙骨科多年附生蕨类植物槲蕨 Drynaria fortunei (Kunze) J. Sm.的根茎。砂烫去毛，用时捣碎。

处方用名 骨碎补。

性味归经 苦，温。入肝、肾经。

功效应用

1. 补肾固齿止痛：用于肾虚腰痛，脚弱，耳鸣，耳聋，齿痛等症，常与熟地、山茱萸、补骨脂等同用。

2.活血续筋疗伤：用于筋骨折伤，可与续断、乳香、没药等同用。亦可研末外敷。

此外，亦治肾虚久泄。

用量用法 3～10克。煎服。外用适量。

补 骨 脂

为豆科1年生草本植物补骨脂 Psoralea corylifolia L.的种子。晒干，盐水炒用。

处方用名 补骨脂、破故纸。

性味归经 辛、苦，温。入肾、脾经。

功效应用

1. 补肾壮阳，固精缩尿：用于肾阳不足，阳萎，遗精，尿频遗尿，腰膝冷痛等症，常与菟丝子、续断、山药、仙灵脾等同用。

2. 温脾止泻：用于脾肾阳虚，五更泄泻，肠鸣腹痛，泻后则安，常与肉豆蔻同用。

此外，又治虚寒喘咳，每与胡桃肉、蜂蜜等配伍。

用量用法 3～10克。煎服。

使用注意 阴虚有火及大便燥结者忌用。

益 智 仁

为姜科多年生草本植物益智 Alpinia oxyphylla Miq.的成熟果实。去壳取仁，盐水拌炒用。

处方用名 益智仁。

性味归经 辛，温。入脾、肾经。

功效应用

1. 补肾固精，缩小便：用于肾虚遗精，遗尿尿频及白浊等症，常与菟丝子、桑螵蛸及山药、乌药等同用。

2. 温脾止泻，摄涎唾：用于脾胃虚寒，腹中冷痛，吐泻食少或时唾清涎，常与党参、白术、干姜、砂仁等同用。

用量用法 3～10克。煎服。

使用注意 阴虚火旺及症属湿热者忌用。

冬虫夏草

为麦角菌科植物冬虫夏草菌 Cordyceps sinensis（Serk.）Sacc.的子座及其寄主蝙蝠蛾科昆虫绿蝙蝠蛾 Hepialus varians staudinger 幼虫尸体等的复合体。晒干或烘干。生用。

处方用名 冬虫草、冬虫夏草。

性味归经 甘，温。入肾、肺经。

功效应用 滋肺补肾，止血化痰：用于劳嗽痰血，阳萎遗精及病后虚损不复等症，均可单用持续服用。治阴虚劳嗽，咳血胸痛，常与川贝、麦冬、阿胶、沙参等同用。若治阳萎遗精，腰酸腿软，可与杜仲、淫羊藿、肉苁蓉等同用。

用量用法 6～10 克。煎服。研末服，每次 1.5～3 克。

蛤蚧

为守宫科动物蛤蚧 Gekko gecko（L.）除去内脏的干燥品。用时去头足，洗去鳞皮间之不洁物，炙酥研粉用。

处方用名 蛤蚧、蛤蚧尾。

性味归经 咸，平，有小毒。入肺、肾、心经。

功效应用 补肺益肾，纳气定喘：用于肺肾两虚，肾不纳气之久喘或虚劳咳嗽，痰中带血等症，常与人参、胡桃肉、百部、紫菀及五味子、川贝母等同用；若治肾虚阳萎，遗精尿频等，可单用研末服或与人参、五味子、胡桃肉、巴戟天等同用。

用量用法 研末服，每次 1～1.5 克。制丸散或浸酒服均可。不宜入煎。

使用注意 咳喘由风寒外邪及实热所致者均忌用。

胡桃肉

为胡桃科落叶乔木胡桃 Juglans regia L.果实的核仁。生用或炒用。

处方用名　胡桃肉、核桃肉、胡桃仁。

性味归经　甘，温。入肾、肺、大肠经。

功效应用

1. 补肾强腰：用于肾虚腰痛，常与补骨脂、杜仲等补肾药同用。

2. 敛肺定喘：用于肺肾虚喘，常与人参、蛤蚧或紫菀、冬花等同用。

此外，又可用于老人或病后肠燥便秘，可单用或与肉苁蓉、火麻仁、当归等同用。近年亦常与金钱草、鸡内金、滑石、海金沙等配伍，治疗肾结石腰痛。

用量用法　10～30克。煎服。以烤熟嚼服为宜，每次可嚼食3～5枚。

使用注意　不宜与浓茶同服。

紫　河　车

为健康产妇的胎盘。研粉用。

处方用名　胎盘粉、紫河车。

性味归经　甘、咸，温。入肺、肝、肾经。

功效应用

1. 补肾益精：用于肝肾不足，虚损劳伤，阳萎遗精，潮热盗汗等症，单用研末服，或与熟地、龟板等同用。

2. 补血益气：用于气血亏虚，消瘦乏力，面色萎黄以及产后体弱乳少，单用研末服，或与人参、熟地等其他补益气血药同用。

3. 补肺止咳：用于肺肾阴亏，喘嗽咯血，单用研末服，或与川贝母、百部、天冬、五味子等同用。

用量用法　每次1.5～3克。入丸散或片剂。

菟丝子

为旋花科1年寄生蔓草菟丝子 Cuscuta chinensis Lam.或大菟丝子 Cuscuta japonica Choisy 的种子。原药酒浸用，或捣烂制成饼用。

处方用名 菟丝子、菟丝饼。

性味归经 甘、辛，平。入肝、肾经。

功效应用

1. 补肾益精：用于肾虚阳萎，遗精耳鸣，腰膝酸痛，小便频数等症，常与枸杞子、覆盆子、五味子或补骨脂、杜仲等配伍，若兼肾阴不足，可配熟地、山药等同用。

2. 养肝明目：用于肝肾不足，视力减退，目暗，目眩等症，可与熟地、枸杞子、桑椹子、女贞子等同用。

3. 益脾止泻：用于脾肾两虚，食欲不振，大便溏泻，可与山药、莲子、党参、茯苓等配伍。

此外，与补肾、调经药配伍，亦可用治肾虚胎动、先兆流产及月经不调等症。

用量用法 10～15克。煎服。

使用注意 阴虚火旺，大便燥结者忌用。

沙苑子

为豆科1年生草本植物扁茎黄芪 Astragalus complanatus R. Br.的成熟种子。生用或盐水炒过用。

处方用名 沙苑子、潼蒺藜。

性味归经 甘，温。入肾、肝经。

功效应用

1. 补肾固精：用于肾虚不足，腰膝酸痛，遗精早泄，小便不禁等症，常与山药、莲须及鱼鳔胶等同用。

2. 养肝明目：用于肝肾不足，目暗不明，头晕眼花，可单用为散，或与熟地、枸杞子、女贞子等配伍。

用量用法 10～15克。煎服。

使用注意 阴虚火旺及小便不利者忌服。

17.3 养血药

养血药主要用于血虚的病症。血虚的一般症状是：面色无华，唇甲苍白，眩晕，心悸，女子月经不调等。养血药主要用于上述诸症。应用时，如血虚而兼气虚者，宜配用补气药；血虚而兼阴虚者，须配以补阴药；脾胃虚弱者，应与健脾胃药合用。

本类药物性多粘腻，如湿滞中满，食少便溏者忌用。

熟 地

为玄参科多年生草本植物地黄 Rehmannia glutinosa (Gaertn.) Libosch 的块根经蒸制而成。切片用。

处方用名 熟地、熟地黄。

性味归经 甘，微温。入心、肝、肾经。

功效应用

1. 补血调经：用于心肝血虚，头晕心悸及妇女崩漏，月经不调等症，常与当归、白芍、川芎等同用。

2. 滋肾育阴：用于肾阴不足，骨蒸潮热、盗汗、遗精、腰膝酸软及消渴等症，常与山茱萸、山药或知母、龟板等同用。

用量用法 15～30克，大剂量可用30～60克。煎服。

使用注意 惟药性粘腻，易于助湿碍胃，凡脾弱有湿及痰多气郁患者忌服。

何 首 乌

为蓼科多年生缠绕草本植物何首乌 Polygonum multiflorum Thunb.的块根。切片生用或制用。

处方用名 制首乌、生首乌。

性味归经 苦、甘、涩，微温。入肝、肾经。

功效应用

1. 补肝肾，益精血（制用）：用于肝肾不足，血虚阴亏，心悸失眠，头晕耳鸣，腰膝酸软，崩带遗精等症，常与枣仁、白芍、熟地、当归、龙骨等随症选用；若血虚精亏，须发早白，脱发等症，可与熟地、生侧柏、女贞子等同用，或与熟地、当归、羌活等同用。

2. 通便治疮，截疟（生用）：用于血虚津亏，肠燥便秘，可单用煎服，鲜者更佳；用于阴虚瘰疬，痈肿疮毒，可随症配伍；若治血虚风疹，可与生地、当归、蝉蜕、白蒺藜等配合；如治疮癣瘙痒，可与艾叶煎汤外洗；用于久疟不止，属气血两虚者，可与党参、当归等煎服。

此外，本品能治精子生成不良症，单用制首乌常服。

用量用法 10～15克。煎服。补血益精宜制用，通便治疮宜生用。

附药 夜交藤：为何首乌的藤，又名首乌藤。味甘，性平。入心、肝经。功能养心安神，止痒通络。可用于不寐，多汗，血虚肢体酸痛，并可单用外洗皮肤痒疹者。用量15～30克。煎汤服。外用适量，煎汤洗。

当 归

为伞形科多年生草本植物当归 Angelica sinensis（Oliv.）Diels的根。生用或酒炒用。

处方用名 当归、全当归、当归身、当归尾、酒当归。

性味归经 甘、辛、苦，温。入肝、心、脾经。

功效应用

1. 补血调经：用于心肝血虚，月经不调、经闭痛经等症，常与川芎、白芍、地黄等同用；若上症属血滞者，可再配活血行气药同用。

2. 活血止痛：用于跌打损伤，痈疽疮疡，风湿痹痛，及经产血滞疼痛等症，常与乳香、没药或桃仁、红花、穿山甲等同用。

3. 润肠通便：用于血虚肠燥便秘，常与火麻仁、生首乌、肉苁蓉等同用。

用量用法 6～15克。煎服。补血宜用当归身，活血宜用当归尾，和血宜用全当归。补血润肠可生用，通络活血可酒炒。

使用注意 湿盛中满，大便泄泻者不宜用。

白芍药

为毛茛科多年生草本植物芍药 Paeonia lactiflora Pall.的根。晒干切片。生用或酒炒、清炒用。

处方用名 白芍、生白芍、酒芍、炒杭芍。

性味归经 苦、酸，微寒。入肝、脾经。

功效应用

1. 补血敛阴：用于血虚月经不调，痛经，崩漏等症，常与当归、川芎、熟地等同用；用于外感风寒，表虚自汗而恶风，可与桂枝同用，以调和营卫，亦可用于盗汗。

2. 柔肝止痛：用于肝气不和所致之胸、肋、胃、腹疼痛等症，常与柴胡、香附等疏肝解郁药同用；用于脘腹疼痛，四肢拘挛疼痛，常与甘草同用；用于泻痢腹痛，常与黄连、黄芩、木香等同用。

3. 养阴平肝：用于肝阴不足，肝阳亢盛之头痛，眩晕等症，常与生地、石决明、钩藤、菊花等同用。

用量用法 6～12克。煎服。敛阴平肝治痢多生用，柔肝和脾止痛多炒用，酒炒减其寒性。

阿胶

为马科动物驴 Eguus asinus L.的皮，经漂泡去毛后熬制而成的胶块。原药打碎用，或用蛤粉、蒲黄粉炒成珠用。

处方用名 生阿胶、阿胶珠。

性味归经 甘，平。入肝、肺、肾经。

功效应用

1. 补血止血：用于虚性失血，吐血，咳血等症，常与生地、麦冬等配伍；若治胎产崩漏，又常与艾叶、当归、白芍等同用。

2. 滋阴润燥：用于阴虚心烦失眠，常与黄连、鸡子黄，黄芩、白芍、生地等同用；用于肺虚有热之燥咳，常与杏仁、马兜铃、牛蒡子等同用；用于阴血亏虚，不能养筋所致之痉厥抽搐，可与龟板、牡蛎、鸡子黄等同用。

用量用法 6～15 克。滋阴润燥可生用，烊化冲服；止血宜蒲黄炒，清肺宜蛤粉炒用。

使用注意 生阿胶能腻胃，凡脾胃虚弱，消化不良者均不宜用。

龙 眼 肉

为无患子科常绿乔木龙眼树 Euphoria longan (Lour.) Steud.的成熟果实。取肉去核，晒干用。

处方用名 桂园肉、龙眼肉、元肉。

性味归经 甘，平。入心、脾经。

功效应用 养血安神：用于心血不足的失眠、健忘、惊悸怔忡等症，常与酸枣仁、远志、茯苓等同用。

用量用法 6～12 克。煎服。

17.4 滋阴药

凡具有养阴、增液、润燥等作用，适用于阴虚液亏诸症者称为滋阴药，亦称养阴药。如肺阴伤多见干咳、咯血、虚热，烦渴；胃阴伤多见舌红欲饮，甚或呕哕；肝阴虚多见视力减退，夜盲、头晕、耳鸣、指甲干枯、睡眠不宁；肾阴伤则潮热、盗汗等。滋阴药各有专长，可随症选用。

北 沙 参

为伞形科多年生草本植物珊瑚菜 Glehnia littoralis F. Schmidt ex Miq.的根。切段或切片生用。

处方用名　北沙参。

性味归经　甘、微苦，微寒。入肺、胃经。

功效应用

1. 润肺止咳：本品能清肺热，补肺阴，可用于肺热燥咳，干咳少痰或久咳声哑，常与麦冬、玉竹、花粉等同用。

2. 养胃生津：用于热病伤津，咽干口渴之症，常与麦冬、玉竹等同用。

用量用法　10～15克。煎服。

麦 门 冬

为百合科多年生草本植物沿阶草 Ophiopogon japonicus Ker–Gawl.或大叶麦冬 Liriope spicata Lour.的块根。晒干，原药生用。

处方用名　麦门冬、麦冬、寸冬。

性味归经　甘、微苦，微寒。入肺、心、胃经。

功效应用　润肺清心，养胃生津：用于肺胃阴伤之虚劳咳嗽，咽干口燥，干咳痰稠，常与半夏、党参等同用，或与天冬等分，加蜂蜜收膏，每次用开水冲服1～2匙，日3次，饭前服；用于津伤口渴，常与沙参、生地黄等同用；用于热性病邪热犯心，心烦不寐，常与犀角、生地、丹参等同用；用于津液不足，肠燥便秘，常与生地、玄参同用。

用量用法　6～12克。煎服。

使用注意　虚寒泄泻及外感咳嗽均忌用。

天 门 冬

为百合科攀援状多年生草本植物天门冬 Asparagus cochinchinensis (Lour.) Merr.的块根。切段生用。

处方用名 天门冬、天冬。

性味归经 甘、微苦，寒。入肺、肾经。

功效应用 润肺滋肾，清热化痰：用于肺热燥咳，痰稠难咯，或咳血等症，常与麦冬同用；用于阴虚津亏口渴之症，常与熟地、人参等同用；用于肠燥便秘，可与生地、当归、火麻仁、玄参等同用。

用量用法 6～12克。煎服。

石 斛

为兰科多年生常绿草本植物金钗石斛 Dendrobium nobile Lindll.或其多种同属植物的茎。切段生用或鲜用。

处方用名 金石斛、川石斛、霍石斛、鲜石斛。

性味归经 甘，寒。入肺、胃、肾经。

功效应用 养胃生津，滋阴除热：用于热病伤津，口燥烦渴，常与鲜生地、鲜麦冬、天花粉、玉竹等同用；用于胃痛干呕，常与藿香、丹皮、橘皮等同用；用于阴虚发热，常与麦冬、生地、玄参等同用。

用量用法 6～12克，鲜者15～30克。煎服。鲜石斛清热生津之力尤大，干石斛较差，所以热病伤津，舌绛烦渴当用鲜石斛，一般阴虚舌干可用干石斛，宜久煎。

使用注意 本品能恋邪助湿，故温热病尚未化燥者不宜早用，而湿温尤当忌用。

玉 竹

为百合科多年生草本植物玉竹 Polygonatum odoratum

(Mill.) Druce var. pluriflorum (Miq.) Ohwi 的根茎。晒干，切片蒸后用。

处方用名 玉竹、葳蕤。

性味归经 甘，微寒。入肺、胃经。

功效应用 养阴润燥，生津止渴：用于肺燥咳嗽，咽干痰稠，常配沙参、麦门冬等同用；用于肺胃燥热，津伤口渴，或胃热炽盛，烦渴之症，常配沙参、麦冬、甘草等同用；用于阴虚感冒，头痛发热，咳嗽，口干，咽痛等症，常与白薇、桔梗、薄荷、葱白等同用。

用量用法 10～30 克。煎服。

黄　精

为百合科多生草本植物黄精 Polygonatum sibiricum Redoute 或囊丝黄精 Polygonatum cyrtonema Hua 以及同属多种植物的根茎。切段黄酒蒸熟用。

处方用名 黄精。

性味归经 甘，平。入脾、肺、肾经。

功效应用

1. 滋阴润肺：用于肺阴不足，干咳无痰，可单用熬膏服，或与沙参、知母、川贝母等清养润肺药同用；用于肾精亏损，腰膝酸软，须发早白，可与天冬、侧柏叶、苍术、地骨皮等共研，制蜜丸服。

2. 补中益气：用于脾胃虚弱，倦怠食少，或病后虚羸，体倦乏力等症，常与党参、黄芪同用；若气虚精亏，可与熟地、枸杞配伍。

用量用法 10～30 克。煎服。

百　合

为百合科多年生草本植物百合 Lilium brownii F. E. Brown

var. colchesteri Wils.或细叶百合 Lilium pumilum DC.的肉质鳞茎。生用或蜜炙用。

处方用名 生百合、炙百合。

性味归经 甘，微寒。入心、肺经。

功效应用

1. 润肺止咳：用于肺燥咳嗽，痰中带血之症，可与冬花熬膏服，或与生地、麦冬、川贝、玄参等同用。

2. 清心安神：用于热病后期，余热未清，虚烦惊悸，失眠多梦等症，常与知母或生地同用。

用量用法 10～30克。煎服。清心宜生用，润肺宜炙用。

枸 杞 子

为茄科多年生落叶灌木枸杞 Lycium chinense Mill.或宁夏枸杞 Lycium barbarum L.的果实。生用。

处方用名 枸杞、甘枸杞、枸杞子。

性味归经 甘，平。入肝、肾经。

功效应用

1. 滋补肝肾：用于肾虚精亏，腰脊酸痛等症，可与黄精同用。

2. 养肝明目：用于肝肾阴虚，头晕目眩，视力减退者，常与菊花、熟地等同用。

用量用法 10～15克。煎服。

女 贞 子

为木樨科常绿大灌木或小乔木女贞 Ligustrum lucidum Ait 的果实。黄酒蒸熟晒干用。

处方用名 女贞子、女贞实。

性味归经 甘、苦，凉。入肝、肾经。

功效应用 滋肾益肝，乌发明目：用于肝肾阴虚，骨蒸劳热，腰膝酸软，须发早白等症，常与旱莲草同用；用于肝肾阴亏之目暗不明，常与生地、枸杞子、菊花、沙苑子等同用。

用量用法 10～15克。煎服。

桑 椹 子

为桑科落叶乔木桑树 Morus alba L.的成熟果穗。生用，或加蜜熬膏用。

处方用名 桑椹子、黑桑椹、桑椹膏。

性味归经 甘、酸，寒。入心、肝、肾经。

功效应用 滋阴补血：用于阴血虚少，眩晕、失眠等，可与女贞子、旱莲草各等分，研末蜜丸用；用于津少口渴或消渴，常与生地、麦冬、花粉等同用；用于阴亏血虚之肠燥便秘，可单用熬膏用，或与地黄水煎，加蜂蜜少许冲服。

用量用法 10～15克。煎服。桑椹膏15～30克，冲服。

旱 莲 草

为菊科1年生草本植物鳢肠草 Eclipta alba（L.）Hassk.的全草。切段生用。

处方用名 旱莲草、墨旱莲。

性味归经 甘、酸，寒。入肝、肾经。

功效应用 养肝益肾，凉血止血：用于肝肾阴虚，头昏目眩，须发早白等症，常与女贞子、桑椹子等同用；用于阴虚血热所致各种出血症，如咯血，衄血，便血，尿血及妇女崩漏等。单用即有效；也常与滋阴凉血止血药配伍同用。

此外，外伤出血，可用鲜品捣敷。

用量用法 6～15克。煎服。外用适量。

龟 板

为脊椎动物龟科乌龟 Chinemys reevesii（Gray）的腹甲。

生用或醋炙用。

处方用名 生龟板、炙龟板。

性味归经 咸、甘，平。入肾、肝经。

功效应用

1. 滋阴潜阳：用于阴虚火旺，骨蒸劳热，盗汗，常与黄柏、知母、熟地等同用；用于阴虚阳亢，头晕目眩之症，常与天冬、玄参、龙骨、牡蛎等同用；用于温热病后，热邪伤阴，筋脉拘挛，手足抽动之症，常与白芍、麦冬、生地等同用。

2. 益肾强骨：用于肾阴亏虚，腰脚痿弱，筋骨不健，及小儿囟门不合等症，常与虎骨、熟地、白芍等同用。

3. 固经止崩：用于阴虚血热，月经过多，崩漏带下等症，常与白芍、黄柏、椿根皮、香附等同用。

用量用法 10～30克。煎服。滋阴煎服宜生用；入丸散宜炙用。入汤剂宜先煎。

使用注意 凡脾胃虚寒，外感邪气未解者均忌用。

鳖　甲

为脊椎动物鳖 Amyda sinensis（Weigmann）的背甲。生用或醋炙用。

处方用名 生鳖甲、炙鳖甲。

性味归经 咸，寒。入肝、脾经。

功效应用

1. 滋阴退蒸：用于阴虚劳热，骨蒸盗汗，常与秦艽、地骨皮、知母等同用；亦可用于温热病后期阴液耗伤，夜热早凉等症，常与青蒿、丹皮、生地等同用；若温邪伤阴，深入下焦，舌干齿黑，手指蠕动。本品能滋阴潜阳，可与生地、阿胶、白芍、牡蛎等同用。

2. 软坚散结：用于肝脾肿大及腹中瘀块等症，常与香附、青皮、三棱、莪术等同用。

用量用法 10～30 克。煎服。滋阴煎服宜生用；软坚散结或入丸散宜炙用。入汤剂宜先煎。

18 收涩药

凡以收敛固涩为主要作用的药物，称为收涩药。又称固涩药。

本类药物大多具有酸、涩的性味，有收敛固涩之功，可以治疗各种滑脱的病证。

滑脱的症证，主要有自汗盗汗，久咳虚喘，遗精滑精，溲多遗尿，久泻脱肛，失血崩漏，带下日久等症。

应用收涩药的目的在于及时敛其耗散，防止因滑脱不禁而致正气渐衰，变生它症。本类药物仅能治病之标，不能治病之本。滑脱证的病因是正气虚弱，所以临床需与相应的补益药配伍，以期标本兼顾。

本类药物具有敛汗、止嗽、固精，缩小便，止泻，止血，止带等作用。凡外感实邪未解，或泻痢，咳嗽初起时不宜早用，以免留邪。

五 味 子

为木兰科多年生落叶木质藤本植物五味子 Schisandra chinensis（Turcz.）Baill.的成熟果实。捣碎用。

处方用名 五味子、北五味。

性味归经 酸，温。入肺、心、肾经。

功效应用

1. 敛肺止咳：用于肺虚喘咳，常与党参、麦冬、杏仁等同用。

2. 固表敛汗：用于阴虚盗汗或阳虚自汗，常与牡蛎、白术、麻黄根等同用。

3. 涩精止泻：用于肾虚精滑不固，常与桑螵蛸、附子、龙骨等同用；用于脾肾虚寒，五更泄泻，常与肉豆蔻、吴茱萸等同用。

4. 生津止渴：用于津液不足，口干作渴，常与党参、麦冬同用。

5. 宁心安神：用于心肾阴血亏损所致的虚烦心悸，失眠多梦，可与生地、麦冬、丹参、枣仁等同用。

此外，本品研末内服，对慢性肝炎转氨酶升高者，有降低作用。

用量用法 3～10克。煎服。用于敛肺镇咳量宜少（1.5～3克），用于滋补益阴量可稍大（6～10克）。

使用注意 凡表邪未解，麻疹初起咳喘者，均当忌服。

乌　梅

为蔷薇科落叶小乔木梅 Prunus mume（sieb.）Sieb. et Zucc. 未成熟的绿色果实（青梅）。生用或炒炭用。

处方用名 乌梅肉、乌梅炭。

性味归经 酸、涩，平。入肺、脾、大肠经。

功效应用

1. 敛肺止咳：用于肺虚久咳，可与罂粟壳、杏仁、阿胶等同用。

2. 涩肠止泻：用于久泻久痢，可与肉豆蔻、党参、木香等同用。

3. 生津止渴：用于虚热消渴，可与麦冬、花粉、葛根等同用。

4. 和胃安蛔：用于肠蛔虫病腹痛、呕吐等症，常与黄连、黄柏、干姜、川椒等同用；用于胆道蛔虫病，可与乌梅、茵陈各30克，水煎，每剂分为两次服，每2小时1次，连服4次。

5. 固下止血：用于大便下血，尿血，崩漏不止等，乌梅炭研末，醋丸梧子大，每次30丸，日服3次，或配方煎服。

此外，又可用于牙关紧闭，以乌梅擦之；用于痈疽溃后胬肉外突，以乌梅炭为末，外敷；治胼胝，鸡眼，可用生梅肉配轻粉研末，醋调敷。

用量用法 3～10克，大剂量可用至30克。煎服。外用适量。止血宜炒炭。

五 倍 子

为倍蚜科昆虫角倍蚜 Melaphis chinensis（Bell）或倍蛋蚜 Melaphis paitan Tsai et Tang 寄生于漆树科落叶灌木或小乔木盐肤木、青麸扬和红麸扬叶上虫瘿。生用或煅用。

处方用名 五倍子。

性味归经 酸、咸，寒。入肝、胃、大肠经。

功效应用

1. 敛肺降火：用于肺虚久咳，常与五味子、罂粟壳等敛肺药同用。

2. 涩肠止泻：用于久泻久痢、脱肛等症，可单用，或与诃子、五味子等同用。

3. 涩精缩尿：用于遗精、遗尿，可与茯苓同用。

4. 敛汗生津：用于盗汗，取五倍子末，水调为膏，敷肚脐上，纱布固定，晚敷晨去，治消渴，可单用内服。

5. 收敛止血：用于崩漏下血、便血等，常与乌梅、艾叶炭等收敛止血药同用。

此外，研末外敷或煎汤熏洗，可用于疮癣肿毒，皮肤湿烂，脱肛不收，子宫下垂等症。

用量用法 3～6克。煎服。宜入丸散剂。外用适量。

麻 黄 根

为麻黄科多年生草本状小灌木草麻黄 Ephedra sinica Stapf

或木贼麻黄 E. eguisetina Bge.的根。切段用。

处方用名 麻黄根。

性味归经 甘；平。入肺经。

功效应用 止汗：用于自汗，盗汗等症，可随症配用。若治表虚自汗，可与黄芪、白术等补气药同用；治阳虚自汗，可与人参、附子等补阳药同用；治阴虚盗汗，可与熟地、山茱萸、龙骨、牡蛎等滋阴收敛药同用；治产后虚汗，可与当归、黄芪等养血固表药同用。

用量用法 3～10 克。煎服。外用适量，研末作扑粉。

使用注意 有表邪者忌用。

浮 小 麦

为禾本科 1 年生草本植物小麦 Tritcum aestivum L.的干燥瘪瘦的果实。生用或炒用。

处方用名 浮小麦。

性味归经 甘，凉。入心经。

功效应用 益气除热止汗：用于盗汗，可用浮小麦适量炒为末，米汤送服，或煎服；用于自汗，可与黄芪、牡蛎、麻黄根等同用；用于骨蒸虚热，可用浮小麦 30 克，地骨皮 10 克，水煎服。

用量用法 15～30 克。煎服。入散剂内服可炒用。

附药 小麦：为生长成熟的小麦。味甘，性凉。入心经。功能养心除烦。适用于妇女脏躁，悲伤欲哭之症，常与甘草、大枣同用。用量 30～60 克。煎汤服。

椿 皮

为楝科植物落叶乔木椿树（香椿）Toona sinensis（A. Juss.）Roem.或樗树（臭椿）Ailanthus altissima（Mill.）Swingle 的根皮。生用或炒用。

处方用名 椿根皮、樗根皮。

性味归经 苦、涩，寒。入胃、大肠经。

功效应用

1. 燥湿清热：用于赤白带下，常与黄柏、高良姜、白芍、当归等同用；若治湿热带下，可与芍药、黄柏、贯众等同用。

2. 涩肠止泻：用于久泻久痢，可与诃子、木香、丁香等同用。

3. 固下止血：用于妇女阴虚火旺，月经过多，经色紫黑等症，可与龟板、黄柏等同用；治便血，亦可单味为末服。

此外，煎汤外洗可治疥癣湿疮，有燥湿清热之功。

用量用法 3～10克。煎服。

诃　子

为使君子科落叶乔木诃子树 Terminalia chebula Retz.的成熟果实。生用或煨用。

处方用名 诃子、诃子皮、诃子肉、煨诃子。

性味归经 酸、苦，平。入肺、大肠经。

功效应用

1. 涩肠止泻：用于久泻久痢，可与黄连、木香等同用；或与罂粟、干姜等同用。

2. 敛肺止咳：用于肺虚喘咳或久咳失音，可用诃子、桔梗9克，甘草6克，水煎服。

用量用法 3～10克。敛肺降火宜生用，涩肠止泻宜煨熟用。

肉豆蔻

为肉豆蔻科高大乔木植物肉豆蔻树 Myristica fragrans Houtt.的成熟种仁。面裹煨去油用。

处方用名 肉豆蔻、肉果、玉果、煨肉果。

性味归经　辛，温。入脾、胃、大肠经。

功效应用

1. 涩肠止泻：用于脾胃虚寒，久泻不止，脱肛等症，可与诃子、罂粟、党参、白术、肉桂等同用；若治脾肾虚寒，五更泄泻，可与补骨脂、吴茱萸、五味子同用。

2. 温中行气：用于脾胃虚寒，脘腹胀痛，食欲不振，呕吐等症，可与木香、姜半夏等同用。

用量用法　3～10克。煎服。

赤　石　脂

为单斜晶系的多水高领土 Halloysite。研粉水飞或火煅水飞用。

处方用名　赤石脂。

性味归经　甘、酸、涩，温。入肾、大肠经。

功效应用

1. 涩肠止泻：用于久泻久痢不止，或便血等症，可与干姜、粳米、或党参、白术、龙骨等同用。

2. 敛血止血：用于便血及妇女月经过多，崩漏带下属于虚寒者，常与侧柏叶、乌贼骨烧煅为末服。

3. 生肌收口：用于痈疮溃疡，疮口不敛，常与象皮、龙骨、血竭等同用。

用量用法　10～20克。煎服。

禹　余　粮

为斜方晶系褐铁矿的矿石。打碎火煅用。

处方用名　禹余粮、余粮石。

性味归经　甘、涩，平。入胃、大肠经。

功效应用

1. 涩肠止泻：用于久泻久痢不止，常与赤石脂同用。

2. 敛血止血：用于便血，痢血及崩漏，带下等症，可与赤石脂、乌贼骨、伏龙肝、煅牡蛎、肉桂等分为末，每次6克，日2次，黄酒送服。

用量用法 10～24克。煎服。

罂粟壳

为罂粟科1年生或2年生草本植物罂粟 Papaver somniferum L.的成熟蒴果的外壳。醋炒或蜜炙用。

处方用名 罂粟壳、御米壳、炙米壳。

性味归经 酸、涩，平。入肺、大肠、肾经。

功效应用

1. 敛肺止咳：用于久咳虚嗽等症，可与乌梅同用。

2. 涩肠止泻：用于泄泻不止，可与大枣同用；用于久痢及血痢等症，可与木香、黄连、生姜等同用。

3. 止痛；用于胃腹及筋骨肌肉疼痛，可单用，或随症配用。

用量用法 3～10克。煎服。止咳可蜜炙用，止泻，止痛可醋炒用。

使用注意 咳嗽及泻痢初起忌服。本品有毒，不可过量及持续服用。

莲子

为睡莲科多年生水生草本植物莲 Nelumbo nucifera Gaertn.的种仁。去心，打碎用。

处方用名 莲子、莲子肉。

性味归经 甘、涩，平。入脾、肾、心经。

功效应用

1. 补脾止泻：用于脾虚泄泻，常与茯苓、白术、山药、砂仁等同用。

2. 养心安神：用于心肾不交，心悸失眠，可与酸枣仁、远志、茯苓等同用。

3. 益肾固精：用于肾亏遗精，崩漏带下等症，可与沙苑子、芡实、龙骨、牡蛎、莲须等同用。

用量用法 10～15克。煎服。

附药

1. 莲须：为莲花中的花蕊，又称莲蕊。味甘涩，性平。入心肾，功能清心固肾，涩精止血。可用于梦遗滑精，尿频，遗尿，吐血，崩漏等症。用量3～6克。

2. 莲房：为莲蓬壳。味苦涩，性温。入心肝血分，功能消瘀止血。可治一切下血、溺血、血崩等症。炙炭用，用量6～10克。

3. 莲子心：为莲子中的青嫩胚芽。味苦，性寒。功能清心安神。可用于温热病邪陷心包，神昏谵语，常与元参、竹叶心、连翘等同用；用于心烦不寐，遗精等，可与安神、止遗药随症配用。用量1.5～3克。

4. 荷叶：为莲的叶片。味苦、涩，性平。功能清暑利湿，升清醒脾，化瘀止血。可治暑热病症及脾虚泄泻和一切血症。用量10～15克。鲜者用1角（1张的1／4），煎服。清热解暑，用鲜荷叶；升清醒脾，宜用干荷叶；化瘀止血，干荷叶、荷叶炭均可。

芡　实

为睡莲科1年生水生草本植物芡 Euryale ferox Salisb.的种仁。用时捣碎。

处方用名 芡实、芡实米。

性味归经 甘、涩，平。入脾、肾经。

功效应用

1. 健脾止泻：用于脾虚泄泻，日久不止者，常与党参、白术、山药、茯苓等同用。

2. 益肾固精：用于肾虚梦遗滑精，小便不禁等症，常与金樱子同用。

3. 祛湿止带：用于湿热带下，常与山药、黄柏、白果、车前子等同用；用于白带，可以芡实粉、茯苓粉等量，炼蜜为丸，每次10克，淡盐水送服。

用量用法 10～15克。煎服。

山茱萸

为山茱萸科落叶小乔木山茱萸 Cornus officinalis Sieb. et Zucc.的成熟果肉。晒干用。

处方用名 山茱萸、山萸肉。

性味归经 酸、涩，微温。入肝、肾经。

功效应用

1. 补益肝肾，涩精缩尿：可用于肝肾亏虚，阳萎遗精，腰酸眩晕，耳鸣耳聋，小便频数等症，常与补骨脂、当归等同用。

2. 固经止血：用于妇女体虚，月经过多，或漏下不止等症，常与乌贼骨、棕炭、茜草根等同用。

3. 敛汗固脱：用于大汗欲脱或久病虚脱之证，可与党参、龙骨、牡蛎等同用。

用量用法 6～10克。大剂量可用至30克。煎服。

使用注意 凡肾阳偏亢，素有湿热，小便不利者均忌服。

金樱子

为蔷薇科常绿攀援灌木金樱子 Rosa laevigata Michx.的成熟果实。除去刺、核，生用。

处方用名 金樱子。

性味归经 酸、涩，平。入肾、膀胱、大肠经。

功效应用

1. 固精缩尿：用于肾虚遗精，遗尿，白带等症，可单用，或与芡实等量，研末为丸，每次6克，米汤送服。

2. 涩肠止泻：用于脾虚泄泻，日久不止，常与山药、芡实、白术、茯苓、五味子等同用。

用量用法 6～15克。煎服。熬膏或为丸服。

桑螵蛸

为螳螂科昆虫大刀螂 Paratilia maculata Thunb.的卵鞘。杀死虫卵后晒干用。

处方用名 桑螵蛸。

性味归经 甘、咸，平。入肝、肾经。

功效应用 补肾助阳，固精缩尿：用于肾阳不足，遗尿，小便频数，遗精，早泄等症。治遗尿、尿频，常与党参、龙骨、牡蛎等同用；治遗精，早泄，常与五味子、煅龙骨等同用。

用量用法 3～10克。煎服。宜入丸散剂。

覆盆子

为蔷薇科落叶灌木植物掌叶覆盆子 Rubus chingii Hu 的未成熟果实。酒拌蒸熟，晒干入药。

处方用名 覆盆子。

性味归经 甘、酸，微温。入肝、肾经。

功效应用

1. 益肾缩尿：用于小便频数，遗尿等症，常与桑螵蛸、益智仁、菟丝子、山茱萸等同用。

2. 益肾涩精：用于遗精，阳萎等症，常与枸杞子、菟丝子、五味子、车前子等同用。

用量用法 6～12克。煎服。

乌 贼 骨

为乌贼科软体动物无针乌贼 Sepiella maindroni de Rochebrune.或金乌贼 Sepia esculenta Hoyle 的内壳。炙黄用。

处方用名 乌贼骨、海螵蛸。

性味归经 咸、涩，微温。入肝、肾经。

功效应用

1. 收敛止血：用于妇女崩漏，常与茜草、棕榈炭、五倍子、黄芪、山茱萸等同用；用于便血，痔血等症，可单用炙黄，研末，每服 6 克，温开水送服；用于肺胃出血，可单用本品研末，温开水送服，每次 6 克，日 3 次，或与白及共研细末，每服 6 克，日 3 次；用于创伤出血，可单用研粉外用。

2. 固精止带：用于遗精早泄之症，可与其他益肾固精药配用；若治妇女赤白带下，可与白芷、血余炭同用。

3. 制酸止痛：用于胃炎，溃疡病胃酸过多者，可用乌贼骨 240 克，浙贝母 60 克，共研为末，每次 3 克，日 3 次，饭前吞服；若治溃疡穿孔，亦可与白及等同用。

4. 生肌祛湿：用于疮面多浓，皮肤湿疹、下肢溃疡等症，单用为末外敷，或酌配石膏、血竭、枯矾等同用。

用量用法 6～10 克。煎服。外用适量。

19 外用药及其他

凡在人体外部使用的药物，均称为外用药。虽然有些外用药可以内服，但以外用为主。

外用药一般具有杀虫解毒，消肿定痛，化腐生肌，收敛止血等不同作用，故应用范围较广，可分别用于各种疮疡肿毒，疥癣，以及目、耳、喉、鼻等疾患。由于这些疾患发生的部位及发现不同，所以用药形式与方法也是多种多样的。如膏贴，掺敷，涂抹，熏，洗等等。

本类药物大都具有不同程度的毒性，使用时应慎重，特别是剧毒药，如水银、砒石、斑蝥等，在外用时亦不能过量，并不宜在头部、五官涂布，以免局部刺激过强引起反应或吸收中毒。如可内服的药物，亦多制成丸剂或散剂；即使外用，也大都配制后用，很少原药单独使用。制剂时应严格遵照一定法度，不可任意操作，以保证用药安全。

铅　丹

为黑铅与硫黄、硝、盐、矾等炼制而成的铅化合物，成橙红色或橙黄色的粉末。原药用。

处方用名　铅丹、樟丹、黄丹。

性味归经　辛，微寒，有毒。入心、脾、肝经。

功效应用

1. 拔毒生肌：主要与植物油化合为制外贴膏药的基础剂。

2. 坠痰镇惊：用于惊痫，心悸，胸闷，失眠等症，可与龙骨、牡蛎、柴胡、黄芩等同用。

用量用法　1.5～4.5 克。煎服；入丸散剂 1 次服量不超过

0.6 克。外用适量。

使用注意 不可过量或持续内服，以防蓄积中毒。

砒 石

为砷矿中的砷华 Arsenolite 矿石的加工品。商品有红砒、白砒两种，市售以红砒为多。将砒石升华精制成白色粉末为砒霜，毒性更剧。与绿豆同煮减其毒性，研末用。

处方用名 红砒、白砒、砒霜。

性味归经 辛、酸，大热，有大毒。入肺、脾、胃经。

功效应用

1.外用蚀疮祛腐：用于牙疳，可与红枣炭、硼砂、青黛等同用；治痔疮，常与枯矾、朱砂等同用；治瘰疬，以本品为末合浓墨汁为丸如梧子大，锅内炒干，每用针刺破患处，将药半丸贴之，蚀尽为度。

2. 劫痰平喘：用于痰饮遇寒即发，哮喘气急，不能平卧，可与豆豉为丸用。

3. 截疟：治疟疾，白砒、硫黄（醋煮）、绿豆各 15 克共研细末，水丸绿豆大，每次 3～5 丸，疟发前 2 小时，温开水送服。

用量用法 外用适量，研末撒，调敷或入膏药中贴之。内服每次 0.002～0.004 克，入丸散。

使用注意 不能持续和大剂量服用，以防中毒。孕妇忌用。

轻 粉

为水银与食盐、胆矾用升华法制成的白色粉末（氯化亚汞结晶）。原药用。

处方用名 轻粉。

性味归经 辛，寒，有小毒。入肺、大肠、小肠经。

功效应用

1. 杀虫止痒：用于皮肤疥癣，瘙痒，可与其它解毒止痒药同用。

2. 逐水消肿：用于臌胀水肿，二便不通，形气俱实者，可与甘遂、芫花、大戟等同用。

3. 攻毒医疮：用于冻疮溃疡及梅毒等症，可与其它解毒化腐药同用。

用量用法 外用适量，研末调涂或干撒。内服1日量0.1～0.2克，分3次服，入丸散剂。不入煎剂。

使用注意 本品毒性强烈，内服宜慎，不可过量和持续服用，以免中毒；内服后需立即漱口，以防口腔、牙龈糜烂。

升 药

为水银、火硝、明矾各等分混合升华而成。红色者称红升，黄色者称黄升。研细末入药，陈久者良。

处方用名 升药。

性味归经 辛，热。有大毒。

功效应用 拔毒去腐：用于痈疽溃后，脓去不畅，或腐肉不去，新肉难生。常与煅石膏研末外用。煅石膏与升药的比例为9∶1者称为九一丹，拔毒力较轻；1∶1者称五五丹，拔毒之力较强；而1∶9者则称九转丹，拔毒力尤强。可视病情需要选用，掺于患处，亦可将药粘附于纸捻上插入脓腔中。

用量用法 不可内服。外用适量。不用纯品。

使用注意 本品拔毒去腐作用强烈，故疮疡腐肉已去或脓水已净者及手足、背部、口眼附近、乳头、脐中、关节部位与阴蚀、下疳等均不宜用。

硫 黄

为天然硫黄矿 Sulphur 的提炼加工品。原药研末用或与豆腐同煮后用（称鱼子黄）。

处方用名 硫黄、制硫黄、鱼子黄。

性味归经 酸、温，有毒。入命门、心包、大肠经。

功效应用

1. 外用杀虫止痒：用于湿疥癣痒及顽硬阴疽，可与轻粉、雄黄、冰片等同用。

2. 内服壮阳通便：用于命门火衰所致的腰膝冷痛，阳萎及肾不纳气的喘逆等症，可与附子、肉桂等助阳药同用；用于脏寒引起之大便冷秘，常与半夏同用制丸服。

用量用法 1日量1.5～6克。宜入丸散。外用适量。生者外用，制者内服。

使用注意 阴虚阳亢及孕妇忌服。

雄　黄

为含砷的结晶矿石雄黄 Realgar（二硫化二砷 AS_2S_2）。研细或水飞用。

处方用名 雄黄、雌黄、雄精、腰黄。

性味归经 苦、辛，温，有毒。入肝、胃经。

功效应用

1. 解毒杀虫：用于痈疮疔毒，湿疹疥癣等症，可与乳香、没药或黄柏、牡蛎等同用；治毒蛇咬伤，可与五灵脂等分为末，酒调服6克，并以药末掺患处。

2. 燥湿祛痰：用于急性咽喉肿痛，喉痹极危之症，及小儿惊痫痰涎壅盛者，雄黄、郁金各30克，巴豆（去壳去净油）14粒，研末，醋煮面糊为丸，如绿豆大，每次2～5丸（小儿酌减），温开水送服。

用量用法 1次量0.2～0.4克，日服1～2次，入丸散剂。外用适量。不入煎剂。

使用注意 不宜持续服用。

炉 甘 石

为天然的菱锌矿石 Smithsonite（碳酸锌 $ZnCO_3$）。火煅研末水飞用或与黄连水拌用。

处方用名 炉甘石、飞甘石。

性味归经 甘，平。

功效应用

1. 退翳明目：用于目赤翳障，常与硼砂、冰片等同用。

2. 收湿生肌：用于慢性溃疡，脓水淋漓，久不收口，及皮肤湿疹等症，常与煅石膏、煅牡蛎等同用。

用量用法 外用适量。水飞点眼，研末撒或调敷。

硼 砂

为硼砂矿石 Borax 提炼出的结晶体。生用或火煅用。

处方用名 硼砂。

性味归经 甘、咸，凉。入肺、胃经。

功效应用

1. 外用消肿解毒：用于咽喉肿痛，口舌生疮，常与冰片、玄明粉、朱砂同用；若治目赤肿痛，可浸水冲洗。

2. 清热化痰：用于痰热壅滞，咳痰不畅，可与桑皮、苏子等同用。

用量用法 1.5～3 克。煎服。入丸散剂每次服 0.6～1.5 克。外用适量。化痰可生用，外敷宜煅用。

明 矾

为明矾石 Alunite 的提炼品。生用或煅用，（煅后称枯矾）。

处方用名 白矾、明矾、枯矾。

性味归经 酸，寒。入肺、肝、脾、胃、大肠经。

功效应用

1. 解毒医疮：用于痈疽疮毒，口舌生疮，耳内流脓等症。治痈疽红肿及湿疹，可用白矾、雄黄各等分，共研细末，浓茶调患处；治耳内流脓，可用枯矾、黄丹各等分，研细末，少许吹耳内；治小儿口舌生疮，流涎气臭者，可用枯矾、朱砂各等分，研细末，敷患处。

2. 收湿止痒：用于皮肤湿疹，疥癣，可与硫黄、冰片等外用。

3. 敛泻止血：用于久泻不止，及便血、崩漏，带下等症，可与五倍子、诃子皮等同用；若治肺吐血，可与儿茶各等分，为末，每次 1～1.5 克，温开水送服。

4. 祛痰开闭：用于中风痰厥，神识昏迷，口噤痰壅，白矾、皂角各等分，研末，每次 1.5 克，温开水调灌，取吐痰涎；用于癫痫，常与郁金配用。

此外，本品有清热退黄之功，单用研末内服，可治湿热黄疸。

用量用法 外用适量。内服每次 1～3 克。入丸散剂服。

斑 蝥

为芫青科昆虫南方大斑蝥 Mylabris phalerata Pall.和黄黑小斑蝥 Mylabris cichorii L.的干燥虫体。原药去头足两翅，用糯米同炒至米黄黑为度，或用麸皮炒过再用醋煮，研末用。

处方用名 斑蝥、斑猫。

性味归经 辛，寒。有大毒。入大、小肠、肝、肾经。

功效应用

1. 攻毒蚀疮：用于痈疽顽强不破，或破而肿硬无脓，以本品为末和蒜捣膏，用少许贴患处，脓出即去药；用于各种顽癣，可与土槿皮、蜈蚣、全蝎、肉桂、细辛等同用；用于瘰疬瘘疮，可与白砒、草乌、黄连等同用；或与江米同炒用；用于狂犬咬伤，斑蝥（去头足翅）3 个，黄连、江米各 9 克，共炒黄，研末，每次1.5克，黄酒送服，日1次。

2. 破血散结：用于经闭不通，可配桃仁、大黄为丸服。

此外，近代用于多种癌肿有一定疗效。如《中药大辞典》方，用鸡蛋打一小孔放入去头、足、翅的斑蝥1～3枚，烤熟去斑蝥，食蛋，每日1只，治肝癌、胃癌有效。又本品尚能发泡生毛，浸酒可搓擦头部，治秃发。

用量用法 0.03～0.06，3次分服。只入丸散，不入煎剂。外用适量。

使用注意 本品外涂皮肤，能使皮肤发红起泡，所以内服宜慎。若内服中毒，可出现口咽部烧灼感，恶心呕吐，腹部绞痛及尿血，中毒性肾炎等症状。严格掌握内服剂量。孕妇禁用。

蟾　酥

为蟾蜍科动物中华大蟾蜍 Bufo bufo gargarizans Cantor 和黑眶蟾蜍 B. melanostictus Schneider 等的耳后腺及皮肤腺所分泌的白色浆液，经加工而成的饼状干燥品。原药研末用。

处方用名 蟾酥。

性味归经 甘、辛，温，有毒。入心、胃经。

功效应用

1. 拔毒消肿：用于一切痈疽疮疡疔毒，肿硬疼痛等症，常与轻粉、冰片、麝香、乳香、没药、朱砂等同用。

2. 开窍醒神：用于中暑昏厥，呕吐泄泻，腹中绞痛，胸腹胀满等症，常与雄黄、天麻、苍术、丁香等同用。

3. 杀虫止痛：用于风虫牙痛，可用蟾酥少许，与胡椒共研末，取粟米大，用药棉包裹，放于牙痛处，咬定，吐涎，每日1～2次。

用量用法 内服1日量0.01～0.02克，只入丸散，不入煎剂。本品有毒，不宜久服。外用适量。

马　钱　子

为马钱子科乔木马钱 Strychnos nux-vomica L.及同科木质大藤本皮氏马钱（云南马钱）Strychnospierriana A. W. Hill 的成熟种子。马钱子又称番木鳖。经炮制后入药。

处方用名　马钱子。

性味归经　苦，寒，有大毒。入肝、脾经。

功效应用

1. 通经络止疼痛：用于风寒湿痹，全身关节拘急疼痛或麻木等症，可与麻黄、苍术、乳香、没药、地龙等同用。

2. 散结消肿：用于跌仆骨折之瘀血肿痛，可与土鳖、制乳香、制没药、自然铜、骨碎补等为末外敷；用于喉痹肿痛，可与青木香、山豆根等分研末吹之。

此外，现有用本品治癌肿者，虽有疗效，但尚在试验中。

用量用法　内服 0.3～0.6 克（1 日量），入丸散剂，不入煎剂。外用适量。

使用注意　本品有毒，内服必须炮制得宜，严格掌握剂量，且不可持续服用过久，以防中毒。若服用过量，可出现肢体颤动，甚至麻痹，不省人事，或造成肢体长期拘缩不展。孕妇忌服。

蛇　床　子

为伞形科 1 年生草本植物 Cnidium monnieri（L.）Cusson 的成熟果实。原药生用。

处方用名　蛇床子。

性味归经　辛、苦，温。入肾经。

功效应用

1. 温肾壮阳：用于肾虚阳痿及女子不孕之症。常与菟丝子、五味子等补肾益精药同用。

2. 杀虫止痒：用于女子阴道滴虫，男子阴囊湿痒及风疹疥癣，皮肤瘙痒等症。治滴虫阴痒，可与苦参、花椒、百部等煎水熏洗，坐浴；或用蛇床子15克，明矾少许研末以水调和，用纱布纳入阴道内，日换1次；治外阴瘙痒，也可用蛇床子15克配明矾3克、花椒6克、土槿皮12克，煎汤外洗；如治湿疹瘙痒，可与苦参、地肤子、苍术等同用。

用量用法 3～10克。煎服。外用15～30克。一般多以外用为主。

露蜂房

为胡蜂科昆虫大黄蜂 Polistes mandarinus Saussure 或同属近缘昆虫的巢。酒洗用或焙黄研末用。

处方用名 蜂房、露蜂房。

性味归经 微甘，平。入肝、肾、胃经。

功效应用

1. 解毒疗疮；用于痈疽恶疮，发背，瘰疬等症，可与其他解毒药同用；如治乳痈初起尚未化脓者，将蜂房撕碎，文火焙焦(忌焦黑)，研细末，每次1.8～3克，温黄酒30克冲服，每4小时1次，服药期间，多饮井水；如治脱疽，用蜂房焙研为末，醋调敷患处，每日一换；如治瘰疬成瘘，可用末和猪油调膏外涂。

2. 祛风除痹：用于风湿性或类风湿性关节肿痛、僵直，甚至变形者，可与土鳖、全蝎、蜈蚣等配服；用于风疹瘙痒，可与蝉衣、浮萍、地肤子等配服。

3. 兴阳益肾：用于遗尿失禁，蜂房（焙黄）、桑螵蛸各等分，研细末，每次3～6克（小儿酌减），1日2次，黄酒送服。

此外，还可用治胃癌、乳癌、肺癌及癌肿转移引起的淋巴结肿大等，常与蜈蚣、全蝎、守宫等同用，效果显著。

用量用法 外用适量，研末调敷或煎水冲洗。内服入煎6～12克；研末服用每次1.5～3克。外用适量。

血　竭

为棕榈科常绿藤本蔓茎植物麒麟竭 Daemonorops draco Bl. 的红色树脂。布包入热水中软化成团，取出放冷待干。研末用。

处方用名　血竭、麒麟竭。

性味归经　微甘、咸，平。入心、肝经。

功效应用

1. 行瘀止痛：用于跌打损伤，筋断骨折之瘀血肿痛，常与乳香、没药、儿茶、红花等同用。

2. 生肌敛疮：用于痈疽溃疡，疮面久不愈合，常与象皮、乳香、没药、赤石脂、龙骨等同用；若治骨结核，可与松香、蓖麻子、木鳖子、轻粉等同用；用于鼻衄、齿衄、刀伤出血等症，可与蒲黄等分为末，敷患处。

用量用法　外用适量，研末敷。内服每次 1～1.5 克。入丸散剂，不入煎剂。

使用注意　无瘀血者不宜服。

大 风 子

为大风子科常绿乔木大风子树 Hydnocarpus anthelmintica Pier 的成熟种仁。去壳研泥用，或熬油用。

处方用名　大风子、大枫子。

性味归经　辛、热，有毒。

功效应用　燥湿杀虫：用于疥疮、皮癣、麻风等症。治疥疮，常与胡桃仁、水银等同用；治顽癣，可与松香、苦参等同用；治牛皮癣，可与木鳖仁、巴豆仁、水银等同用；治各型麻风，可用大风子油 30 克，苦参（研末）90 克，加酒少许，糊为丸，如梧子大，每次 50 丸，空腹温酒送下。并以苦参煎汤洗患处，或用大风子 10 克（煅存性），轻粉 4.5 克，共研细末，香油调涂，治麻风疮烂及梅毒疮。

用量用法　外用适量。内服1次量0.3～1克，不入煎剂。

常　山

为虎耳草科落叶小灌木黄常山 Dichroa febrifuga Lour.的根。切片生用，醋炒或酒蒸用。

处方用名　黄常山、鸡骨常山、酒常山、醋常山。

性味归经　苦、辛，微寒，有小毒。入肺、心、肝经。

功效应用

1. 吐痰行水：用于胸中痰饮，可用醋常山9克，甘草4.5克，水煎，入蜜温服。取吐，不吐再服。

2. 杀虫截疟：用于疟疾，偏于痰湿者，常与槟榔、草果等同用；偏于痰热者，可与草果，知母、贝母、槟榔等同用。

用量用法　3～10克。煎服。生用力猛，醋炒则催吐更剧；若酒蒸酒炒则性和缓，少用不致呕吐，故治疟疾都经酒制。

丝　瓜　络

为葫芦科1年生攀援草本植物丝瓜 Luffa cylindrica （L.）Roem.老熟果实的网状纤维或粤丝瓜 L. acutangula Roxb.的枯老果实。切段生用。

处方用名　丝瓜络。

性味归经　甘，平。入肺、胃、肝经。

功效应用　凉血解毒，行血通络：用于气血阻滞的胸肋疼痛，筋骨酸痛及乳痈肿痛等症，可随症配伍。

用量用法　10～15克。煎服。

孩　儿　茶

为豆科落叶乔木植物儿茶树 Acacia catechu（L.）Willd.的枝干及心材煎汁浓缩而成，称儿茶膏、黑儿茶。

处方用名　儿茶、孩儿茶。

性味归经 苦、涩，微寒。入肺经。

功效应用 清热收湿，敛疮止血：用于湿疮、口疳、牙疳及金疮出血等症。治湿疮，可与龙骨、轻粉等同用；治口疳，牙疳，可与人中白、黄柏、青黛等同用；若治下疳，可用儿茶 3 克，轻粉 0.3 克，冰片 0.015 克，共研末，敷患处；治金疮出血，可用本品为末擦之。

用量用法 外用适量，研末撒或调敷。内服 0.1～1 克。入丸散，不入煎剂。

瓦 楞 子

为海产软体动物蚶科魁蚶 Arca inflata Reeve.泥蚶 A.granosa L.或毛蚶 A.subcrenata Lischke.的贝壳。打碎生用或煅用。

处方用名 瓦楞子、煅瓦楞。

性味归经 甘、咸，平。入肺、胃、肝、脾经。

功效应用

1. 消痰软坚：用于顽痰积结，稠粘难咯，可与海浮石、贝母、旋复花等同用。

2. 化瘀散结：用于妇女症瘕痞块，可与三棱、莪术、桃仁、鳖甲等同用。

3. 制酸止痛：用于气滞血瘀之胃脘疼痛，常与香附、木香、五灵脂等同用；若用于溃疡病、胃痛泛吐酸水，煅瓦楞 150 克，生甘草 30 克，共研末，每次 9 克，日服 3 次，饭前服。

用量用法 10～15 克。煎服。消痰散结宜生用，制酸止痛宜煅用。

THE ENGLISH–CHINESE ENCYCLOPEDIA OF PRACTICAL TCM

(Booklist)

英汉实用中医药大全

（书目）

VOLUME	TITLE	书名
1	ESSENTIALS OF TRADITIONAL CHIN ESE MEDICINE	中医学基础
2	THE CHINESE MATERIA MEDICA	中药学
3	PHARMACOLOGY OF TRADITION–AL CHINESE MEDICAL FORMULAE	方剂学
4	SIMPLE AND PROVEN PRESCRIPTION	单验方
5	COMMONLY USED CHINESE PATENTMEDICINES	常用中成药
6	THERAPY OF ACUPUNCTURE AND MOXIBUSTION	针灸疗法
7	*TUINA* THERAPY	推拿疗法
8	MEDICAL *QIGONG*	医学气功
9	MAINTAINING YOUR HEALTH	自我保健
10	INTERNAL MEDICINE	内科学

11	SURGERY	外科学
12	GYNECOLOGY	妇科学
13	PEDIATRICS	儿科学
14	ORTHOPEDICS	骨伤科学
15	PROCTOLOGY	肛门直肠病学
16	DERMATOLOGY	皮肤病学
17	OPHTHALMOLOGY	眼科学
18	OTORHINOLARYNGOLOGY	耳鼻喉科学
19	EMERGENTOLOGY	急症学
20	NURSING	护理
21	CLINICAL DIALOGUE	临床会话

(京)112 号

The English-Chinese

Encyclopedia of Practical TCM

Chief Editor Xu Xiangcai

2

THE CHINESE MATERIA MEDICA

English Chief Editor Huang Kuiming

Chinese Chief Editor Zou Jilong

英汉实用中医药大全

主编 徐象才

2

中 药 学

中文主编 邹积隆

英文主编 黄奎铭

*

高等教育出版社出版

新华书店总店科技发行所发行

化学工业出版社印刷厂印刷

*

开本 850×1168 1/32 印张 27.25 字数 700 000

1994 年12月第1版 1994 年12月第1次印刷

印数 0001—5040

ISBN7-04-004849-3/R·30

定价 23.70 元